Breast Cancer

Contemporary Cancer Research

SERIES EDITOR: JAC A. NICKOLOFF

Breast Cancer

*Molecular Genetics, Pathogenesis,
and Therapeutics*

Edited by

Anne M. Bowcock

*Department of Pediatrics
and McDermott Center for Human Growth and Development
University of Texas Southwestern Medical Center, Dallas, TX*

Humana Press ✳ Totowa, New Jersey

Acknowledgments

Robert Dickson (Lombardi Cancer Research Center, Georgetown University) and Tony Brown (Cornell University and the Strang Center Research Laboratory, Rockefeller University) provided invaluable suggestions regarding the content of this book.
This book would not have been completed without the dedication and competence of Colleen Campbell.
To all the authors of individual chapters, I am profoundly grateful, as I am to reviewers who provided valuable and incisive criticism and suggestions.
Finally, to my husband, Michael Lovett, I am constantly appreciative of his tireless support, patience, and a sense of humor that never wanes.

© 1999 Humana Press Inc.
999 Riverview Drive, Suite 208
Totowa, New Jersey 07512

This publication is printed on acid-free paper. ∞
ANSI Z39.48-1984 (American Standards Institute) Permanence of Paper for Printed Library Materials.

Cover design by Patricia F. Cleary.

For additional copies, pricing for bulk purchases, and/or information about other Humana titles, contact Humana at the above address or at any of the following numbers: Tel: 973-256-1699; Fax: 973-256-8341; E-mail: humana@humanapr.com, or visit our Website: http://humanapress.com

Printed in the United States of America. 10 9 8 7 6 5 4 3 2 1

Library of Congress Cataloging in Publication Data

Breast cancer: molecular genetics, pathogenesis, and therapeutics / edited by Anne M. Bowcock.
        p.   cm.—(Contemporary cancer research)
   Includes index.
   ISBN 0-89603-560-3 (alk. paper)
   1. Breast—cancer. 2. Breast—Cancer—Genetic aspects. I. Bowcock, Anne M. II. Series.
       [DNLM: 1. Breast Neoplasms—genetics. WP 870 B8211342 1998]
   RC280.B8B66555   1998
   616.99'449—dc21   98-21525
   DNLM/DLC   CIP
   for Library of Congress

Preface

Breast cancer is the leading type of cancer in women in the United States, and affects almost one million women worldwide at any given time. The incidence of this disease in the United States has risen steadily since 1930, with an average increase of 1.2% per year. Today, one in eight American women will develop breast cancer at some point in their lifetimes, and, of these women, approximately 30% will develop the metastatic form of the disease, which is ultimately fatal.

The emotional, social, and healthcare costs of this disease are enormous. The financial cost is estimated to be $6 billion within the United States alone. The psychological toll is inestimable. Unfortunately, unraveling the causes and cures for this disease is not a simple task. Breast cancer, in common with many other cancers, is complex and involves multiple genetic changes within both somatically occurring and heritable cases. Nevertheless, major strides have been made in the last few years in understanding some of the molecular events that give rise to human breast cancer, and we are beginning to develop a conceptual framework of what specific processes are involved. Our expanding knowledge of these genetic alterations is beginning to provide us with the material for translating scientific discovery into clinical practice for both treatment and detection.

Historically, breast cancer treatment falls into four distinct periods. The first was the "era of the incurable disease" that ended with the close of the 19th century. Before the development of modern medicine, countless numbers of women died in fear and shame from untreated, disfiguring tumors. By the mid-20th century, the second period had begun and was influenced and dominated by the surgical treatments of William S. Halsted. Radical surgeries saved some lives and prolonged others, but women continued to suffer fear, disfigurement, and shame into the mid-1970s. The early 1970s saw the introduction of life-saving multimodal treatments, including surgery and radiotherapy, generally combined with chemotherapy or monotherapy. We are now at the junction between this third phase and a new period in which a more targeted and proactive approach will be possible through our insights into the molecular pathogenesis of the disease.

The pace of gene and mutation identification is rapidly accelerating and has begun to have a profound impact on our understanding and treatment of disease. It is likely that many additional genes that are important in the genesis and progression of breast cancer will be identified in the next decade. These will be used to determine breast cancer risk in women in the general population, and will be accompanied by prevention programs involving targeted screening or the avoidance of predisposing environmental factors. Newly discovered genes will also permit the tailoring of therapeutic regimes to individual cancers and individual women with breast cancer. They should also lead to a more precise understanding of the natural history of breast cancer and to the possibility of identifying populations at risk.

Breast Cancer: Molecular Genetics, Pathogenesis, and Therapeutics is geared toward both clinicians and basic researchers working on breast cancer and is intended to provide insight into basic issues from a genetic standpoint. The first section deals with known genetic changes associated with breast cancer. These changes include genes that are somatically mutated in breast cancer, as distinct from heritable genetic defects. I have used the term "Etiology" to cover the broad topics in this section. The second section is devoted to hereditary breast cancer. It is estimated that 5% of breast cancers in the general US population arise from alterations in the dominantly inherited breast cancer genes, BRCA1 or BRCA2. This second section also includes a discussion of the psychological issues related to testing for *BRCA1/2* alterations. The contribution of genes with weaker effects than *BRCA1* or *BRCA2* is not currently well understood, but the identification of further predisposing alleles represents a challenge for future genetic research. These still-to-be-discovered mutations may be in genes that are involved in the metabolism of environmental contaminants (e.g., the production of procarcinogens or the failure to detoxify or extrude carcinogenic intermediates) or in DNA repair.

Virtually all deaths from breast cancer result from invasion and metastasis of the tumor. Therefore, the third section deals with this important process of tumor progression. The next section deals with diagnostics, therapeutics, drug resistance, and risk factors, and the concluding section explores some less well trodden paths in breast cancer risk and includes discussions of the roles of selected nutrients, of physicochemistry, of pesticides and pollutants, and of smoking in breast cancer.

It is not possible in one small volume to cover all topics related to breast cancer in general. Nevertheless, it is hoped that these chapters will provide an introduction to current thinking in the field of breast cancer genetics and a background of ideas on which future breast cancer research can be built.

Anne M. Bowcock

Contents

Contributors

CHRISTINE B. AMBROSONE • *Division of Molecular Epidemiology, National Center for Toxicological Research, Jefferson, AR*

CARLOS L. ARTEAGA • *Division of Medical Oncology, Department of Medicine, Vanderbilt University School of Medicine, Nashville, TN*

SIMON M. BARRATT-BOYES • *Department of Molecular Genetics and Biochemistry, University of Pittsburg, Pittsburg, PA*

LYNDA B. BENNETT • *Department of Pediatrics, University of Texas Southwestern Medical Center, Dallas, TX*

IVAN BERGSTEIN • *Department of Hematology–Medical Oncology, Cornell University, New York, NY*

CATERINA BIANCO • *Laboratory of Tumor Immunology and Biology, National Cancer Institute, National Institutes of Health, Bethesda, MD*

ANNE M. BOWCOCK • *Department of Pediatrics, University of Texas Southwestern Medical Center, Dallas, TX*

ANGELA BRODIE • *Department of Pharmacology and Experimental Therapeutics, University of Maryland, Baltimore, MD*

ANTHONY M. C. BROWN • *Strang Center Research Laboratory, Cornell University, New York, NY*

NILS BRÜNNER • *Finsen Laboratory, Rigshospitalet, Copenhagen, Denmark*

HELEN K. CHEW • *Department of Molecular Medicine, Institute of Biotechnology, University of Texas, San Antonio, TX*

PAWEL CIBOROWSKI • *Department of Molecular Genetics and Biochemistry, University of Pittsburgh, Pittsburgh, PA*

SUSAN E. CLARE • *National Cancer Institute, Bethesda, MD*

ROBERT CLARKE • *Lombardi Cancer Center, Georgetown University, Washington, DC*

KENNETH H. COWAN • *National Cancer Institute, National Institutes of Health, Bethesda, MD*

MARTA DE SANTIS • *Laboratory of Tumor Immunology and Biology, National Cancer Institute, National Institutes of Health, Bethesda, MD*

ROBERT B. DICKSON • *Lombardi Cancer Research Center, Georgetown University, Washington, DC*

KENDALL E. DONALDSON HERSCHLER • *Department of Pharmacology and Experimental Therapeutics, University of Maryland, Baltimore, MD*

MATTHEW J. ELLIS • *Lombardi Cancer Research Center, Georgetown University, Washington, DC*

ZHEN FAN • *M. D. Anderson Cancer Center, University of Texas, Houston, TX*

ANDREW A. FARMER • *Department of Molecular Medicine, Institute of Biotechnology, University of Texas, San Antonio, TX*

OLIVERA J. FINN • *Department of Molecular Genetics and Biochemistry, University of Pittsburgh, Pittsburgh, PA*

THOMAS L. FRANDSEN • *Finsen Laboratory, Rigshospitalet, Copenhagen Denmark*

SUZANNE A. W. FUQUA • *Health Science Center, University of Texas, San Antonio, TX*

PRISCILLA A. FURTH• *Institute of Human Virology, Medical Biotechnology Center, University of Maryland, Baltimore, MD*

GIAMPIETRO GASPARINI • *Department of Oncology, St. Bortolo Hospital, Bassano del Grappa, Italy*

R. K. HANSEN • *Health Science Center, University of Texas, San Antonio, TX*

MELANIE T. HARTSOUGH • *National Cancer Institute, Bethesda, MD*

SVERRE HEIM • *Department of Medical Genetics, Institute for Cancer Research, The Norwegian Radium Hospital, Oslo, Norway*

LEENA HILAKIVI-CLARKE • *Lombardi Cancer Research Center, Georgetown University, Washington, DC*

ELISABETH M. HILTBOLD • *Department of Molecular Genetics and Biochemistry, University of Pittsburgh, Pittsburgh, PA*

CLAUS HOLST-HANSEN • *Finsen Laboratory, Rigshospitalet, Copenhagen, Denmark*

FRANCIS G. KERN • *Southern Research Institute, Birmingham, AL*

KATRI M. KOLI • *Department of Virology, Haartman Institute, University of Helsinki, Helsinki, Finland*

WEN-HWA LEE • *Department of Molecular Medicine, Institute of Biotechnology, University of Texas, San Antonio, TX*

CARYN LERMAN • *Lombardi Cancer Research Center, Georgetown University, Washington, DC*

JOHN R. MACDOUGALL • *Department of Cell Biology, Vanderbilt University, Nashville, TN*

ISABEL MARTINEZ-LACACI • *Laboratory of Tumor Immunology and Biology, National Cancer Institute, National Institutes of Health, Bethesda, MD*

LYNN M. MATRISIAN • *Department of Cell Biology, Vanderbilt University, Nashville, TN*

JOHN MENDELSOHN • *M. D. Anderson Cancer Center, University of Texas, Houston, TX*

BOYE SCHNACK NIELSEN • *Finsen Laboratory, Rigshospitalet, Copenhagen, Denmark*

NIKOS PANDIS • *The Norwegian Radium Hospital, Institute for Cancer Research, Oslo, Norway*

DEVCHAND PAUL • *National Cancer Institute, National Institutes of Health, Bethesda, MD*

ANDERS N. PEDERSEN • *Finsen Laboratory, Rigshospitalet, Copenhagen, Denmark*

BETH N. PESHKIN • *Lombardi Cancer Research Center, Georgetown University, Washington, DC*

GEORGE N. PETERS • *University of Texas Southwestern Medical Center for Breast Care, Dallas, TX*

EDWARD C. ROSFJORD • *Lombardi Cancer Research Center, Georgetown University, Washington, DC*

DAVID S. SALOMON • *Laboratory for Tumor Immunology and Biology, National Cancer Institute, National Institutes of Health, Bethesda, MD*

PETER G. SHIELDS • *Laboratory for Human Carcinogenesis, Division of Basic Sciences, National Cancer Institute, Bethesda, MD*

GEORGE W. SLEDGE, JR. • *Hematology/Oncology Division, Department of Medicine, Indiana University, Indianapolis, IN*

PATRICIA S. STEEG • *National Cancer Institute, Bethesda, MD*

ROSS W. STEPHENS • *Finsen Laboratory, Rigshospitalet, Copenhagen, Denmark*

JOEL D. TAUROG • *Department of Internal Medicine, Harold C. Simmons Arthritis Research Center, University of Texas Southwestern Medical Center, Dallas, TX*

MANUEL R. TEIXEIRA • *Department of Medical Genetics, Institute for Cancer Research, The Norwegian Radium Hospital, Oslo, Norway*

ERIK W. THOMPSON • *Department of Surgery, Victorian Breast Cancer Research Consortium Unit, St. Vincent's Institute for Medical Research, Melbourne University, Australia*

BRUCE TROCK • *Lombardi Cancer Research Center, Georgetown University, Washington, DC*

I
Etiology
Genetic Changes Associated with Breast Cancer

The Estrogen Receptor and Breast Cancer

R. K. Hansen and S. A. W. Fuqua

1. INTRODUCTION

Estrogens are steroid hormones that play important roles in the growth and development of the mammary gland. In addition, estrogens are thought to significantly contribute to breast carcinogenesis. For example, women treated with the estrogen diethylstilbestrol have a significantly increased risk of developing breast cancer *(1)*. In addition, it is well established that the growth of breast cancer cell lines in culture or in ovariectomized nude mice is stimulated by estrogens *(2,3)*. Thus, estrogens appear to not only be associated with normal cell growth, but also breast cancer cell growth, leading to the development and/or progression of this disease.

The proliferative effects of estrogens are mediated through an intracellular receptor, the estrogen receptor (ER) *(4,5)*. Estrogens (Fig. 1A,E) pass through the cell membrane and bind the ER, transforming the receptor into an active transcription factor, which binds DNA as a dimer at specific estrogen response elements (EREs), and regulates the expression of a variety of genes (Fig. 1A). Since the ER mediates estrogen activity, its role has been extensively studied in clinical breast cancer. These investigations have provided strong evidence that ER status is a very important factor in the management of breast cancer. First, the ER is useful in predicting patient outcome *(6,7)*. In general, ER-negative tumors are associated with early recurrence and poor patient survival, compared with ER-positive tumors. Second, and more important, the ER is useful in predicting response to endocrine therapy *(8–10)*. Patients with ER-negative tumors rarely respond to endocrine therapy, and there appears to be a correlation between the level of ER expression and endocrine response *(8)*.

1.1. Antiestrogen Mechanism of Action

Endocrine therapy targets estrogen-mediated growth pathways, and several estrogen antagonists have proven successful in the clinic *(11,12)*. However, the mechanism of action of these agents is not fully understood, and their effectiveness varies in individual patients. Some antiestrogens, such as the steroidal compounds ICI 164,384 and ICI 182,780, are very efficient antagonists, both in vitro *(13)* and in vivo *(14,15)*, without apparent agonist activities; other antiestrogens, such as the nonsteroidal agent tamoxifen, have mixed agonist/antagonist effects, depending on the cell type *(16–18)*. Initial models of antiestrogen action involved simple competition of antiestrogen with

From: Breast Cancer: *Molecular Genetics, Pathogenesis, and Therapeutics*
Edited by: A. M. Bowcock © Humana Press Inc., Totowa, NJ

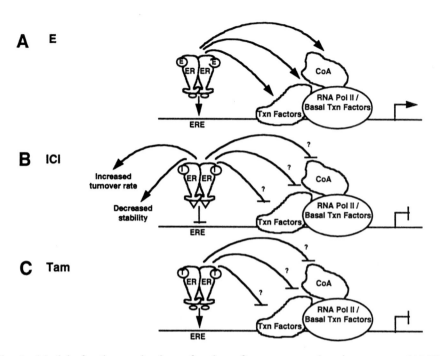

Fig. 1. Models for the mechanism of action of estrogens and antiestrogens. **(A)** The ER dimer (ER) bound to estrogen (E) may act by binding to an estrogen responsive element (ERE) upstream of an estrogen-regulated gene. Transcription is activated by direct interaction with components of the RNA polymerase II transcription complex and basal transcription factors (RNA Pol II/Basal Txn Factors), sequence-specific transcription factors (Txn Factors), and/or additional coactivator proteins (CoA). **(B)** Steroidal antiestrogens (ICI or I) may act by increasing the turnover rate of ER or by decreasing the stability of the ER. They may also interfere with DNA binding or interactions of the ER with components of the RNA Pol II/Basal Txn Factor complex. **(C)** Nonsteroidal antiestrogen (Tam or T) bindings result in an altered conformation, which interferes with ER's interaction with transcription factors.

estrogen for the ligand-binding site of the ER. When bound to antiestrogen, the receptor would be unable to bind estrogen and stimulate cell growth. However, additional studies have shown that the mechanism of action of antiestrogens is much more complex, as will be discussed in this subheading.

Steroidal antiestrogens have been developed to circumvent the mixed agonist/antagonist activity of nonsteroidal antiestrogens, and have been postulated to work through a different mechanism of action than that of nonsteroidal antiestrogens. Current models of steroidal antiestrogen mechanism of action (Fig. 1B) suggest that these compounds may increase the turnover rate of the ER, and alter the conformation of the ER, so that it is either unstable, or exhibits reduced DNA binding ability *(19–21)*. An area of active research is how steroidal antiestrogen-occupied ER interacts with other important transcription factors.

Delineating the mechanism of action of the nonsteroidal antiestrogens has proven more problematic because of their mixed activities. Although tamoxifen blocks estrogen-stimulated growth and gene transcription, this effect varies, depending on the species, the cell type, and the promoter used for the analysis *(22,23)*. Recent data suggest that tamoxifen alters ER conformation, changing its interaction with specific accessory proteins (Fig. 1C, CoA), thereby resulting in their differential recruitment to the basal transcriptional machinery (Fig. 1.C, Basal Txn Factors) *(24)*. There appear to be a number of different accessory protein interactions important in the ER signaling pathway, which we will discuss in detail in Subheading 4.

1.2. Antiestrogen Resistance

A major problem with the clinical use of antiestrogens is the development of resistance to these compounds. A minority of patients are resistant, *de novo*, to tamoxifen, with the majority of ER-positive patients exhibiting a response in the metastatic setting *(10)*. Invariably, tumors become resistant to the drug, although hormone resistance is reversible. For example, tamoxifen-resistant patients, switched to a different type of therapy, may later once again respond to tamoxifen *(25)*. Therefore, mechanisms of resistance are probably multifactorial, and understanding these mechanisms might provide clues for new strategies for preventing or reversing the emergence of resistant cells. From the preceding subheading on antiestrogen mechanisms of action, it is apparent that there are a number of potential routes by which resistance could be achieved.

Potential mechanisms of resistance, excluding that involving differential ER accessory protein recruitment, have been extensively reviewed by others, and will only be briefly discussed here. First, loss of the ER or alterations in the ER can result in hormone resistance. These changes can occur, but explain only a minority of cases *(26–28)*. Second, metabolic tolerance as a result of altered systemic metabolism, and altered uptake or metabolism by the tumor itself, have been studied as potential mechanisms. Recent studies, however, have discounted the importance of tamoxifen metabolism in experimental mouse models of tamoxifen resistance *(29–31)*. And finally, expression of antiestrogen binding sites *(32)*, or the altered production of autocrine growth factors, have been studied as mechanisms of antiestrogen resistance *(33–35)*.

Here is reviewed some of the most significant ER research of the past few years, which contributed to understanding of antiestrogen resistance. The followiing topics will be discussed: refined detail of the ligand-binding domain (LBD) deduced from crystal structures; the cell- and promoter-specificity of the transcriptional activation domains of the ER; the role of receptor phosphorylation and crosstalk between different signal transduction pathways in ER function; the discovery of a new ER subtype (called ERβ); and, finally, the interaction of accessory proteins (either coactivators or corepressors) with the ER, and their influence on the transcriptional response to estrogens and antiestrogens.

2. ORGANIZATIONAL STRUCTURE AND DOMAIN FUNCTION OF THE ER

2.1. Structure/Functional Domains

The ER is a member of a superfamily of nuclear receptors that includes the steroid hormone, the thyroid hormone (TR), the vitamin D (VDR) and the retinoic acid receptors (RXR, RAR), as well as orphan receptors with as-yet unknown ligands (reviewed

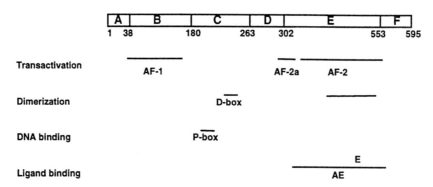

Fig. 2. Schematic representation of ER. The structural domains of ER (A–F) are shown with amino acid numbers below the figure corresponding to domain boundaries. The functional domains of the receptor are indicated below the structural figure.

in refs. *4* and *5*). The cloning and sequencing of the cDNAs for each of these receptors reveals that, although there is considerable diversity in molecular size, they share a common structural and functional organization. The receptors are commonly organized in functional domains termed A–F *(36,37)*; the human ER is shown in Fig. 2. The amino-terminal A/B-domain exhibits the most variation in both sequence and length. The A/B-domain also contains a hormone-independent transcription activation function (AF-1), which may be important for the agonist activity of antiestrogens *(16,23)*, as will be discussed in detail in Subheading 2.1.2. The central C-domain is highly conserved among the nuclear receptors, and is the site of the DNA-binding domain (DBD). This domain contains eight cysteine residues, which are arranged in two zinc-finger motifs, each of which is followed by an extended α-helix, forming two subdomains *(38–40)*. These helices are positioned along regions of DNA that are found within the promoter of estrogen-responsive target genes; these DNA regions are called EREs, and are inverted repeats of the sequence GGTCA, separated by three variant bases *(41–43)*. The recognition site for EREs, called the P-box, is contained within three residues (glutamate 203, glycine 204, alanine 207) directly carboxy-terminal of the first zinc domain in the ER *(44)*. Another element in the DBD, the D-box, consists of five residues (222–226) located downstream of the P-box in the second zinc-finger domain, and is at least partially responsible for cooperative binding (dimerization) of ER DBDs to EREs *(45)*. Recently the crystal structure of the ER was solved both in solution and as a complex with DNA *(46,47)*. These structures confirmed the models of the DBD developed from the NMR structure of the ER *(48)* and models predicted from mutational analysis *(45,49)*. Carboxy-terminal to the C-domain is the D-domain, which appears to function as a hinge region, and may be an important binding site for coaccessory proteins *(24)*, as discussed in Subheading 4. Finally, the E- and F-domains are less conserved among family members, and contain the LBD, which was recently crystallized for three of the nuclear receptors, as will be discussed in Subheading 2.1.1. In addition, the E- and F-domains contain the ligand-dependent transcription activation functions-2 and -2a (AF-2 and AF-2a), and another dimerization domain.

2.1.1. Structure of the LBD

In 1995, the crystal structures for the LBDs of three nuclear receptors (RXRα, RARγ, and TRα) were solved *(50–52)*. The structure of RXRα in the absence of ligand was the first to be reported *(50)*. It was followed by the structures for RARγ and TRα, which were crystallized in the presence of ligand *(51,52)*. Although the LBD of the ER is not identical to these three receptors, it is a good assumption that the overall structures are similar *(53,54)*. Furthermore, by aligning the sequences of the entire family of nuclear receptors, Wurtz et al. *(54)* identified a region that contains most of the conserved residues important for stabilizing the LBD core, thus defining what constitutes a nuclear receptor LBD. This also suggests that the residues, which differ among the various family members, may be the residues involved in conveying ligand-binding specificity.

The structures of the LBDs of RXRα, RARγ, and TRα consist of 12 α-helices, arranged in an antiparallel sandwich formation, in which the α-helical elements are linked by short loops *(50–52)*. In the ligand-bound RARγ and TRα structures, the ligand is buried in a pocket, forming part of the hydrophobic core of the molecule. The most notable difference between the ligand-bound RARγ and TRα and the unliganded RXRα concerns the position of one of the carboxy-terminal helices, helix 12. It extends beyond the core in the absence of ligand *(50)*, but is repositioned across the core in the presence of ligand *(51,52)*. This suggests that the receptor undergoes extensive conformational changes upon ligand binding *(51,52)*. In addition, the RARγ and TRα structures reveal that helix 12 makes direct contact with the ligand, and is positioned in close proximity to α-helices 3 and 4. This creates a three-dimensional structure involving the surface and binding pocket, which may affect how the receptor interacts with both the ligand and other proteins.

Translation of the structural information from RXRα, RARγ, and TRα into a structure for the ER in the absence of ligand, and the presence of different ligands is an issue of current interest *(55,56)*. That helix 12 is involved in the conformational realignment is particularly exciting, since this region is critical for ligand-dependent AF-2 transcriptional activation of a number of nuclear receptors *(57–60)*. Mutations in this region can block AF-2 activity without affecting ligand binding, suggesting that helix 12 is not part of the binding pocket, but is instead involved in interactions with other proteins. This is supported by studies in which mutations of residues in helix 12 appear to disrupt the interaction of the ER with various coactivators, such as RIP140, TIF1, and mSUG1 *(61–63)*. However, other helices may also be important in transcriptional activation, including helices 3 and 4, since helix 12 is lodged between these helices in the ligand-bound structure. In support of this idea, mutation of lysine 366 in the mouse ER, which maps to the helix 3/4 region, reduces transcriptional activation without affecting hormone or DNA-binding activity *(64)*. Furthermore, helix 12 alone is insufficient for binding some coactivators, such as TIF1 *(65)*.

In summary, the LBD crystal structures of RXRα, RARγ, and TRα have provided exciting new insights into ER structure and function. The conformational changes that appear to occur upon ligand binding provide an explanation for observations from previous functional studies that residues located in separate regions of the receptor are important for transcriptional activation, as will be discussed in Subheading 2.1.2. Furthermore, when the crystal structure of the ER is solved with bound antiestrogens, one should finally be able to see how the structure differs upon binding estrogen vs antiestrogens, and perhaps more accurately predict how specific mutations affect interactions of the receptor with different ligands.

2.1.2. Activation Functions

Two, possibly three, transcription activation functions have been defined in the ER, as shown in Fig. 2 *(66–70)*. AF-2 is found in the carboxy-terminal region of the LBD, and is highly conserved among members of the nuclear receptor family; AF-1 is less conserved among members of the family *(5)*. AF-2 requires ligand for activity, but AF-1 exhibits constitutive activity, and can stimulate transcription in the absence of estrogen, and, in some cells, even in the absence of AF-2. In most cell types, however, both AF-1 and AF-2 appear to function together for optimal transcriptional activity. Recently, a third AF, AF-2a, was identified in the amino-terminal portion of AF-2 while screening for ER mutants in yeast *(68)*. AF-2a functions in a ligand-independent manner in the absence of both AF-1 and AF-2 *(67)*.

Some of the most enlightening studies of the past few years have demonstrated that the activities of the ER AFs vary, depending on the cell type and gene promoter. In these studies, truncated forms of the wild-type ER, lacking either AF-1 or AF-2, were cotransfected with different estrogen-responsive reporter constructs into ER-negative cell lines, such as human ovarian cancer cells (HeLa) and chicken embryo fibroblasts (CEF) *(16,37,69)*. The reporter constructs were either complex promoter regions containing upstream elements of the thymidine kinase, globin, or pS2 gene promoters, in addition to an ERE and a TATA box, or a minimal promoter composed of an ERE inserted upstream of the TATA region of the adenovirus-2 major late promoter. The carboxy-terminal truncated ER containing the AF-1-domain stimulated transcription only poorly (2–12% of wild-type activity) from all these promoters in HeLa cells, but it functioned efficiently (20–94% of wild-type activity) irrespective of the promoter utilized in CEF cells. In contrast, an amino-terminal truncated ER containing AF-2 stimulated transcription from the complex promoters (20–100% of activity), but not the minimal promoter (only 1–8% of activity) in these cells. Similar results were obtained with cotransfection of the truncated forms of the ER and another complex ER-inducible reporter (containing one copy of an ERE upstream of the thymidine kinase promoter) into several different ER-negative cell lines *(23)*, again emphasizing the importance of both cell- and promoter-type specific factors in the estrogen activation of the ER.

Cell-type and gene promoter context also affects the agonist activity of nonsteroidal antiestrogens. The partial agonist effect of tamoxifen is caused, at least in part, by two factors: the cell- and promoter-type specific activity of AF-1, and the carboxy-terminal F-domain. First, there is a strong correlation between AF-1 activity and tamoxifen agonism. One of the studies described above also analyzed transcriptional activation of wild-type and truncated ERs in the presence of antiestrogens, finding that tamoxifen was an efficient agonist in CEF cells, irrespective of the promoter used, but it had very little agonist effect in HeLa cells *(16)*. The agonist effect of tamoxifen is probably through the AF-1-domain, since AF-1 was active with tamoxifen treatment, and AF-2 activity was not induced but inhibited by tamoxifen. Furthermore, the AF-1-dependent effect of tamoxifen resides within a specific region (amino acids 41–64) of the AF-1-domain *(71)*. Second, the F-domain affects the agonist (and antagonist) activities of nonsteroidal antiestrogens, and this may depend on the cell-type-dependent activity of both AF-1 and AF-2 *(72)*. This was shown via transient transfection of mutants lacking the F-domain into MDA-MB-231 and Chinese hamster ovary (CHO) cells, in which estrogen was equally effective in stimulating transcription from the reporters with both the wild-type and F-domain-truncated ERs; antiestrogens exhibited reduced agonist, but higher antagonist, activities with the F-domain mutant. In HeLa and 3T3 cells, however, estrogen stimulated higher levels of transcription from the wild-type ER, compared to the F-domain-truncated ER. Antiestrogens had no agonist activity with either ER construct, consistent with the previous observation that antiestrogens are unable to stimulate transcription in HeLa cells, because the AF-1-domain exhibits very low activity in these cells *(16)*. Despite the general lower transcriptional activity of the F-domain-truncated ER in response to estrogen, it was less sensitive than wild-type ER to antiestrogen antagonist activity, supporting a potential role for the F-domain in antiestrogen resistance. It is unknown whether the effect of the F-domain is dependent on the activity of the other ER regions. One hypothesis is that the F-domain simply enhances the effectiveness of transactivation by the AF-1- and AF-2-domains *(72)*.

The effectiveness of transcriptional activation by the AF-1- and AF-2-domains depends on a conformational change in the ER with ligand binding, possibly resulting in a physical interaction between the AFs. This physical interaction was demonstrated again, using transient transfection of truncated ERs containing either AF-1 or AF-2, separately, or simultaneously *(73)*. AF-1 and AF-2 interacted synergistically, resulting in the transcriptional activation of reporters in the presence of estrogen, but not tamoxifen, again suggesting that the ER undergoes distinct conformational changes upon binding by different ligands. Additional studies involving proteolytic digestion of ER in the presence of different ligands directly confirm that receptor conformation differs in a ligand-dependent manner, and illustrate that these differences reside in the carboxy-terminus of the receptor *(74–76)*.

Mutagenesis studies have identified residues in the LBD, near the AF-2-domain, important for the discrimination between different ligands. Specifically, amino acids 515–535 (corresponding to α-helix 11) appear to be involved in ligand recognition, because mutations in some of these residues (amino acids 521, 522, 524, 525, 528, 529, 531, and 532) reduce ER affinity or sensitivity for estrogen, reduce ER affinity for the antiestrogen tamoxifen (amino acids 515, 516, 521, and 525), or reduce the agonist activity of tamoxifen (amino acids 520, 522, 532, and 535) *(77–80)*. These mutants also show altered transcriptional activity, suggesting that these residues play an important role in receptor conformation. Other residues carboxy-terminal of this region (corresponding to α-helix 12), appear to be most important for discriminating between estrogen and antiestrogen activity. Mutation of amino acid 540 from a leucine to a glutamine produces an activity inversion; this receptor is activated by antiestrogens (tamoxifen or ICI 164,384), but not by estrogens *(81)*. The inversion activity of this mutant requires the AF-1- and F-domains, and does not appear to be promoter specific, although it is cell-type specific, occurring in MDA-MB-231 and MCF-10A cells, but not in CHO or 3T3 cells. Furthermore, the introduction of two additional amino acid changes in this mutant (residues 542 and 545) produces a receptor that can discriminate between different antiestrogens, because it retains inversion activity with tamoxifen, but not the pure steroidal antiestrogen ICI 164,384. These studies emphasize the importance of receptor conformation in ligand interpretation, and again demonstrate that cell-type-specific factors play significant roles in ER function.

Thus, the transcriptional activity of the ER in response to estrogen and antiestrogen binding depends on a number of factors. Estrogen binding promotes a productive interaction between AF-1 and AF-2 (and coaccessory protein interactions as will be discussed in Subheading 4.), leading to transcriptional activation (agonism); antiestrogen binding leads to an association between AF-1 and AF-2, but may or may not result in transcriptional activation (agonism or antagonism), depending on the antiestrogen bound. Nonsteroidal antiestrogens (such as tamoxifen) block AF-2, but not AF-1 activity, and steroidal antiestrogens (such as ICI 164,384) inhibit the activity of both of the AF-domains. Finally, additional regions of the ER, such as the F-domain, also influence the response to antiestrogens.

2.2. Regulation of Function

The activity of many transcription factors is regulated by phosphorylation and dephosphorylation, which involves various signal transduction pathways. Phosphorylation of members of the nuclear receptor superfamily occurs in vivo *(82–85)* and is known to be involved in receptor function, as suggested by several lines of evidence (reviewed in refs. *86* and *87*). First, hormone binding increases the level of receptor phosphorylation, and, second, certain growth factors activate nuclear receptors in the absence of hormone. The precise role of phosphorylation in nuclear receptor function is still unclear, although hormone binding, DNA binding, dimerization, and transactivation have all been proposed as functional targets of phosphorylation, as will be discussed in Subheading 2.2.1. for the ER.

2.2.1. Phosphorylation

Similar to other nuclear receptor superfamily members, the ER exhibits enhanced phosphorylation in response to hormone treatment *(88–90)*. Tyrosine 537 (Tyr537) was one of the first residues implicated as an important ligand-induced phosphorylation site within the ER LBD *(91–93)*, and is located near the amino-terminal end of helix 12 *(54)*; replacement of Tyr537 with other amino acids suggests that phosphorylation of this residue is important to hormone binding and transcriptional activation of the ER. Castoria et al. *(92)* mutated all five tyrosine residues within the LBD of the ER to phenylalanine, a residue with a hydrophobic side chain similar in size and structure to tyrosine, which cannot be phosphorylated, and was able to demonstrate that only phosphorylation at Tyr537 conferred efficient hormone-binding ability. Phosphorylation of Tyr537 may influence the structural conformation of the receptor required for activation, since mutations of this site to alanine, serine, aspartate, and glutamate produce a constitutively active ER, which interacts with the coactivators RIP140 and SRC-1 in the absence of hormone *(94,95)*. Recently, the authors have also identified an ER cDNA with a substitution of Tyr537 with asparagine (Asn), while screening metastatic breast tumors for mutations in the ER *(96)*. The Tyr537Asn mutant exhibits constitutive activity in the absence of estrogen, which is only minimally affected by antiestrogens. The authors favor a model in which the Tyr537Asn mutation produces a conformational change in the receptor that mimics hormone binding. As a result, the mutant ER only weakly binds estrogen and antiestrogens, explaining their limited effects on mutant ER activity.

Serine (Ser)118, located within the AF-1-domain, has also been identified as a major phosphorylation site within the ER *(88,90,97)*. Using site-directed mutagenesis, Ali et al. *(88)* demonstrated that mutation of Ser118 to alanine reduced the transcriptional activity of the receptor by up to 75%. In contrast, Le Goff et al. *(90)* found that mutation of Ser118 alone only marginally affected activity, but mutation of three serines, including serines 104, 106, and 118, reduced transcriptional activity to about 50%. Taken together, these studies do suggest that phosphorylation of Ser118 is important to ER transcriptional activity. This conclusion is also supported by recent data demonstrating that Ser118 can be phosphorylated in vitro and in vivo by the mitogen-activated protein kinase pathway, which enhances both estrogen-dependent and estrogen-independent ER activity *(98–100)*.

In addition to transcriptional activation, phosphorylation may also be important for DNA binding and dimerization. Phosphatase treatment decreases general DNA binding *(89)*; phosphorylation of Tyr537 is implicated in DNA binding and dimerization *(91,98,101)*. A study by Arnold and Notides *(101)* suggests that ER dimerization interactions involve both Tyr537 and a Src homology 2-domain located between residues 424 and 524. Recently, it was also proposed that Tyr537 phosphorylation, receptor dimerization, and hormone-binding events are intimately connected, so that phosphorylation increases dimerization, which then results in an enhanced hormone-binding capacity *(102)*. This proposed mechanism involves the cooperative binding of estrogen, which is induced by conformational changes in the dimeric receptor, and is an important area for future research.

2.2.2. Crosstalk with Other Signal Transduction Pathways

ER activity can be regulated by phosphorylation through various signaling pathways. Since the discovery that crosstalk between receptors and cell signaling pathways occurs, a number of studies have focused on dissecting these communication networks (reviewed in refs. *56, 87,* and *103*). Crosstalk involves a variety of interactions, including those that do not require DNA or ligand binding by the ER. Although the mechanisms of action are still largely unknown, advances of the past few years have identified some of the participants in ER crosstalk, and suggest that crosstalk may also influence the agonist activity of antiestrogens.

Agents that activate the ER include growth factors such as epidermal growth factor (EGF) and insulin growth factor I *(104–106)*, cAMP *(104,107)*, neurotransmitters (dopamine) *(108)*, phosphatase inhibitors (vanadate) *(109)*, and cyclin D1 *(110–111)*. Initial studies involving EGF suggested that this growth factor might stimulate hormone-independent activation of the ER through signaling pathways involving protein kinases *(105,106)*. Subsequent investigations demonstrated that phosphorylation of Ser118 in the AF-1-domain via the mitogen-activated protein kinase pathway is important for EGF-induced activation of the ER *(99,107)*.

Several other agents that activate the ER also work through phosphorylation pathways. Cyclic AMP activation of the ER involves protein kinase A (PKA) phosphorylation of the AF-2-domain *(107)*; the neurotransmitter dopamine activates the ER through the dopamine receptor, which signals via both the PKA and protein kinase C pathways *(108)*. Studies involving phosphatase inhibitors, such as vanadate, provide further evidence for the involvement of protein kinases and phosphatases in the activation process *(109)*. Studies with insulin growth factor I emphasize that, although various agents activate the ER, increased phosphorylation does not always correlate with increased transcriptional activation *(104)*. But the in vivo consequences of these events in breast cancer cells are poorly understood. In contrast to agents activating the ER through phosphorylation pathways, cyclin D1 stimulates the hormone-independent activation of the ER without activation of its cyclin-dependent kinase (CDK4) *(110,111)*.

In addition to regulating ER transcriptional activity, crosstalk may alter the effects of antiestrogens in cells. Support for this hypothesis comes mostly from the work of the Katzenellenbogen group (reviewed in ref. *112*). In these studies, the ER-positive breast cancer cell line MCF-7 was transfected with different estrogen-responsive promoter constructs, and treated with either estrogen or antiestrogens, in combination with agents that stimulated intracellular cAMP levels, such as isobutylmethylxanthine and cholera toxin *(113)*. Treatment of cells with these agents resulted in stronger agonist (and a weaker antagonist) activity with tamoxifen, while not affecting the antagonist activity of ICI 164,384. Furthermore, stimulation of tamoxifen's agonist activity was promoter-specific, because it occurred with some promoters (TATA and pS2), but not others (thymidine kinase). These results suggest that changes in the cAMP level of a cell could contribute to the development of resistance to antiestrogen therapy, which is an interesting hypothesis that awaits confirmation in vivo.

Finally, alternative pathways of ER action involving protein–protein interactions, instead of the classical ERE binding, may contribute to the agonist effect of antiestrogens in some cell types and tissues. One example of an alternative pathway of ER action is the ER-mediated stimulation of transcription from a promoter lacking an ERE, but containing the binding site for the transcription factors Jun and Fos (an AP-1 site) *(114–116)*. This AP-1 directed method of ER action is believed to involve direct protein–protein interactions between the ER and Jun and Fos. Furthermore, a recent report demonstrated that tamoxifen can stimulate ER-mediated transcription at AP-1 sites, providing a possible mechanism for the agonist effects of tamoxifen in some tissues *(117)*. A second example of an alternative pathway of ER action involves ER binding of certain antiestrogens, such as raloxifene, an antiestrogen with mixed agonist/antagonist activity *(118)*. The raloxifene-bound ER can stimulate transcription of transforming growth factor-3, a gene important in bone cells, to a higher level than estrogen-bound ER *(119)*. This transcriptional effect is mediated, at least in part, by a DNA element distinct from an ERE, called a raloxifene response element, that does not require the DBD of the raloxifene-bound ER, but may be mediated through protein–protein interactions between the ER and a cellular adapter protein.

3. A NEW ER GENE: ERβ

Most of the work described in this chapter concerns the first ER cDNA identified, now called ERα throughout, which was cloned more than 10 yr ago *(120,121)*. Although other members of the nuclear receptor superfamily are expressed in multiple forms from distinct genes (for example, RAR's α, β, and γ, or TR's α and β), none were found for the ER (reviewed in ref. *87*), although numerous splice variants have been described for ER *(122–125)*. The identification of a second ER (ERβ) from rat *(126)*, however, has broadened the view of ER functions, as described below.

3.1. ERβ Structure

3.1.1. Tissue Distribution

ERβ was cloned from both human and rat tissues using degenerate primers based on conserved regions of the DBDs and LBDs of members of the nuclear receptor super-family *(126,127)*; the mouse ERβ was cloned using degenerate primers specific for the rat ERβ LBD *(128)*. Examination of the tissue distribution of ERα and ERβ suggests that the two receptors may have distinct physiological roles. Kuiper et al. *(129)* used RT-PCR of RNA from a variety of rat tissues and found that some tissues, especially the ovary, expressed relatively equal amounts of both subtypes. Other tissues appeared to express more ERα (uterus, pituitary, epididymis, and testis) or more ERβ (prostate and bladder); some tissues expressed exclusively ERα (kidney and liver) or ERβ (lung and brain). That ERβ may have a distinct physiological role in some tissues is also implied by *in situ* hybridization studies demonstrating rat ERβ cell-specific localization in the hypothalamus, ovary, and prostate *(126,130,131)*. Using Northern blot analysis, Mosselman et al. *(127)* showed that human ERβ was expressed in the thymus, testis, ovary, and spleen, and that human ERα was expressed in the testis, ovary, prostate, and skeletal muscle. Tremblay et al. *(128)* also detected mouse ERβ in the ovary. There were multiple ERβ ovarian transcripts, but only one transcript of ERα was detected *(128,130)*. Recently, ERβ expression was detected in human breast tumor biopsy samples, with the level of expression varying among samples and not correlated with ERα expression *(132)*. The tissue distribution of ERβ protein, as opposed to RNA, has not yet been reported, and awaits the development of specific antibodies.

3.1.2. Homology Between ERα and ERβ

Protein sequence comparisons of ERβ with members of the nuclear hormone receptor superfamily indicate that it is most related to ERα *(126–128)*. The region of highest homology is in the ER DBD, with 96, 95, and 97% for human, rat, and mouse, respectively, which is not surprising, since the DBD is the most conserved region among nuclear receptor family members *(4)*. The high degree of homology between the DBDs of ERβ and ERα suggests that they can both bind EREs, and conservation in regions within the DBD required for dimer formation suggests that the two receptors may heterodimerize, as will be discussed in Subheading 3.2. Therefore, ERβ and ERα may influence or affect each other's transcriptional activity if expressed in the same cells. The LBD is also highly conserved between ERβ and ERα, with 58, 54, and 60% for human, rat, and mouse, respectively, indicating that they might bind similar ligands, also discussed in Subheading 3.2. In contrast, the A- and B-domains and the hinge region are not as conserved. Since the putative transactivation domains are not homologous, especially in the amino-terminal AF-1-domain, ERβ and ERα may therefore activate different genes. Furthermore, since ERβ appears to lack the carboxy-terminal F-domain *(127)*, which has a specific modulatory function that affects the agonist/antagonist balance of certain antiestrogens *(72)*, it might contribute to antiestrogen resistance by interfering with antiestrogen inhibition of tumor growth.

Thus, the balance of ERβ and ERα expression in tumors might prove to be an important biomarker for tumor progression.

3.2. ERβ Function

3.2.1. DNA Binding and Dimerization

ERβ binds DNA in a manner similar to ERα, as a homodimer interacting with EREs *(133–135)*. Furthermore, as predicted by protein sequence comparisons, ERβ and ERα form functional heterodimers on EREs. The DNA binding ability of the heterodimer is dependent on both receptors *(135)*, and the binding affinity of the ERα/ERβ heterodimer is similar to ERα homodimers, but greater than that of ERβ homodimers *(133)*. Thus, although these results clearly demonstrate an interaction of ERβ homodimers and ERα/ERβ heterodimers with EREs, they do not exclude the possibility that there may also be interactions with novel response elements, different from the known EREs. Finally, using ERα mutants with mutations in a region of the LBD required for both dimerization and DNA binding, it was shown that the amino acid residues involved in ERα/ERβ heterodimerization overlap, but are not identical to those involved in ERα homodimerization *(133)*.

3.2.2. Ligand-Binding Affinity

The binding affinity of ERβ for estradiol is similar to that of ERα, although ERβ may have a slightly lower affinity *(126–128)*. Kuiper et al. *(129)* determined the binding affinities of 36 compounds, in addition to estradiol, for ERα and ERβ. For most ligands, the overall binding affinities were very similar, although there were some differences between affinities for both synthetic and naturally occurring compounds. The stilbene estrogens, a group of synthetic estrogens with a composite diphenolic ring structure, bind with high affinity to both ER subtypes, but the order of competition is different (diethylstilbestrol > hexestrol > dienestrol > [estradiol] for ERα and dienestrol > diethylstilbestrol > hexestrol > [estradiol] for ERβ). Another estrogen, moxestrol, which is used as a radioligand in ER functional assays, binds ERα with a higher affinity than ERβ. The same order of affinity for both ER receptors was found for the triphenylethylene (anti)estrogens, although ERβ has about twice the affinity for 4-OH-tamoxifen and ICI 164,384, compared to estradiol as ERα. Finally, genistein and coumestrol, plant-derived compounds, also exhibit a higher affinity for ERβ. These examples suggest that ERβ may preferentially bind some ligands, and ERβ binds others. However, as the authors suggest, these compounds need to be tested in functional transactivation assay systems using different cellular backgrounds before definitive conclusions can be reached.

3.2.3. Transcriptional Activation

Although ERα and ERβ have similar DBDs and LBDs, it is important to determine if they preferentially activate transcription of the same genes. Preliminary studies testing whether ERβ could bind an ERE and activate transcription from ERE-containing promoters in CHO cells *(126,127)*, Cos-1, or HeLa cells *(128)* demonstrated that ERβ could indeed activate transcription in these cells, although the levels of induction were higher for ERα *(127,133)*. Furthermore, ERα antagonists (tamoxifen and the ICI compounds) were also potent antagonists for ERβ *(127)*, although Tremblay et al. *(128)*

found that tamoxifen exhibited agonist activity against mouse ERα, but not mouse ERβ, in Cos-1 and HeLa cells. The authors suggest that the differences in tamoxifen activities may be the result of differences in the AF-1 region, since mouse ERβ lacks a portion of the ERα AF-1 region (amino acids 41–64) which has been shown to be important for tamoxifen agonism *(71)*. Cotransfection of human ERα and ERβ into Cos-1 and HeLa cells resulted in a level of transcription intermediate between the level with either ERα or ERβ alone *(133)*; cotransfection of human ERα and mouse ERβ into human fetal kidney 293 cells resulted in a level of transcription which was not significantly different from that with ERα alone *(135)*. Studies testing whether ERβ can activate transcription from AP-1-containing promoters in HeLa cells indicates that ERβ can also activate transcription from this response element, although the transactivation properties of ERβ and ERα differ in a ligand-dependent manner *(136)*. Although estradiol was an agonist, and tamoxifen and ICI 164,384 were antagonists of ERα-mediated transactivation at an AP-1 response element, these compounds had the opposite effect on ERβ-mediated transactivation, providing additional evidence that the two ERs signal in different ways, suggesting they play different roles in gene regulation.

Do the same coactivators that upregulate ligand-dependent ERα transcriptional activation (like SRC-1) *(137,138)* also influence ERβ activity? Tremblay et al. *(128)* demonstrated that SRC-1 upregulates the ligand-dependent transcriptional activity of ERβ by about two- to threefold in Cos-1 and HeLa cells. These observations correlated with GST pull-down experiments in which the ERβ LBD interacted with SRC-1 in a hormone-dependent manner *(128)*, although a separate study suggested that SRC-1 may also interact with ERβ in the absence of hormone *(133)*. SRC-1 coexpression increased basal levels of ERβ transcriptional activity, and ICI 182,780, but not tamoxifen, blocked this effect *(128)*. The clinical significance of this observation, and whether there are other ERβ specific accessory proteins, is not known. Finally, ERα and ERβ heterodimers also interact with SRC-1 *(133)*.

4. REGULATION OF TRANSCRIPTIONAL ACTIVATION AT GENE PROMOTERS

Nuclear receptor regulation of gene expression involves not only ligand and DNA binding, but also interactions with basal and general transcription factors (*see* Subheading 4.1.; reviewed in refs. *103* and *139*). However, additional factors are also necessary for gene activation, as was first suggested from squelching experiments in which the overexpression of one nuclear receptor interfered with the transcriptional activity of another nuclear receptor *(140,141)*. It was hypothesized that both receptors required common interacting proteins (also called coaccessory proteins), which were present in limiting amounts, resulting in transcriptional interference. A number of coaccessory proteins have recently been identified that interact with the ER (Subheadings 4.2. and 4.3.), and appear to act as bridging factors with the general transcriptional machinery (reviewed in refs. *103,139,* and *142*). These proteins are called coactivators if they enhance, and corepressors if they inhibit, the transcriptional activity of nuclear receptors. As reviewed by Horwitz et al. *(139)*, the complete definition of these transcriptional effectors is not yet refined. Alternate terms may be more appropriate to distinguish whether a specific factor influences the ligand-activated and/or basal transcriptional activity of a receptor, or whether there is direct contact with the receptor and/or basal transcription factors, and whether ligands alter the interaction of the factor with the receptor. Other proteins involved in interactions with nuclear receptors include chromatin factors *(143–145)* and sequence-specific transcription factors *(146,147),* which will not be discussed in this chapter.

4.1. Basal Transcription Factors

Transcription by RNA polymerase II requires the assembly of basal and general transcription factors. In addition to interacting with each other, these proteins form direct contacts with nuclear receptors (reviewed in refs. *103* and *139*); for the ER, these include TFIID and TFIIB. One of the first events in the assembly of the basal transcription complex involves the binding of TFIID, which is composed of the TATA box-binding protein (TBP) and TBP-associated factors (TAFIIs), to a sequence within the promoter called the TATA box *(148).* Both ER activation functions AF-1 and AF-2 interact with TBP in vitro, and overexpression of TBP enhances ER transactivation in HeLa cells *(149).* Another component of TFIID, TAFII30, also interacts with the ER in vitro *(150).* TAFII30 is required for transactivation by the ER in HeLa cells, and this interaction involves the amino-terminal end of the E-domain, corresponding to the location of AF-2a. Following binding of TFIID to the TATA box, binding of TFIIB, RNA polymerase II, and TFIIF are required for the assembly of the minimal transcription initiation complex *(151).* TFIIB makes contact with DNA sequences both upstream and downstream of the TATA box, and interacts with TBP, TFIIF, and RNA polymerase II *(152-154),* in addition to interacting with nuclear receptors, such as the ER *(103,139).* Although TFIIB interacts with the ER AF-2-domain *(155),* contacts formed with other nuclear receptors involve other domains. The significance of these differences remains to be established, although it may be an important factor in the regulation of nuclear receptor function.

4.2. Coactivators

Coactivators function as bridging proteins between nuclear receptors and basal transcription factors in the preinitiation complex (reviewed in refs. *139* and *142*). Numerous factors that associate with the activated ER have been identified using in vitro protein interaction assays, yeast two-hybrid systems with different nuclear receptor LBDs as bait, or expression library screening. These include CBP/p300, SRC-1, TIF2, GRIP-1, ERAP160, TIF1, and RIP140, as discussed in this subheading. In addition, there are a few other putative coactivators of the ER, including SPT6 *(156),* RAP46 *(157),* ARA70 *(158),* and TRIP1/SUG1 *(63),* which will not be discussed.

4.2.1. CBP/p300

A coactivator of the cAMP response element binding protein (CREB), called CBP (for CREB binding protein) *(159),* also interacts with RNA polymerase II and TFIIB, as well as a number of other proteins *(152-154;* reviewed in refs. *103* and *142*). CBP and a closely related protein, p300, associate with several members of the nuclear receptor superfamily *(160),* and stimulate the transcriptional activity of the ER *(161).* Furthermore, cotransfection of CBP/p300 with another coactivator, SRC-1, stimulates

ER activity in a synergistic manner in HeLa cells, suggesting that they may function cooperatively. In a separate study, Hanstein et al. *(162)* used immunoprecipitation to demonstrate that CBP/p300 is part of a complex of proteins, including ERAP160 and possibly SRC-1 (*see* Subheading 4.2.2.), which all influence ER activity. A direct interaction between SRC-1 and CBP/p300 has also been demonstrated using yeast two-hybrid analyses *(163)*; thus, it appears that CBP/p300 play key regulatory roles in the cell. Since CBP/p300 are coactivators for a number of different transcription factors, it has been proposed that they function as coordinators or cointegrators for nuclear receptors with other signaling pathways *(160,162,164)*.

4.2.2. SRC-1 and Related Coactivators

Several coactivators have been identified as a family of related proteins, and include SRC-1 and related isoforms *(138,165)*, TIF2 *(166)*, GRIP1 *(167,168)*, and ERAP160 (or p160) *(160,169)*. The amino-terminal region of the SRC-1 family of proteins contains a PAS A/helix–loop–helix domain, which is a dimerization interface that has been identified in several other nuclear proteins, including period (PER), the aryl hydrocarbon receptor (AHR), and single-minded (SIM) (reviewed in ref. *170*). This dimerization interface may allow for interactions between the SRC-1 coactivator family and the PAS A/helix–loop–helix family, providing a link between steroid receptors and other nuclear proteins. SRC-1, isolated in a yeast two-hybrid screen, using the progesterone receptor (PR) as bait, stimulates the transcriptional activation of a number of nuclear receptors, including the ER, in transient transfection analyses *(138)*. TIF2 was isolated by screening an expression library with ligand-bound ER *(166)*. Although TIF2 enhances the transcriptional activation of the ER, it fails to stimulate the activity of a number of other nuclear receptors (glucocorticoid receptor, GR; RXR; RAR; TR; vitamin D receptor, VDR). Since TIF2 does bind these receptors in vitro, the authors propose that it may function in conjunction with other factors, or in a cell-type-specific manner. GRIP1 is a mouse protein isolated in a yeast two-hybrid screen, using glucocorticoid receptor as the bait *(168)*. Based on homology to TIF2 (94%), GRIP1 is probably the mouse version of TIF2. Finally, ERAP160 was originally identified by in vitro biochemical assays as a protein whose binding to the LBD of the ER was stabilized by estrogen and destabilized by antiestrogens *(169)*. ERAP160 was subsequently cloned from an expression library based on its interaction with both CBP and ligand-bound ER, revealing that it encodes an SRC-1-related protein(s) *(160)*.

Recent studies have focused on the ER domains and specific amino acids involved in its interactions with SRC-1 and related coactivators. Replacement of lysine 366 (Lys366) in the mouse ER (predicted to be at the carboxy-terminal end of helix 3) reduces both AF-2 activity and SRC-1 binding *(64)*. This mutation, however, does not affect the binding of the RIP140 coactivator, and ligand or DNA binding, indicating that Lys366 (and possibly helix 3) is found in an ER region important for interactions with coactivators, but distinct from the regions important for ligand binding. When another residue, Tyr537, is mutated, SRC-1 binds in the absence of ligand, but in the wild-type receptor, SRC-1 requires ligand to bind *(94,95)*. Using ER LBDs with mutations eliminating AF-2 activity, it was found that the interaction between GRIP1 and the ER requires an intact AF-2-domain *(168)*. The interaction between ERAP160 and the ER also requires an intact, functionally active AF-2-domain, and occurs in the presence of estrogens, but not antiestrogens *(169)*. Finally, McInerney et al. *(137)* proposed that SRC-1 interacts with specific ER residues that enhance transcriptional activity by facilitating the interaction of the two ER activation functions, AF-1 and AF-2. Thus, amino acids located in both the AF-1- and AF-2-domains are important for interactions of the SRC-1 family members with the ER.

4.2.3. TIF1 and RIP140

Mouse TIF1 (mTIF1) was identified in a yeast genetic screen as a protein that stimulated RXRγ activity *(61)*; human TIF1 (hTIF1) and human RIP140 were cloned from expression libraries using the mouse ER LBD *(65,171)*. mTIF1 and hTIF1 are about 93% homologous, and hTIF1 and RIP140 contain a low degree of homology (35%) between their nuclear receptor binding sites. mTIF1, hTIF1, and RIP140 all bind the ER AF-2-domain *(61,65,171)*, and the interaction between RIP140 and the ER is dependent on an intact α-helix, predicted to be helix 12 *(62)*. A short sequence of 26 residues, which is homologous to two receptor binding sites characterized on RIP140 *(62)*, is sufficient for the in vitro binding of hTIF1 to the ER *(65)*. This implies that TIF1 and RIP140 may interact with the same interface on nuclear receptors, although Henttu et al. *(64)* suggest that there are some differences in their binding sites, since mutation of Lys366 blocks TIF1, but not RIP140 binding.

Whether or not TIF1 and RIP140 are true coactivators is uncertain, because overexpression of mTIF1 in Cos-1 cells *(61)*, or overexpression of RIP140 in CEF and MCF-7 cells *(171)*, inhibits rather than stimulates ligand-dependent transactivation by the ER. This is in contrast to the activity of mTIF1 in yeast, in which it potentiates RXR-dependent transcription *(61)*. At first, it is paradoxical that coactivators suppress transcriptional activity when they are overexpressed in cells. However, TIF1 and RIP140 may be components of a complex in which the relative levels of the different interacting proteins is the critical parameter *(142)*, so that overexpression of one factor leads to transcriptional inhibition if the other components of the complex are not also overexpressed.

4.3. Corepressors

Fewer corepressors than coactivators have been reported to date. One corepressor, SMRT, was isolated as a human protein that bound RXRα in the absence of ligand *(172,173)*; mouse N-CoR (mN-CoR) was isolated in a similar manner, using TRβ *(174)*. These corepressors appeared to interact specifically with unliganded TR/RAR/RXRs. Recently, the human homolog of mN-CoR, hN-CoR, was also isolated, but in a slightly different manner, using antiprogestin-occupied PR hinge/LBD as the bait in two-hybrid studies *(24)*. hN-CoR is 99% homologous to mN-CoR, and binds not only the LBD of the PR, but also the LBD of the ER *(24)*. This interaction depends on the type of antagonist bound to the receptor. The interaction is strong with receptors bound to antagonists having mixed agonist/antagonist activity (for the PR, RU486 or ZK112993, and for the ER, tamoxifen), but weak with receptors bound to pure antagonists (for the PR, ZK98299, and for the ER, ICI 164,384). To analyze the effect of corepressors on the activity of mixed antagonists, Jackson et al. *(24)* transfected mN-CoR or SMRT with either the PR or the ER, and found that both corepressors suppress the agonist

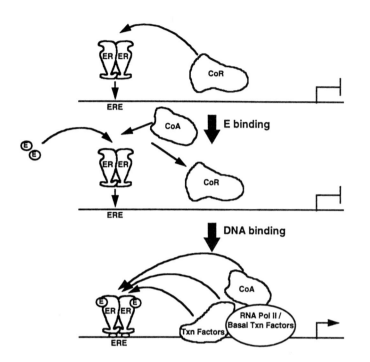

Fig. 3. A proposed model for the interactions of ER with corepressors and coactivators. The unliganded ER may interact with corepressors (CoR). When estrogen (E) is added, coactivators (CoA) are recruited to the ER, potentially displacing CoR, so that the receptor interacts with components of the RNA polymerase II transcription complex and basal transcription factors (RNA Pol II/Basal Txn Factors), and sequence-specific transcription factors (Txn Factors) to initiate transcription (arrow).

activity of antagonists, but that coexpression of the PR hinge and LBD relieves this suppression. These corepressors have disparate effects on agonist-dependent transcription: mN-CoR represses and SMRT enhances transcription.

In the same yeast two-hybrid screen with the PR hinge/LBD, another receptor-interacting protein, called L7/SPA, was identified *(24)*. Similar to hN-CoR, the interaction of L7/SPA with either the PR or the ER depends on the type of antagonist present. L7/SPA binds the hinge region, rather than the LBD, of these receptors. Furthermore, L7/SPA enhances, rather than suppresses, the agonist activity of mixed antagonists, but does not affect the activity of pure antagonists or pure agonists. Thus, L7/SPA is not, by definition, a corepressor, but is a coactivator of antagonist-mediated transcription.

Recent data indicates that, similar to coactivators, corepressors are components of multiprotein complexes. Furthermore, these complexes appear to repress transcription through histone deacetylation *(175,176)*. These findings predict a mechanism of action of corepressors (and coactivators) *(177)*, as shown in Fig. 3. The unliganded receptor may interact with a corepressor (Fig. 3., CoR) complex. Addition of ligand may result in the dissociation of the corepressor complex, which could then be replaced by a coactivator complex (Fig. 3., CoA). However, this model does not predict what the role of ligand antagonists might be, or whether all receptors, such as the ER, are involved in the same type of interactions.

4.4. Coregulation of Transcription

Since coactivators and corepressors are found in the same cells and involved in the regulation of the transcriptional response to antagonists, as well as agonists, what determines whether mixed antagonists will have agonist or antagonist activity? To address this question, Jackson et al. *(24)* cotransfected HeLa cells with the GR and either L7/SPA, SMRT, or both L7/SPA and SMRT, and then treated the cells with the mixed antagonist, RU486. L7/SPA alone enhances, and SMRT alone inhibits, transcriptional activity of the RU486-bound GR; transfection of both only slightly inhibit transcription from the receptor. In a similar study, Smith et al. *(178)* cotransfected HepG2 cells with the ER and either SRC-1, SMRT, or both SRC-1 and SMRT, then treated with the mixed antagonist tamoxifen. SRC-1 alone stimulates, and SMRT alone inhibits, the agonist activity of tamoxifen, and, again, both SRC-1 and SMRT slightly inhibit tamoxifen agonist activity. Taken together, these studies demonstrate that the effect of one coregulator can neutralize or override the effect of another coregulator, and suggest that antagonist-driven transcription depends on the relative levels of coregulators within the cell.

5. CONCLUDING REMARKS

The purpose of this chapter was to review some of the most significant recent advances in ER research, and to discuss current ideas or mechanisms for the mixed agonist/antagonist activity of steroidal antiestrogens and the development of resistance to antiestrogen therapy. What determines whether tamoxifen will have agonist or antagonist activity? Based on the discussion above, the effect of tamoxifen on ER transcriptional activation depends both upon the availability and activity of coaccessory proteins for a particular cell type and promoter. What types of changes can result in hormone resistance? Proposed models of hormone resistance are shown in Fig. 4. Although this review has concentrated on the ER and ER signal transduction pathways, it must be emphasized that many other mechanisms are most certainly involved in the development of antiestrogen resistance. As discussed in the introduction, hormone resistance can result from the impaired uptake, increased degradation, or altered metabolism of the antiestrogen, and the loss or mutation of the ER. Additional mechanisms that may be even more important in the development of hormone resistance include other ERs (ERβ), and changes in receptor effectors (for example, phosphorylation, signal transduction pathways, growth factors, and coaccessory proteins), as discussed below.

How could ERβ contribute to antiestrogen resistance? First, since ERβ lacks the carboxy-terminal F-domain, it may interfere with antiestrogen inhibition of growth through the ERα. Second, ERβ may interact with specific coaccessory proteins through the AF-1 and hinge regions, since these regions of ERβ are not conserved with ERα, to induce gene transcription even in the presence of antiestrogens. Third, ERβ may compete with ERα for binding antiestrogens, freeing ERα to bind estrogen and activate transcription. Fourth, ERβ and ERα may heterodimerize, and thus stimulate, rather than inhibit, transcription with antiestrogen binding. Finally, ERβ might be involved in crosstalk with different signal transduction pathways than ERα, circumventing the effects of antiestrogens. Alternatively, ERβ may not contribute

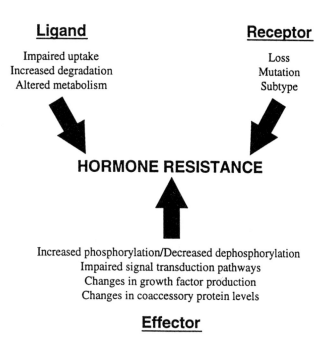

Fig. 4. The development of hormone resistance is probably multifactorial. Resistance to hormone can occur by changes at the level of ligand, receptor, or other effectors.

to antiestrogen resistance, since it has a higher affinity for tamoxifen and ICI 164,384 *(129)*, but exhibits limited agonist activity with tamoxifen, at least in primary studies *(128)*.

How might coaccessory proteins contribute to antiestrogen resistance? Both coactivators and corepressors are present at the same time in the same cells. Under these conditions, a number of factors could influence whether activation or inhibition of transcription might occur. Changes in the relative levels of coactivators to corepressors could result in antiestrogen resistance by determining whether an antagonist (like tamoxifen) stimulates or inhibits transcription. The interaction of coactivators and corepressors with receptor may also be influenced by the type of ligand bound (and the structural conformation of the ligand-bound receptor). In addition, different receptors, for example ERα or ERβ, might favor interactions with different coactivators and corepressors, resulting in transcriptional activation and antiestrogen resistance. Furthermore, the chromatin structure at the promoter might favor the interaction of certain coaccessory proteins with the receptor, also resulting in resistance to antiestrogens. Finally, the influence of the previous four factors may vary, depending on the types and levels of coactivators and corepressors present in different cell types.

Effective therapy is essential for the control of breast cancer. Clearly, although the current group of steroidal and nonsteroidal antiestrogens have proven to be valuable clinically, these agents have their limitations. So, what are the goals in developing new antiestrogens? Very simply, the ideal antiestrogen will block estrogen-stimulated growth of mammary carcinoma cells, but not interfere with estrogen activity in nontarget tissues. In addition, there should not be the development of resistance to this antiestrogen similar to that now seen, or at least there should be an increased length of time before resistance is formed. Hopefully, continual re-examination of what is known about the basic biology of the ERs (ERα, ERβ, and more?) and the specific coaccessory proteins that interact with them, will provide the answers necessary to design new, more effective antiestrogens.

ACKNOWLEDGMENTS

The authors would like to thank Julia Perkins for secretarial support. R. K. H. is supported by DAMD 17-95-1-5025 and NIH CA 30195 awarded to S. A. W. F.

REFERENCES

1. Henderson, B. E., R. Ross, and L. Bernstein. 1988. Estrogens as a cause of human cancer: the Richard and Hinda Rosenthal Foundation award lecture. *Cancer Res.* **48:** 246–253.
2. Katzenellenbogen, B. S., K. L. Kendra, M. J. Norman, and Y. Berthois. 1987. Proliferation, hormone responsiveness and estrogen receptor content of MCF-7 human breast cancer cells grown in the short-term and long-term absence of estrogens. *Cancer Res.* **47:** 4355–4360.
3. Osborne, C. K., K. Hobbs, and G. M. Clark. 1985. Effect of estrogens and antiestrogens on growth of human breast cancer cells in athymic nude mice. *Cancer Res.* **45:** 584–590.
4. Beato, M. 1989. Gene regulation by steroid hormones. *Cell* **56:** 335–344.
5. Evans, R. M. 1988. The steroid and thyroid hormone receptor superfamily. *Science* **240:** 889–895.
6. Clark, G. M. and W. L. McGuire. 1988. Steroid receptors and other prognostic factors in primary breast cancer. *Semin. Oncol.* **15:** 20–25.
7. Clark, G. M., C. K. Osborne, and W. L. McGuire. 1984. Correlations between estrogen receptor, progesterone receptor, and patient characteristics in human breast cancer. *J. Clin. Oncol.* **2:** 1102–1109.
8. Bezwoda, W. R., J. D. Esser, R. Dansey, I. Kessel, and M. Lange. 1991. The value of estrogen and progesterone receptor determinations in advanced breast cancer. Estrogen receptor level but not progesterone receptor level correlates with response to tamoxifen. *Cancer* **68:** 867–872.
9. Bloom, N. D., E. H. Tobin, B. Schreibman, and G. A. Degenshein. 1980. The role of progesterone receptors in the management of advanced breast cancer. *Cancer* **45:** 2992–2997.
10. Osborne, C. K., M. G. Yochmowitz, W. A. Knight, 3d, and W. L. McGuire. 1980. The value of estrogen and progesterone receptors in the treatment of breast cancer. *Cancer* **46:** 2884–2888.
11. Henderson, M. 1993. Current approaches to breast cancer prevention. *Science* **259:** 630–631.
12. Jordan, V. C. 1992. The strategic use of antiestrogens to control the development and growth of breast cancer. *Cancer* **70:** 977–982.
13. Wakeling, A. E. 1990. Novel pure antiestrogens. Mode of action and therapeutic prospects. *Ann. NY Acad. Sci.* **595:** 348–356.
14. DeFriend, D. J., A. Howell, R. I. Nicholson, E. Anderson, M. Dowsett, R. E. Mansel, et al. 1994. Investigation of a new pure antiestrogen (ICI 182,780) in women with primary breast cancer. *Cancer Res.* **54:** 408–414.
15. Howell, A., D. DeFriend, J. Robertson, R. Blamey, and P. Walton. 1995. Response to a specific antioestrogen (ICI 182,780) in tamoxifen-resistant breast cancer. *Lancet* **345:** 29–30.
16. Berry, M., D. Metzger, and P. Chambon. 1990. Role of the two activating domains of the oestrogen receptor in the cell-type and promoter-context dependent agonistic activity of the anti-oestrogen 4-hydroxytamoxifen. *EMBO J.* **9:** 2811–2818.

17. Jordan, V. C. and C. S. Murphy. 1990. Endocrine pharmacology of antiestrogens as antitumor agents. *Endocr. Rev.* **11:** 578–610.

18. Wolf, D. M. and S. A. W. Fuqua. 1995. Mechanisms of action of antiestrogens. *Cancer Treatment Rev.* **21:** 247–271.

19. Dauvois, S., P. S. Danielian, R. White, and M. G. Parker. 1992. Antiestrogen ICI 164,384 reduces cellular estrogen receptor content by increasing its turnover. *Proc. Natl. Acad. Sci. USA* **89:** 4037–4041.

20. Dauvois, S., R. White, and M. G. Parker. 1993. The antiestrogen ICI 182,780 disrupts estrogen receptor nucleocytoplasmic shuttling. *J. Cell Sci.* **106:** 1377–1388.

21. Fawell, S. E., R. White, S. Hoare, M. Sydenham, M. Page, and M. G. Parker. 1990. Inhibition of estrogen receptor-DNA binding by the "pure" antiestrogen ICI 164,384 appears to be mediated by impaired receptor dimerization. *Proc. Natl. Acad. Sci. USA* **87:** 6883–6887.

22. Bocquel, M. T., V. Kumar, C. Stricker, P. Chambon, and H. Gronemeyer. 1989. The contribution of the N- and C-terminal regions of steroid receptors to activation of transcription is both receptor and cell-specific. *Nucleic Acids Res.* **17:** 2581–2595.

23. Tzukerman, M. T., A. Esty, D. Santiso-Mere, P. Danielian, M. G. Parker, R. B. Stein, J. W. Pike, and D. P. McDonnell. 1994. Human estrogen receptor transactivational capacity is determined by both cellular and promoter context and mediated by two functionally distinct intramolecular regions. *Mol. Endocrinol.* **8:** 21–30.

24. Jackson, T. A., J. K. Richer, D. L. Bain, G. S. Takimoto, L. Tung, and K. B. Horwitz. 1997. The partial agonist activity of antagonist-occupied steroid receptors is controlled by a novel hinge domain-binding coactivator L7/SPA and the corepressors N-CoR or SMRT. *Mol. Endocrinol.* **11:** 693–705.

25. Vassilomanolakis, M. E., S. Tsoussis, K. Kandylis, E. Hajichristou, and A. P. Efredmidis. 1991. Rechallenge by tamoxifen in metastatic breast cancer: prospective study of different dose levels. *Breast Dis.* **4:** 129–134.

26. Fuqua, S. A. W. 1996. Estrogen and progesterone receptors and breast cancer, in *Diseases of the Breast* (Harris, J. R., Lippman, M. E., Morrow, M., Hellman, S., eds.), Lippincott-Raven, Philadelphia, PA, pp. 261–271.

27. Karnik, P. S., S. Kulkarni, X. P. Liu, G. T. Budd, and R. M. Bukowski. 1994. Estrogen receptor mutations in tamoxifen-resistant breast cancer. *Cancer Res.* **54:** 349–353.

28. Roodi, N., L. R. Bailey, W. Y. Kao, C. S. Verrier, C. J. Yee, W. D. Dupont, and F. F. Parl. 1995. Estrogen receptor gene analysis in estrogen receptor-positive and receptor-negative primary breast cancer. *J. Natl. Cancer Inst.* **87:** 446–451.

29. Osborne, C. K. 1995. Tamoxifen metabolism as a mechanism for resistance. *Endocr.-Related Cancer* **2:** 53–58.

30. Osborne, C. K., M. Jarman, R. McCague, E. B. Coronado, S. G. Hilsenbeck, and A. E. Wakeling. 1994. The importance of tamoxifen metabolism in tamoxifen-stimulated breast tumor growth. *Cancer Chemother. Pharmacol.* **34:** 89–95.

31. Wolf, D. M., S. M. Langan-Fahey, C. J. Parker, R. McCague, and V. C. Jordan. 1993. Investigation of the mechanism of tamoxifen-stimulated breast tumor growth with nonisomerizable analogues of tamoxifen and metabolites. *J. Natl. Cancer Inst.* **85:** 806–812.

32. Pavlik, E. J., K. Nelson, S. Srinivasan, D. E. Powell, D. E. Kenady, P. D. DePriest, H. H. Gallion, and J. R. van Nagell, Jr. 1992. Resistance to tamoxifen with persisting sensitivity to estrogen: possible mediation by excessive antiestrogen binding site activity. *Cancer Res.* **52:** 4106–4112.

33. Arteaga, C. L., A. R. Hanauske, G. M. Clark, C. K. Osborne, P. Hazarika, R. L. Pardue, F. Tio, and D. D. Von Hoff. 1988. Immunoreactive α transforming growth factor activity in effusions from cancer patients as a marker of tumor burden and patient prognosis. *Cancer Res.* **48:** 5023–5028.

34. Kern, F. G., S. W. McLeskey, L. Zhang, J. Kurebayashi, Y. Liu, I. Y. Ding, et al. 1994. Transfected MCF-7 cells as a model for breast cancer progression. *Breast Cancer Res. Treatment* **31:** 153–165.

35. Knabbe, C., A. Kopp, W. Hilgers, D. Lang, V. Muller, G. Zugmaier, and W. Jonat. 1996. Regulation and role of TGFβ production in breast cancer. *Ann. NY Acad. Sci.* **784:** 263–276.

36. Green, S. and P. Chambon. 1986. A superfamily of potentially oncogenic hormone receptors. *Nature* **324:** 615–617.

37. Kumar, V., S. Green, G. Stack, M. Berry, J. R. Jin, and P. Chambon. 1987. Functional domains of the human estrogen receptor. *Cell* **51:** 941–951.

38. Freedman, L. P., B. F. Luizi, Z. R. Korszun, R. Basavappa, P. B. Sigler, and K. R. Yamamoto. 1988. The function and structure of the metal coordination sites within the glucocorticoid receptor DNA binding domain. *Nature* **334:** 543–546.

39. Hollenberg, S. M. and R. M. Evans. 1988. Multiple and cooperative trans-activation domains of the human glucocorticoid receptor. *Cell* **55:** 899–906.

40. Severne, Y., S. Wieland, W. Schaffner, and S. Rusconi. 1988. Metal binding "finger" structures in the glucocorticoid receptor defined by site-directed mutagenesis. *EMBO J.* **7:** 2503–2508.

41. Klein-Hitpass, L., G. U. Ryffel, E. Heitlinger, and A. C. Cato. 1988. A 13 bp palindrome is a functional estrogen responsive element and interacts specifically with estrogen receptor. *Nucleic Acids Res.* **16:** 647–663.

42. Martinez, E., F. Givel, and W. Wahli. 1987. The estrogen-responsive element as an inducible enhancer: DNA sequence requirements and conversion to a glucocorticoid-responsive element. *EMBO J.* **6:** 3719–3727.

43. Walker, P., J. E. Germond, M. Brown-Luedi, F. Givel, and W. Wahli. 1984. Sequence homologies in the region preceding the transcription initiation site of the liver estrogen-responsive vitellogenin and apo-VLDLII genes. *Nucleic Acids Res.* **12:** 8611–8626.

44. Mader, S., V. Kumar, H. de Verneuil, and P. Chambon. 1989. Three amino acids of the oestrogen receptor are essential to its ability to distinguish an oestrogen from a glucocorticoid-responsive element. *Nature* **338:** 271–274.

45. Mader, S., P. Chambon, and J. H. White. 1993. Defining a minimal estrogen receptor DNA binding domain. *Nucleic Acids Res.* **21:** 1125–1132.

46. Schwabe, J. W., L. Chapman, J. T. Finch, and D. Rhodes. 1993. The crystal structure of the estrogen receptor DNA-binding domain bound to DNA: how receptors discriminate between their response elements. *Cell* **75:** 567–578.

47. Schwabe, J. W. R., L. Chapman, J. T. Finch, D. Rhodes, and D. Neuhaus. 1993. DNA recognition by the oestrogen receptor: from solution to the crystal. *Structure* **1:** 187–204.

48. Schwabe, J. W., D. Neuhaus, and D. Rhodes. 1990. Solution structure of the DNA-binding domain of the oestrogen receptor. *Nature* **348:** 458–461.

49. Kumar, V. and P. Chambon. 1988. The estrogen receptor binds tightly to its responsive element as a ligand-induced homodimer. *Cell* **55:** 145–156.

50. Bourguet, W., M. Ruff, P. Chambon, H. Gronemeyer, and D. Moras. 1995. Crystal-structure of the ligand-binding domain of the human nuclear receptor RXR-α. *Nature* **375:** 377–382.

51. Renaud, J. P., N. Rochel, M. Ruff, V. Vivat, P. Chambon, H. Gronemeyer, and D. Moras. 1995. Crystal structure of the RAR-γ ligand-binding domain bound to all-trans retinoic acid. *Nature* **378:** 681–689.

52. Wagner, R. L., J. W. Apriletti, M. E. McGrath, B. L. West, J. D. Baxter, and R. J. Fletterick. 1995. A structural role for hormone in the thyroid hormone receptor. *Nature* **378:** 690–697.

53. Anstead, G. M., K. E. Carlson, and J. A. Katzenellenbogen. 1997. The estradiol pharmacophore: ligand structure-estrogen receptor binding affinity relationships and a model for the receptor binding site. *Steroids* **62:** 268–303.

54. Wurtz, J. M., W. Bourguet, J. P. Renaud, V. Vivat, P. Chambon, D. Moras, and H. Gronemeyer. 1996. A canonical structure for the ligand-binding domain of nuclear receptors. *Nat. Struct. Biol.* **3:** 87–94.

55. Katzenellenbogen, J. A. and B. S. Katzenellenbogen. 1996. Nuclear hormone receptors: ligand-activated regulators of transcription and diverse cell responses. *Chem. Biol.* **3:** 529–536.

56. Katzenellenbogen, J. A., B. W. O'Malley, and B. S. Katzenellenbogen. 1996. Tripartite steroid hormone receptor pharmacology: interaction with multiple effector sites as a basis for the cell- and promoter-specific action of these hormones. *Mol. Endocrinol.* **10:** 119–131.

57. Barettino, D., M. M. VivancoRuiz, and H. G. Stunnenberg. 1994. Characterization of the ligand-dependent transactivation domain of thyroid hormone receptor. *EMBO J.* **13:** 3039–3049.

58. Danielian, P. S., R. White, J. A. Lees, and M. G. Parker. 1992. Identification of a conserved region required for hormone dependent transcriptional activation by steroid hormone receptors. *EMBO J.* **11:** 1025–1033.

59. Durand, B., M. Saunders, C. Gaudon, B. Roy, R. Losson, and P. Chambon. 1994. Activation function 2 (AF-2) of retinoic acid receptor and 9-cis retinoic acid receptor: presence of a conserved autonomous constitutive activating domain and influence of the nature of the response element on AF-2 activity. *EMBO J.* **13:** 5370–5382.

60. Saatcioglu, F., P. Bartunek, T. Deng, M. Zenke, and M. Karin. 1993. A conserved C-terminal sequence that is deleted in v-ErbA is essential for the biological activities of c-ErbA (the thyroid hormone receptor). *Mol. Cell. Biol.* **13:** 3675–3685.

61. LeDouarin, B., C. Zechel, J. M. Garnier, Y. Lutz, L. Tora, B. Pierrat, et al. 1995. The N-terminal part of TIF1, a putative mediator of the ligand-dependent activation function (AF-2) of nuclear receptors, is fused to B-raf in the oncogenic protein T18. *EMBO J.* **14:** 2020–2033.

62. L'Horset, F., S. Dauvois, D. M. Heery, V. Cavailles, and M. G. Parker. 1996. RIP-140 interacts with multiple nuclear receptors by means of two distinct sites. *Mol. Cell. Biol.* **16:** 6029–6036.

63. vom Baur, E., C. Zechel, D. Heery, M. J. Heine, J. M. Garnier, V. Vivat, et al. 1996. Differential ligand-dependent interactions between the AF-2 activating domain of nuclear receptors and the putative transcriptional intermediary factors mSUG1 and TIF1. *EMBO J.* **15:** 110–124.

64. Henttu, P. M., E. Kalkhoven, and M. G. Parker. 1997. AF-2 activity and recruitment of steroid receptor coactivator 1 to the estrogen receptor depend on a lysine residue conserved in nuclear receptors. *Mol. Cell. Biol.* **17:** 1832–1839.

65. Thenot, S., C. Henriquet, H. Rochefort, and V. Cavailles. 1997. Differential interaction of nuclear receptors with the putative human transcriptional coactivator hTIF1. *J. Biol. Chem.* **272:** 12,062–12,068.

66. Lees, J. A., S. E. Fawell, and M. G. Parker. 1989. Identification of two transactivation domains in the mouse oestrogen receptor. *Nucleic Acids Res.* **17:** 5477–5488.

67. Norris, J. D., D. Fan, S. A. Kerner, and D. P. McDonnell. 1997. Identification of a third autonomous activation domain within the human estrogen receptor. *Mol. Endocrinol.* **11:** 747–754.

68. Pierrat, B., D. M. Heery, P. Chambon, and R. Losson. 1994. A highly conserved region in the hormone-binding domain of the human estrogen receptor functions as an efficient transactivation domain in yeast. *Gene* **143:** 193–200.

69. Tora, L., J. White, C. Brou, D. Tasset, N. Webster, E. Scheer, and P. Chambon. 1989. The human estrogen receptor has two independent nonacidic transcriptional activation functions. *Cell* **59:** 477–487.

70. Webster, N. J., S. Green, J. R. Jin, and P. Chambon. 1988. The hormone-binding domains of the estrogen and glucocorticoid receptors contain an inducible transcription activation function. *Cell* **54:** 199–207.

71. McInerney, E. M. and B. S. Katzenellenbogen. 1996. Different regions in activation function-1 of the human estrogen receptor required for antiestrogen- and estradiol-dependent transcription activation. *J. Biol. Chem.* **271:** 24,172–174,178.

72. Montano, M. M., V. Muller, A. Trobaugh, and B. S. Katzenellenbogen. 1995. The carboxy-terminal F domain of the human estrogen receptor: role in the transcriptional activity of the receptor and the effectiveness of antiestrogens as estrogen antagonists. *Mol. Endocrinol.* **9:** 814–825.

73. Kraus, W. L., E. M. McInerney, and B. S. Katzenellenbogen. 1995. Ligand-dependent, transcriptionally productive association of the amino- and carboxyl-terminal regions of a steroid hormone nuclear receptor. *Proc. Natl. Acad. Sci. USA* **92:** 12,314–12,318.

74. Allan, G. F., X. Leng, S. Y. Tsai, N. L. Weigel, D. P. Edwards, M. J. Tsai, and B. W. O'Malley. 1992. Hormone and antihormone induce distinct conformational changes which are central to steroid receptor activation. *J. Biol. Chem.* **267:** 19,513–19,520.

75. Beekman, J. M., G. F. Allan, S. Y. Tsai, M. J. Tsai, and B. W. O'Malley. 1993. Transcriptional activation by the estrogen receptor requires a conformational change in the ligand binding domain. *Mol. Endocrinol.* **7:** 1266–1274.

76. McDonnell, D. P., D. L. Clemm, T. Hermann, M. E. Goldman, and J. W. Pike. 1995. Analysis of estrogen receptor function *in vitro* reveals three distinct classes of antiestrogens. *Mol. Endocrinol.* **9:** 659–669.

77. Danielian, P. S., R. White, S. A. Hoare, S. E. Fawell, and M. G. Parker. 1993. Identification of residues in the estrogen receptor that confer differential sensitivity to estrogen and hydroxytamoxifen. *Mol. Endocrinol.* **7:** 232–240.

78. Ekena, K., K. E. Weis, J. A. Katzenellenbogen, and B. S. Katzenellenbogen. 1996. Identification of amino acids in the hormone binding domain of the human estrogen receptor important in estrogen binding. *J. Biol. Chem.* **271:** 29,953–29,059.

79. Ekena, K., K. E. Weis, J. A. Katzenellenbogen, and B. S. Katzenellenbogen. 1997. Different residues of the human estrogen receptor are involved in the recognition of structurally diverse estrogens and antiestrogens. *J. Biol. Chem.* **272:** 5069–5075.

80. Pakdel, F. and B. S. Katzenellenbogen. 1992. Human estrogen receptor mutants with alter estrogen and antiestrogen ligand discrimination. *J. Biol. Chem.* **267:** 3429–3437.

81. Montano, M. M., K. Ekena, K. D. Krueger, A. L. Keller, and B. S. Katzenellenbogen. 1996. Human estrogen receptor ligand activity inversion mutants: receptors that interpret antiestrogens as estrogens and estrogens as antiestrogens and discriminate among different antiestrogens. *Mol. Endocrinol.* **10:** 230–242.

82. Jones, B. B., P. W. Jurutka, C. A. Haussler, M. R. Haussler, and G. K. Whitfield. 1991. Vitamin D receptor phosphorylation in transfected ROS 17/2.8 cells is localized to the N-terminal region of the hormone-binding domain. *Mol. Endocrinol.* **5:** 1137–1146.

83. Rochette-Egly, C., M. P. Gaub, Y. Lutz, S. Ali, I. Scheuer, and P. Chambon. 1992. Retinoic acid receptor-β: immunodetection and phosphorylation on tyrosine residues. *Mol. Endocrinol.* **6:** 2197–2209.

84. Sheridan, P. L., M. D. Francis, and K. B. Horwitz. 1989. Synthesis of human progesterone receptors in T47D cells. Nascent A- and B-receptors are active without a phosphorylation-dependent post-translational maturation step. *J. Biol. Chem.* **264:** 7054–7058.

85. van Laar, J. H., C. A. Berrevoets, J. Trapman, N. D. Zegers, and A. O. Brinkmann. 1991. Hormone-dependent androgen receptor phosphorylation is accompanied by receptor trans-

formation in human lymph node carcinoma of the prostate cells. *J. Biol. Chem.* **266:** 3734–3438.

86. Tsai, M. J. and B. W. O'Malley. 1994. Molecular mechanisms of action of steroid/thyroid receptor superfamily members. *Annu. Rev. Biochem.* **63:** 451–486.

87. Weigel, N. L. 1996. Steroid hormone receptors and their regulation by phosphorylation. *Biochem. J.* **319:** 657–667.

88. Ali, S., D. Metzger, J. M. Bornert, and P. Chambon. 1993. Modulation of transcriptional activation by ligand-dependent phosphorylation of the human oestrogen receptor A/B region. *EMBO J.* **12:** 1153–1160.

89. Denton, R. R., N. J. Koszewski, and A. C. Notides. 1992. Estrogen receptor phosphorylation: hormonal dependence and consequence on specific DNA binding. *J. Biol. Chem.* **267:** 7263–7268.

90. Le Goff, P., M. M. Montano, D. J. Schodin, and B. S. Katzenellenbogen. 1994. Phosphorylation of the human estrogen receptor. Identification of hormone-regulated sites and examinations of their influence on transcriptional activity. *J. Biol. Chem.* **269:** 4458–4466.

91. Arnold, S. F., J. D. Obourn, H. Jaffe, and A. C. Notides. 1995. Phosphorylation of the human estrogen receptor on tyrosine 537 *in vivo* and by src- family tyrosine kinases *in vitro*. *Mol. Endocrinol.* **9;** 24–33.

92. Castoria, G., A. Migliaccio, S. Green, M. Di Domenico, P. Chambon, and F. Auricchio. 1993. Properties of a purified estradiol-dependent calf uterus tyrosine kinase. *Biochemistry* **32:** 1740–1750.

93. Migliaccio, A., A. Rotondi, and F. Auricchio. 1986. Estradiol receptor: phosphorylation on tyrosine in uterus and interaction with anti-phosphotyrosine antibody. *EMBO J.* **5:** 2867–2872.

94. Weis, K. E., K. Ekena, J. A. Thomas, G. Lazennec, and B. S. Katzenellenbogen. 1996. Constitutively active human estrogen receptors containing amino acid substitutions for tyrosine 537 in the receptor protein. *Mol. Endocrinol.* **10:** 1388–1398.

95. White, R., M. Sjoberg, E. Kalkhoven, and M. G. Parker. 1997. Ligand-independent activation of the oestrogen receptor by mutation of a conserved tyrosine. *EMBO J.* **16:** 1427–1435.

96. Zhang, Q. X., A. Borg, D. M. Wolf, S. Oesterreich, and S. A. W. Fuqua. 1997. An estrogen receptor mutant with strong hormone-independent activity from a metastatic breast cancer. *Cancer Res.* **57:** 1244–1249.

97. Joel, P. B., A. M. Traish, and D. A. Lannigan. 1995. Estradiol and phorbol ester cause phosphorylation of serine 118 in the human estrogen receptor. *Mol. Endocrinol.* **9:** 1041–1052.

98. Arnold, S. F., D. P. Vorojeikina, and A. C. Notides. 1995. Phosphorylation of tyrosine 537 on the human estrogen receptor is required for binding to an estrogen response element. *J. Biol. Chem.* **270:** 30,205–30,212.

99. Bunone, G., P. A. Briand, R. J. Miksicek, and D. Picard. 1996. Activation of the unliganded estrogen receptor by EGF involves the MAP kinase pathway and direct phosphorylation. *EMBO J.* **15:** 2174–2183.

100. Kato, S., H. Endoh, Y. Masuhiro, T. Kitamoto, S. Uchiyama, H. Sasaki, et al. 1995. Activation of the estrogen receptor through phosphorylation by mitogen-activated protein kinase. *Science* **270:** 1491–1494.

101. Arnold, S. F. and A. C. Notides. 1995. An antiestrogen: a phosphotyrosyl peptide that blocks dimerization of the human estrogen receptor. *Proc. Natl. Acad. Sci. USA* **92:** 7475–7479.

102. Arnold, S. F., M. Melamed, D. P. Vorojeikina, A. C. Notides, and S. Sasson. 1997. Estradiol-binding mechanism and binding capacity of the human estrogen receptor is regulated by tyrosine phosphorylation. *Mol. Endocrinol.* **11:** 48–53.

103. Beato, M. and A. Sanchez-Pacheco. 1996. Interaction of steroid hormone receptors with the transcription initiation complex. *Endocr. Rev.* **17:** 587–609.

104. Aronica, S. M. and B. S. Katzenellenbogen. 1993. Stimulation of estrogen receptor-mediated transcription and alteration in the phosphorylation state of the rat uterine estrogen receptor by estrogen, cyclic adenosine monophosphate, and insulin-like growth factor-I. *Mol. Endocrinol.* **7:** 743–752.

105. Ignar-Trowbridge, D. M., K. G. Nelson, M. C. Bidwell, S. W. Curtis, T. F. Washburn, J. A. McLachlan, and K. S. Korach. 1992. Coupling of dual signaling pathways: epidermal growth factor action involves the estrogen receptor. *Proc. Natl. Acad. Sci. USA* **89:** 4658–4662.

106. Ignar-Trowbridge, D. M., C. T. Teng, K. A. Ross, M. G. Parker, K. S. Korach, and J. A. McLachlan. 1993. Peptide growth factors elicit estrogen receptor-dependent transcriptional activation of an estrogen-responsive element. *Mol. Endocrinol.* **7:** 992–998.

107. El-Tanani, M. K. and C. D. Green. 1997. Two separate mechanisms for ligand-independent activation of the estrogen receptor. *Mol. Endocrinol.* **11:** 928–937.

108. Smith, C. L., O. M. Conneely, and B. W. O'Malley. 1993. Modulation of the ligand-independent activation of the human estrogen receptor by hormone and antihormone. *Proc. Natl. Acad. Sci. USA* **90:** 6120–6124.

109. Auricchio, F., M. Di Domenico, A. Migliaccio, G. Castoria, and A. Bilancio. 1995. The role of estradiol receptor in the proliferative activity of vanadate on MCF-7 cells. *Cell Growth Differ.* **6:** 105–113.

110. Neuman, E., M. H. Ladha, N. Lin, T. M. Upton, S. J. Miller, J. DiRenzo, et al. 1997. Cyclin D1 stimulation of estrogen receptor transcriptional activity independent of cdk4. *Mol. Cell. Biol.* **17:** 5338–5347.

111. Zwijsen, R. M. L., E. Wientjens, R. Klompmaker, J. van der Sman, R. Bernards, and R. J. A. M. Michalides. 1997. CDK-independent activation of estrogen receptor by cyclin D1. *Cell* **88:** 405–415.

112. Katzenellenbogen, B. S., M. M. Montano, K. Ekena, M. E. Herman, and E. M. McInerney. 1997. Antiestrogens: mechanisms of action and resistance in breast cancer. *Breast Cancer Res. Treatment* **44:**23–38.

113. Fujimoto, N. and B. S. Katzenellenbogen. 1994. Alteration in the agonist/antagonist balance of antiestrogens by activation of protein kinase A signaling pathways in breast cancer cells: antiestrogen selectivity and promoter dependence. *Mol. Endocrinol.* **8:** 296–304.

114. Gaub, M. P., M. Bellard, I. Scheuer, P. Chambon, and C. P. Sassone. 1990. Activation of the ovalbumin gene by the estrogen receptor involves the fos-jun complex. *Cell* **63:** 1267–1276.

115. Philips, A., D. Chalbos, and H. Rochefort. 1993. Estradiol increases and anti-estrogens antagonize the growth factor-induced activator protein-1 activity in MCF7 breast cancer cells without affecting c-fos and c-jun synthesis. *J. Biol. Chem.* **268:** 14,103–14,108.

116. Umayahara, Y., R. Kawamori, H. Watada, E. Imano, N. Iwama, T. Morishima, et al. 1994. Estrogen regulation of the insulin-like growth factor I gene transcription involves an AP-1 enhancer. *J. Biol. Chem.* **269:** 16,433–16,442.

117. Webb, P., G. N. Lopez, R. M. Uht, and P. J. Kushner. 1995. Tamoxifen activation of the estrogen receptor/AP-1 pathway: potential origin for the cell-specific estrogen-like effects of antiestrogens. *Mol. Endocrinol.* **9:** 443–456.

118. Jones, C. D., M. G. Jevnikar, A. J. Pike, M. K. Peters, L. J. Black, A. R. Thompson, J. F. Falcone, and J. A. Clemens. 1984. Antiestrogens. 2. Structure-activity studies in a series of 3-aroyl-2-arylbenzo[b]thlophene derivatives leading to [6-hydroxy-2-(4-hydroxyphenyl)benzo[b]thienyl] [4-[2-(1-piperidinyl)ethoxy]phenyl]methanone hydrochloride (LY156758), a remarkably effective estrogen antagonist with only minimal intrinsic estrogenicity. *J. Med. Chem.* **27:** 1057–1066.

119. Yang, N. N., M. Venugopalan, S. Hardikar, and A. Glasebrook. 1996. Identification of an estrogen response element activated by metabolites of 17beta-estradiol and raloxifene. *Science* **273:** 1222–1225.

120. Green, S., P. Walter, V. Kumar, A. Krust, J. M. Bornert, P. Argos, and P. Chambon. 1986. Human oestrogen receptor cDNA: sequence, expression and homology to v-erb-A. *Nature* **320:** 134–139.

121. Greene, G. L., P. Gilna, M. Waterfield, A. Baker, Y. Hort, and J. Shine. 1986. Sequence and expression of human estrogen receptor complementary DNA. *Science* **231:** 1150–1154.

122. Leygue, E., A. Huang, L. C. Murphy, and P. H. Watson. 1996. Prevalence of estrogen receptor variant messenger RNAs in human breast cancer. *Cancer Res.* **56:** 4324–4327.

123. Leygue, E. R., P. H. Watson, and L. C. Murphy. 1996. Estrogen receptor variants in normal human mammary tissue. *J. Natl. Cancer Inst.* **88:** 284–290.

124. Pfeffer, U., E. Fecarotta, G. Arena, A. Forlani, and G. Vidali. 1996. Alternative splicing of the estrogen receptor primary transcript normally occurs in estrogen receptor positive tissues and cell lines. *J. Steroid Biochem. Mol. Biol.* **56:** 99–105.

125. Zhang, Q. X., S. G. Hilsenbeck, S. A. W. Fuqua, and A. Borg. 1996. Multiple splicing variants of the estrogen receptor are present in individual human breast tumors. *J. Steroid Biochem. Mol. Biol.* **59:** 251–260.

126. Kuiper, G. G., E. Enmark, M. Pelto-Huikko, S. Nilsson, and J. A. Gustafsson. 1996. Cloning of a novel estrogen receptor expressed in rat prostate and ovary. *Proc. Natl. Acad. Sci. USA* **93:** 5925–5930.

127. Mosselman, S., J. Polman, and R. Dijkema. 1996. ERβ: identification and characterization of a novel human estrogen receptor. *FEBS Lett.* **392:** 49–53.

128. Tremblay, G. B., A. Tremblay, N. G. Copeland, D. J. Gilbert, N. A. Jenkins, F. Labrie, and V. Giguere. 1997. Cloning, chromosomal localization, and functional analysis of the murine estrogen receptor β. *Mol. Endocrinol.* **11:** 353–365.

129. Kuiper, G. G., B. Carlsson, K. Grandien, E. Enmark, J. Haggblad, S. Nilsson, and J. A. Gustafsson. 1997. Comparison of the ligand binding specificity and transcript tissue distribution of estrogen receptors α and β. *Endocrinology* **138:** 863–870.

130. Byers, M., G. G. Kuiper, J. A. Gustafsson, and O. K. Park-Sarge. 1997. Estrogen receptor-β mRNA expression in rat ovary: down-regulation by gonadotropins. *Mol. Endocrinol.* **11:** 172–182.

131. Shughrue, P. J., B. Komm, and I. Merchenthaler. 1996. The distribution of estrogen receptor-β mRNA in the rat hypothalamus. *Steroids* **61:** 678–681.

132. Dotzlaw, H., E. Leygue, P. H. Watson, and L. C. Murphy. 1997. Expression of estrogen receptor-beta in human breast tumors. *J. Clin. Endocrinol. Metab.* **82:** 2371–2374.

133. Cowley, S. M., S. Hoare, S. Mosselman, and M. G. Parker. 1997. Estrogen receptors α and β form heterodimers on DNA. *J. Biol. Chem.* **272:** 19,858–19,862.

134. Pace, P., J. Taylor, S. Suntharalingam, R. C. Coombes, and S. Ali. 1997. Human estrogen receptor β binds DNA in a manner similar to and dimerizes with estrogen receptor α. *J. Biol. Chem.* **272:** 25,832–25,838.

135. Pettersson, K., K. Grandien, G. G. J. M. Kuiper, and J. A. Gustafsson. 1997. Mouse estrogen receptor β forms estrogen response element-binding heterodimers with estrogen receptor α. *Mol. Endocrinol.* **11:** 1486–1496.

136. Paech, K., P. Webb, G. G. J. M. Kuiper, S. Nilsson, J. A. Gustafsson, P. J. Kushner, and T. S. Scanlan. 1997. Differential ligand activation of estrogen receptors ERα and ERβ at AP1 sites. *Science* **277:** 1508–1510.

137. McInerney, E. M., M. J. Tsai, B. W. O'Malley, and B. S. Katzenellenbogen. 1996. Analysis of estrogen receptor transcriptional enhancement by a nuclear hormone receptor coactivator. *Proc. Natl. Acad. Sci. USA* **93:** 10,069–10,073.

138. Onate, S. A., S. Y. Tsai, M. J. Tsai, and B. W. O'Malley. 1995. Sequence and characterization of a coactivator for the steroid hormone receptor superfamily. *Science* **270:** 1354–1357.

139. Horwitz, K. B., T. A. Jackson, D. L. Bain, J. K. Richer, G. S. Takimoto, and L. Tung. 1996. Nuclear receptor coactivators and corepressors. *Mol. Endocrinol.* **10:** 1167–1177.

140. Meyer, M. E., H. Gronemeyer, B. Turcotte, M. T. Bocquel, D. Tasset, and P. Chambon. 1989. Steroid hormone receptors compete for factors that mediate their enhancer function. *Cell* **57:** 433–442.

141. Tasset, D., L. Tora, C. Fromental, E. Scheer, and P. Chambon. 1990. Distinct classes of transcriptional activating domains function by different mechanisms. *Cell* **62:** 1177–1187.

142. Glass, C. K., D. W. Rose, and M. G. Rosenfeld. 1996. Nuclear receptor coactivators. *Curr. Opin. Cell Biol.* **9:** 222–232.

143. Khavari, P. A., C. L. Peterson, J. W. Tamkun, D. B. Mendel, and G. R. Crabtree. 1993. BRG1 contains a conserved domain of the SWI2/SNF2 family necessary for normal mitotic growth and transcription. *Nature* **366:** 170–174.

144. Muchardt, C. and M. Yaniv. 1993. A human homologue of *Saccharomyces cerevieiae* SNF2/SWI2 and *Drosophila-brm* genes potentiates transcriptional activation by the glucocorticoid receptor. *EMBO J.* **12:** 4279–4290.

145. Yoshinaga, S. K., C. L. Peterson, I. Herskowitz, and K. R. Yamamoto. 1992. Roles of SWI1, SWI2, and SWI3 proteins for transcriptional enhancement by steroid receptors. *Science* **258:** 1598–1604.

146. Bruggemeier, U., M. Kalff, S. Franke, C. Scheidereit, and M. Beato. 1991. Ubiquitous transcription factor OTF-1 mediates induction of the mouse mammary tumour virus promoter through synergistic interaction with hormone receptors. *Cell* **64:** 565–572.

147. Rigaud, G., J. Roux, R. Pictet, and T. Grange. 1991. *In vivo* footprinting of rat TAT gene: dynamic interplay between the glucocorticoid receptor and a liver-specific factor. *Cell* **67:** 977–986.

148. Greenblatt, J. 1991. Roles of TFIID in transcriptional initiation by RNA polymerase-II. *Cell* **66:** 1067–1070.

149. Sadovsky, Y., P. Webb, G. Lopez, J. D. Baxter, P. M. Fitzpatrick, E. Gizang-Ginsberg, et al. 1995. Transcriptional activators differ in their responses to overexpression of TATA-box-binding protein. *Mol. Cell. Biol.* **15:** 1554–1563.

150. Jacq, X., C. Brou, Y. Lutz, I. Davidson, P. Chambon, and L. Tora. 1994. Human TAFII30 is present in a distinct TFIID complex and is required for transcriptional activation by the estrogen receptor. *Cell* **79:** 107–117.

151. Buratowski, S. 1994. The basics of basal transcription by RNA polymerase II. *Cell* **77:** 1–3.

152. Lee, S. and S. Hahn. 1995. Model for binding of transcription factor TFIIB to the TBP-DNA complex. *Nature* **376:** 609–612.

153. Nikolov, D. B., H. Chen, E. D. Halay, A. A. Usheva, K. Hisatake, D. K. Lee, R. G. Roeder, and S. K. Burley. 1995. Crystal structure of TFIIB-TBP-TATA-element ternary complex. *Nature* **377:** 119–128.

154. Usheva, A., E. Maldonado, A. Goldring, H. Lu, C. Houbavi, D. Reinberg, and Y. Aloni. 1992. Specific interaction between the nonphosphorylated form of RNA polymerase-II and the TATA-binding protein. *Cell* **69:** 871–881.

155. Ing, N. H., J. M. Beekman, S. Y. Tsai, M. J. Tsai, and B. W. O'Malley. 1992. Members of the steroid hormone receptor superfamily interact with TFIIB (S300-II). *J. Biol. Chem.* **267:** 17,617–17,623.

156. Baniahmad, C., Z. Nawaz, A. Baniahmad, M. A. Gleeson, M. J. Tsai, and B. W. O'Malley. 1995. Enhancement of human estrogen receptor activity by SPT6: a potential coactivator. *Mol. Endocrinol.* **9:** 34–43.

157. Zeiner, M. and U. Gehring. 1995. A protein that interacts with members of the nuclear hormone receptor family: identification and cDNA cloning. *Proc. Natl. Acad. Sci. USA* **92:** 11,465–11,469.

158. Yeh, S. and C. Chang. 1996. Cloning and characterization of a specific coactivator, ARA70, for the androgen receptor in human prostate cells. *Proc. Natl. Acad. Sci. USA* **93:** 5517–5521.

159. Chrivia, J. C., R. P. Kwok, N. Lamb, M. Hagiwara, M. R. Montminy, and R. H. Goodman. 1993. Phosphorylated CREB binds specifically to the nuclear protein CBP. *Nature* **365:** 855–859.

160. Kamei, Y., L. Xu, T. Heinzel, J. Torchia, R. Kurokawa, B. Gloss, et al. 1996. A CBP integrator complex mediates transcriptional activation and AP-1 inhibition by nuclear receptors. *Cell* **85:** 403–414.

161. Smith, C. L., S. A. Onate, M. J. Tsai, and B. W. O'Malley. 1996. CREB binding protein acts synergistically with steroid receptor coactivator-1 to enhance steroid receptor-dependent transcription. *Proc. Natl. Acad. Sci. USA* **93:** 8884–8888.

162. Hanstein, B., R. Eckner, J. DiRenzo, S. Halachmi, H. Liu, B. Searcy, R. Kurokawa, and M. Brown. 1996. p300 is a component of an estrogen receptor coactivator complex. *Proc. Natl. Acad. Sci. USA* **93:** 11,540–11545.

163. Yao, T. P., G. Ku, N. Zhou, R. Scully, and D. M. Livingston. 1996. The nuclear hormone receptor coactivator SRC-1 is a specific target of p300. *Proc. Natl. Acad. Sci. USA* **93:** 10,626–10,631.

164. Chakravarti, D., V. J. LaMorte, M. C. Nelson, T. Nakajima, I. G. Schulman, H. Juguilon, M. Montminy, and R. M. Evans. 1996. Role of CBP/p300 in nuclear receptor signalling. *Nature* **383:** 99–103.

165. Takeshita, A., P. M. Yen, S. Misiti, G. R. Cardona, Y. Liu, and W. W. Chin. Molecular cloning and properties of a full-length putative thyroid hormone receptor coactivator. *Endocrinology* **137:** 3594–3597.

166. Voegel, J. J., M. J. Heine, C. Zechel, P. Chambon, and H. Gronemeyer. 1996. TIF2, a 160 kDa transcriptional mediator for the ligand-dependent activation function AF-2 of nuclear receptors. *EMBO J.* **15:** 3667–3675.

167. Hong, H., K. Kohli, M. J. Garabedian, and M. R. Stallcup. 1997. GRIP1, a transcriptional coactivator for the AF-2 transactivation domain of steroid, thyroid, retinoid, and vitamin D receptors. *Mol. Cell. Biol.* **17:** 2735–2744.

168. Hong, H., K. Kohli, A. Trivedi, D. L. Johnson, and M. R. Stallcup. 1996. GRIP1, a novel mouse protein that serves as a transcriptional coactivator in yeast for the hormone binding domains of steroid receptors. *Proc. Natl. Acad. Sci. USA* **93:** 4948–4952.

169. Halachmi, S., E. Marden, G. Martin, H. MacKay, C. Abbondanza, and M. Brown. 1994. Estrogen receptor-associated proteins: possible mediators of hormone-induced transcription. *Science* **264:** 1455–1458.

170. Hankinson, O. 1995. The aryl hydrocarbon receptor complex. *Annu. Rev. Pharmacol. Toxicol.* **35:** 397–340.

171. Cavailles, V., S. Dauvois, F. L'Horset, G. Lopez, S. Hoare, P. J. Kushner, and M. G. Parker. 1995. Nuclear factor RIP140 modulates transcriptional activation by the estrogen receptor. *EMBO J.* **14:** 3741–3751.

172. Horlein, A. J., A. M. Naar, T. Heinzel, J. Torchia, B. Gloss, R. Kurokawa, et al. 1995. Ligand-independent repression by the thyroid hormone receptor mediated by a nuclear receptor co-repressor. *Nature* **377:** 397–404.

173. Kurokawa, R., M. Soderstrom, A. Horlein, S. Halachmi, M. Brown, M. G. Rosenfeld, and C. K. Glass. 1995. Polarity-specific activities of retinoic acid receptors determined by a co-repressor. *Nature* **377:** 451–454.

174. Chen, J. D. and R. M. Evans. 1995. A transcriptional co-repressor that interacts with nuclear hormone receptors. *Nature* **377:** 454–457.

175. Alland, L., R. Muhle, H. Hou, Jr., J. Potes, L. Chin, N. Schreiber-Agus, and R. A. DePinho. 1997. Role for N-CoR and histone deacetylase in Sin3-mediated transcriptional repression. *Nature* **387:** 49–55.

176. Heinzel, T., R. M. Lavinsky, T. M. Mullen, M. Soderstrom, C. D. Laherty, J. Torchia, et al. 1997. A complex containing N-CoR, mSin3 and histone deacetylase mediates transcriptional repression. *Nature* **387:** 43–48.

177. Wolffe, A. P. 1997. Transcriptional control. Sinful repression. *Nature* **387:** 16–17.

178. Smith, C. L., Z. Nawaz, and B. W. O'Malley. 1997. Coactivator and corepressor regulation of the agonist/antagonist activity of the mixed antiestrogen, 4-hydroxytamoxifen. *Mol. Endocrinol.* **11:** 657–666.

2

Epidermal Growth Factor-Related Peptides and Their Cognate Receptors in Breast Cancer

Isabel Martinez-Lacaci, Caterina Bianco, Marta De Santis, and David S. Salomon

1. INTRODUCTION

The regulation of normal breast development is dependent on several hormones. Among these hormones, estrogens are the most well-characterized and they perform an essential role in the control of normal mammary development and in the etiology and progression of breast cancer. In addition, normal and malignant mammary epithelial and stromal cells synthesize locally acting growth factors that function through autocrine, juxtacrine, and paracrine pathways. Several studies have demonstrated that estrogens influence mammary epithelial-cell growth both directly and indirectly by modulating growth-factor production and growth-factor receptor expression *(1)*. The epidermal growth factor (EGF)-family of peptides, in combination with their cognate receptors, is significantly involved in the regulation of mammary-gland development, morphogenesis and lactation, and also plays a pivotal role in the pathogenesis of human breast cancer *(2)* (Table 1 and Fig. 1). In fact, the morphological changes during mammary-gland development are accompanied by changes in the pattern of expression of EGF-related peptides in mammary epithelial and stromal cells. EGF, amphiregulin (AR), transforming growth factor α (TGF-α), cripto-1 (CR-1), and heregulin α (HRG-α) are expressed in the virgin mouse mammary gland in ductal epithelial cells (EGF, AR) and in the cap stem cells (TGF-α, CR-1) of the growing terminal end buds. In contrast, HRG-α expression is detected during pregnancy and lactation in a subpopulation of mesenchymal cells *(3,4)*. In addition, experiments using slow-release Elvax pellets containing EGF, TGF-α, HRG-α, or β1 implanted in the virgin mammary gland of ovariectomized mice have shown that these peptides stimulate lobulo-alveolar development *(5)*. Recent experiments have shown that transformation of mammary epithelial cells might result from increased production or response to stimulatory growth factors. In fact, TGF-α can act as a transforming gene when overexpressed in mouse and human mammary epithelial cells in vitro or in vivo *(6,7)*. In addition, activation of cellular proto-oncogenes such as c-Ha-*ras* and c-*erb*B-2 in mouse and human mammary epithelial cells leads to cellular transformation and to the up-regulation of expression of several different EGF-related peptides *(8)*. Finally, direct

From: Breast Cancer: *Molecular Genetics, Pathogenesis, and Therapeutics*
Edited by: A. M. Bowcock © Humana Press Inc., Totowa, NJ

Table 1
**Epidermal Growth Factor (EGF) Family of Growth Factors
and Type 1 *erb*B Receptor Tyrosine Kinases**

Ligand	Receptor
Epidermal growth factor (EGF)	EGF receptor (EGFR/*erb*B)
Transforming growth factor α (TGF-α)	
Amphiregulin (AR)	
Epiregulin (EP)	
Betacellulin (BTC)	EGFR and *erb*B-4
Heparin-binding EGF-line growth factor (HB-EGF)	
?	*erb*B-2
Neuregulins-1	
Heregulin (HRG-α and -β)-1	*erb*B-3 and *erb*B-4
Glial cell growth factor (GGF)	
Sensory motor neuron-derived growth factor (SMDGF)	
Acetylcholine receptor-inducing activity (ARIA)	
Neuregulins-2 (α and β)	*erb*B-3 and *erb*B-4
Cripto-1 (CR-1)	?

evidence of the role of these growth factors in neoplastic progression of the mammary gland is provided by transgenic mouse studies, because transgenic mice overexpressing TGF-α or HRG under the control of tissue-specific promoters develop, in a stochastic fashion, mammary hyperplastic lesions and focal adenocarcinomas *(6,9)*.

The purpose of this chapter is to describe the role of EGF-related growth factors and their receptors in the control of proliferation and differentiation of human mammary epithelial cells and in the pathogenesis of human breast cancer. An accurate knowledge of how these growth factors affect normal and malignant mammary cell growth may also help to focus and improve the efficacy of the many growth factor/receptor-targeted therapies that are currently under clinical investigation in cancer patients (reviewed in Chapter 19).

2. EPIDERMAL GROWTH FACTOR FAMILY IN BREAST CANCER

2.1. EGF

EGF is a 6-kDa polypeptide of 53 amino acid that is encoded by a 4.8 kb mRNA transcript. The human EGF gene is 110 kb long, contains 24 exons, and is located on human chromosome 4 (4q25) *(20)*. It was originally isolated from the male mouse submaxillary gland as a factor that caused eyelid opening *(11)* and later from human urine as urogastrone *(12)*. EGF is synthesized as a larger transmembrane precursor of 128 kDa that contains a total of 9 EGF units. The EGF unit that is located closest to the transmembrane domain gives rise to the mature EGF protein; the other 8 EGF units do not have a known function *(13)*. The EGF precursor is a transmembrane glycosylated protein that is biologically active as it can bind to and activate EGF receptors in adjacent cells through a juxtacrine mode of action *(14)*. EGF is the main milk-derived growth factor *(15)*. EGF has been detected in human breast-cancer cells *(16)*. In par-

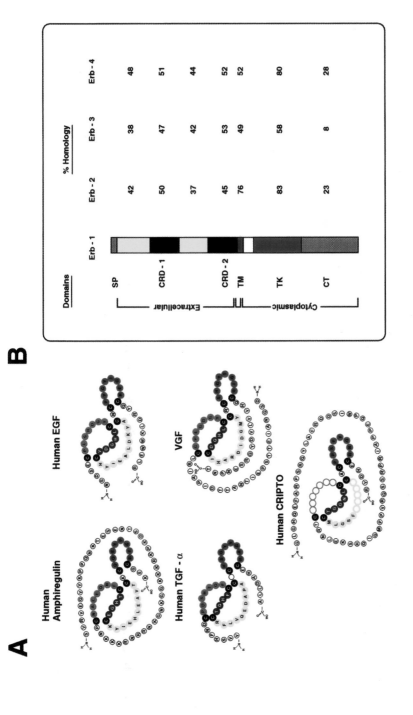

Fig. 1. Schematic diagram of EGF-related peptide structures (**A**) in which common amino acids within comparable domains are shaded the same color, whereas lack of sufficient regional homology are denoted by open circles and the domains of the type 1 receptor *erb*B tyrosine kinase receptors (**B**) that exhibit regional homology, SP, signal peptide; CRD, cysteine rich domain; TM, transmembrane domain; TK, tyrosine kinase, CT, cytoplasmic tail; Domain III, ligand-binding region (B).

ticular, EGF mRNA levels are more abundant in estrogen-responsive, estrogen receptor (ER) positive human breast-cancer cell lines (T-47D) and can be increased with progestins, while 17-β-estradiol (E$_2$) has no effect on regulating EGF levels in these cells *(17)*. EGF can promote the anchorage-dependent growth of both rodent and human mammary epithelial cells *(18,19)* and is mitogenic for several human breast-cancer cells that retain EGF receptors *(20,21)*. EGF is a crucial regulator of growth and differentiation in the mouse mammary gland *(22,23)*, especially during pregnancy and lactation *(24)* and during the spontaneous formation of mammary tumors *(25)*. EGF mRNA has been detected in 83% of human breast tumors *(26)*. Additionally, EGF protein has been detected in 15-30% of human primary invasive breast carcinomas *(27)*.

2.2. Transforming Growth Factor-alpha

TGF-α was first identified in the culture media of virus-transformed cells and of human tumors cells. This factor, in combination with TGF-β, has the ability to transform and confer anchorage-independence to normal fibroblasts. TGF-α is a 50-amino-acid polypeptide that has a M$_r$ of ~5.6 kDa and is encoded by a 4.8 kb mRNA. The human TGF-α gene of 100 kb contains 6 exons and is located on chromosome 2 (2p11–13) *(28)*. TGF-α shares 42% homology with human EGF. Its tertiary structure is identical to EGF and is able to bind to the EGF receptor with the same affinity. Like all the EGF-related polypeptides, it contains 6 conserved cysteine residues that form 3 disulfide bonds. Human TGF-α is derived from a larger membrane-bound glycosylated precursor of 160 amino-acids (M$_r$ ~22 kDa) that is biologically active. Like EGF, proTGF-α is able to activate the EGF receptor of neighboring cells *(29)*. The 50 amino-acid low molecular weight form of TGF-α corresponds to the NH2-terminal domain of the precursor and is cleaved by an elastase-like enzyme. In fact, several secreted forms of TGF-α that are biologically active can be found in the conditioned-media of various tumor cells *(30)*. TGF-α is expressed in mammary epithelial and breast-cancer cells *(31)* and it appears to have qualitatively the same biological effects as EGF. In particular, TGF-α is a potent mitogen for normal and malignant mammary epithelial cells in vitro *(32,33)* and is able to induce development of the mammary gland in vivo *(176)*. The basal levels of TGF-α are higher in ER-positive, estrogen responsive cell lines *(133)* and it can be regulated by estrogens. Specially, TGF-α mRNA and protein levels are induced by physiological concentrations of E$_2$ *(35)*. The mechanism of induction seems to be transcriptional because several imperfect estrogen response elements (EREs) that are located in the promoter are thought to be active, as determined by an increase in CAT activity of transiently transfected cells *(36)*. This induction is mediated by a 53 bp sequence that can function as an ERE *(37)* and can be blocked with antiestrogens, suggesting that this effect is mediated through the ER. In addition, TGF-α mRNA levels can be induced by progestins *(38)* and by phorbol esters such as 12-O-tetradecanoylphorbol-13-acetate (TPA) *(39)* in human breast-cancer cells. Similarly, EGF can induce expression of TGF-α. The mechanism of induction by TPA and EGF in human breast-cancer cells operates at the transcriptional level, suggesting that these two agents utilize a common regulatory mechanism that involves protein kinase C *(40)*. TGF-α functions as an autocrine growth factor in human mammary epithelial cells that have been transformed with an activated form of the c-Ha-*ras* proto-oncogene *(8)*. TGF-α mRNA and protein levels have been detected in 40–70% of human breast tumors *(41)*. The majority of the tumors that express higher levels of TGF-α also express higher levels of the EGF receptor, suggesting that an autocrine loop may be operative. However, TGF-α has also been found in milk, indicating that it may be secreted by normal mammary epithelial cells. Additionally, TGF-α mRNA has been detected during the proliferative, lobular development of both the rat and human mammary gland and its expression is enhanced during pregnancy and lactation *(3)*. Interestingly, TGF-α is predominantly expressed in the proliferative and terminal end bud cap cells, whereas EGF is expressed in ductal epithelial cells *(42)*. Several studies using TGF-α transgenic mouse models have shown that TGF-α may be important in facilitating the onset of early stages of mouse mammary tumorigenesis *(1)*. However, a definite role of TGF-α in the induction of human breast cancer has not been established.

2.3. Amphiregulin

Amphiregulin (AR) is a heparin-binding glycoprotein that is structurally related to EGF, but it has lower affinity for the EGF receptor than EGF or TGF-α *(43)*. However, it has been shown that AR acts only through the EGF receptor, even though it can transphosphorylate c-*erb*B-2 *(44)*. AR was originally isolated from conditioned media of the human breast-carcinoma cell line, MCF-7, treated with the phorbol ester tumor promoter TPA *(45)*. AR is synthesized from a 252 amino-acid membrane-bound glycosylated precursor (M_r ~34–36 kDa) *(43)* and it is secreted into the conditioned-media as a monomer of 78 or 84 amino-acids (~22–26 kDa) after proteolytic cleavage of the precursor. The processing of AR is not well understood. AR can be found in the conditioned-media in different isoforms that vary in the degree of glycosylation and the length of the peptide core *(46)*. A novel ~55–60 kDa form has been found in the conditioned-media of TPA-treated MCF-7 cells *(47)*. The AR protein is encoded by a 1.4 kb mRNA, and the AR gene is located on chromosome 4 (4q13–4q21) and contains 6 exons spanning a region of 10.2 kb *(48)*. AR has a bifunctional mode of action. Depending on the concentration, presence of other growth factors and target cells, it can either stimulate or inhibit cell proliferation *(49)*. In this regard, AR can inhibit the growth of a variety of human breast-cancer cells, but stimulates the growth of fibroblasts, keratinocytes, mammary epithelial cells, and some tumor cells *(45,50,51)*. AR has been detected in several breast-cancer cell lines and the levels of expression are higher in ER positive, estrogen-responsive cell lines. It has been found that E_2 stimulates transcription of AR. The mechanism of induction of AR by TPA, however, is different because TPA is able not only to stimulate transcription of the AR gene but also to further stabilize AR mRNA *(52)*. Additionally, AR is expressed in normal and nontransformed mammary epithelial cells. Similar to TGF-α, AR can function as an autocrine factor in these cells *(53,54)*. Moreover, AR expression is enhanced in nonmalignant, immortalized MCF-10A mammary epithelial cells that have been transformed with a point mutated form of the c-Ha-*ras* proto-oncogene or with c-*erb*B-2 *(54)*. AR protein has been detected in 80% of human primary breast carcinomas by immunocytochemistry *(55)* and AR mRNA has been detected in 60% of primary human breast carcinomas *(56)*. However, in a different study, AR expression was detected in only 37% of human primary breast carcinomas *(57)*. The discrepancy could be owing to the use of different antibodies utilized for immunocytochemistry.

The carboxyl-terminal half of the AR molecule shares high homology with other EGF family members. AR has 38% amino-acid sequence homology with EGF and 32% homology with TGF-α and it contains the characteristic six-cysteine motif common to all EGF family members. Preceding the EGF-like domain, AR contains two stretches of basic, hydrophilic residues which resemble nuclear targeting sequences *(48)*. In fact, AR has been found in the nucleus of a variety of breast carcinoma cell lines, as well as in paraffin-embedded tissue sections of breast- and colon-carcinoma cells by immunocytochemical staining *(49,51,54,58,59)*. Interestingly, it is predominantly localized to the nucleus of MCF-7 cells that have been treated with E_2 *(47)*. It has been shown that these nuclear targeting signals are necessary for Schwannoma-derived growth factor, the AR rat homolog, to exert its mitogenic activity *(60)* and that AR is able to bind to nuclear phosphoproteins *(61)*. The role of growth factors in the nucleus, however, is still controversial. In contrast with the other members of the EGF family, AR binds to heparin and its mitogenic activity can be regulated by heparin *(50)*. In fact, the basic-rich regions contained in the amino-terminal domain, which resemble nuclear-targeting sequences, may also confer heparin regulation *(48)*. It has been shown that heparin can inhibit the EGF-independent autocrine stimulation of normal mammary epithelial cells, suggesting a role of AR in this mechanism *(62)* and that heparin-like glycosaminoglycans can regulate the AR-dependent growth of keratinocytes *(63)*. Moreover, heparan sulfate can modulate the binding of AR to the EGF receptor *(64)*, similar to the effect that heparan sulfate proteoglycans exhibit on the binding of fibroblast growth factors (FGF) to their receptor(s).

2.4. Heparin-binding EGF-like Growth Factor

Heparin-binding EGF-like growth factor (HB-EGF) is a novel growth factor that binds to and phosphorylates the EGF receptor, with lower affinity than EGF or TGF-α. It was originally isolated from conditioned-media of macrophage-like U-937 cells treated with TPA *(65)*. HB-EGF is synthesized as a 208 amino-acid transmembrane glycoprotein composed of a putative signal peptide and heparin-binding, EGF-like, transmembrane and cytoplasmic domains *(66)*. Several secreted forms of the mature, fully processed HB-EGF protein can be found in the conditioned media of U-937 cells ranging from 19–23 kDa *(66)*. Similar to AR, these forms differ in truncations of the NH2-terminal domain. HB-EGF protein is encoded by a 2.5 kb mRNA transcript that is expressed in several tissues *(67–69)*. The human HB-EGF gene is located on chromosome 5 (5q23), contains six exons and spans a region of 14 kb *(67)*. The HB-EGF precursor can function as the bacterial diphteria toxin receptor *(70)*. The membrane-anchored HB-EGF precursor can form a complex with DRAP27/CD9 that mediates sensitivity to diphteria toxin *(71)* and the juxtacrine mitogenic activity of proHB-EGF *(72)*. Furthermore, CD9 is coexpressed with proHB-EGF and proAR *(73)*. The HB-EGF precursor is also synthesized by the ER negative, estrogen-independent human breast-cancer cells, MDA-MB-231, and can be processed and secreted into the conditioned media after TPA treatment *(74)*. Processing of proHB-EGF results in loss of juxtacrine activity with a concomitant increase in soluble HB-EGF mitogenic activity in cells that overexpress recombinant HB-EGF *(75)*. Furthermore, it has been shown that processing of the NH2-terminal domain of human proHB-EGF induces the juxtacrine activity of HB-EGF, but not its paracrine activity *(76)*. HB-EGF is closely related to AR and it can also bind heparin. The biological activity of HB-EGF can be stimulated by heparin *(77)* owing to the leucine$_{76}$ present in the carboxyl-terminal domain of the molecule that is absent in AR *(78)*. Whereas heparin agonists or inhibitors of proteoglycan sulfation are able to inhibit the mitogenic activity of AR, the bioactivity of HB-EGF is unaffected, suggesting that AR and HB-EGF act in a different manner *(79)*. HB-EGF activates the EGF receptor, but it can also induce tyrosine phosphorylation of c-*erb*B-4 *(80)*.

HB-EGF is a potent mitogen for smooth muscle cells, macrophages, fibroblasts, and keratinocytes, but not for endothelial cells *(65)*. It has been suggested that HB-EGF may participate in wound healing *(81)* and atheroscelerosis *(82)*. HB-EGF mRNA levels can be induced by TPA in both rat aortic and human smooth-muscle cells *(83,84)*. Likewise, HB-EGF mRNA levels can be regulated by progesterone and E$_2$ in rat uterine epithelial cells *(85)*. Conversely, HB-EGF expression is only regulated by estrogen in the epithelium, whereas both estrogen and progesterone regulate HB-EGF expression in the stroma of ovariectomized mouse uterus *(86)*. However, the role of HB-EGF and its regulation in breast cancer is unknown and is under investigation in our laboratory.

2.5. Betacellulin

Betacellulin (BTC) is a newly discovered member of the EGF family of growth factors. BTC was originally identified in the conditioned media of cell lines derived from a transgenic mouse expressing the SV40 large T antigen under the control of the insulin promoter *(87–89)*. More recently, the human BTC cDNA has been cloned from MCF-7 cells *(90)*. The mature BTC protein of 80 amino-acids (M$_r$ of ~32 kDa) is heavily glycosylated and is derived from larger precursors of 177 and 178 amino-acids, respectively, that are 79% homologous *(41)*. BTC is a mitogen for mouse fibroblasts and smooth-muscle cells. BTC binds to the EGF receptor with much lower affinity than EGF or TGF-α and it has been recently shown that BTC can bind to and activate c-*erb*B-4 *(80,91)*. BTC mRNA is expressed in several tissues in the mouse and several transcripts can be detected (4.3, 3,0, 1.2, and 0.9 kb). Additionally, BTC mRNA has been detected in several mouse cell lines, MCF-7 human breast-cancer cells, and in HT1080 human fibrosarcoma cells. Human BTC is highly expressed in the pancreas and small intestine *(92)*. The expression and function of BTC in breast cancer is an area of current investigation in our laboratory.

2.6. Neuregulins (Heregulins)

Rat *neu* differentiation factor (NDF) and the human homolog heregulin (HRG) are members of the neuregulin-1 (NRG-1) subfamily *(93)*. Additionally, peptides that also belong to the NRG-1 subfamily include glial growth factors, sensory motor neuron-derived growth factor, and acetylcholine receptor-inducing activity (Table 1) *(94)*. There are at least 15 known structural variants. All these forms are derived from the same gene by alternative mRNA splicing. Recently, a new NRG-like gene, the NRG-2 gene, has been cloned *(95,96)*. NRG-2 has an alternative splicing site in the EGF-like domain that results in α and β isoforms. Similar to NRG-1, NRG-2 binds to and activates both c-*erb*B-3 and c-*erb*B-4. In addition, NRG-2 preferentially promotes heterodimerization of c-*erb*B-3 with the EGF receptor, whereas NRG-1 favors heterodimerization of c-*erb*B-3 or c-*erb*B-4 with c-*erb*B-2 *(96)*.

NDF was originally identified and purified from the conditioned medium of Rat-1 fibroblasts transformed with c-Ha-*ras* *(97)*, whereas HRG, the human homolog, was purified from the conditioned medium of MDA-MB-231 cells *(98)*. HRG is a 44 kDa membrane-associated glycoprotein that lacks a hydrophobic signal peptide, contains an EGF-like repeat, an immunoglobulin-like domain in the NH2-terminal region, and a long cytoplasmic tail *(99)*. Most of the HRG isoforms can bind to heparin by virtue of the basic, hydrophobic stretches that resemble nuclear-targeting sequences and that are also present in AR and HB-EGF. HRG is synthesized from a larger transmembrane precursor. It has been shown recently that transmembrane NDF molecules can undergo processing after phorbol ester treatment and can be secreted into the culture media, similar to TGF-α, AR or HB-EGF *(100)*. All the cell-associated and secreted HRG isoforms and the different HRG mRNA transcripts (6.7, 2.6, and 1.8 kb) are derived from the same gene that is located on chromosome 8 (8p12–21) *(101)*. The cDNAs encode proteins of different lengths termed HRG-1, HRG-2 and HRG-3, with a and b isoforms of each *(97)*. HRG mRNA has been detected in 25-30% of primary breast carcinomas *(51,102)* and in some breast-cancer cell lines *(118)*. HRG expression is induced in MCF-10A cells following transformation with a point mutated form of c-Ha-*ras*, c-*erb*B-2 or c-*neu* and may function as an autocrine growth factor in these cells, as well as in some human breast-cancer cell lines *(103)*. Its distribution, however, is more restricted than TGF-α or AR, because only ER negative, estrogen-independent cell lines express HRG *(51)*. Unlike TGF-α or AR, but similar to HB-EGF *(104)*, HRG expression is not affected by E_2. However, HRG seems to inhibit the effect of estrogen in ER positive estrogen-responsive breast-cancer cells *(105)*. Furthermore, overexpression of HRG-1 in MCF-7 cells can down-regulate ER expression *(106)*. The effect of HRG on proliferation or differentiation of human breast-cancer cells and in development of the mammary gland is not yet clear. It has been shown that NRG can stimulate lobulo-alveolar development and the production of milk proteins in the mouse mammary gland and that antisense oligonucleotides against NDF can abolish branching morphogenesis and lobulo-alveolar differentiation of the mammary gland *(4,107)*. Additionally, HRG can induce the expression of milk proteins, such as β-casein in mouse mammary epithelial HC-11 cells and whey acidic protein in mouse mammary-gland explant cultures *(108,109)*. Although NDF/HRG was originally thought to be the ligand for c-*erb*B-2, it is now known that HRG binds to and activates c-*erb*B-3 and c-*erb*B-4. However, HRG can phosphorylate c-*erb*B-2 in the presence of c-*erb*B-4 *(110)* or c-*erb*B-3 *(21)*. In addition, HRG-α and β1 can bind to c-*erb*B-3 and stimulate phosphorylation of p185*erb*B-2/*neu* in cells that coexpress both receptors *(111)*. Recent reports have shown that NDF/HRG isoforms differ in their ability to induce heterodimer formation *(112)* and that depending on the cellular context, NDF/HRG has a differential requirement for c-*erb*B-2 *(80,113)*.

2.7. Cripto-1

The human cripto-1 (CR-1) gene, also known as teratocarcinoma-derived growth factor-1, was isolated by screening a cDNA library obtained from a human teratocarcinoma cell line *(114)*. The human CR-1 gene is 4.8 kb long, is organized into 6 exons, with exon 4 containing the EGF/TGF-α-like segment, and is located on chromosome 3 (3p21.3). The human CR-1 cDNA encodes an mRNA of 2.2 kb and codes for a 24-28 kDa glycoprotein of 188 amino-acids that contains a potential N-glycosylation site, five potential myristylation sites, and three sites for phosphorylation by protein kinase C *(115)*. CR-1 has an EGF-like domain that contains 6 cysteine residues but, unlike the other EGF-related peptides, CR-1 lacks an A loop and the B loop is truncated. In addition, CR-1 lacks a conventional hydrophobic signal peptide and a hydrophobic transmembrane domain *(116)*. A recombinant CR-1 protein is secreted by cells that were transiently transfected with human CR-1 cDNA. The recombinant protein, as well as refolded peptides that correspond to the EGF-like repeat, are weakly mitogenic for nontransformed and malignant human mammary epithelial cells. Furthermore, mouse NIH-3T3 fibroblasts, nontransformed mouse NOG-8 or human MCF-10A mammary epithelial cells transfected with the full-length human CR-1 cDNA exhibit the ability to form colonies in soft agar, although these cells fail to form tumors in nude mice *(114,117,118)*. CR-1 mRNA and protein expression has been detected in several human breast-cancer cell lines *(51)*. In addition, CR-1 protein has been detected by immunocytochemistry in 83% of human primary infiltrating breast carcinomas and in 45% of ductal carcinomas *in situ (55)*. An additional study has demonstrated expression of CR-1 protein in 55% of human breast ductal carcinomas *in situ (119)*. However, no correlation was found between CR-1 expression and clinicopathologial parameters. CR-1 does not bind to or activate the EGF receptor, c-*erb*B-2, c-*erb*B-3 or c-*erb*B-4 either alone or in different pairwise combinations *(120)*. However, CR-1 can interact with a specific high-affinity, saturable binding site on HC-11 mouse mammary epithelial cells and various human breast-cancer cell lines. Additionally, CR-1 induces tyrosine phosphorylation of the SH2-adaptor protein Shc, the association of Grb2-mSos with Shc, and the activation of mitogen-activated protein kinase (MAPK) *(120)*. These data suggest that CR-1 acts through a receptor that activates the *ras/raf*/MEK/MAPK pathway. CR-1 can function as a differentiation factor as it stimulates proliferation and differentiation in mouse mammary epithelial HC-11 cells and primary mouse mammary explant cultures *(109)*.

3. TYPE 1 *ERBB* RECEPTOR TYROSINE KINASES IN BREAST CANCER

3.1. Type 1 ErbB Receptor Family

At present, four distinct members of the *erb*B type 1 growth factor-receptor family have been characterized, although the existence of a fifth candidate was recently suggested *(121)*. The first type 1 growth factor receptor to be cloned was the EGF receptor (EGFR) or c-*erb*B-1, which showed considerable homology to the avian erythroblastosis virus-transforming protein, v-*erb*B. The other three family members that have been identified are: *erb*B-2 or HER-2, *erb*B-3 or HER-3, and *erb*B-4 or HER-4 *(122)*. A rat homolog of *erb*B-2, termed *neu*, has also been cloned and characterized. This family of receptors is of particular interest owing to their frequent involvement in human cancer. Aberrant expression of *erb*B-1 has been observed in various human tumors *(41,123)*. Overexpression of *erb*B-2 in the presence or absence of gene amplification is frequently found in tumors arising at many sites, especially the breast and ovary, where it correlates with poor patient prognosis *(124)*. High levels of *erb*B-3, and to a lesser extent *erb*B-4, have been described both in breast tumor cell lines *(125)* and in primary human breast cancer *(102,126)*. All of these receptors were identified by low-stringency screening of human (or rat) cDNA libraries with a v-*erb*B probe or degenerate oligonucleotides to conserved regions of receptors (for *erb*B-3 and *erb*B-4). These receptor proteins are glycosylated and share a similar primary structure consisting of an extracellular, ligand-binding domain (which has two cysteine-rich regions), a single transmembrane region, a short juxtamembrane sequence, and an intracellular domain that contains a tyrosine-kinase domain flanked by a large hydrophilic carboxyl-tail (Fig. 1B). The carboxyl-tail displays sequence heterogeneity and carries several tyrosine autophosphorylation sites *(110,127)*. The latter serve as docking sites for various cytoplasmic signaling proteins that share a Src homology 2 (SH*2*)-domain. Signal transduction by type 1 receptor-tyrosine kinases is initiated by ligand-induced dimerization, which is followed by receptor autophosphorylation and recruitment of specific SH2-domain-containing signaling proteins *(1,128,129)*. Besides differences in the receptor structures and potential docking sites for SH2-containing proteins, the intrinsic catalytical activities of each *erb*B protein differ remarkably. Whereas *erb*B-2 is characterized by a constitutively active kinase, *erb*B-3 possesses an impaired kinase *(130)*.

3.2. Homo- and Heterodimerization of ErbB: Receptor Activation

Despite the absence of a direct ligand for *erb*B-2, EGF can elevate tyrosine phosphorylation of *erb*B-2. This transphosphorylation reaction is preceded by the formation of noncovalent heterodimers between the ligand-occupied EGFR and *erb*B-2. Moreover, coexpression of EGFR and *erb*B-2 results in synergistic transformation of fibroblasts owing to the appearance of high-affinity binding sites for EGF *(129)*. Similarly, NRGs stimulate tyrosine transphosphorylation of *erb*B-2, presumably through formation of *erb*B-3/*erb*B-2 or *erb*B-4/*erb*B-2 heterodimers *(131)*. An important consequence of heterodimerization of NRG receptors with *erb*B-2 is also a dramatic increase in affinity for the respective ligand for binding to *erb*B-3 or *erb*B-4 *(80)*. Thus, *erb*B-2 appears to be the preferred heterodimerizing coreceptor partner of the other three *erb*B receptors. This observation is supported by the fact that heterodimerization with *erb*B-2 impairs internalization, greatly prolonging the duration of signaling *(132)*. Although less prominent, the other types of heterodimers, such as EGFR/*erb*B-1, EGFR/*erb*B-3 and EGFR/*erb*B-4, exist, being more easily detectable in the absence of *erb*B-2 *(129)*. Several other lines of evidence indicate that NRG and EGFR interact with each other. Thus, NRG binding to certain tumor cells can inhibit EGF binding in a temperature-independent manner *(133)*, and EGF-dependent recruitment of phosphatidylinositol 3'-kinase to *erb*B-3 has been demonstrated in certain cell lines *(134,135)*. Moreover, it has been shown that NRG-induced dimers are more stable than EGF-induced complexes. Thus, in the absence of *erb*B-2 (breast carcinoma MDA-MB468 cell line) or in the presence of overexpressed *erb*B-1 (epidermoid carcinoma A-431 cell line), the NRG-induced formation of *erb*B-1/*erb*B-3 heterodimer can be detected by coimmunoprecipitation, whereas the EGF-induced EGFR/*erb*B-3 heterodimers are less stable. Likewise, NRG-induced formation of *erb*B-4 (NRG)/EGFR heterodimers is readily detectable, whereas EGF-induced EGFR/*erb*B-4 heterodimers are undetectable by affinity labeling *(129)*. In contrast, it has been shown recently that HB-EGF and BTC were significantly more efficacious in inducing *erb*B-3 phosphorylation and association of phosphatidylinositol 3'-kinase activity with *erb*B-3 than either EGF or TGF-α in the breast tumor cell line T47D *(80)*. This implies that ligand-binding affinities vary between different EGF agonists and that there is a hierarchical degree of association between different *erb*B receptor tyrosine kinases. Finally, there is evidence that a secondary dimerization between *erb*B receptors occurs. Growth factor-induced dimerization and receptor transphosphorylation results in the dissociation of the original receptor dimer. Each phosphorylated monomer then interacts with a new receptor partner to form a secondary dimer. EGF leads to *erb*B-2/*erb*B-3 secondary dimers and NRG to EGFR/*erb*B-2 dimers *(136)*. This second wave of signals might elongate or terminate the effects induced by the first wave, providing a means for control and for fine-tuning of the primary signals. All this evidence implies that a very complex network of inter-*erb*B crosstalks exists, leading to signal diversification, but the details of such interactions remain to be elucidated.

3.3. Signaling Through the erbB Receptor

Signal transduction through the *erb*B type 1 receptor tyrosine kinases mediates the effects on: ion fluxes, gene expression, DNA repair, and, probably, malignant growth *(19)*. Once the *erb*B receptors become activated, their first substrates are several of the tyrosine residues in their C-termini, which can then act as docking sites for proteins with SH2 domains. One of these proteins is the adapter protein Shc. Once phosphorylated, it can bind to another adapter protein, Grb2, which binds to its target proteins, the most important partner of which is Sos-1. Sos-1 is a guanine nucleotide-exchange factor that activates one of the most important effectors in the proliferative cascade, the p21ras protein. p21ras is a membrane-bound small G-protein *(137)*. p21ras-GTP recruits proteins to the membrane, where they are activated by phosphorylation. In the proliferation cascade the most important of these appears to be a serine-threonine kinase, *raf*. *Raf* activation probably requires both *ras* localization at the membrane and activation of an appropriate *raf* kinase *(138)*. The activated *raf* kinase serves to activate a subsequent phosphorylation cascade termed the MAP cascade. The kinase at the top of the cascade is termed MEK (a MAPK kinase). Once MEK is phosphorylated, it activates MAPK, leading to nuclear translocation where MAPK can modulate expression of genes such as *fos* and *cyclin D_1* by phosphorylation of transcription factors *(60)*. MAPK phosphorylates the nuclear-transcription factors *c-myc* and *c-ets*. Phosphorylation of these three nuclear proto-oncogenes is thought to modulate their transcription activity. A separate MAPK activation pathway is known to activate the product of *c-jun*. Ras activates MEKK, which then activates the stress-activated JNK kinase. JNK kinase then can phosphorylate *c-jun (1)*. The *ras-raf*-MEK-MAPK cascade is an important pathway for regulation of proliferation. The JNK stress-activated pathway also starts with small G-proteins *(138)*, and proceeds through a serine/threonine kinase. Effectors within MAPK and JNK pathways are very similar. With the exception of MEK-MAPK activation step, there is probably considerable crosstalk between those pathways. The *ras* cascade is not the only pathway to the nucleus. As mentioned previously, neither the EGFR nor *erb*B-2 has a consensus for the SH2 domains of the lipid-activated phosphatidylinositol 3'-kinase. However, heterodimerization with *erb*B-3 allows both proto-oncogenes the ability to fully activate this second messenger pathway *(139)*. The signal transducer and activator of transcription (STAT) pathway to the nucleus is mainly but not exclusively used by hematopoietic lymphokines and inflammatory cytokines and it involves the cytoplasmic JAK family kinases *(140)*. However, the EGFR can activate STAT1 as well as STAT3. Once phosphorylated, STAT proteins dimerize and translocate to the nucleus and regulate genes containing growth arrest specific (GAS) and interferon stimulated response element (ISRE) sequences in their promoters *(1,140)*. STAT1 is hypothesized to be a necessary component of the EGF-induced DNA-binding activity that recognizes the c-sis-inducible element (SIE) in the *c-fos* gene promoter. Moreover, it has been shown that the EGFR can catalyze the tyrosine phosphorylation of STAT1 without activating JAK *(141)*. Also, the EGFR can increase the levels of cyclic AMP (cAMP), thereby activating protein kinase A (PKA) and the PKA-dependent cyclic AMP response binding element (CRBE) *(1,128)*. Finally, cellular adhesion receptors appear to have a negative effect on cellular proliferation *(128)*. The phosphorylation substrates of the EGFR and *erb*B-2 include a large number of proteins directly or indirectly involved in adhesion. Radixin and ezrin are substrates for the EGFR, and tyrosine phosphorylation of these proteins is associated with the disruption of focal adhesions. ZO-1 is also tyrosine phosphorylated by the EGFR, leading to a major redistribution and the disruption of tight junctions *(128)*. Perhaps the most significant of these phosphorylations are β-catenin and plakoglobin/γ-catenin *(143)*. The catenins are involved in the formation of adherens junctions with the cadherins between epithelial cells. Catenins bind to the EGFR, *erb*B-2 *(143)*, E-cadherin *(143)*, and adenomatous polyposis coli protein (APC) *(128,142)*. These observations suggest that one of the functions of these receptors is to prepare the cells for mitogenesis by disrupting their contact with neighboring cells and substratum, and to relieve the proliferative-suppressive signals that many of these contacts engender. EGFR-mediated dispersion of E-cadherin from the adherens junctions *(143)* leads to transformation *(125)* and may also facilitate metastasis. Transfection of α-catenin into some tumors leads to restoration of E-cadherin activity and reversal of the transformed phenotype.

4. EGF-LIKE PEPTIDES AND THEIR RECEPTORS AS TARGETS FOR THERAPY IN BREAST CANCER

Breast cancer represents the most prevalent malignancy in women of Western countries. The strategies used to treat breast cancer were developed several decades ago and include surgery and radiation therapy to control local disease, and chemotherapy and hormonal therapy to eliminate metastatic disease. The failure to achieve a complete eradication of the tumor in the majority of patients is owing primarily to acquired resistance to drug and hormonal therapy. In addition, chemotherapeutic agents act by killing rapidly proliferating cells, without any selectivity for malignant cells, which results in high toxicity for the patient. For these reasons, there have been increasing efforts to more fully understand the biology of this disease and to translate the advances in basic biological knowledge into translational improvements in diagnosis and therapy. A promising area involves growth factors and their receptors. Several studies have demonstrated that cancer cells synthesize different families of growth factors and their specific receptors, which act in a cooperative fashion to modulate tumor growth, angiogenesis, and metastasis *(145)*. Among the various families of growth factors, the

EGF family of peptides with their cognate receptors are important growth modulators of breast-cancer cells. Frequent coexpression of the ligand and its cognate receptor is often detected in primary human breast carcinomas, suggesting that EGF-related peptides in combination with their receptors may perform an important role in the pathogenesis of human-breast cancer *(56)*.

Differential expression of EGF-related peptides along with their receptors in breast cancer suggests that they may be utilized as novel diagnostic and prognostic tumor markers. For example, CR-1 expression may be used as a tumor marker for early detection of breast cancer, because this protein is differentially expressed in normal breast tissue, in ductal carcinoma *in situ*, and in infiltrating breast cancer *(55,119)*. In addition, the possible detection of TGF-α or EGF in the urine and in pleural effusions from metastatic breast-cancer patients suggests that these proteins may be useful in the monitoring of tumor progression or recurrence *(146,147)*. Furthermore, EGFR and *erb*B-2 expression in human primary breast carcinomas has been shown to correlate with several known prognostic factors. In fact, EGFR and/or *erb*B-2 overexpression is associated with an estrogen-independent phenotype that correlates with poor prognosis *(123,124,148)*. EGFR expression is also an important prognostic marker for shorter relapse free survival and overall survival in lymph-node-positive patients, second only to lymph node involvement. EGFR is also a predictive marker of recurrence and overall survival in lymph node-negative patients *(149–152)*. In addition, EGFR expression has been associated with a multi-drug resistant phenotype with a lack of response to endocrine therapy *(153)*.

Several approaches that are attempting to interfere with the function of growth factors and their receptors have been identified and are being tested in vitro and in vivo in cancer patients. The complex ligand/receptor can be attacked in several fashions, by using agents that block or prevent ligand binding (monoclonal antibodies; MAbs) or by using ligands or antibodies directed against the extracellular domain of the receptor that are linked to chemotherapeutic agents, to toxins such as *P. aeruginosa* and *Diphtheria* toxins, or to radionuclides *(154–156)*. In addition, the tyrosine-kinase domain of growth-factor receptors represents another potential target for therapy with specific tyrosine-kinase inhibitors *(157)*. Finally, antisense oligodeoxynucleotides or ribozyme-based vectors that block growth factor or growth factor-receptor gene expression are also of potential utility *(158)*.

There are several MAbs that have been generated against the EGFR, such as MAbs 528 and 225, and that block ligand binding and prevent activation of the EGFR tyrosine kinase *(154,159,160)*. These anti-EGFR antibodies have been shown, in vitro and in human-tumor xenografts, to inhibit the growth of tumor cells overexpressing the EGFR and responding in culture to TGF-α, such as A431 vulvar-carcinoma cell line and MDA-MB-468 breast-carcinoma cell line, providing convincing evidence that EGFR blockade is worthy of clinical trials *(161,162)*. The first clinical studies have been conducted with MAb 225 labeled with ^{111}In and MAb 528 labeled with ^{131}I in patients with advanced carcinomas, to determine the toxicity and the pharmacokinetics of the labeled antibodies *(163,164)*. These studies have shown that concentrations in the blood of radiolabeled MAbs saturating for EGFR are without any toxicity and these MAbs are able to image primary tumors and metastases 1 cm or larger in diameter. To avoid human antimouse antibody production that can interfere with the therapeutic efficacy of the MAbs in humans, a human-murine chimeric MAb 225 (C225) that contains the human immunoglobulin G1 constant region has been developed using recombinant molecular technology *(165)*. Two multi-center dose-escalation studies with the humanized MAb 225 have been completed in patients with EGFR overexpressing tumors, including breast cancer *(166)*. Blockade of the EGFR with C225 appears to be safe without any toxicity and feasible in patients with advanced tumors. However, the results of these series of studies in vitro and in vivo demonstrate that the EGFR blockade alone is not sufficient to completely eradicate the tumor. Because the majority of cancer patients with advanced breast cancer have large tumor masses, this treatment alone was not curative. Therefore, to improve the antitumor activity of receptor-blocking antibodies, a combined therapy with standard chemotherapeutic agents has been explored. The combination therapy has shown synergistic activity in xenograft models. A431 squamous carcinoma and MDA-MB-468 breast adenocarcinoma xenografts, resistant to the maximum tolerated doses of doxorubicin or cisplatin, can be completely eradicated when these chemotherapeutic agents are combined with anti-EGFR 225 and 528 MAbs *(167,168)*. Similar synergistic responses have been observed with the combination of anti-EGFR MAbs and taxol against breast-cancer cells *(169)*. Following this promising preclinical data, a clinical trial of humanized C225 MAb in combination with taxol in patients with metastatic breast cancer is in progress *(170)*. The mechanism(s) by which sensitization to chemotherapy can be induced by EGFR blocking antibodies has not be determined and several explanations have been postulated. Receptor blockade with MAbs could alter drug uptake or metabolism, or could interfere with the repair of drug-induced DNA damage. In addition, the combined therapy could interfere with cell proliferation at two different levels. Tumor cells may not be able to survive concomitant damage to DNA and growth-factor deprivation and may therefore be more sensitive to this dual attack, thereby triggering apoptotic cell death *(171)*.

Several MAbs directed against p185*erb*B-2 have also been produced and have been shown to inhibit proliferation of human breast-cancer cell lines overexpressing p185*erb*B-2 in vitro *(172,173)*. The monoclonal anti-*erb*B-2 MAb 4D5 is able to eradicate well-established tumors overexpressing *erb*B-2 in nude mice bearing human xenografts *(173)*. Phase I clinical studies in patients with tumors overexpressing *erb*B-2 have demonstrated the safety of administration of anti-*erb*B-2 MAbs, and a phase II study in women with metastatic breast cancer has documented objective partial responses in 10% of patients as well one complete response *(174,175)*. In order to enhance the antitumor activity of anti-*erb*B-2 MAbs, a phase II clinical trial has been conducted with anti-*erb*B-2 MAbs administered in combination with cisplatin in patients with overexpressing *erb*B-2 breast tumors and a history of resistance to chemotherapy. A synergistic activity of the combined therapy was observed with objective responses in 25% of patients with cisplatin resistance *(176)*. Another phase II clinical study is testing the efficacy of a doxorubicin-containing regimen in combination with an anti-*erb*B-2 chimeric antibody in patients who were not pretreated with standard chemotherapy for metastatic disease *(170)*.

Another emerging approach to interfere with uncontrolled proliferation of cancer cells is immunotoxin therapy. An antibody directed against a cell-membrane receptor or a ligand with specificity for tumor cells is linked to a potent toxin. When injected in cancer patients, the ligand or antibody carries the toxin to the tumor cells that are overexpressing the receptor. Once bound to the cells, the toxin is internalized by the receptor and kills the cell *(156)*. Recombinant fusion proteins containing EGF, HB-EGF, TGF-α or HRG and a bacterial toxin, such as a modified version of *P. aeruginosa* exotoxin A (PE) or *Diphtheria* toxin (DT), have been generated. The chimeric toxin TGF-α-PE40 causes regression of subcutaneous tumors overexpressing EGFR in nude mice *(177)*. This agent has been used in a phase-I clinical study for the regional therapy of superficial bladder cancer, with encouraging evidence of biological activity of TGF-α-PE40 *(178)*.

Specific inhibitors of tyrosine kinases that are part of growth factor receptors, such as specific tyrphostins, have shown antitumor activity in vitro and in vivo *(157,179)*. Another approach to block the expression of specific growth factors and growth factor receptors may be the use of antisense oligodeoxynucleotides containing genes or gene fragments in the antisense orientation or hammerhead ribosyme-based vectors. This strategy has been shown to be effective in blocking the expression of TGF-α, AR, CR-1, EGFR and *erb*B-2 in colon and breast-cancer cell lines, and in significantly inhibiting tumor cell growth in vitro and tumorigenicity in nude mice *(180–182)*. The use of modified oligodeoxynucleotides as antisense inhibitors of gene expression in cancer patients is appealing, but their development as novel, specific antineoplastic therapies is still in the early preclinical trial stages.

These different technologies that can impair or compromise growth factor-activated signal transduction pathways can offer new opportunities in breast-cancer treatment and can lead to new therapies. In fact, clinical trials have demonstrated the safe administration of these agents with specific targeting of tumor cells and have reported clinical responses in women who have failed to respond to conventional chemotherapy. In addition, alteration in the expression or activation of receptor tyrosine kinases may affect the sensitivity of cancer cells to conventional chemotherapy, offering the opportunity to enhance their antitumor activity, not by increasing drug doses to supertoxic levels, but by using maximum tolerated doses of standard drugs in combination with agents perturbing a signal-transduction pathway. A major goal over the next several years will be to link these novel biological strategies to conventional cytotoxic drug therapy in human breast-cancer treatment, thereby improving the therapeutic efficacy of well-known antineoplastic agents and hopefully changing the clinical outcome of breast cancer.

5. CONCLUSIONS

From the tenor of this chapter, we hoped to provide a small yet succinct overview of those EGF-related peptides and their receptors that have been implicated at some level in the pathogenesis of human breast cancer. To appreciate their potential role in breast-cancer development, we feel that it is important to delineate the function that these cytokines and the *erb*B type 1 receptor tyrosine kinases might perform in regulating the growth and differentiation of the normal mammary gland. In this context, assessment of their site of synthesis and their level of expression during development of the mammary gland in the adult mouse has been instructive. In addition, the development of different transgenic mouse lines in which these EGF-related growth factors (e.g., TGF-α and HRG-α) or their *erb*B tyrosine kinase receptors (e.g., c-*erb*B-2*)* have been selectively overexpressed in the mammary gland using mammary epithelial cell specific promoters (e.g., mouse mammary tumor virus [MMTV] or whey acidic protein [WAP]) has provided invaluable information relating to their ability to function as dominantly transforming oncogenes in mammary epithelial cells in an in vivo setting. An alternative approach that has proved equally as informative is the ex vivo transduction of growth factor or growth factor-receptor genes directly into primary cultures of mouse mammary epithelial cells in vitro and the subsequent repopulation of a cleared mammary fat pad in virgin syngeneic mice with these transduced cells. In vitro studies utilizing nontransformed mammary epithelial cells and breast-cancer cell lines have also been useful in delineating the intracellular signaling pathways that are engaged by these growth factors through their cognate receptors. Using various mammary epithelial cells in vitro, it has become clear that all four *erb*B receptor tyrosine kinases can heterodimerize among themselves in a possible hierarchical order and that the ability of different EGF-like ligands (e.g., heregulins, BTC, and HB-EGF) to bind to multiple receptors within this family contributes to the generation of a complex level of signal diversification as determined by the repertoire and level of *erb*B receptor expression in different mammary epithelial cell types. Finally, from a therapeutic perspective, the differential overexpression of some of these growth factors or their receptors in breast cancer cells provides potential novel targets for both immunotherapy and for the application of selective and specific biological response modifiers (e.g., specific tyrosine kinase inhibitors). A combination of these approaches with conventional chemotherapeutic modalities that are routinely used in breast-cancer management (e.g., doxorubicin or taxol) has already demonstrated significant synergistic antitumor activity in preclinical and phase-II trials.

REFERENCES

1. Dickson, R. B., and M. E. Lippman. 1995. Growth factors in breast cancer. *Endocrine Rev.* **16**: 559–589.
2. Normanno, N. and F. Ciardiello. 1997. EGF related peptides in the pathophysiology of the mammary gland. *J. Mam. Gland Biol. Neoplasia* **2(2)**: 143–151.
3. Liscia, D. S., G. Merlo, F. Ciardiello, N. Kim, G. H. Smith, R. H. Callahan, and D. S. Salomon. 1990. Transforming growth factor-α messenger RNA localization in the developing adult rat and human mammary gland by in situ hybridization. *Dev. Biol.* **140**: 123–131.
4. Yang, Y., E. Spitzer, D. Meyer, M. Sachs, C. Niemann, G. Hartmann, K. M. Weidner, and W. Birchmeier. 1995. Sequential requirement of hepatocyte growth factor and neuregulin in the morphogenesis and differentiation of the mammary gland. *J. Cell. Biol.* **131**: 215–226.
5. Vonderhaar, B. K. 1987. Local effect of EGF, TGF-α and EGF-like growth factors on lobuloalveolar development of the mouse mammary gland *in vivo. J. Cell. Physiol.* **132**: 581–584.
6. Sandgren, E. P., N. C. Luetteke, R. D. Palmiter, R. L. Brinster, and D. C. Lee. 1990. Overexpression of TGFα in transgenic mice: induction of epithelial hyperplasia, pancreatic metaplasia, and carcinoma of the breast. *Cell* **61**: 1121–1135.
7. Shankar, V., F. Ciardiello, N. Kim, R. Derynck, D. S. Liscia, G. Merlo, B. C. Langton, D. Sheer, R. Callahan, R. H. Bassin, M. E. Lippman, N. Hynes, and D. S. Salomon. 1989. Transformation of an established mouse mammary epithelial cell line following transfection with a human transforming growth factor alpha cDNA. *Mol Carcinogenesis* **2**: 1–11.

8. Ciardiello, F., M. L. McGeady, N. Kim, F. Basolo, N. Hynes, B. C. Langton, H. Yokozaki, T. Saeki, J. W. Elliott, H. Masui, J. Mendelsohn, H. Soule, J. Russo, and D. S. Salomon. 1990. Transforming growth factor-α expression is enhanced in human mammary epithelial cells transformed by an activated c-Ha-ras proto-oncogene, and overexpression of the transforming growth factor-α complementary DNA leads to transformation. *Cell Growth Diff.* **1:** 407–420.

9. Matsui, Y., S. A. Halter, J. T. Holt, B. L. Hogan, and R. J. Coffey. 1990. Development of mammary hyperplasia and neoplasia in MMTV-TGFα transgenic mice. *Cell* **61:** 1147–1155.

10. Carpenter, G. and S. Cohen. 1990. Epidermal growth factor. *J. Biol. Chem.* **265:** 7709–7712.

11. Cohen, S. 1962. Isolation of a mouse submaxillary gland protein accelerating incisor eruption and eyelid opening in the new-born animal. *J. Biol. Chem.* **237:** 1555–1562.

12. Gregory, H. 1975. Isolation and structure of urogastrone and its relationship to epidermal growth factor. *Nature* **257:** 325–327.

13. DiAugustine, R. P. 1994. The epidermal growth factor family in the mammary gland and other target organs for ovarian steroids, in *Mammary Tumorigenesis and Malignant Progression* (Lippman M. E. and R. B. Dickson, eds.), Kluwer, Boston, MA, pp. 131–160.

14. Mroczkowski B., M. Reich, K. Chen, G. I. Bell, and S. Cohen. 1989. Recombinant human EGF precursor is a glycosylated membrane protein with biological activity. *Mol. Cell Biol.* **9:** 2771–2778.

15. Carpenter, G. 1980. Epidermal growth factor is a major growth-promoting agent in human milk. *Science* **210:** 198–199.

16. Murphy, L. C., H. Dotzlaw, M. S. J. Wong, T. Miller, B. Mrockowski, Y. Gong, and L. J. Murphy. 1990. Epidermal growth factor: receptor and ligand expression in human breast cancer. *Sem. Cancer Biol.* **1:** 305–315.

17. Murphy, L. C., L. J. Murphy, D. Dubik, G. I. Bell, and R. P. C. Shiu. 1988b. Epidermal growth factor gene expression in human breast cancer cells: regulation of expression by progestins. *Cancer Res.* **48:** 4555–4560.

18. Taketani, Y. and T. Oka. 1983. Biological action of epidermal growth factor and its functional receptors in human mammary epithelial cells. *Proc. Natl. Acad. Sci. USA* **80:** 2647–2650.

19. Stampfer, M. R. 1985. Isolation and growth of human mammary epithelial cells. *J. Tissue Cult. Methods* **9:** 107–115.

20. Osborne, C. K., B. Hamilton, G. Titus, and R. B. Livingston. 1980. Epidermal growth factor stimulation of human breast cancer cells in culture. *Cancer Res.* **40:** 2361–2366.

21. Imai, Y., C. K. H. Leung, H. G. Friesen, and R. P. C. Shiu. 1982. Epidermal growth factor receptors and effect of epidermal growth factor on growth of human breast cancer cells in long term tissue culture. *Cancer Res.* **42:** 4394–4398.

22. Vonderhaar, B. K. 1988. Regulation of development of the normal mammary gland by hormones and growth factors, in *Breast Cancer: Cellular and Molecular Biology* (Lippman, M. E. and R. B. Dickson, eds.), Kluwer, Boston, MA, pp. 251–266.

23. Oka, T., O. Tsutsumi, Kurachi, and S. Okamoto. 1988. The role of epidermal growth factor in normal and neoplastic growth of mouse mammary epithelial cells, in *Breast Cancer: Cellular and Molecular Biology* (Lippman, M. E. and R. B. Dickson, eds.), Kluwer Press, Boston, MA, pp. 343–362.

24. Okamoto, S. and T. Oka. 1984. Evidence for physiological function of epidermal growth factor: progestational sialoadenectomy of mice decrease milk production and increases offspring mortality during lactation period. *Proc. Natl. Acad. Sci. USA* **81:** 6059–6063.

25. Tsutsumi O., A. Tsutsumi, and T. Oka. 1987. Importance of epidermal growth factor in implantation and growth of mouse mammary tumor in female mice. *Cancer Res.* **47:** 4651–4653.

26. Dotzlaw, H., T. Miller, J. Karvelas, and L. C. Murphy. 1990. Epidermal growth factor gene expression in human breast cancer biopsy samples: relationship to estrogen and progesterone receptor gene expression. *Cancer Res.* **50:** 4204–4208.

27. Mizukami, Y., A. Nonomura, M. Noguchi, T. Taniya, N. Koyasaki, Y. Saito, T. Hashimoto, F. Matsubara, and N. Yanaihara. 1991. Immunohistochemical study of oncogene product Ras p21, c-Myc, and growth factor EGF in breast carcinomas. *Anticancer Res.* **11:** 1485–1494.

28. Derynck, R. 1992. The physiology of transforming growth factor-α. Adv. *Cancer Res.* **58:** 27–52.

29. Massagué, J. 1990. Transforming growth factor-α. *J. Biol. Chem.* **265:** 21,393–21,396.

30. Massagué, J. and A. Pandiella. 1993. Membrane-anchored growth factors. *Annu. Rev. Biochem.* **62:** 515–541.

31. Salomon, D. S., J. A. Zwiebel, M. Bano, I. Losonczy, P. Fehnel, and W. R. Kidwell. 1984. Presence of transforming growth factors in human breast cancer cells. *Cancer Res.* **44:** 4069–4077.

32. Valverius, E. M., S. Bates, M. R. Stampfer, R. Clark, F. McCormick, D. S. Salomon, M. E. Lippman, and R. B. Dickson. 1989. Transforming growth factor alpha production and epidermal growth factor receptor expression in normal and oncogene transformed human mammary epithelial cells. *Mol. Endocrinol.* **3:** 203–214.

33. Bates, S. E., E. M. Valverius, B. W. Ennis, D. A. Bronzert, J. P. Sheridan, M. R. Stampfer, J. Mendelsohn, M. E. Lippman, and R. B. Dickson. 1990. Expression of TGF-alpha/EGF receptor pathway in normal human breast epithelial cells. *Endocrinology* **126:** 596–607.

34. Perroteau, I., D. S. Salomon, M. DeBortoli, W. R. Kidwell, P. Hazarika, R. Pardue, J. Dedman, and J. Tam. 1986. Immunological detection and quantitation of alpha transforming growth factors in human breast carcinoma cells. *Breast Cancer Res. Treat.* **7:** 201–210.

35. Bates, S. E., N. E. Davidson, E. M. Valverius, C. E. Freter, R. B. Dickson, J. E. Kudlow, M. E. Lippman, and D. S. Salomon. 1988. Expression of transforming growth factor-α and its messenger ribonucleic acid in human breast cancer: its regulation by estrogen and its possible functional significance. *Mol. Endocrinol.* **2:** 543–555.

36. Saeki, T., A. Cristiano, M. Lynch, M. Brattain, N. Kim, N. Normanno, N. Kenney, F. Ciardiello, and D. S. Salomon. 1991. Regulation by estrogen through the 5'-flanking region of the transforming growth factor-α gene. *Mol. Endocrinol.* **5:** 1955–1963.

37. El-Ashry, D., S. Chrysogelos, M. E. Lippman, and F. G. Ker. 1996. Estrogen induction of TGF-α is mediated by an estrogen response element composed of two imperfect palindromes. *J. Steroid Biochem.* **59:** 261–269.

38. Murphy, L. C. and H. Dotzlaw. 1989. Regulation of transforming growth factor α and transforming growth factor β messenger ribonucleic acid abundance in T-47D human breast cancer cells. *Mol. Endocrinol.* **3:** 611–616.

39. Bjorge, J. D., A. J. Paterson, and J. E. Kudlow. 1989. Phorbol ester or epidermal growth factor (EGF) stimulates the concurrent accumulation of mRNA for the EGF receptor and its ligand transforming growth factor-α in a breast cancer cell line. *J. Biol. Chem.* **264:** 4021–4027.

40. Kudlow, J. E. and J. D. Bjorge. 1990. TGF-α in normal physiology. *Sem. Cancer Biol.* **1:** 293–302.

41. Salomon, D. S., R. Brandt, F. Ciardiello, and N. Normanno. 1995. Epidermal growth factor-related peptides and their receptors in human malignancies. *Critical Rev. Oncol./ Hematol.* **19:** 183–232.

42. Snedeker, S. M., C. F. Brown, and R. P. DiAugustine. 1991. Expression and functional properties of TGFα and EGF during mouse mammary gland ductal morphogenesis. *Proc. Natl. Acad. Sci. USA* **88:** 276–280.

43. Shoyab, M., G. D. Plowman, V. L. McDonald, J. G. Bradley, and G. J. Todaro. 1989. Structure and function of human amphiregulin: a member of the epidermal growth factor family. *Science* **243:** 1074–1076.

44. Johnson, G. R., B. Kannan, M. Shoyab, and K. Stromberg. 1993a. Amphiregulin induces tyrosine phosphorylation of the epidermal growth factor receptor and p185[erbB2] *J. Biol. Chem.* **268:** 2924–2931.

45. Shoyab, M., V. L. McDonald, J. G. Bradley, and G. J. Todaro. 1988. Amphiregulin: a bifunctional growth-modulating glycoprotein produced by the phorbol 12-myristate 13-acetate-treated human breast adenocarcinoma cell line MCF-7. *Proc. Natl. Acad. Sci. USA* **85:** 6528–6532.

46. Johnson, G. R., S. A. Prigent, W. J. Gullick, and K. Stromberg. 1993. Characterization of high and low molecular forms of amphiregulin that differ in glycosylation and peptide core length. *J. Biol. Chem.* **268:** 18,835–18,843.

47. Martínez-Lacaci, I., G. Johnson, D. S. Salomon, and R. B. Dickson. 1996. Characterization of a novel amphiregulin-related molecule in 12-O-tetradecanoylphorbol–13-acetate-treated breast cancer cells. *J. Cell. Physiol.* **169:** 497–508.

48. Plowman, G. D., J. M. Green, V. L. McDonald, M. G. Neubauer, C. M. Disteche, G. J. Todaro, and M. Shoyab. 1990. The amphiregulin gene encodes a novel epidermal growth factor-related protein with tumor inhibitor activity. *Mol. Cell Biol.* **10:** 1969–1981.

49. Johnson G. R., T. Saeki, N. Auersperg, A. W. Gordon, M. Shoyab, D. S. Salomon, and K. Stromberg. 1991. Response to and expression of amphiregulin by ovarian carcinoma and normal ovarian surface epithelial cells: nuclear localization of endogenous amphiregulin. *Biochem. Biophys. Res. Commun.* **180:** 481–488.

50. Cook, P. W., P. A. Mattox, W. W. Keeble, M. R. Pittelkow, G. D. Plowman, M. Shoyab, J. P. Adelman, and G. D. Shipley. 1991. A heparin sulfate-regulated human keratinocyte autocrine growth factor is similar or identical to amphiregulin. *Mol. Cell Biol.* **11:** 2547–2557.

51. Normanno, N., C.-F. Qi, W. J. Gullick, G. Persico, Y. Yarden, D. Wen, G. Plowman, N. Kenney, G. Johnson, N. Kim, R. Brandt, I. Martínez-Lacaci, R. B. Dickson, and D. S. Salomon. 1993. Expression of amphiregulin, cripto–1, and heregulin in human breast cancer cells . *Intl. J. Oncol.* **2:** 903–911.

52. Martínez-Lacaci, I., M. Saceda, G. Plowman, G. R. Johnson, N. Normanno, D. S. Salomon, and R. B. Dickson. 1995. Estrogen and phorbol esters regulate amphiregulin expression by two separate mechanisms in human breast cancer cells. *Endocrinology* **136:** 3983–3992.

53. Kenney, N., G. R. Johnson, M. P. Selvan, N. Kim, C.-F. Qi, T. Saeki, R. Brandt, B. Wallace-Jones, F. Ciardiello, M. Shoyab, G. Plowman, A. Day, and D. S. Salomon. 1993. Transforming growth factor α (TGF-α) and amphiregulin (AR) as autocrine growth factors in nontransformed, immortalized 184A1N4 human mammary epithelial cells. *Mol. Cell. Differ.* **1:** 163–184.

54. Normanno, N, P. Selvam, C.-F. Qi, T. Saeki, G. Johnson, N. Kim, F. Ciardiello, M. Shoyab, G. Plowman, R. Brandt, G. Todaro, and D. S. Salomon. 1994a. Amphiregulin as an autocrine growth factor for c-Ha-*ras* and c-*erb*B-2-transformed human mammary epithelial cells. *Proc. Natl. Acad. Sci. USA* **91:** 2790–2794.

55. Qi, C., D. S. Liscia, N. Normanno, G. Merlo, G. R. Johnson, W. J. Gullick, F. Ciardiello, T. Saeki, R. Brandt, N. Kim, N. Kenney and D. S. Salomon. 1994. Expression of transforming growth factor α, amphiregulin and cripto-1 in human breast carcinomas. *Br. J. Cancer* **69:** 903–910.

56. Normanno, N., F. Ciardiello, R. Brandt, and D. S. Salomon. 1994. Epidermal growth factor-related peptides in the pathogenesis of human breast cancer. *Breast Cancer Res. Treat.* **29:** 11–27.

57. LeJeune, S., R. Leek, E. Horak, G. D. Plowman, M. Greenall, and L. Harris. 1993. Amphiregulin, epidermal growth factor receptor, and estrogen receptor expression in human primary breast cancer. *Cancer Res.* **53:** 3597–3602.

58. Saeki, T., K. Stromberg, C.-F. Qi, W. Gullick, E. Tahara, N. Normanno, F. Ciradello, N. Kenney, G. R. Johnson, and D. S. Salomon. 1991. Differential immunohistochemical localization of amphiregulin and cripto in human normal colon and colorectal tumors. *Cancer Res.* **52:** 3467–3473.

59. Cook, P. W., M. R. Pittelkow, W. W. Keeble, R. Graves-Deal, R. J. Coffey, and G. D. Shipley. 1992. Amphiregulin messenger RNA is elevated in psoriatic epidermis and gastrointestinal carcinomas. *Cancer Res.* **52:** 3224–3227.

60. Kimura, H. 1993. Schwannoma-derived growth factor must be transported into the nucleus to exert its mitogenic activity. *Proc. Natl. Acad. Sci. USA* **90:** 2165–2169.

61. Modrell, B., V. L. McDonald, and M. Shoyab. 1992. The interaction of amphiregulin with nuclei and putative nuclear localization sequence binding proteins. *Growth Factors* **7:** 305–314.

62. Li, S., G. D. Plowman, S. D. Buckley, and G. D. Shipley. 1992. Heparin inhibition of autonomous growth implicates amphiregulin as an autocrine growth factor for normal human mammary epithelial cells. *J. Cell Physiol.* **153:** 103–111.

63. Piepkorn, M., C. Lo, and G. D. Plowman. 1994. Amphiregulin-dependent proliferation of cultured human keratinocytes: autocrine growth, the effects of exogenous recombinant cytokine, and apparent requirement for heparin-like glycosaminoglycans. *J. Cell Physiol.* **159:** 114–120.

64. Johnson, G. R. and L. Wong. 1994. Heparan sulfate is essential to amphiregulin-induced mitogenic signaling by the epidermal growth factor receptor. *J. Biol. Chem.* **269:** 27,149–27,154.

65. Higashiyama, S., J. A. Abraham, J. Miller, J. C. Fiddes, and M. Klagsbrun. 1991. A heparin-binding growth factor secreted by macrophage-like cells that is related to EGF. *Science* **251:** 936–939.

66. Higashiyama, S., K. Lau, G. E. Besner, J. A. Abraham, and M. Klagsbrun. 1992. Structure of heparin-binding EGF-like growth factor. *J. Biol. Chem.* **267:** 6205–6212.

67. Fen, Z., M. S. Dhadly, M. Yoshizumi, R. J. Hilkert, T. Quertermous, R. L. Eddy, T. B. Shows, and M.-E. Lee. 1993. Structural organization and chromosomal assignment of the gene encoding the human heparin-binding epidermal growth factor-like growth factor/ diphtheria toxin receptor. *Biochemistry* **32:** 7932–7938.

68. Abraham, J. A., D. Damm, A. Bajardi, J. Miller, M. Klagsbrun, and A. B. Ezekowitz. 1993. Heparin-binding EGF-like growth factor: characterization of rat and mouse cDNA clones, protein domain conservation across species, and transcript expression in tissues. *Biochem. Biophys. Res. Commun.* **190:** 125–133.

69. Vaughan T. J., J. C. Pascall, and K. D. Brown. 1992. Tissue distribution of mRNA for heparin-binding epidermal growth factor. *Biochem. J.* **287:** 681–684.

70. Naglich, J. G., J. E. Metherall, D. W. Russel, and L. Eidels. 1992. Expression cloning of a diphtheria toxin receptor: identity with a heparin-binding EGF-like growth factor precursor. *Cell* **69:** 1051–1061.

71. Iwamoto, R., S. Higashiyma, T. Mitamura, N. Taniguchi, M. Klagsbrun, and E. Mekada. 1994. Heparin-binding EGF-like growth factor, which acts as the diphtheria toxin receptor, forms a complex with the membrane protein DRAP27/CD9, which up-regulates functional receptors and diphtheria toxin sensitivity. *EMBO J.* **13:** 2322–2330.

72. Higashiyama, S., R. Iwamoto, K. Goishi, G. Raab, N. Taniguchi, M. Klagsbrun, and E. Mekada. 1995. The membrane protein DRAP27/CD9 potentiates the juxtacrine growth

factor αctivity of the membrane-anchored heparin-binding EGF-like growth factor. *J. Cell Biol.* **128:** 929–938.

73. Inui, S., S. Higashiyama, K. Hashimoto, M. Higashiyama, K. Yoshikawa, and N. Taniguchi. 1997. Possible role of coexpression of CD9 with membrane-anchored heparin-binding EGF-like growth factor and amphiregulin in cultured human keratinocyte growth. *J. Cell. Physiol.* **171:** 291–298.

74. Raab, G., S. Higashiyama, S. Hetelekidis, J. A. Abraham, D. Damm, M. Ono, and M. Klagsbrun. 1994. Biosynthesis and processing by phorbol ester of the cell surface-associated precursor form of heparin-binding EGF-like growth factor. *Biochem. Biophys. Res. Commun.* **204:** 592–597.

75. Goishi, K., S. Higashiyama, M. Klagsbrun, N. Nakano, T. Umata, M. Ishikawa, E. Mekada, and N. Taniguchi. 1995. Phorbol ester induces rapid processing of cell surface heparin-binding EGF-like growth factor: conversion from juxtacrine to paracrine growth factor activity. *Mol. Cell Biol.* **6:** 967–980.

76. Nakagawa, T., S. Higashiyama, T. Mitamura, E. Mekada, and N. Taniguchi. 1996. Amino-terminal processing of cell surface heparin-binding epidermal growth factor-like growth factor up-regulates its juxtacrine but not its paracrine growth factor activity. *J. Biol. Chem.* **271:** 30,858–30,863.

77. Besner, G. E., D. Whelton, M. A. Crissman-Combs, C. L. Steffen, G. Y. Kim, and D. R. Brigstock. 1992. Interaction of heparin-binding EGF- like growth factor (HB-EGF) with the epidermal growth factor receptor: modulation by heparin, heparinase, or synthetic heparin-binding HB-EGF fragments. *Growth Factors* **7:** 289–296.

78. Cook, P. W., D. Damm, B. L. Garrick, K. M. Wood, C. E. Karkaria, S. Higashiyama, M. Klagsbrun and J. A. Abraham. 1995a. Carboxyl-terminal truncation of leucine$_{76}$ converts heparin-binding EGF-like growth factor from a heparin-enhancible to a heparin-suppressible growth factor. *J. Cell. Physiol.* **163:** 407–417.

79. Cook, P. W., N. M. Ashton, C. E. Karkaria, D. C. Siess and G. D. Shipley. 1995b. Differential effects of a heparin antagonist (hexadimethrine) or chlorate on amphiregulin, basic fibroblast growth factor, and heparin-binding EGF- like growth factor activity. *J. Cell. Physiol.* **163:** 418–429

80. Beerli, R. R. and N. H. Hynes. 1996. Epidermal growth factor-related peptides activate distinct subsets of erbB receptors and differ in their biological activities. *J. Biol. Chem.* **271:** 6071–6076.

81. Marikovsky, M., K. Breiung, P. Y. Liu, E. Eriksson, S. Higashiyama, P. Farber, J. Abraham, and M. Klagsbrun. 1993. Appearance of heparin- binding EGF-like growth factor in wound fluid as a response to injury. *Proc. Natl. Acad. Sci. USA* **90:** 3889–3893.

82. Yoshizumi, M., S. Kourembanas, D. H. Temizer, R. P. Cambria, T. Quertermous, and M.-E. Lee. 1992. Tumor necrosis factor increases transcription of the heparin-binding epidermal growth factor gene in vascular endothelial cells. *J. Biol. Chem.* **267:** 9467–9469.

83. Temizer, D. H., M. Yoshizumi, M. A. Perrella, E. E. Susanni, T. Quertermous, and M.-E. Lee. 1992. Induction of heparin-binding epidermal growth factor-like growth factor mRNA by phorbol ester and angiotensin II in rat aortic smooth muscle cells. *J. Biol. Chem.* **267:** 24,892–24,896.

84. Dluz, S. M., S. Higashiyama, D. Damm, J. A. Abraham, and M. Klagsbrun. 1993. Heparin-binding epidermal growth factor-like growth factor expression in cultured fetal human vascular smooth muscle cells. *J. Biol. Chem.* **268:** 18,330–18,334.

85. Zhang, Z., C. Funk, D. Roy, S. Glasser, and J. Mulholland. 1994. Heparin-binding epidermal growth factor-like growth factor is differentially regulated by progesterone and estradiol in rat uterine epithelial and stromal cells. *Endocrinology* **134:** 1089–1094.

86. Wang, X.-N., S. K. Das, D. Damm, M. Klagsbrun, J. A. Abraham, and S. K. Dey. 1994. Differential regulation of heparin-binding epidermal growth factor-like growth factor in the adult ovariectomized mouse uterus by progesterone and estrogen. *Endocrinology* **135**: 1264–1271.

87. Shing, Y., G. Christofori, D. Hanahan, Y. Ono, R. Sasada, K. Igarashi, and J. Folkman. 1993. Betacellulin: a mitogen from pancreatic cell tumors. *Science* **259**: 1604–1607.

88. Hanahan, D. 1985. Heritable formation of pancreatic beta-cell tumours in transgenic mice expressing recombinant insulin/simian virus 40 oncogenes. *Nature* **315**: 115–122.

89. Folkman J., K. Watson, D. Ingber, and D. Hanahan. 1989. Induction of angiogenesis during the transition from hyperplasia to neoplasia. *Nature* **339**: 58–61.

90. Sasada, R., Y. Ono, Y. Taniyama, Y. Shing, J. Folkman, and K. Igarashi. 1993. Cloning and expression of cDNA encoding betacellulin, a new member of the EGF family. *Biochem. Biophys. Res. Commun.* **190**: 1173–1179.

91. Riese, D. J., II, Y. Bermingham, T. M. van Raaij, S. Buckley, G. D. Plowman, and D. F. Stern. 1996. Betacellulin activates the epidermal growth factor receptor and erbB-4, and induces cellular response patterns distinct from those stimulated by epidermal growth factor or neuregulin-beta. *Oncogene* **12**: 345–353.

92. Seno, M., H. Tada, M. Kosaka, R. Sasada, K. Igarashi, Y. Shing, J. Folkman, M. Ueda, and H. Yamada. 1996. Human betacellulin, a member of the EGF family dominantly expressed in pancreas and small intestine, is fully active in a monomeric form. *Growth Factors* **13**: 181–191.

93. Peles, E. and Y. Yarden. 1993. Neu and its ligands: from an oncogene to neural factors. *Bioessays* **15**: 815–824.

94. Pinkas-Kramarski, R., R. Eilam, O. Spiegler, S. Lavi, N. Liu, D. Chang, D. Wen, A. Schwartz, and Y. Yarden. 1994. Brain neurons and glial cells express neu differentiation factor/heregulin: a survival factor for astrocytes. *Proc. Natl. Acad. Sci. USA* **91**: 9387–9391.

95. Chang, H., D. J. Riese II, W. Gilbert, D. F. Stern, and U. J. McMahan. 1997. Ligands for erbB-family receptors encoded by a neuregulin-like gene. *Nature* (London) **387**: 509–512.

96. Carraway, K. L., III, J. L. Weber, M. J. Unger, J. Ledesma, N. Yu, M. Gassmann, and C. Lai. 1997. Neuregulin-2, a new ligand of erbB3/erbB4-receptor tyrosine kinases. *Nature* (London) **387**: 512–516.

97. Yarden Y. and E. Peles. 1991. Biochemical analysis of the ligand for the neu oncogenic receptor. *Biochemistry* **30**: 3543–3550.

98. Holmes, W. E., M. X. Sliwkowski, R. W. Akita, W. J. Henzel, J. Lee, J. W. Park, D. Yansura, N. Abadi, H. Raab, G. D. Lewis, M. Shepard, W.-J. Kuang, W. I. Wood, D. V. Goeddel, and R. L. Vandlen. 1992. Identification of heregulin, a specific activator of p185^{erbB2}. *Science* **256**: 1205–1210.

99. Peles, E., S. S. Bacus, R. A. Koski, H. S. Lu, D. Wen, S. G. Ogden, R. Ben-Levy and Y. Yarden. 1992. Isolation of the Neu/HER-2 stimulatory ligand: a 44 kd glycoprotein that induces differentiation of mammary tumor cells. *Cell* **69**: 205–216.

100. Burgess, T. L., S. L. Ross, Y.-X. Qian, D. Brankow, and S. Hu. 1995. Biosynthetic processing of the *neu* differentiation factor. *J. Biol. Chem.* **270**: 19,188–19,166.

101. Peles, E., R. Ben-Levy, E. Tzahar, N. Liu, and Y. Yarden. 1993. Cell- type specific interaction of Neu differentiation factor (NDF/heregulin) Neu/HER-2 suggests complex ligand receptor relationships. *EMBO J.* **12**: 961–971.

102. Bacus, S. S., A. V. Gudkov, C. R. Zelnik, D. Chin, R. Stern, I. Stancovski, E. Peles, H. Ben-Baruch, H. Farbstein, R. Lupu, D. Wen., M. Sela, and Y. Yarden. 1993. Neu differentiation factor (heregulin) induces expression of intracellular adhesion molecule 1: implications for mammary tumors. *Cancer Res.* **53**: 5251–5261.

103. Mincione, G., C. Bianco, S. Kannan, G. Collettaa, F. Ciardiello, M. Sliwkowski, Y. Yarden, N. Normanno, A. Pramaggiore, N. Kim, and D. S. Salomon. 1996. Enhanced expression of heregulin in c-erbB-2 and c-Ha-ras transformed mouse and human mammary epithelial cells. *J. Cell. Biochem.* **60:** 437–446.

104. Martínez-Lacaci, I., D. S. Salomon, and R. B. Dickson. Unpublished results.

105. Grunt. T. W., M. Saceda, M. Martin, R. Lupu, E. Dittrich, G. Krupitza, H. Harant, H. Huber, and C. Dittrich. 1995. Bidirectional interactions between the estrogen receptor and the c-erbB–2 signalling pathways: heregulin inhibits estrogenic effects in breast cancer cells. *Int. J. Cancer* **63:** 560–567.

106. Pietras, R. J., J. Arboleda, J. D. Riese II, N. Wongvipat, M. D. Pegram, L. Ramos, C. M. Gorman, M. G. Parker, M. X. Sliwkowski, and D. J. Salmon. 1995. HER-2 tyrosine kinase pathway targets estrogen receptor and promotes estrogen-independent growth in human breast cancer cells. *Oncogene* **10:** 2435–2447.

107. Jones, F. E., D. J. Jerry, B. C. Guarino, G. C. Andrews, and D. F. Stern. 1996. Heregulin induces in vivo proliferation and differentiation of mammary epithelium into secretory lobuloalveoli. *Cell Growth Diff.* **7:** 1031–1038.

108. Marte, B. M., D. Graus-Porta, M. Jeschke, D. Fabbro, N. E. Hynes, and D. Taverna. 1995. NDF/heregulin activates MAP kinase and p70/p85 S6 kinase during proliferation and differentiation of mammary epithelial cells. *Oncogene* **10:** 167–175.

109. DeSantis M., S. Kannan, G. H. Smith, M. Seno, C. Bianco, N. Kim, I. Martinez-Lacaci, B. Wallace-Jones, and D. S. Salomon. 1997. Cripto-1 inhibits β-casein expression in mammary epithelial cells through a p21*ras*- and phosphatidylinositol-3 kinase-dependent pathway. *Cell Growth and Differentiation* **8:** 1257–1266.

110. Plowman, G. D., J. M. Green, J.-M. Culouscou, G. W. Carlton, V. M. Rothwell, and B. Sharon. 1993. Heregulin induces tyrosine phosphorylation of HER4/p180erbB–4. *Nature* (London) **366:** 473–475.

111. Carraway K. L., III, M. X. Sliwkowski, R. Akita, J. V. Platko, P. M. Guy, A. Nuijens, A. J. Diamonti, R. L. Vandlen, L. C. Cantley, and R. A. Cerione. 1994. The erbB3 gene product is a receptor for heregulin. *J. Biol. Chem.* **269:** 14,303–14,306.

112. Pinkas-Kramarski, R., M. Shelly, S. Glathe, B. J. Ratzkin, and Y. Yarden. 1996. Neu differentiation factor/neuregulin isoforms activate distinct receptor combinations. *J. Biol. Chem.* **271:** 19,029–19,032.

113. Beerli, R. R., D. Graus-Porta, K. Woods-Cook, X. Chen, Y. Yarden, and N. E. Hynes. 1995. Neu differentiation factor activation of erbB-3 and erbB-4 is cell specific and displays a differential requirement for erbB-2. *Mol. Cell. Biol.* **15:** 6496–6505.

114. Ciccodiocola, A., R. Dono, S. Obici, A. Simeone, M. Zollo, and M. G. Persico. 1989. Molecular characterization of a gene of the EGF family expressed in undifferentiated human NTERA–2 teratocarcinoma cells. *EMBO J.* **8:** 1987–1989.

115. Dono, R., N. Montuori, M. Rocchi, L. De Ponti-Zilli, A. Ciccodiocola, and M. G. Persico. 1991. Isolation and characterization of the CRIPTO autosomal gene and its X-linked related sequence. *Am. J. Hum. Genet.* **49:** 555–565.

116. Brandt, R., N. Normanno, W. J. Gullick, J.-H. Lin, R. Harkins, D. Schneider, B.-W. Jones, F. Ciardiello, M. G. Persico, F. Armenante, N. Kim, and D. S. Salomon. 1994. Identification and biological characterization of an epidermal growth factor gene-related protein: cripto-1. *J. Biol. Chem.* **269:** 17,320–17,328.

117. Ciardiello, F., R. Dono, N. Kim, M. G. Persico, and D. S. Salomon. 1991. Expression of cripto, a novel gene of the epidermal growth factor gene family leads to *in vitro* transformation of a normal mouse mammary epithelial cell line. *Cancer Res.* **51:** 1051–1054.

118. Normanno, N. and Salomon D. Unpublished results.

119. Panico, L., A. D'Antonio, G. Salvatore, E. Mezza, G. Tortora, M. De Laurentis, S. De Placido, T. Giordano, M. Merino, D. S. Salomon, W. J. Gullick, G. Pettinato, S. J. Schnitt,

A. R. Bianco, and F. Ciardiello. 1996. Differential immunohistochemical detection of transforming growth factor α, amphiregulin and cripto in human normal and malignant breast tissues. *Int. J. Cancer* **65**: 51–56.

120. Kannan, S., M. De Santis, M. Lohmeyer, D. J. Riese II., G. H. Smith, N. Hynes, M. Seno, R. Brandt, C. Bianco, G. Persico, N. Kenney, N. Normanno, I. Martínez-Lacaci, F. Ciardiello, D. F. Stern, W. J. Gullick, and D. S. Salomon. 1997. Cripto enhances the tyrosine phosphorylation of Shc and activates mitogen-activated protein kinase (MAPK) in mammary epithelial cells. *J. Biol. Chem.* **272**: 3330–3335.

121. Panneerselvam, K., P. Kanakaraj, S. Raj, M. Das, and S. Bishayee. 1995. Characterization of a novel epidermal-growth-factor-receptor-related 200-kDa tyrosine kinase in tumor cells. *Eur. J. Biochem.* **230**: 951–957.

122. Mason, S. and W. J. Gullick. 1995. Type 1 growth factor receptors: an overview of recent developments. *The Breast* **4**: 11–18.

123. Gullick, W. J. 1991. Prevalence of aberrant expression of the epidermal growth factor receptor in human cancers. *Br. Med. Bull.* **47**: 87–98.

124. Hynes, N. H. and D. F. Stern. 1994. The biology of erbB–2/neu/HER–2 and its role in cancer. *Biochim. Biophys. Acta* **1**198: 165–184.

125. Kraus, M. H., P. Fedi, V. Starks, R. Muraro, and S. A. Aaronson. 1993 Demonstration of ligand-dependent signaling by the erbB-3 tyrosine kinase and its constitutive activation in human breast tumor cells. *Proc. Natl. Acad. Sci. USA* **90**: 2900–2904.

126. Lemoine, N. R., D. M. Barnes, D. P. Hollywood, C. M. Hughes, P. Smith, E. Dublin, S. A. Prigent, W. J. Gullick, and H. C. Hurst. 1992. Expression of the ERBB3 gene product in breast cancer. *Br. J. Cancer* **66**: 1116–1121.

127. Peles, E., R. Ben-Levy, E. Tzahar, L. Naili, D. Wen, and Y. Yarden. 1993. Cell-type specific interaction of Neu differentiation factor (NDF/heregulin) with Neu/HER-2. *EMBO J.* **10**: 2077–2086.

128. Bridges, A. J. 1996. The epidermal growth factor receptor family of tyrosine kinases and cancer: can an atypical exemplar be a sound therapeutic target? *Current Med. Chem.* **3**: 167–194.

129. Tzahar, E., H. Waterman, X. Chen, G. Levkowitz, D. Karunagaran, S. Lavi, B. J. Ratzkin, and Y. Yarden. 1996. A hierarchical network of interreceptor interactions determines signal transduction by Neu differentiation factor/neuregulin and epidermal growth factor. *Mol. Cell. Biol.* **16**: 5276–5287.

130. Pinkas-Kramarski, R., L. Soussan, H. Waterman, G. Levkowitz, I. Alroy, L. Klapper, S. Lavi, R. Seger, B. J. Ratzkin, M. Sela, and Y. Yarden. 1996. Diversification of Neu differentiation factor and epidermal growth factor signaling by combinatorial receptor interactions. *EMBO J.* **15**: 2452–2467.

131. Riese, D. J., T. M. van Raaij, G. D. Plowman, G. C. Andrews, and D. F. Stern. 1995. The cellular response to neuregulins is governed by complex interactions of the erbB receptor family. *Mol. Cell. Biol.* **15**: 5770–5776.

132. Sorkin, A., P. P. Difiore, and G. Carpenter. 1993. The carboxyl terminus of epidermal growth factor receptor/erbB-2 chimerae is internalization impaired. *Oncogene* **8**: 3021–3028.

133. Karunagaran, D. E., E. Tzahar, N. Liu, D. Wen, and Y. Yarden. 1995. Neu differentiation factor inhibits EGF binding: a model for trans-regulation within the erbB family of receptor tyrosine kinases. *J. Biol. Chem.* **270**: 9982–9990.

134. Kim, H.-H., S. L. Sierke, and J. G. Koland. 1994. Epidermal growth factor-dependent association of phosphatidylinositol 3'-kinase with the erbB-3 gene product. *J. Biol. Chem.* **269**: 24,747–24,755.

135. Sliwkowski, M. X., G. Schaefer, R. W. Akita, J. A. Lofgren, V. D. Fitzpatrick, A. Nuijens, B. M. Fendly, R. A. Cerione, R. L. Vandlen, and K. L. Carraway. 1994. Coexpression of erbB-2 and erbB-3 proteins reconstitutes a high affinity receptor for heregulin. *J. Biol. Chem.* **269**: 14,661–14,665.

136. Gamett, D. C., G. Pearson, R. A. Cerione, and I. Friedberg. 1997. Secondary dimerization between members of the epidermal growth factor receptor family. *J. Biol. Chem.* **272:** 12,052–12,056.

137. Hall, A. 1994. A biochemical function for ras-at last. *Science* **264:** 1413–1414.

138. Vojtek, A. B. and J. A. Cooper. 1995. Rho family members: activators of MAP kinase cascades. *Cell* **82:** 527–529.

139. Fedi, P., J. H. Pierce, P. P. Difiore, M. H. Kraus. 1994. Efficient coupling with phosphatidylinositol 3-kinase, but not phospholipase C gamma or GTPase-activating protein, distinguishes ErbB-3 signaling from that of other ErbB/EGFr family members. *Mol. Cell Biol.* **264:** 492–500.

140. Sadowski H. B., K. Shuai, J. E. Darnell, M. Z. Gilman. 1993. A common nuclear signal transduction pathway activated by growth factor and cytokine receptors. *Science* **261:** 1739–1743.

141. Quelle, F. W., W. Thierfelder, B. A. Witthuhn, B. Tang, S. Cohen, and J. N. Ihle. 1995. Phosphorylation and activation of the DNA binding activity of purified STAT1 by the Janus protein-tyrosine kinases and the epidermal growth factor receptor. *J. Biol. Chem.* **270:** 20,775–20,780.

142. Shibata, T., M. Gotoh, A. Ochiai, and S. Hirohashi. 1994. Association of plakoglobin with APC, a tumor suppressor gene product, and its regulation by tyrosine phosphorylation. *Biochem. Biophys. Res. Commun.* **203:** 519–522.

143. Ochiai, A., S. Akimoto, Y. Kanai, T. Shibata, T. Oyama, S. Hirohashi. 1994. C-erbB–2 gene product associates with catenins in human cancer cells. Biochim. Biophys. Res. Commun. **205:** 73–78.

144. Ewing, C. M., N. Ru, R. A. Morton, J. C. Robinson, M. J. Wheelock, K. R. Johnson, J. C. Barrett, and W. B. Isaacs. 1995. Chromosome 5 suppresses tumorigenicity of PC3 prostate cancer cells: correlation with re-expression of alpha-catenin and restoration of E-cadherin function. *Cancer Res.* **55:** 4813–4817.

145. Sporn, M. B. and A. B. Roberts. 1992. Autocrine secretion: 10 years later. *Ann. Intern. Med.* **117:** 408–414.

146. Eckert, K., A. Granetzny, J. Fisher, E. Nexo, and R. Grosse. 1990. An Mr 43,000 epidermal growth-factor related protein purified from the urine of breast cancer patients. *Cancer Res.* **50:** 903–910.

147. Arteaga, C. L., A. R. Hanauske, G. M. Clark, C. K. Osborne, P. Harazika, R. L. Pardue, F. Tio, and D. D. Van Hoff. 1988. Immunoreactive α transforming growth factor activity in effusions from cancer patients as a marker of tumor burden and patients' prognosis. *Cancer Res.* **48:** 5023–5028.

148. Fitzpatrick S., J. Brightwell, J. Wittlif, G. Barrows, and G. Schultz. 1984. Epidermal growth factor binding by breast tumor biopsies and relationship to estrogen receptor and progestin receptor levels. *Cancer Res.* **44:** 3448–3453.

149. Sainsbury J. R., J. R. Fardon, G. K. Needham, A. J. Malcolm, and A. L. Harris. 1987. Epidermal growth factor receptor status as predictor of early recurrence of and death from breast cancer. *Lancet* **1:** 1398–1402.

150. Nicholson, S., J. Richard, C. Sainsbury, P. Halcrow, P. Kelly, B. Angus, C. Wright, J. Henry, J. R. Farndon, and A. L. Harris. 1991. Epidermal growth factor receptor (EGFr); results of a six-year follow-up study on operable breast cancer with emphasis on node negative subgroup. *Br. J. Cancer* **63:** 146–150.

151. Klijn, J. G., P. M. Berns, P. I. Schmitz, and J. A. Foekesen. 1992. The clinical significance of epidermal growth factor receptor (EGFr) in human breast cancer: a review on 5,232 patients. *Endocrinol. Rev.* **13:** 3–17.

152. Klijn, J. G., P. M. Berns, P. I. Schmitz, and J. A. Foekesen. 1993. Epidermal growth factor receptor (EGFr) in clinical breast cancer: update 1993. *Endocrinol. Rev. Monographs.* **1:** 171–174.

153. Nicholson, R. I., R. A. McClelland, J. M. Gee, D. L. Manning, P. Cannon, J. F. Robertson, I. O. Ellis, and R. W. Blamey. 1994. Epidermal growth factor receptor expression in breast cancer: association with response to endocrine therapy. *Breast Cancer Res. Treat.* **29:** 117–125.

154. Kawamoto, T., J. D. Sato, A. Le, J. Polikoff, G. H. Sato, and J. Mendelsohn. 1983. Growth stimulation of A431 cells by EGF: identification of high affinity receptors for epidermal growth factor by an anti-receptor monoclonal antibody. *Proc. Natl. Acad. Sci. USA* **80:** 1337–1341.

155. Chaudhary, V. K., D. J. Fitzgerald, S. Adhya, and I. Pastan. 1987. Activity of a recombinant fusion protein between transforming growth factor type α and Pseudomonas toxin. *Proc. Natl. Acad. Sci. USA* **84:** 4538–4542.

156. Fitzgerald, D. and I. Pastan. 1989. Targeted toxin therapy for the treatment of cancer. *J. Natl. Cancer Inst.* **81:** 1455–1463.

157. Levitzki, A. and A. Gazit. 1995. Tyrosine kinase inhibition: an approach to drug development. *Science* **267:** 1782–1787.

158. Stein, C. A. and J. S. Cohen. 1988. Oligodeoxynucleotides as inhibitors of gene expression: a review. *Cancer Res.* **48:** 2659–2688

159. Sato, J. D., T. Kawamoto, A. Le, J. Mendelsohn, J. Polikoff, and G. H. Sato. 1983. Biological effect *in vitro* of monoclonal antibodies to human EGF receptors. *Mol. Biol. Med.* **1:** 511–529.

160. Gill, G. N., T. Kawamoto, C. Cochet, A. Le, J. D. Sato, H. Masui, C. L. MacLeod, and J. Mendelsohn. 1984. Monoclonal anti-epidermal growth factor receptor antibodies which are inhibitors of epidermal growth factor binding and antagonists of epidermal growth factor-stimulated tyrosine protein kinase activity. *J. Biol. Chem.* **259:** 7755–7760.

161. Masui, H., T. Kawamoto, J. D. Sato, B. Wolf, G. H. Sato, and J. Mendelsohn. 1984. Growth inhibition of human tumor cells in athymic mice by anti-EGF receptor monoclonal antibodies. *Cancer Res.* **44:** 1002–1007.

162. Mendelsohn, J. 1989. Potential clinical applications of anti-EGF receptor monoclonal antibodies, in *Cancer Cells* (Furth, M. and M. Greaves, ds.), Cold Spring Harbor Laboratory, Cold Spring Harbor, NY, pp. 359–362.

163. Divgi, C. R., C. Welt, M. Kris, F. X. Real, S. D. J. Yeh, R. Gralla, B. Merchant, S. Schweighart, M. Unger, S. M. Larson, and J. Mendelsohn. 1991. Phase I and imaging trial of indium-111 labeled anti-EGF receptor monoclonal antibody 225 in patients with squamous cell lung carcinoma. *J. Natl. Cancer Inst.* **83:** 97–104.

164. Baselga, J., A. Scott, D. Pfister, M. Kris, C. Divgi, Z. Zhang, S. Larson, H. Oettgen, and J. Mendelsohn. 1993a. Comparative pharmacology in phase I and imaging trials utilizing anti-epidermal growth factor receptor (anti-EGFr) monoclonal antibodies (MAbs) labeled with ^{131}I or [111]In. *Proc. Amer. Soc. Clin. Oncol.* **12:** 368.

165. Goldstein, N. I., M. Prewett, K. Zuklys, P. Rockwell, and J. Mendelsohn. 1995. Biological efficacy of a chimeric antibody to the epidermal growth factor receptor in a human tumor xenograft model. *Clin. Cancer Res.* **1:** 1311–1318.

166. Bos, M., J. Mendelsohn, D. Bowden, et al. 1996. Phase I studies of anti-epidermal growth factor receptor (EGFr) chimeric monoclonal antibody C225 in patients with EGFr overexpressing tumors. *Proc. Am. Soc. Clin. Oncol.* **15:** A1381.

167. Baselga, J., L. Norton, H. Masui, A. Pandiello, K. Coplan, W. H. Miller, and J. Mendelsohn. 1993. Antitumor effects of doxorubicin in combination with anti-epidermal growth factor receptor monoclonal antibodies. *J. Natl. Cancer Inst.* **85:** 1327–1332.

168. Fan, Z., J. Baselga, H. Masui, and J. Mendelsohn. 1993. Antitumor effect of anti-EGF receptor monoclonal antibodies plus cis-Diamminedichloroplatinum (cis-DDP) on well-established A431 cell xenografts. *Cancer Res.* **53:** 4637–4642.

169. Baselga, J., L. Norton, K. Coplan, R. Shalaby, and J. Mendelsohn. 1994. Antitumor activity of paclitaxel in combination with anti-growth factor receptor monoclonal antibodies in breast cancer xenografts. *Proc. AACR* **35:** 380.

170. Baselga, J. and J. Mendelsohn. 1997. Type I receptor tyrosine kinase as target for therapy in breast cancer. *J. Mam. Gland Biol. Neoplasia* **2(2):** 165–174.

171. Wu, X., Z. Fan, H. Masui, H. Rosen, and J. Mendelsohn. 1994. Apoptosis induced by blocking epidermal growth factor receptors is rescued by insulin-growth factor receptor. *Proc. AACR* **35:** 3.

172. Hudziak, R. M., G. D. Lewis, M. Winget, B. M. Fendly, H. M. Shepard, and A. Ulrich. 1989. p185^{HER2} monoclonal antibody has antiproliferative effects *in vitro* and sensitizes human breast tumor cells to tumor necrosis factor. *Mol. Cell. Biol.* **9:** 1165–1172.

173. McKenzie, S. J., P. J. Marks, T. Lam, et al. 1989. Generation and characterization of monoclonal antibodies specific for the human neu oncogene product, p185. *Oncogene* **4:** 543–548.

174. Baselga, J., D. Tripathy, J. Mendelsohn et al. 1996. Phase II study of weekly intravenous recombinant humanized anti-p185^{HER}2 monoclonal antibody in patients with HER2/neu overexpressing metastatic breast cancer. *J. Clin. Oncol.* **14:** 737–744.

175. Carter, P., L. Presta, C. M. Gorman et al. 1992. Humanization of an anti-p185 HER2 antibody for human cancer therapy. *Proc. Natl. Acad. Sci. USA* **89:** 4285–4289.

176. Pegram, M., A. Lipton, R. Pietras, et al. 1995. Phase II study of intravenous recombinant humanized anti-p185 HER-2 monoclonal antibody (rhuMAb HER-2) plus Cisplatin in patients with HER-2/neu overexpressing metastatic breast cancer. *Proc. Am. Soc. Clin. Oncol.* (abstract) **1282:** 7812–7711.

177. Theuer, C. P., D. J. Fitzgerald, and I. Pastan. 1993. A recombinant form of pseudomonas exotoxin A containing transforming growth factor alpha near its carboxyl terminus for the treatment of bladder cancer. *J. Urol.* **149:** 1626–1632.

178. Theuer, C. P. and I. Pastan. 1993. Immunotoxin and recombinant toxins in the treatment of solid carcinomas. *Am. J. Surg.* **166:** 284–288.

179. Osherov, N., A. Gazit, C. Gilon, and A. Levitzki. 1993. Selective inhibition of the epidermal growth factor and Her2/neu receptors by tyrphostins. *J. Biol. Chem.* **268:** 11,134–11,142.

180. Moroni, M. C., M. C. Willingham, and L. Beguinot. 1992. EGF-R antisense RNA blocks expression of the epidermal growth factor receptor and suppresses the transforming phenotype of a human carcinoma cell line. *J. Biol. Chem.* **267:** 2714–2722.

181. Ciardiello, F., C. Bianco, N. Normanno, G. Baldassarre, S. Pepe, G. Tortora, A. R. Bianco, and D. S. Salomon. 1993. Infection with a transforming growth factor α anti-sense retroviral expression vector reduces the in vitro growth and transformation of a human colon cancer cell line. *Int. J. Cancer* **54:** 952–958.

182. Ciardiello, F., G. Tortora, C. Bianco, M. P. Selvam, F. Basolo, G. Fontanini, F. Pacifico, N. Normanno, R. Brandt, M. G. Persico, D. S. Salomon, and A. R. Bianco. 1994. Inhibition of Cripto expression and tumorigenicity in human colon cancer cells by antisense RNA and oligodeoxynucleotides. *Oncogene* **9:** 291–298.

3

The Role of Fibroblast Growth Factors in Breast Cancer Pathogenesis and Progression

Francis G. Kern

1. INTRODUCTION

The potential importance of growth factor signaling in human breast cancer pathogenesis was brought to light by the finding that overexpression of members of the erbB family of transmembrane tyrosine kinase receptors had an impact on outcome [1–3]. Since that time, there have been numerous studies attempting to clarify the relationship of expression of this family of receptors to treatment response, time to relapse, and overall survival. The fibroblast growth factor family of ligands and receptors share a number of similarities with the erbB family of ligands and receptors. For both families, there are multiple ligands, multiple receptors, and the clear potential for complex interactions, which presumably fine-tune the response of a cell to the signals emanating from receptor activation. However, for the FGF family, relationships of receptor signaling to either pathogenesis or progression have not been established, and whether FGFs and FGF-receptors have any impact at all in either of these processes should probably still be considered an open question. Nonetheless, there have been a number of reports that together suggest a possible role for FGF signaling in these processes, and this review will attempt to provide an overview of the available information on this topic.

2. THE FGF FAMILY OF LIGANDS

To date, 10 different genes [4–12] have been found that encode proteins that are capable of binding to at least one of four different transmembrane tyrosine kinase receptors [9,13–18], and it is quite likely that the massive cDNA sequencing efforts ongoing in a number of laboratories have identified at least four additional FGF-related proteins [19]. The most widely studied proteins are commonly known as acidic and basic FGF, but this review will adhere to the accepted nomenclature and refer to these proteins as FGF-1 and FGF-2, respectively. Both of these proteins, as well as FGF-9, (glial activating factor, or GAF), lack typical secretory signal peptides, but all three proteins can be found outside of expressing cells, where they can then interact with cell surface receptors. There have been numerous suggestions of alternative mechanisms for release or export of these three proteins [10,20–25]. Both FGF-1 and FGF-2 have

From: Breast Cancer: *Molecular Genetics, Pathogenesis, and Therapeutics*
Edited by: A. M. Bowcock © Humana Press Inc., Totowa, NJ

strong mitogenic potential for mesodermally or ectodermally derived cell types *(7)*. Both are mitogenic for epithelial cells, as well *(26)*. Both FGF-1 and FGF-2 are strong transforming genes when signal peptides are artificially fused to the coding sequences *(27–30)*, and three of the FGF members that naturally encode secretory signal peptides, FGF-3 (int-2), FGF-4 (hst-1/KFGF, or Kaposi fibroblast growth factor), and FGF-5, were originally discovered as oncogenes *(31–33)*. At least four of the five remaining FGF proteins also have transforming potential. FGF-6 (hst-2), was isolated, based on sequence homology to FGF-4, and is similarly transforming when overexpressed in NIH 3T3 cells *(34,35)*. Transfecting the same cells with an FGF-9 cDNA will result in morphological transformation *(36)*. FGF-7 (keratinocyte growth factor, or KGF) and FGF-8 (androgen induced growth factor, or AIGF) can also both cause transformation. Completion of an autocrine loop by transfection of FGF-7-expressing NIH 3T3 cells with the receptor for this factor results in transformed foci *(37)*. The gene for FGF-8 encodes at least seven different proteins as a result of alternative splicing of the primary transcript. Transfection of NIH 3T3 cells with vectors for the FGF-8b isoform leads to their tumorigenic conversion; transfection with the FGF-8a and FGF8c isoforms leads to a moderately transformed phenotype in vitro, and the transformed cells are weakly tumorigenic *(38,39)*. Transforming activity has not yet been reported for FGF-10, but the gene has only recently been discovered. Thus, at least nine of the 10 identified FGF family members possess transforming potential.

The primary transcripts of other FGF family members also have the potential of encoding multiple forms. The transcripts for FGF-3 and FGF-2 both contain CUG codons located upstream of the AUG initiation codon, which can be used as alternative start sites for translation. The extended proteins can have different biological properties from the AUG-initiated forms, as a result of their being directed to the nucleus *(40–43)*. The genes for at least some of the FGF family members have been shown to have multiple promoters and polyadenylation signals, which presumably can affect the efficiency of transcription initiation and mRNA stability in different cell types *(44–47)*. The efficiency of translation of some FGF transcripts can also be tightly regulated by upstream open-reading frames and upstream untranslated regions capable of forming extensive inhibitory secondary structures, and by the level of expression of translation initiation factors, such as eIF-4, which appears to be elevated in some breast cancers *(48–50)*. Thus, there are a number of levels at which the expression and biological function of FGF family members can be regulated; attempts at associating expression of mRNA for a particular family member with disease outcome or other prognostic or predictive parameters of breast cancer may ultimately prove to be far too simplistic.

3. FGF-RECEPTOR COMPLEXITY

The potential for generation of complex signaling networks also exists at the receptor level. FGFs interact with two classes of receptors. Four high-affinity transmembrane tyrosine kinase receptors have been identified *(5,9,14,15,18)*. A fifth cysteine-rich nontyrosine kinase receptor has also been described, but its expression currently has unknown consequences regarding the transmission of growth signals *(51)*. Heparan sulfate proteoglycans (HSPGs) on the cell surface function as a reservoir for released heparin-binding FGFs. They also act as low-affinity receptors that are required for efficient ligand binding to the high-affinity tyrosine kinase receptors via the formation of a ternary complex *(52–55)*. Various FGFs can have different affinities for the same HPSG, which presumably can affect the rate of formation of such a complex *(56,57)*.

The primary transcripts of the high-affinity receptors can be alternatively spliced to yield numerous secreted and cell-bound isoforms *(15,16,18,58,59)*. The extracellular domains of FGFR-1 and FGFR-2 can consist of either two or three immunoglobulin-like regions, but FGFR-3 and FGFR-4 appear to be limited to the three Ig-loop form *(60)*. There is some degree of ligand-binding specificity that is conferred by alternative usage of exons that encode the second half of the third immunoglobulin-like domain, but most ligands are capable of binding to multiple receptors *(61,62)*. One FGFR-1 variant results from a splice that replaces the region immediately downstream of the secretory signal peptide with a 144 base-pair sequence having an in-frame termination codon. Reinitiation of translation at a downstream AUG may lead to the production of a cytoplasmic receptor *(58)*. A role for such a receptor in generating an intracrine loop in FGF-producing prostate cells has been proposed *(63)*.

Other splice variants can probably result in the modulation or attenuation of signaling. A juxtamembrane region containing a threonine residue, which is suitably positioned to be a substrate for protein kinase C, is variably present or absent in FGFR-1 *(58)*. Alternative usage of a third possible exon for the second half of the third Ig-like domain of FGFR-1 can introduce a termination codon. The resulting protein lacks a transmembrane domain, and can be efficiently secreted because of the presence of the signal peptide *(59,64)*. The secreted receptor isoform presumably can affect the concentration of extracellular ligand available to bind to full-length functional receptors *(65,66)*. Another variant introduces a termination codon in the tyrosine kinase domain, to produce a kinase-defective protein *(58)*. Since FGF-receptor signaling appears to require dimerization with another functional wild-type receptor *(54,67)*, the kinase-defective variant can presumably attenuate signaling by pairing with wild-type receptors and acting in a dominant-negative manner *(68,69)*.

Different FGFRs are frequently coexpressed in the same cell *(70–72)*. Hetero-dimerization of FGFRs has been shown to occur *(73)*, but effects on affinities for the various family members remain to be elucidated. In some sense, then, the situation with the FGF family of ligands and receptors may be very similar to that suggested for the erbB family of ligands and receptors, in which multiple ligands can differentially bind to multiple receptor pairs, and in such a manner amplify the number of potential cellular responses to receptor activation *(74)*. It is thus apparent that the FGF signaling system is one that is extremely complex, even before one starts to consider the signaling events that occur after receptor activation. Given this complexity, it may again be too simplistic to expect an association of expression of a particular receptor with breast cancer prognosis or phenotype to be readily apparent.

4. EXPRESSION OF FGFS IN NORMAL, PREMALIGNANT, AND MALIGNANT BREAST TISSUES AND CELL LINES

4.1. MMTV Proviral Activation of FGF Loci in Mouse Mammary Tumors

A role for FGFs in breast cancer pathogenesis was originally suggested by the finding that the mouse FGF-3 locus was frequently transcriptionally activated by insertion of MMTV proviral sequences in mammary tumors of strains of susceptible mice *(32)*.

Subsequently, it was found that the FGF-4 locus was also activated by the same mechanism in some MMTV-induced mammary tumors *(75)*. Both genes are located on chromosome seven, and are separated by only 17 kb in the mouse. The syntenic region in the human is 11q13, which is frequently amplified in a number of human malignancies, including breast cancer, in which the region is amplified in 15–20% of tumors *(76–78)*. Although earlier studies using *in situ* hybridization did suggest FGF-3 or FGF-4 might be expressed in tumors with 11q13 amplification *(78,79)*, subsequent studies attempting to identify either FGF-3 or FGF-4 transcripts in human breast tumors failed to detect either mRNA with any appreciable frequency, even in tumors where the locus was amplified *(70,77,80,81)*. It was subsequently found that the gene for cyclin D1 is located in the same chromosomal region *(82,83)*. Cyclin D1 is overexpressed in tumors and cell lines with 11q13 amplification, and the resulting growth advantage conferred by the overexpression is therefore commonly presumed to be the driving force behind the amplification process *(84,85)*. However, EMS-1, another coampiflied gene, is also overexpressed in tumors with 11q13 amplifications *(86)*. The product of this gene is cortactin, a protein that is found in association with Src family member proteins. Both Src and cortactin are tyrosine-phosphorylated in response to FGF-receptor activation *(87)*. Therefore, although one may see reports associating int-2/hst-1 amplification with a poor prognosis in breast cancer *(88–90)*, one should bear in mind that this has no relation to the expression of either gene in human breast cancers, despite the previous association with MMTV-induced mammary tumors. However, there remains the possibility of a relationship of 11q13 amplification to enhanced FGF signaling, mediated by other FGFs that are expressed in human breast tumors.

FGF signaling is also implicated in mammary gland tumorigenesis by the observation that MMTV proviral activation of FGF-3, FGF-4, or FGF-8 can accelerate mammary gland tumorigenesis in Wnt-1 transgenic mice *(91,92)*. The Wnt-1 locus is another site for MMTV proviral integration that can lead to mammary tumors in infected mice *(93)*, but either Wnt-1 or FGF-3/Int-2 transgenic animals typically develop mammary hyperplasias, and tumors only occur in a stochastic manner after a long latency period *(94,95)*. However, crossing Wnt-1 and FGF-3/Int-2 transgenic mice results in earlier tumor formation in bitransgenic animals *(96)*, and the two genes are frequently coactivated in mammary tumors that arise from MMTV infection *(97)*. This indicates that FGF and Wnt signaling pathways can cooperate in the process of mammary gland tumorigenesis. It has recently been found that there is preferential activation of FGF-8 in the mammary tumors of MMTV-infected Wnt-1 transgenic mice, compared to MMTV-infected normal mice, suggesting that Wnt-1 sensitizes mammary epithelial cells to further stimulation by FGF-8 *(98)*.

4.2. FGF Expression During Mouse Mammary Gland Development and Tumorigenesis

Although aberrant FGF-3 expression in transgenic mice can result in mammary gland hyperplasias *(94)*, the gene itself is not expressed during normal mammary gland development *(99,100)*. FGF-1 and FGF-2 were the most highly expressed FGFs observed throughout mammary development, with FGF-1 being primarily expressed in the luminal epithelial cells of the ducts, and FGF-2 being expressed primarily in the stroma. FGF-4 was found to be expressed only in the glands of virgin animals undergoing ductal development. FGF-5 was not expressed at any developmental stage, and the pattern of FGF-7 expression was consistent with it being a mesenchymally produced factor that acts on epithelial tissues. FGF-1 and FGF-2 mRNA were also present in hyperplastic alveolar nodules (HAN) and tumors derived from these outgrowths, but there was no indication of overproduction of either factor in any of these tissues. FGF-7 mRNA was detected in the tumors that arise from the HAN outgrowths, but was not present in the HAN. FGF-4 transcripts were not detected in either the preneoplastic or tumor outgrowths *(99)*. FGF-6, -8, and -9 were not analyzed in this study, but another study reported high levels of FGF-10 mRNA being present in normal mouse mammary gland tissue *(6)*.

4.3. FGF Expression in Normal and Tumor-Derived Mammary Epithelial Cell Lines

Various FGFs are found to be expressed in many normal and tumor-derived mammary epithelial cells in culture. FGF-2 transcripts were found in four strains of human mammary epithelial cells, and in the SV-40-immortalized HBL-100 cell line derived from luminal epithelial cells. FGF-2 was also detected in the HS578T cell line, but not in the MCF-7 or T47-D tumor cell lines, by Northern or Western blot analyses *(101)*. Other studies also found FGF-2 expressed in epithelial cell lines derived from normal breast *(102)*, or in SV40 or spontaneously transformed cells of normal origin *(103)*. However, in the latter study, FGF-2 expression levels were much higher in cells having myoepithelial characteristics *(103)*. This is in line with results from a study on separated populations of epithelial and myoepithelial cells from normal human breast, in which FGF-2 mRNA was found only in the myoepithelial cells *(104)*. FGF-2 mRNA and protein are also found in the MDA-MB-231 breast cancer cell line *(105,106)*, and can be induced in MCF-7 cells by overexpression of PKC *(107)*. The increased sensitivity afforded by RT-PCR analysis indicated FGF-2 was expressed in six of seven breast cancer cell lines examined, including cell lines previously reported to be negative for expression when less-sensitive assays were used *(81)*.

FGF-1 mRNA and protein are also frequently detected in cell lines derived from normal breast tissue, and in the MDA MB-231 cell line *(106,108,109)*. When extremely sensitive RT-PCR analyses for FGF-1 are performed, FGF-1 mRNA can also be detected in the MCF-7 cell line and BT-20 cell line, but five other breast cancer cell lines examined were still negative *(81,109)*. However, a third study using the same assay found FGF-1 mRNA in all 14 breast cancer cell lines examined *(108)*. Reports of screens for expression of other FGF family members in normal, immortalized, or breast cancer cell lines are limited. FGF-5 mRNA was found in the MDA MB-231 cell line by RT-PCR or RNAse protection. FGF-6 mRNA was found in the MDA-MB-453 cell line, but the six other breast cancer cell lines examined in this screen were negative for both, suggesting that neither is commonly expressed in breast cancer cell lines. FGF-8 mRNA could be detected in the MDA-MB-231 cell line and in the SK-BR-3 cell line by RT-PCR, but was not found in five other cell lines examined. FGF-8 mRNA could be induced by dihydrotestosterone in the androgen receptor-positive MDA-MB-231 cell line, but not in the androgen receptor-negative SK-BR-3 cells *(110)*. FGF-7 and FGF-9 mRNA could not be detected in any of the seven breast cancer cell lines tested in a different study *(81)*.

4.4. FGF Expression in Human Breast Tumor Tissues

In determining the significance of the results of the different screens of normal breast and breast cancer cell lines for expression of various FGFs, one should bear in mind that cultures of both types of breast tissue are difficult to establish, and, once cell lines become established, gene expression can be altered by culture conditions *(109,111)*. Thus, results from screening cell lines may not accurately reflect the expression pattern observed in patients with breast cancer, or in the breasts of normal women. In addition, breast cancer tissue is very heterogeneous, and the screens of epithelial cell lines may fail to indicate the potential importance of interactions between tumor and stromal cells that might be mediated by FGFs produced by the stroma, or in response to FGFs released by tumor cells. In most cases in which FGF expression has been examined in actual breast cancer tissue, it has not been possible to first dissociate the tumor cells from the stroma. Frequently, the expression seen in normal areas adjacent to tumor tissue has been taken as indicative of the expression pattern that exists in the nondiseased tissue, which may negate the contribution of possible field effects. When assays have been used to attempt to localize the site of expression, the effects of fixation and differences in antibody affinities and avidities on the sensitivity of the immunohistochemical assays may sometimes lead to what appears to be conflicting results in separate studies.

Although all these factors may make it difficult to assess the potential importance of FGF expression, it is readily apparent that multiple FGFs are indeed expressed in breast tumor tissues. FGF-1 and FGF-2 appear to be the most ubiquitously expressed, with detectable mRNA being present in virtually all samples examined when sensitive RT-PCR assays are used *(81,102,108)*. Northern blotting and RNAse protection assays for RNA expression, and Western blotting and ELISA assays for both FGF-1 and FGF-2 protein expression, also support the contention that these family members are widely expressed in normal and malignant breast tumor tissue *(50,70,105,108,112–115)*. As mentioned above in Subheading 4.1., most studies have failed to find evidence of either FGF-3 or FGF-4 being expressed in either normal or cancerous breast tissue, but expression of FGF-6 and FGF-9 has been reported in 15 and 37% of 103 breast tumor samples analyzed using RT-PCR *(81)*. In this same study, FGF-7 was expressed in 30% of the samples, but a second study, also using RT-PCR, found FGF-7 mRNA in 12 of 15 samples analyzed, and in all five of the normal tissues examined *(116)*. FGF-5 was detected in 59% of the 103 samples analyzed by RT-PCR *(81)*, but was not detected in appreciable amounts in any of the 31 cases analyzed with a RNAse protection assay *(70)*, suggesting the levels of FGF-5 mRNA present may be very low, and can only be detected with a very sensitive assay.

In addition to being found in breast tumors, mRNA for FGF-1, FGF-2, FGF-7, and FGF-9 can all be detected in samples from normal breast tissue *(81,116)*. In many breast cancers, the level of expression of FGF-1 and FGF-2 may actually be lower that seen in benign or normal tissue *(105,108,114)*, causing some investigators to question the significance of the FGF expression found in tumors as a causal factor of increased malignancy. However, another study found that levels of FGF-2 protein detected with an ELISA assay to be significantly higher in tumors, compared to normal tissue controls from reduction mammoplasties or nonmalignant tissue from mastectomies *(112)*.

An earlier immunohistochemical study with a FGF-2 antibody, using paraffin-embedded material, found strong immunostaining in the myoepithelial cells lining normal ducts, and no staining in cancerous epithelial cells *(117)*. This led some investigators to suggest that the majority of the FGF-2 found in tumor samples with assays for RNA or total protein was the result of contamination of the sample with normal tissue. However, subsequent studies by the same group, using frozen sections, found FGF-2 immunostaining in luminal epithelial cells, as well as in myoepithelial cells *(114)*. In general, the level of expression was reduced in cancer tissues, compared to nonmalignant tissues, but some tumors had levels of RNA or protein expression similar to that seen in some nonmalignant tissues *(114)*. In this study, higher levels of FGF-2 expression were associated with improved overall and disease-free survival. FGF-2 expression is high in myoepithelial cells, which are lost during the progression of invasive breast cancer. Therefore, this association may reflect the lower number of myoepithelial cells present in more advanced breast cancers. However, a second immunohistochemical study of 79 breast carcinomas, which used acetone-fixed cryostat sections, found an association of disease recurrence with stronger FGF-2 immunostaining of either the cancerous epithelial cells or the stromal cells localized to the tumor–host interface *(118)*. In this study, strong epithelial cell staining was observed in 38% of the tumors, and strong stromal staining was found in 37%. Thus, it would appear that the significance of FGF-2 expression in breast tumors remains an open question. For this question to be rigorously addressed, antibodies capable of detecting variable amounts of FGF-2 in archival samples of paraffin-embedded material from patients with extensive follow-up information may still need to be developed.

The same situation appears to hold true for FGF-1, in which the expression seen in both nonmalignant and malignant breast tissue makes the issue of determining its role in breast cancer pathogenesis one that is difficult to address. It would seem that levels of FGF-1 expression are generally higher in nonmalignant breast tissue, compared to malignant breast tissue, and in cell lines derived from normal breast, compared to lines derived from cancerous breast. This finding has led to the suggestion that FGF-1 may be a differentiation factor, rather than a growth factor, and may act to suppress the proliferation of breast cells. However, the same study indicated that there remain a significant proportion of tumors in which the levels of expression appear to be as high as, or higher than, that seen in the nonmalignant tissue *(108)*. There is also the issue of what constitutes an appropriate control for purposes of comparison, since one study reported FGF-1 to be undetectable by Western blotting in benign or reduction mammoplasty normal tissue, but present in the normal tissue adjacent to some breast tumors *(113)*. This result raises the possibility of field effects of the tumor on the adjacent normal areas, or the presence of predisposing molecular lesions in the normal-appearing adjacent tissue that may alter gene expression. Immunohistochemical analyses of FGF-1 expression in breast tumors are limited to three reports, all using small numbers of samples. In studies using a monoclonal antibody and frozen sections, FGF-1 staining is detected in the basement membrane and stromal cells surrounding the malignant epithelial cells, but not in the stroma or membranes surrounding nonmalignant epithelial cells *(108,119)*. When protease inhibitors are utilized, the stromal staining is intense, suggesting the existence of a cancer-specific protease that acts to release FGF-1 from stromal storage sites, and allows the ligand to interact with receptors on the surface of carcinoma cells *(119)*. Another study, using a polyclonal antiserum and formalin-fixed and paraffin-embedded material, reported strong staining of stromal or malignant epithelial cells in approximately one-third of the samples analyzed *(120)*. Thus, although it is still not entirely clear what the source of FGF-1 is in breast tumors, there are certainly indications that sufficient FGF-1 is present in the immediate vicinity of cancerous epithelial cells, or in normal epithelial cells adjacent to the cancer, for autocrine or paracrine effects to be exerted.

5. EXPRESSION OF FGF-RECEPTORS IN NORMAL AND MALIGNANT BREAST TISSUES AND CELL LINES

Both high- and low-affinity receptors for FGFs are expressed in normal and malignant breast tissue. The heparan sulfate proteoglycan perlecan has been suggested as the predominant low-affinity FGF-receptor *(121)*, and this molecule has been immunolocalized to myoepithelial cells of the breast, and to stromal cells in breast tumors *(122,123)*. Other heparan sulfate-containing proteoglycans may also function as low-affinity receptors *(57)*. Both high- and low-affinity receptors for FGF-2 can be detected by binding experiments on MCF-7 cells *(124)*, although only one class of receptor was detected with this cell line when membrane preparations were used *(125)*. HSPGs capable of binding FGF-2 can be isolated in varying amounts from the culture medium and cell layers of HBL-100, MDA-MB-231, and MCF-7 cells *(126)*. A number of breast cancer cell lines produce mRNA and protein for all four of the transmembrane-type tyrosine kinase receptors *(71,72,127)*. Evidence for expression of multiple-receptor family members can also be found when primary breast tumors are examined *(70,81,102)*.

Amplification of FGFR-1 and FGFR-2 has been seen in 9–15% of human breast cancers *(128–130)*. Overexpression of FGFR-1 and amplification were positively correlated, but there is not a strict overlap, since there are examples of tumors with amplification without overexpression, and examples of overexpression without amplification *(129,130)*. Amplification of FGFR-1 was associated with nodal involvement, estrogen receptor (ER) positivity, and 11q13 amplification; FGFR-2 amplification was associated with patients >50 yr and patients with tumors having myc amplification *(128)*. There is evidence that the 8p12 FGFR-1 locus and the FGF-3- and FGF-4-containing 11q13 locus may be coamplified, since both are present on a homogeneously staining region (HSR) present in the MDA-MB-134 breast cancer cell line *(131)*. The frequent detection of both amplicons in the same tumors has led to the suggestion that such coamplification may accentuate an autocrine loop, but, as previously stated, neither FGF-3 nor FGF-4 are expressed in these tumors. There remains the possibility that overexpression of cyclin D or cortactin resulting from 11q13 amplification may further accentuate the enhanced FGF signaling resulting from FGFR-1 amplification and overexpression.

Two- to fourfold amplification of FGFR-4 is detected in three of 30 primary breast tumors examined *(132)*, and FGFR-4 mRNA is expressed at higher levels than FGFR-1 mRNA in the majority of the 14 breast cancer cell lines examined *(133)*. Despite the reports of amplification and overexpression of FGFR-1 and FGFR-4, an immunohistochemical analysis found no apparent difference in staining intensity of either receptor between normal and malignant breast epithelial cells *(119)*. There is some controversy regarding the expression of FGFR-3 in breast tumors. FGFR-3 expression was not detected in any of the 103 breast tumor samples analyzed by RT-PCR, despite the use of three different sets of primers spanning the whole sequence *(81)*. In contrast, FGFR-3 mRNA can be detected in breast cancer cell lines using a RNAse protection assay *(72)* or a RT-PCR assay *(127)*, and protein can be detected with an FGFR-3-specific antibody in an immunofluorescence assay *(127)*. The authors have also used a RNAse protection assay with RNA from primary breast tumors, and can readily detect FGFR-3 mRNA in eight of the 14 tumors tested (I. Ding and F.G. Kern, unpublished results). There is also evidence for expression of an unusual splice variant of FGFR-3 in immortalized normal breast and breast cancer cell lines. RT-PCR analysis indicates exons 7 and 8 can be removed in these cell lines. The resulting transcript encodes a protein that is missing the second half of the third Ig loop and the transmembrane domain, but possesses an intact kinase domain, since the coding sequences after the deletion remain in frame. It is postulated that this shortened form of FGFR-3 receptor represents an intracellular form that predominately localizes in the nucleus *(127)*. There is also evidence that FGFR-1 localizes to the peripheral nuclear matrix upon treatment of Swiss 3T3 cells with FGF-2, in which it appears to retain tyrosine kinase activity *(134)*. However, the biological consequences of having a nuclear localized receptor with potential tyrosine kinase activity are unknown at this point.

As stated, the extracellular domain of FGFR-1 can contain either two or three Ig loops. The two-Ig loop form (FGFR-1β) has a higher affinity for FGF-1, FGF-2, and heparin than the three-Ig loop form (FGFR-1α) *(135)*. In some systems, an increase in the ratio of FGFR-1β to FGFR-1α is observed, which is associated with increased malignancy. As astrocytomas progress from a benign to a malignant phenotype, there is an increase in the ratio of FGFR-1β to FGFR-1α *(136)*. A similar situation is seen in pancreatic cancers, in which the two forms are present in equal proportions in pancreatic acinar cells. Overall FGFR-1 expression is elevated in pancreatic ductal carcinoma cells, and it is the FGFR-1β isoform that predominates *(137)*.

When a monoclonal antibody is used for immunohistochemistry, intense staining for FGFR-1 protein is observed in normal ductal and lobular epithelium of the breast. FGFR-1 was also detectable in seven of the 10 breast tumors examined *(138)*. An earlier study with a rabbit polyclonal antibody against an FGFR-1 peptide, which was confined to examining normal tissues, found strong staining of myoepithelial cells *(139)*. Using an RT-PCR assay, which can discriminate the two- and three-loop forms of FGFR-1, it was found that, in the normal breast, there is typically more of the two-loop form, compared to three, but, in both invasive and noninvasive cancerous breast tissues, the ratio of FGFR-1β to FGFR-1α was even higher. When individual tumors were compared, patients with tumors having a higher ratio of FGFR-1β to FGFR-1α than the median had reduced relapse-free survival *(140)*. This study also found that the combined overall amount of FGFR-1 transcripts was not statistically different between normal and cancerous breast, but it was also observed that ER-negative patients had a significantly higher level of FGFR-1 than ER-positive. Another study has found that the FGFR-1β present in breast fibroblasts and myoepithelial cells contains a carboxy terminal truncation, resulting in a protein that is 106 kDa in size, instead of 115 kDa. Normal breast epithelial cells express equal amounts of the 115 kDa and 106 kDa forms. In contrast, expression of the 106 kDa form is not detectable in breast cancer cells, suggesting that its loss may be associated with the acquisition of a malignant pheno-type *(141)*.

FGFR-1, FGFR-2, and FGFR-3 also undergo differential splicing of multiple exons which encode the second half of the third Ig loop. The affinity of the receptor for indi-vidual FGF family members can be significantly affected as a consequence. With FGFR-2, it was thought that the splicing event was mutually exclusive, and that epithe-lial cells primarily utilized exon IIIb, which allows FGF-7 to bind with high affinity, but mesenchymal cells used exon IIIc, which allows high-affinity binding of FGF-2 *(142,143)*. A rat bladder carcinoma cell line undergoes an epithelial-to-mesenchymal transition in response to treatment with FGF-1, and associated with this transition is a change in the utilization of the IIIb to the IIIc form *(144)*. This suggests that the switch may be associated with a more invasive or motile phenotype, which also occurs with the transition. In a rat prostate progression model, a switch in the utilization of IIIb to IIIc is also observed when the cells progress from an androgen-sensitive, well-differ-entiated tumor to one that is androgen-insensitive, undifferentiated, and more malig-nant *(143)*. This transition is accompanied by an increase in the expression of FGFR-1 and reintroduction of FGFR-2 IIIb isoform restored epithelial cell differentiation *(145)*. Loss of the FGFR-2 IIIb isoform also correlated with the loss of androgen sensitivity in three human prostate cancer cell lines, and in three metastatic human prostate tumors that were maintained as xenografts in athymic nude mice *(146)*. This suggests that loss of responsiveness to FGF-7, and establishment of new autocrine loops between FGF ligands and their receptors, may allow autonomous growth.

FGF-7 is found in breast tumors, but, in breast cancer cell lines, it is expressed only at very low levels that require a sensitive RT-PCR assay for detection *(116,147)*. This is consistent with earlier results, indicating that FGF-7 is produced by fibroblasts, but not epithelial cells *(148)*. Thus, if one were to extend by analogy to breast cancer the observations made in the rat bladder and prostate progression models, a paracrine loop could be envisaged whereby epithelial cells may initially respond to FGF-7 produced by stromal fibroblasts, and, as a consequence, change the exon utilized to allow a sub-sequent response to FGF-2. However, this does not appear to be the case in breast cancer. RT-PCR was used to investigate which of the alternative forms of FGFR-2 were present in normal and malignant breast cancers, and in breast cancer cell lines. It was found that levels of FGFR-2 were present in widely varying amounts in both nor-mal and breast cancer tissues, and there was no difference in the relative amounts of either splice variant between these tissues. However, patients with advanced clinical staging did have a higher proportion of IIIc to IIIb. Somewhat surprising was the num-ber of breast cancer cell lines that expressed the IIIc form of the receptor, since this was previously thought to be expressed by mesenchymal cells. However, the majority of the cell lines did express much more of the IIIb form than the IIIc form, but two cell lines did express approximately equal amounts of both mRNAs *(149)*.

6. BIOLOGICAL EFFECTS OF FGF SIGNALING

6.1. *Implications of Alternative Mechanisms of FGF-Receptor Activation*

Because the biological response mediated by an individual FGF will in large part probably be determined by the repertoire of high- and low-affinity receptors expressed by a particular cell, it should be readily apparent that the degree of complexity involved in FGF signaling will make it difficult to develop generalized predictions as to how individual FGFs can influence the processes of pathogenesis or progression. In addition, it is now evident that FGF-receptor activation can occur independent of interaction with a ligand. Mutations have been reported for FGFR-2 and FGFR-3 that can constitutively activate the tyrosine kinase activity of the receptor *(150–153)*. When these mutations are inherited through the germ line, they are associated with skeletal and cranial malformation disorders *(153–156)*. Although constitutively active mutants of FGFR-3 negatively regulate the growth of long bones *(157)*, the effects on PC12 rat pheochromocytoma cells appear to be the same as those exerted by FGFR-1, in that activation of both types of receptors can lead to a differentiated neuronal phenotype *(158)*. The same activating FGFR-3 mutations have been found in multiple myeloma cell lines and tumors *(159)* and constructs directing the plasma membrane to the localization of kinase-activated FGFR3 receptors with deletions of the extracellular domain can morphologically transform NIH 3T3 cells *(160)*.

Constitutive activation of FGFR-2 through mutation in the transmembrane domain can also lead to oncogenic transformation of NIH 3T3 cells stably transfected with either of two mutants tested *(150)*. Deletions of the carboxy terminal region of FGFR-2, or engineered point mutations of tyrosine residues within this region, can also result in receptors with ligand independent transforming activity, when they are transfected into NIH 3T3 cells *(161)*. Interaction of wild-type receptors with either heparin or cell adhesion molecules can also activate FGF-receptors in the absence of FGF *(162–164)*. Constitutively activated FGF-receptors have not yet been described in breast cancer cell lines or tumors. Nonetheless, these results indicate that the consequences of functional FGF signaling on the processes of breast cancer pathogenesis or progression do not necessarily have to be considered solely within the context of association with expression of an individual FGF.

6.2. Effects of FGF Signaling in Normal and Immortalized Breast Epithelial Cells

It has been possible to associate both growth-stimulatory and growth-inhibitory effects of various FGFs on malignant and nonmalignant breast epithelial cells. FGF-2 was first shown to be capable of stimulating the growth of rat mammary epithelial and stromal cell lines *(165,166)*. Subsequent reports indicated that FGF-2 addition to serum-free media could also stimulate the proliferation of breast epithelial cell cultures derived from fresh tissue fragments from human breast carcinomas, or histologically normal areas away from the cancer *(26)*. FGF-1 at a dose of 1 ng/mL had no significant effect on the growth of either type of cells in the same study, but the growth factor was supplied at the time of cell plating, and there is no indication that heparin was included to stabilize the protein. A later report, using mouse mammary epithelial cells cultured within collagen gels in serum-free media containing insulin, demonstrated that multifold growth stimulation by FGF-1 required heparin, but that stimulation of the same cells by FGF-7 did not *(167)*.

Systemic administration of FGF-7 will cause hyperplasia of mammary ductal epithelial cells in either rats or mice *(168,169)*. In mice, the hyperplasia was more pronounced when the ovariectomized mice were also treated with estrogen and progesterone. FGF-7 administration to mice also resulted in cystic dilation of the mammary ducts, but this effect was not observed in FGF-7-treated rats in which 1 wk of daily intraperitoneal injections resulted in severe hyperplasia. The hyperplasia was not observed in postpartum lactating rats, which is of interest, because of the epidemiological evidence indicating a protective effect by pregnancy and the greatly reduced incidence of breast cancer in dairy cows.

As mentioned previously, a MMTV-driven FGF-3 transgene will result in pregnancy-dependent mammary gland hyperplasia *(94)*. The stochastic appearance of tumors, and the long latency period required for mammary tumors to develop in these transgenic mice, suggests that secondary events are required for tumorigenesis. When the differential display RT-PCR technique was applied to identify genes that were specifically expressed in a cell line derived from a transgenic FGF-3 mammary tumor, it was found that FGF-7 was one of the genes that were differentially expressed. However, while subsequent development of MMTV-driven FGF-7 transgenic mice did demonstrate that this FGF could also lead mammary gland hyperplasia in pregnant mice, the tumors that developed also appeared in a stochastic manner, with long latency, suggesting that still-unidentified secondary events were again required *(170)*.

Although the expression of FGF-3 is limited to certain stages in the embryonic development of the mouse *(171,172)*, and is not expressed in normal mammary glands or mammary tumors, addition of purified FGF-3 to two mouse mammary epithelial cell lines increases tritiated thymidine incorporation in a dose-dependent manner *(173)*. Although FGF-1 exhibits similar potency for both cell lines with an ED_{50} of ~0.1 nM, they show differences in their sensitivity to the added growth factor, which is related to the expression of different isoforms of FGFR-1 and FGFR-2. The HC11 cell line expressing the IIIb exon variant of both receptors is more sensitive than the C57MG cell line expressing the IIIc variant of these receptors. Infection of HC11 cells with an FGF-3 retroviral vector stimulates both anchorage-dependent and anchorage-independent growth of this cell line, and abrogates a requirement for priming by either FGF-2 or EGF, for differentiation to be observed in response to the addition of dexamethasone, insulin, and prolactin *(174)*. Infection of the MCF-10A immortalized human mammary epithelial cell line with the same retroviral vector will increase the growth rate in serum-free media, and also results in the cells acquiring the ability to form colonies in soft agar or methyl cellulose *(175)*.

FGF-2 stimulates the growth of mouse mammary epithelial cells in serum-free collagen gel cultures containing insulin *(176)*, and also acts as an autocrine growth factor for the SV-40 immortalized HBL-100 human breast epithelial cell line. This cell line expresses FGF-2 mRNA, and releases FGF-2 protein into the media. Growth of HBL-100 cells in serum-free media is inhibited in a dose-dependent manner by the addition of neutralizing antibodies against FGF-2. Exogenous FGF-2 has no effect on HBL-100 growth in serum-free media, but addition of 20 ng/mL of FGF-1 stimulated growth, suggesting that the two factors were acting through separate FGFRs *(177)*. Both FGF-1 and FGF-2 will also increase the anchorage-independent growth of human mammary epithelial cells overexpressing either SV40 Large T antigen or c-*myc* *(178)*.

6.3. Effects of FGF Signaling in Breast Cancer Cell Lines

It is apparent that the effects of FGFs may differ, depending on the malignant potential of the treated cells. Either FGF-1 or FGF-2 will induce membrane ruffling in some breast cancer cell lines, but not in normal epithelial cells purified from breast organoid cultures. Membrane ruffling involves the formation of many short actin filaments at the edges of cells. The effect could be blocked by transfection with dominant-negative-acting mutants of either FGFR-3 or the p21 Rac GTP-binding protein (179). Membrane ruffling is thought to have a role in growth and directional migration locomotion. This process could be induced by FGF-1 or FGF-2 treatment of COS-7 cells transiently transfected with FGFR-4, but not by FGFR-1, FGFR-2, or FGFR-3 (179).

The information available regarding the effects of FGF-2 on the growth of breast carcinoma cells is in some ways contradictory. A dose-dependent inhibition of MDA-MB-134 cell anchorage-dependent and -independent growth is seen with either FGF-1 or FGF-2 (72), but this may be related to the amplification of FGFR-1 or overexpression of FGFR-4 that is observed in this cell line, since similar growth-inhibitory effects are observed in the EGFR-amplified and overexpressing MDA-MB-468 cell line in response to EGF addition (180). A number of investigators have reported mitogenic or growth-stimulatory effects of FGF-2 addition to MCF-7 or T47-D ER-positive human breast cancer cells (181–185). In many cases, the studies are difficult to compare directly, since different culture conditions were utilized. One study observed that, in the absence of estrogen, there was little effect of FGF-2, unless IGF-1 was present, in which case an additive effect over IGF-1 treatment alone was observed. In the presence of estrogen, FGF-2 had an additive effect over that seen with estrogen alone, but when both estrogen and IGF-1 were present, FGF-2 acted as an antagonist of IGF-1 (185).

In a second study, the combination of insulin, EGF, and FGF-2 inhibited growth, compared to the effects of added insulin or IGF-1 alone (183). In a third study, the stimulatory effects of FGF-2 on MCF-7 cell growth in serum-free media were abolished, if the cells were first treated with heparinase or chlorate. Sodium chlorate decreases proteoglycan sulfation and, in the absence of this treatment, the ER-negative MDA-MB-231 cell line does not show a mitogenic response to FGF-2 treatment. However, the same cells became responsive to FGF-2 when treated with chlorate. This study therefore suggests that the amount of heparan sulfate proteoglycans present, and their degree of sulfation, can both positively and negatively regulate the growth-promoting effects of FGF-2 on breast cancer cells, and again emphasizes the degree of complexity involved in FGF-signaling (182).

In apparent contrast to these reports of stimulatory effects of FGF-2 on breast cancer cell lines, another group has observed inhibitory effects of FGF-2 on MCF-7 cell growth and other breast cancer cell lines (186). However, this effect may be related to the antagonistic effects of FGF-2 on IGF-1 or insulin action referred to in the studies mentioned above. Even though growth inhibition was observed, many of the events elicited by FGF-2 treatment, such as MAPK kinase activation (186) and increases in cyclin D, cyclin E, and cyclin-dependent kinase 4 (cdk4) proteins levels (187), are more typically associated with mitogenesis. However, these investigators have also observed a time- and dose-dependent increase in p21WAF1/CIP1 mRNA and protein levels in response to FGF-2 treatment *(187)*. This result suggests that the conflicting signal resulting from the increased level of this cdk inhibitor is capable of blocking the opposing mitogenic effects of increased MAPK activity and cyclin and cdk protein levels *(187)*. These results also point out that the effects of FGFs may vary, depending on the extent of costimulation resulting from other hormones or factors present in the microenvironment.

6.4. Effects of FGF Overexpression in an Immortalized Breast Epithelial Cell Line

A transfection study examining the effects of FGF-4 overexpression in an immortalized breast epithelial cell line strongly suggests a role for FGFs in breast cancer pathogenesis. Although the studies described above, looking at the effects of FGF-3 overexpression on HC11 mouse mammary epithelial cells or MCF-10A human breast epithelial cells both showed effects on soft agar growth, there was no indication that these infections increased the tumorigenicity of either cell line *(174,175)*. In contrast, transfection of the HBL-100 SV40 immortalized human breast epithelial cell line with an FGF-4 expression vector, not only increases the growth rate in serum-free media and in soft agar, but also results in these cells acquiring the capability of forming rapidly growing tumors that are highly vascularized and invasive *(188)*.

6.5. Effects of FGF Overexpression on Breast Cancer Hormone Dependence and Antiestrogen Sensitivity

Transfection studies demonstrating the increased malignant phenotype of MCF-7 cells overexpressing either FGF-1 or FGF-4 have suggested FGFs may also have a role in breast cancer progression. Control empty-vector transfected cells remain estrogen-responsive in vitro and estrogen-dependent in vivo, in that they only form small tumors in ovariectomized mice, when the mice are supplemented with estrogen. In contrast, FGF-4-transfected cells could form large progressively growing tumors in otherwise untreated ovariectomized mice, or in mice that received tamoxifen pellets *(189)*. FGF-1 transfection has a similar effect on the tumorigenic phenotype *(120)*, suggesting that the results of these transfection studies may have clinical relevance regarding tamoxifen resistance, since this particular FGF family member is expressed in breast tumor tissues *(70,81,102,105,108,113,119,120)*.

Overexpression of either FGF-1 or FGF-4 also increases the frequency of soft agar colony formation in media depleted of estrogens, or in media containing the antiestrogens 4- hydroxytamoxifen or ICI 182,780 *(120,189,190)*. The latter is a pure steroidal antiestrogen that does not have the agonistic properties associated with tamoxifen *(191)*. Consequently, it is currently being considered for use as a second-line therapy for ER-positive patients who have failed on tamoxifen *(192,193)*. FGF-4- or FGF-1-transfected cell tumors will also develop tumors in ovariectomized animals that are treated with ICI 182,780 *(190)*. This result indicates that the growth of FGF-transfected cells in the absence of estrogen is not simply the result of ligand-independent activation of ERs, a process that has been shown by a number of groups to be related to increased mitogen-activated protein kinase (MAPK) activity that results from increased growth factor signaling. Phosphorylation of the ER has been shown to be capable of increasing the agonistic properties of tamoxifen *(194,195)*, but this effect of increased growth factor signaling is abrogated by treatment with the pure antiestrogen *(194–199)*. Thus, although FGF signaling may accentuate the agonistic properties of tamoxifen in the transfected MCF-7 cells, the enhanced in vitro and in vivo growth of these cells in the presence of the pure antiestrogen suggests that the mechanism underlying the estrogen-independent growth of these cells most likely involves FGF signaling providing an alternative or converging growth stimulatory pathway that bypasses the need for ER activation, and its subsequent regulation of the transcription of growth stimulatory genes. This conclusion is further supported by the observation that the FGF-transfected cell lines do not downregulate ER, or show constitutive activation of estrogen-regulated genes, as might be expected if ER were being activated *(190,199)*.

6.6. Potential Importance of Paracrine Effects of FGF-1 in Breast Cancer Progression

The increased in vitro growth of FGF-transfected MCF-7 cells in either estrogen-depleted or antiestrogen-containing media indicates that autocrine or intracrine effects of FGF signaling are at least partially responsible for their increased tumorigenicity. However, both FGF-4 and FGF-1 are strong angiogenic growth factors, and can also affect other mesenchymal cells present in the stroma of the tumor, as well *(200,201)*. Thus, the tumor–stromal interactions resulting from FGF overexpression can presumably provide a paracrine stimulus to tumor growth. It is well documented that tumor growth beyond a volume of a few cubic millimeters requires the development of means of increasing the vascular supply to provide additional nutrients and remove wastes *(202–204)*. The importance of such a paracrine effect of FGF production was suggested by the finding that treatment of mice bearing either FGF-1- or FGF-4-transfected cell tumors with AGM-1470, a specific and potent inhibitor of endothelial cells with low toxicity for breast cancer cells, was capable of restoring some sensitivity to tamoxifen treatment *(205)*.

A second line of experimentation more clearly demonstrates the participation of tumor–stromal interactions resulting from FGF expression in the in vivo phenotype of the transfected cells. Abrogation of functional FGF signaling within FGF-1-overexpressing MCF-7 cells, by retransfection with a dominant-negative FGF-receptor, had the expected effect of eliminating the ability of these cells to form an increased number of soft agar colonies in either estrogen-depleted or antiestrogen-containing media, and to develop tumors in untreated ovariectomized mice, indicating both phenotypes were dependent on the autocrine or intracrine effects of FGF-1 overexpression. However, the tumors that developed in estrogen-supplemented mice were equal in size to those made by control FGF-1-overexpressing cells that were still capable of responding in an autocrine manner. In both cases, the tumors are larger than tumors formed by MCF-7 cells in estrogen-supplemented mice. This result suggests that the paracrine effects of FGF-1 could have additive or synergistic effects with the mitogenic effect of estrogen, and that, in vivo, the autocrine effects of FGF were not additive with the mitogenic effect of estrogen. In addition, the FGF-1-overexpressing cells, transfected with the dominant-negative FGF-receptor, remained capable of forming progressively growing tumors in tamoxifen-treated mice *(206)*. This suggests that the paracrine effects of FGF-1 expression could allow the agonistic properties of tamoxifen to be more readily apparent.

Increased angiogenesis has been shown in other systems to be capable of altering the balance of apoptotic-to-proliferating cells *(207–209)*. It is thus possible that the increased neoangiogenesis resulting from FGF-1 overexpression can reduce the number of cells within a tumor that are undergoing apoptosis in tamoxifen-treated animals, and allow the agonistic properties of tamoxifen to provide a sufficient mitogenic stimulus for tumor growth to be observed. In support of this hypothesis, it was subsequently found that overexpression of the 165 amino acid form of vascular endothelial cell growth factor (VEGF) in MCF-7 cells would also facilitate the development of tumors in tamoxifen-treated mice *(210)*. VEGF is a growth factor that is specific for endothelial cells, and has no mitogenic effect on MCF-7 cells because of the absence of VEGF-receptors. A relationship between tamoxifen resistance or treatment failure and the increased neoangiogenesis resulting from overexpression of FGF or VEGF of any of a number of angiogenic growth factors, shown to be expressed in breast tumors, remains to be established *(112,211)*, but these transfection studies certainly raise this possibility.

6.7. Effects of FGF Overexpression on the Metastatic Phenotype

In a number of types of human cancers, including breast cancer, increased neoangiogenesis has been associated with a poor prognosis and the presence of distant metastases *(212–214)*. Using independently established sublines of a transplantable pregnancy-dependent mammary tumor line, it was found that progression from a nonmetastatic to a metastatic phenotype was associated with activation of the FGF-4 gene *(215)*. Tumor emboli were also present in the lymphatic vessels of mice bearing FGF-4-transfected HBL-100 tumors *(188)*. In the VEGF-, FGF-4-, and FGF-1-transfected MCF-7 cells, detection of the presence of disseminated tumor cells was facilitated by using a MCF-7 cell line stably transfected with the bacterial *lacZ* gene as a recipient for the transfection studies *(120,210,216–218)*. The inclusion of this marker allows the use of the chromogenic substrate X-gal to detect micrometastases of β-galactosidase-expressing cells in organs excised from tumor-bearing mice *(217,218)*. Micrometastases could be detected with high frequency in the lungs and lymph nodes of mice bearing tumors composed of either VEGF-, FGF-1-, or FGF-4-transfected cells, but macrometastases were extremely rare *(120,210,217)*. Micrometastases are not detected with the parental *lacZ*-transfected MCF-7 cells, even when the tumors in estrogen-supplemented mice are of the same size as the FGF-1- or VEGF-transfected cell tumors *(120,210)*, and, since microvessel densities were much higher in either the FGF- or VEGF-transfected cells, there is good reason to believe that the increased ability of the tumor cells to disseminate is related to the increased neoangiogenesis. There is also reason to believe that these results are applicable to human breast cancer, since positive correlations between tumor angiogenesis and the presence of micrometastases in the bone marrow have been observed *(219)*.

Others have associated the presence of long-lived angiogenesis inhibitors, produced by a primary tumor, with inhibition of the development of macrometastases in distant organs. In such a situation, a resection of the primary tumor results in the growth of macroscopic metastatic foci *(220–223)*. However, removal of the primary tumors resulting from inoculation with FGF-1- or VEGF-transfected MCF-7 cells results in the disappearance of micrometastases within three weeks after the resection *(210,224)*. These results suggest that increased neoangiogenesis resulting from expression of FGFs or VEGF can facilitate tumor-cell intravasation and dissemination, but the cells lack the potential to extravasate or proliferate at these distant sites. VEGF overexpression has been associated with a poor patient outcome in breast cancer *(112,225–227)*, and, although the results of these transfection studies suggest that it is possible that expression of FGF-1 may also have an impact on patient survival, they also point out that expression of yet-to-be-discovered cofactors may also be required for this impact to be observed.

7. COMPONENTS OF THE FGF SIGNAL TRANSDUCTION PATHWAY

The results of the transfection studies described above raise the specter that those patients with ER-positive tumors that are nonresponsive to tamoxifen, or those that have acquired resistance to this agent as a result of FGF signal transduction activating an autocrine growth-stimulatory pathway within their tumor cells, would be unlikely to respond to a second-line therapy with a pure antiestrogen *(190)*. However, there remains the possibility that elucidation of the FGF signaling pathways that operate in FGF-responsive breast cancer cells will identify targets upstream of the point where ER and FGFR growth-stimulatory pathways converge *(228)*. Interference with their function might then allow a restoration of sensitivity to the pure antiestrogen. Similarly, the results of the VEGF-transfection studies, and the transfection study examining the specific paracrine effects of FGF-1 production through the use of a dominant-negative FGF-receptor, suggest that a combination therapy, involving an antiangiogenic agent, an FGF signaling inhibitor, and tamoxifen, might also be effective for these patients. Thus, it may be important to gain a better understanding of the mechanism of FGF signal transduction operating in normal and malignant breast epithelial cells.

The studies to date on FGF signaling have primarily involved rat pheochromocytoma cells and mouse fibroblast cell lines. Different FGF-receptors can differ in their ability to induce mitogenesis or differentiation *(229–231)*. Signal transduction requires receptor dimerization, and this process leads to increased intrinsic tyrosine kinase activity and the phosphorylation of multiple tyrosine residues in the cytoplasmic domain of the receptor. For FGFR1, seven tyrosine residues have been definitively identified as sites for phosphorylation. These phosphorylated tyrosine residues presumably participate in the formation of docking sites for other proteins containing SH2 or PTB domains, which transmit the signal resulting from autophosphorylation in response to ligand binding *(67,232,233)*. However, mutation analysis indicates the five tyrosine residues located outside the catalytic domain of the kinase, including one that forms part of a docking site for PLC-γ, are all dispensable for mitogenesis, or the induction of differentiation *(234–236)*. Although a consensus docking site for phosphotidyl inositol-3-OH kinase (PI-3K) is found on all four receptors, PI-3K has not been found in direct association with activated FGF-receptors *(234)*. Similarly, despite the finding that phosphopeptides corresponding to regions of the FGFR-1 cytoplasmic domain can bind to Grb-2 or Shc SH2 domain GST-fusion proteins in an ELISA *(237)*, these, and many of the other proteins frequently found to be complexed with other transmembrane tyrosine kinase receptors, such as Syp and GAP, have also been shown not to be tightly associated with FGF-receptors *(234)*.

Although the direct target proteins involved in signaling through FGF-receptors remains unclear, there is a considerable amount of evidence that FGFR signaling does involve the use of the Ras-Raf1-MEK1-MAPK activation cascade *(231,238–243)*. The mechanism placing Ras in its active GTP-bound form may not involve targeting the SOS guanine nucleotide exchange factor to the membrane through a Shc-Grb-2 complex, but may instead relate to the formation of a complex with a protein that is called either FRS2, or SNT-like protein (SLP) and Grb-2. This protein is phosphorylated immediately after FGFR activation, and migrates with a size of approx 90 kDa. It is also modified by myristylation, which is required for the localization of the complex in the cell membrane *(244–247)*. This protein only weakly associates with the FGF-receptor, but is still rapidly phosphorylated when the five nonessential tyrosine residues in the carboxy terminus of the receptor are all mutated. A 66 kDa protein has recently been identified as a component of the FRS2/SLP/Grb-2 complex in FGFR-3-transfected L6 rat myoblast cells. Because FRS2/SLP is widely expressed and is not phosphorylated in response to EGF, PDGF, or insulin treatment *(245)*, it may represent a potential target for relatively specific inhibition of FGF signaling in breast cancer cells.

Raf-1 activation is clearly a critical step in bringing about the cell proliferation that can result from Ras activation, but in at least one epithelial cell line, Raf activation alone is not sufficient to elicit a transformed phenotype *(248)*. It is now apparent that GTP-bound Ras interacts with multiple effector molecules and that Ras represents a branching point for a number of interacting signaling pathways. The challenge will be to determine which of these interacting pathways are involved in the stimulation of breast cancer cell growth by FGF.

PI-3K is one such direct target of Ras that has recently been demonstrated to be involved in the activation of a serine threonine kinase, variably designated as PKB, RAC-PK, and Akt *(249–251)*. Akt was isolated as an oncogene, and is involved in growth-factor maintenance of cell survival *(252,253)*. Akt activation by FGF-2 in Rat 1 fibroblasts is inhibited by treatment with the PI-3K inhibitor wortmannin *(249)*. A dominant-negative mutant of the p85 subunit of PI-3K inhibits transformation by Ras *(254)*, but it is not clear at this point whether this is caused by downstream inhibition of Akt.

Similarly, the same type of dominant-negative approach has been used to show that transformation by Ras requires members of the Rac/Rho family of small GTP-binding proteins *(255–258)*. As mentioned in Subheading 6.3. above, membrane ruffling in breast cancer cells in response to FGF-1 or FGF-2 treatment is inhibited by a dominant-negative mutant of the p21 Rac protein, but it remains to be determined if this protein is also involved in FGF-stimulated proliferation *(179)*. Thus, there are a number of different signaling pathways that may be related to the activation of small GTP-binding proteins, which might be involved in the estrogen-independent growth of breast cancer cells overexpressing FGFs. This raises the possibility that farnesylation inhibitors targeting the required activation step of membrane localization may ultimately prove to be useful in reversing this phenotype.

There is also evidence that, in addition to these pathways mediated by small GTP-binding proteins, other interacting or parallel signaling pathways might also be stimulated in response to FGFR activation. Pertussis toxin treatment will block the mitogenic effect of FGF on BALB/3T3 *(259)* cells, and will reduce the affinity of FGF for its receptor *(260)*, suggesting that heterotrimeric G proteins might also be involved. Although only one study has reported a direct association of FGF-receptors with the Src kinase *(87)*, there are a number of studies that implicate this family of tyrosine kinases in FGF signal transduction in NIH 3T3 cells *(87)*, lung capillary endothelial cells *(261)*, or human melanoma cells *(262)*. In NIH 3T3 cells, the association of FGF-receptors with c-Src also correlates with an association of c-Src with cortactin and its subsequent tyrosine phosphorylation *(87)*. Cortactin, the product of the *EMS* gene on chromosome 11q13, is amplified in a high proportion of breast tumors, and is overexpressed in a number of breast cancer cell lines *(263)*. Members of the Src family of tyrosine kinases are also expressed at high levels in a number of breast cancer cell lines *(263)*. Cortactin and Src associate with components of the cytoskeleton, and the finding of FGFR-1, PI-3K, PLC-γ, focal adhesion kinase, and Src within focal adhesion complexes *(264)* suggests that this may be a site where the various growth-signaling pathways are integrated.

8. CONCLUDING REMARKS

It is apparent that the exact role of FGFs in breast cancer progression and pathogenesis still remains to be elucidated. However, the expression patterns of the various FGFs and their receptors in normal and cancerous breast tissues, and the demonstrated in vivo or in vitro effects of FGFs on normal breast epithelial cell proliferation and tumorigenicity, and on breast cancer hormone dependence, antiestrogen sensitivity, tumor cell dissemination, and neoangiogenesis, make it clearly evident that this family of growth factors and receptors is potentially important in these disease processes. Because of the complexity of the events likely to be involved in transmitting a growth-stimulatory signal, and the potential role of both autocrine and paracrine effects of FGFs in mediating these observed effects, the response of a cell to a particular growth factor is likely to be controlled by the presence or absence of a number of different ancillary components of the signaling system. Therefore, it may be difficult to simply associate expression of a particular factor or receptor with disease outcome without knowledge of the relative contribution of these various components to the overall process. Since any of these components may also afford a target for intervention, the challenge for the future is clearly defined.

ACKNOWLEDGMENTS

Some of the work described in this review was supported by NIH grants CA 50376, CA 09218, CA 53185, and CA 51008, by the Susan G. Komen Foundation, and by the Adolph Weil Endowed Chair at Southern Research Institute. Thanks also to colleagues at the Lombardi Cancer Center at Georgetown University, particularly Sandra McLeskey, Lurong Zhang, Anton Wellstein, Marc Lippman, Bob Dickson, and Dorraya El-Ashry, who either collaborated on some of the studies mentioned in this review, and/or had helpful comments and discussions on the topics covered.

REFERENCES

1. Harris, A. L., S. Nicholson, J. R. Sainsbury, J. Farndon, and C. Wright. 1989. Epidermal growth factor receptors in breast cancer: association with early relapse and death, poor response to hormones and interactions with neu. *J. Steroid. Biochem.* **34:** 123–131.

2. Sainsbury, J. R., J. R. Farndon, G. K. Needham, A. J. Malcom, and A. L. Harris. 1987. Epidermal-growth-factor receptor status as predictor of early recurrence of and death from breast cancer. *Lancet* **I:** 1398–1402.

3. Slamon, D. J., W. Godolphin, L. A. Jones, J. A. Holt, S. G. Wong, D. E. Keith, et al. 1989. Studies of the HER-2/neu proto-oncogene in human breast and ovarian cancer. *Science* **244:** 707–712.

4. Baird, A. and M. Klagsbrun. 1991. The Fibroblast Growth Factor Family. *Cancer Cells* **3:** 239–243.

5. Basilico, C. and D. Moscatelli. 1992. The FGF family of growth factors and oncogenes. *Adv. Cancer Res.* **59:** 115–165.

6. Beer, H. D., C. Florence, J. Dammeier, L. McGuire, S. Werner, and D. R. Duan. 1997. Mouse fibroblast growth factor 10: cDNA cloning, protein characterization, and regulation of mRNA expression. *Oncogene* **15:** 2211–2218.

7. Burgess, W. H. and T. Maciag. 1989. The heparin-binding (fibroblast) growth factor family of proteins. *Annu. Rev. Biochem.* **58:** 575–606.

8. Emoto, H., S. Tagashira, M. G. Mattei, M. Yamasaki, G. Hashimoto, T. Katsumata, et al. 1997. Structure and expression of human fibroblast growth factor-10. *J. Biol. Chem.* **272:** 23,191–23,194.

9. Hughes, S. E. and P. A. Hall. 1993. Overview of the fibroblast growth factor and receptor families: complexity, functional diversity, and implications for future cardiovascular research. *Cardiovasc. Res.* **27:** 1199–1203.

10. Miyamoto, M., K. Naruo, C. Seko, S. Matsumoto, T. Kondo, and T. Kurokawa. 1993. Molecular cloning of a novel cytokine cDNA encoding the ninth member of the fibroblast growth factor family, which has a unique secretion property. *Mol. Cell. Biol.* **13:** 4251–4259.

11. Tanaka, A., K. Miyamoto, N. Minamino, M. Takeda, B. Sato, H. Matsuo, and K. Matsumoto. 1992. Cloning and characterization of an androgen-induced growth factor essential for the androgen-dependent growth of mouse mammary carcinoma cells. *Proc. Natl. Acad. Sci. USA* **89:** 8928–8932.

12. Yamasaki, M., A. Miyake, S. Tagashira, and N. Itoh. 1996. Structure and expression of the rat mRNA encoding a novel member of the fibroblast growth factor family. *J. Biol. Chem.* **271:** 15,918–15,921.

13. Dionne, C. A., G. Crumley, F. Bellot, J. M. Kaplow, G. Searfoss, M. Ruta, et al. 1990. Cloning and expression of two distinct high-affinity receptors cross-reacting with acidic and basic fibroblast growth factors. *EMBO J.* **9:** 2685–2692.

14. Givol, D. and A. Yayon. 1992. Complexity of FGF receptors: genetic basis for structural diversity and functional specificity. *FASEB J.* **6:** 3362–3369.

15. Johnson, D. E. and L. T. Williams. 1993. Structural and functional diversity in the FGF receptor multigene family. *Adv. Cancer Res.* **60:** 1–41.

16. Keegan, K., D. E. Johnson, L. T. Williams, and M. J. Hayman. 1991. Isolation of an additional member of the fibroblast growth factor receptor family, FGFR-3. *Proc. Natl. Acad. Sci. USA* **88:** 1095–1099.

17. Partanen, J., T. P. Makela, E. Eerola, J. Korhonen, H. Hirvonen, L. Claesson-Welsh, and K. Alitalo. 1991. FGFR-4, a novel acidic fibroblast growth factor receptor with a distinct expression pattern. *EMBO J.* **10:** 1347–1354.

18. Partanen, J., S. Vainikka, J. Korhonen, E. Armstrong, and K. Alitalo. 1992. Diverse receptors for fibroblast growth factors. *Prog. Growth Factor Res.* **4:** 69–83.

19. Smallwood, P. M., I. Munoz-Sanjuan, P. Tong, J. P. Macke, S. H. Hendry, D. J. Gilbert, et al. 1996. Fibroblast growth factor (FGF) homologous factors: new members of the FGF family implicated in nervous system development. *Proc. Natl. Acad. Sci. USA* **93:** 9850–9857.

20. Jackson, A., S. Friedman, X. Zhan, K. A. Engleka, R. Forough, and T. Maciag. 1992. Heat shock induces the release of fibroblast growth factor 1 from NIH 3T3 cells. *Proc. Natl. Acad. Sci. USA* **89:** 10,691–10,695.

21. Jackson, A., F. Tarantini, S. Gamble, S. Friedman, and T. Maciag. 1995. The release of fibroblast growth factor-1 from NIH 3T3 cells in response to temperature involves the function of cysteine residues. *J. Biol. Chem.* **270:** 33–36.

22. Kandel, J., E. Bossy-Wetzel, F. Radvanyi, M. Klagsbrun, J. Folkman, and D. Hanahan. 1991. Neovascularization is associated with a switch to the export of bFGF in the multi-step development of fibrosarcoma. *Cell* **66:** 1095–1104.

23. Mignatti, P., T. Morimoto, and D. B. Rifkin. 1991. Basic fibroblast growth factor released by single, isolated cells stimulates their migration in an autocrine manner. *Proc. Natl. Acad. Sci. USA* **88:** 11,007–11,011.

24. Mignatti, P. and D. B. Rifkin. 1991. Release of basic fibroblast growth factor, an angio-genic factor devoid of secretory signal sequence: a trivial phenomenon or a novel secre-tion mechanism. *J. Cell. Biochem.* **47:** 201–207.

25. Muthukrishnan, L., E. Warder, and P. L. McNeil. 1991. Basic fibroblast growth factor is efficiently released from a cytosolic storage site through plasma membrane disruptions of endothelial cells. *J. Cell. Physiol.* **148:** 1–16.

26. Takahashi, K., K. Suzuki, S. Kawahara, and T. Ono. 1989. Growth stimulation of human breast epithelial cells by basic fibroblast growth factor in serum-free medium. *Int. J. Cancer* **43:** 870–874.

27. Blam, S. B., R. Mitchell, E. Tischer, J. S. Rubin, M. Silva, S. Silver, et al. 1988. Addition of growth hormone secretion signal to basic fibroblast growth factor results in cell trans-formation and secretion of aberrant forms of the protein. *Oncogene* **3:** 129–136.

28. Forough, R., Z. Xi, M. MacPhee, S. Friedman, K. A. Engleka, T. Sayers, R. H. Wiltrout, and T. Maciag. 1993. Differential transforming abilities of non-secreted and secreted forms of human fibroblast growth factor-1. *J. Biol. Chem.* **268:** 2960–2968.

29. Jouanneau, J., J. Gavrilovic, D. Caruelle, M. Jaye, G. Moens, J. P. Caruelle, and J. P. Thiery. 1991. Secreted or nonsecreted forms of acidic fibroblast growth factor produced by transfected epithelial cells influence cell morphology, motility, and invasive potential. *Proc. Natl. Acad. Sci. USA* **88:** 2893–2897.

30. Rogelj, S., A. Weinberg, P. Fanning, and M. Klagsbrun. 1988. Basic fibroblast growth factor fused to a signal peptide transforms cells. *Nature* **331:** 173–175.

31. Delli-Bovi, P., A. M. Curatola, F. G. Kern, A. Greco, M. Ittmann, and C. Basilico. 1987. An oncogene isolated by transfection of Kaposi's sarcoma DNA encodes a growth factor that is member of the FGF family. *Cell* **50:** 729–737.

32. Dickson, C., R. Smith, S. Brookes, and G. Peters. 1984. Tumorigenesis by mouse mam-mary tumor virus: proviral activation of a cellular gene in the common integration region int-2. *Cell* **37:** 529–536.

33. Zhan, X., B. Bates, X. Hu, and M. Goldfarb. 1988. The human FGF-5 oncogene encodes a novel protein related to fibroblast growth factor. *Mol. Cell. Biol.* **8:** 3487–3495.

34. Iida, S., T. Yoshida, K. Naito, H. Sakamoto, O. Katoh, S. Hirohashi, et al. 1992. Human hst-2 (FGF-6) oncogene: cDNA cloning and characterization. *Oncogene* **7:** 303–309.

35. Marics, I., J. Adelaide, F. Raybaud, M. G. Mattei, F. Coulier, J. Planche, O. De Lapeyriere, and D. Birnbaum. 1989. Characterization of the HST-related FGF.6 gene, a new member of the fibroblast growth factor gene family. *Oncogene* **4:** 335–340.

36. Santos-Ocampo, S., J. S. Colvin, A. Chellaiah, and D. M. Ornitz. 1996. Expression and biological activity of mouse fibroblast growth factor-9. *J. Biol. Chem.* **271:** 1726–1731.

37. Miki, T., T. P. Fleming, D. P. Bottaro, J. S. Rubin, D. Ron, and S. A. Aaronson. 1991. Expression cDNA cloning of the KGF receptor by creation of a transforming autocrine loop. *Science* **251:** 72–75.

38. Ghosh, A. K., D. B. Shankar, G. M. Shackleford, K. Wu, A. TÕAng, G. J. Miller, J. Zheng, and P. Roy-Burman. 1996. Molecular cloning and characterization of human FGF8 alternative messenger RNA forms. *Cell Growth Differ.* **7:** 1425–1434.

39. MacArthur, C. A., A. Lawshe, D. B. Shankar, M. Heikinheimo, and G. M. Shackleford. 1995. FGF-8 isoforms differ in NIH3T3 cell transforming potential. *Cell Growth Differ.* **6:** 817–825.

40. Acland, P., M. Dixon, G. Peters, and C. Dickson. 1990. Subcellular fate of the int-2 oncoprotein is determined by choice of initiation codon. *Nature* **343:** 662–665.

41. Kiefer, P., P. Acland, D. Pappin, G. Peters, and C. Dickson. 1997. Competition between nuclear localization and secretory signals determines the subcellular fate of a single CUG-initiated form of FGF3. *EMBO J.* **13:** 4126–4136.

42. Quarto, N., D. Talarico, R. Florkiewicz, and D. B. Rifkin. 1991. Selective expression of high molecular weight basic fibroblast growth factor confers a unique phenotype to NIH 3T3 cells. *Cell Regul.* **2:** 699–708.

43. Rifkin, D. B., D. Moscatelli, M. Roghani, Y. Nagano, N. Quarto, S. Klein, and A. Bikfalvi. 1994. Studies on FGF-2: nuclear localization and function of high molecular weight forms and receptor binding in the absence of heparin. *Mol. Reprod. Dev.* **39:** 102–104.

44. Chiu, I. M., W. P. Wang, and K. Lehtoma. 1990. Alternative splicing generates two forms of mRNA coding for human heparin-binding growth factor 1. *Oncogene* **5:** 755–762.

45. Mansour, S. L. and G. R. Martin. 1988. Four classes of mRNA are expressed from the mouse int-2 gene, a member of the FGF gene family. *EMBO J.* **7:** 2035–2041.

46. Myers, R. L., S. K. Ray, R. Eldridge, M. A. Chotani, and I. M. Chiu. 1995. Functional characterization of the brain-specific FGF-1 promoter, fgf-1.b. *J. Biol. Chem.* **270:** 8257–8266.

47. Smith, R., G. Peters, and C. Dickson. 1988. Multiple RNAs expressed from the int-2 gene in mouse embryonal carcinoma cell lines encode a protein with homology to fibroblast growth factors. *EMBO J.* **7:** 1013–1022.

48. Bates, B., J. Hardin, X. Zhan, K. Drickamer, and M. Goldfarb. 1991. Biosynthesis of human fibroblast growth factor-5. *Mol. Cell. Biol.* **11:** 1840–1845.

49. Forough, R., K. Engleka, J. A. Thompson, A. Jackson, T. Imamura, and T. Maciag. 1991. Differential expression in Escherichia coli of the alpha and beta forms of heparin-binding acidic fibroblast growth factor-1: potential role of RNA secondary structure. *Biochim. Biophys. Acta* **1090:** 293–298.

50. Kevil, C., P. Carter, B. Hu, and A. De Benedetti. 1995. Translational enhancement of FGF-2 by eIF-4 factors, and alternate utilization of CUG and AUG codons for translation initiation. *Oncogene* **11:** 2339–2348.

51. Burrus, L. W., M. E. Zuber, B. A. Lueddecke, and B. B. Olwin. 1992. Identification of a cysteine-rich receptor for fibroblast growth factors. *Mol. Cell. Biol.* **12:** 5600–5609.

52. Kan, M., F. Wang, J. Xu, J. W. Crabb, J. Hou, and W. L. McKeehan. 1993. An essential heparin-binding domain in the fibroblast growth factor receptor kinase. *Science* **259:** 1918–1921.

53. Klagsbrun, M. and A. Baird. 1991. A dual receptor system is required for basic fibroblast growth factor activity. *Cell* **67:** 229–231.

54. Spivak-Kroizman, T., M. A. Lemmon, I. Dikic, J. E. Ladbury, D. Pinchasi, J. Huang, et al. 1994. Heparin-induced oligomerization of FGF molecules is responsible for FGF receptor dimerization, activation, and cell proliferation. *Cell* **79:** 1015–1024.

55. Yayon, A., M. Klagsbrun, J. D. Esko, P. Leder, and D. M. Ornitz. 1991. Cell surface, heparin-like molecules are required for binding of basic fibroblast growth factor to its high affinity receptor. *Cell* **64:** 841–848.

56. Guimond, S., M. Maccarana, B. B. Olwin, U. Lindahl, and A. C. Rapraeger. 1993. Activating and inhibitory heparin sequences for FGF-2 (basic FGF). Distinct requirements for FGF-1, FGF-2, and FGF-4. *J. Biol. Chem.* **268:** 23,906–23,914.

57. Steinfeld, R., H. Van Den Berghe, and G. David. 1996. Stimulation of fibroblast growth factor receptor-1 occupancy and signaling by cell surface-associated syndecans and glypican. *J. Cell Biol.* **133:** 405–416.

58. Hou, J., M. Kan, K. McKeehan, G. McBride, P. Adams, and W. L. McKeehan. 1991. Fibroblast growth factors receptors from liver vary in three structural domains. *Science* **251:** 665–668.

59. Johnson, D. E., J. Lu, H. Chen, S. Werner, and L. T. Williams. 1991. The human fibroblast growth factor receptor genes: a common structural arrangement underlies the mechanisms for generating receptor forms that differ in their third immunoglobulin domain. *Mol. Cell. Biol.* **11:** 4627–4634.

60. Jaye, M., J. Schlessinger, and C. A. Dionne. 1992. Fibroblast growth factor receptor tyrosine kinases: molecular analysis and signal transduction. *Biochim. Biophys. Acta* **1135:** 185–199.

61. Ornitz, D. M., J. Xu, J. S. Colvin, D. G. McEwen, C. A. MacArthur, F. Coulier, G. Gao, and M. Goldfarb. 1996. Receptor specificity of the fibroblast growth factor family. *J. Biol. Chem.* **271:** 15,292–15,297.

62. Zimmer, Y., D. Givol, and A. Yayon. 1993. Multiple structural elements determine ligand binding of fibroblast growth factor receptors. *J. Biol. Chem.* **268:** 7899–7903.

63. Yan, G., F. Wang, Y. Fukabori, D. Sussman, J. Hou, and W. L. McKeehan. 1992. Expression and transforming activity of a variant of the heparin-binding fibroblast growth factor receptor (flg) gene resulting from splicing of the alpha exon at an alternate 3'-acceptor site. *Biochem. Biophys. Res. Commun.* **183:** 423–430.

64. Eisemann, A., J. A. Ahn, G. Graziani, S. R. Tronick, and D. Ron. 1991. Alternative splicing generates at least five different isoforms of the human basic-FGF receptor. *Oncogene* **6:** 1195–1202.

65. Duan, D. R., S. Werner, and L. T. Williams. 1992. A naturally occurring secreted form of fibroblast growth factor (FGF) receptor 1 binds basic FGF in preference over acidic FGF. *J. Biol. Chem.* **267:** 16,076–16,080.

66. Wang, G. and K. A. Thomas. 1994. Purification and characterization of a functional soluble fibroblast growth factor receptor 1. *Biochem. Biophys. Res. Commun.* **203:** 1781–1788.

67. Ullrich, A. and J. Schlessinger. 1990. Signal transduction by receptors with tyrosine kinase activity. *Cell* **61:** 203–212.

68. Shi, E., M. Kan, J. Xu, F. Wang, J. Hou, and W. L. McKeehan. 1993. Control of fibroblast growth factor receptor kinase signal transduction by heterodimerization of combinatorial splice variants. *Mol. Cell. Biol.* **13:** 3907–3918.

69. Ueno, H., M. Gunn, K. Dell, A. Tseng, Jr., and L. Williams. 1992. A truncated form of fibroblast growth factor receptor 1 inhibits signal transduction by multiple types of fibroblast growth factor receptor. *J. Biol. Chem.* **267:** 1470–1476.

70. Ding, I. Y., S. W. McLeskey, K. Chang, Y. M. Fu, J. C. Acol, M. T. Shou, K. Alitalo, and F. G. Kern. 1992. Expression of fibroblast growth factors (FGFS) and receptors (FGFRS) in human breast carcinomas. *Proc. Am. Assoc. Cancer Res.* **33:** A1610(Abstract).

71. Lehtola, L., J. Partanen, L. Sistonen, J. Korhonen, A. Warri, P. Harkönen, R. Clarke, and K. Alitalo. 1992. Analysis of tyrosine kinase mRNAs including four FGF receptor mRNAs expressed in MCF-7 breast-cancer cells. *Int. J. Cancer* **50:** 598–603.

72. McLeskey, S. W., I. Y. F. Ding, M. E. Lippman, and F. G. Kern. 1994. MDA-MB-134 breast carcinoma cells overexpress fibroblast growth factor (FGF) receptors and are growth-inhibited by FGF ligands. *Cancer Res.* **54:** 523–530.

73. Bellot, F., G. Crumley, J. M. Kaplow, J. Schlessinger, M. Jaye, and C. A. Dionne. 1991. Ligand-induced transphosphorylation between different FGF receptors. *EMBO J.* **10:** 2849–2854.

74. Karunagaran, D., E. Tzahar, R. R. Beerli, X. Chen, D. Graus-Porta, B. J. Ratzkin, et al. 1996. ErbB-2 is a common auxiliary subunit of NDF and EGF receptors: implications for breast cancer. *EMBO J.* **15:** 254–264.

75. Peters, G., S. Brookes, R. Smith, M. Placzek, and C. Dickson. 1989. The mouse homolog of the hst/k-FGF gene is adjacent to int-2 and is activated by proviral insertion in some virally induced mammary tumors. *Proc. Natl. Acad. Sci. USA* **86:** 5678–5682.

76. Brison, O. 1993. Gene amplification and tumor progression. *Biochim. Biophys. Acta* **1155:** 25–41.

77. Lammie, G. A., V. Fantl, R. Smith, E. Schuuring, S. Brookes, R. Michalides, et al. 1991. D11S287, a putative oncogene on chromosome 11q13, is amplified and expressed in squamous cell and mammary carcinomas and linked to BCL-1. *Oncogene* **6:** 439–444.

78. Theillet, C., X. Le Roy, O. De Lapeyriere, J. Grosgeorges, J. Adnane, S. D. Raynaud, et al. 1989. Amplification of FGF-related genes in human tumors: possible involvement of HST in breast carcinomas. *Oncogene* **4:** 915–922.

79. Liscia, D. S., G. R. Merlo, C. Garrett, D. French, R. Mariani-Costantini, and R. Callahan. 1989. Expression of int-2 mRNA in human tumors amplified at the int-2 locus. *Oncogene* **4:** 1219–1224.

80. Fantl, V., M. A. Richards, R. Smith, G. A. Lammie, G. Johnstone, D. Allen, et al. 1990. Gene amplification on chromosome band 11q13 and oestrogen receptor status in breast cancer. *Eur. J. Cancer* **26:** 423–429.

81. Penault-Llorca, F., F. Bertucci, J. Adelaide, P. Parc, F. Coulier, J. Jacquemier, D. Birnbaum, and O. deLapeyriere. 1995. Expression of FGF and FGF receptor genes in human breast cancer. *Int. J. Cancer* **61:** 170–176.

82. Motokura, T., T. Bloom, H. B. Kim, H. Juppner, J. V. Ruderman, H. M. Kronenberg, and A. Arnold. 1991. A novel cyclin encoded by a bcl-1-linked candidate oncogene. *Nature* **350:** 512–515.

83. Withers, D. A., R. C. Harvey, J. B. Faust, O. Melnyk, K. Carey, and T. C. Meeker. 1991. Characterization of a candidate bcl-1 gene. *Mol. Cell. Biol.* **11:** 4846–4853.

84. Buckley, M. F., K. J. Sweeney, J. A. Hamilton, R. L. Sini, D. L. Manning, R. I. Nicholson, et al. 1993. Expression and amplification of cyclin genes in human breast cancer. *Oncogene* **8:** 2127–2133.

85. Faust, J. B. and T. C. Meeker. 1992. Amplification and expression of the bcl-1 gene in human solid tumor cell lines. *Cancer Res.* **52:** 2460–2463.

86. Schuuring, E., E. Verhoeven, S. Litvinov, and R. J. Michalides. 1993. The product of the EMS1 gene, amplified and overexpressed in human carcinomas, is homologous to a v-src substrate and is located in cell-substratum contact sites. *Mol. Cell. Biol.* **13:** 2891–2898.

87. Zhan, X., C. Plourde, X. Hu, R. Friesel, and T. Maciag. 1994. Association of fibroblast growth factor receptor-1 with c-src correlates with association between c-src and cortactin. *J. Biol. Chem.* **269:** 20,221–20,224.

88. Lonn, U., S. Lonn, H. Ingelman-Sundberg, B. Nilsson, and B. Stenkvist. 1996. c-erb-B2/int-2 amplification appears faster in breast-cancer patients receiving second-line endocrine treatment. *Int. J. Cancer* **69:** 273–277.

89. Schuuring, E., E. Verhoeven, H. van Tinteren, J. L. Peterse, B. Nunnink, F. B. Thunnissen, et al. 1992. Amplification of genes within the chromosome 11q13 region is indicative of poor prognosis in patients with operable breast cancer. *Cancer Res.* **52:** 5229–5234.

90. Tsuda, H., S. Hirohashi, Y. Shimosato, T. Hirota, S. Tsugane, H. Yamamoto, et al. 1989. Correlation between long-term survival in breast cancer patients and amplification of two putative oncogene-coamplification units: hst-1/int-2 and c-erbB-2/ear-1. *Cancer Res.* **49:** 3104–3108.

91. MacArthur, C. A., D. B. Shankar, and G. M. Shackleford. 1995. FGF-8, activated by proviral insertion, cooperates with the Wnt-1 transgene in murine mammary tumorigenesis. *J. Virol.* **69:** 2501–2507.

92. Shackleford, G. M., C. A. MacArthur, H. C. Kwan, and H. E. Varmus. 1993. Mouse mammary tumor virus infection accelerates mammary carcinogenesis in wnt-1 transgenic mice by insertional activation of int-2/fgf-3 and hst/fgf-4. *Proc. Natl. Acad. Sci. USA* **90:** 740–744.

93. Nusse, R. and H. E. Varmus. 1982. Many tumors induced by the mouse mammary tumor virus contain a provirus integrated in the same region of the host genome. *Cell* **31:** 99–109.

94. Muller, W. J., F. S. Lee, C. Dickson, G. Peters, P. Pattengale, and P. Leder. 1990. The int-2 gene product acts as an epithelial growth factor in transgenic mice. *EMBO J.* **9:** 907–913.

95. Tsukamoto, A. S., R. Grosschedl, R. C. Guzman, T. Parslow, and H. E. Varmus. 1988. Expression of the int-1 gene in transgenic mice is associated with mammary gland hyperplasia and adenocarcinomas in male and female mice. *Cell* **55:** 619–625.

96. Kwan, H., V. Pecenka, A. Tsukamoto, T. G. Parslow, R. Guzman, T. P. Lin, et al. 1992. Transgenes expressing the wnt-1 and int-2 proto-oncogenes cooperate during mammary carcinogenesis in doubly transgenic mice. *Mol. Cell. Biol.* **12:** 147–154.

97. Peters, G., A. E. Lee, and C. Dickson. 1986. Concerted activation of two potential proto-oncogenes in carcinomas induced by mouse mammary tumour virus. *Nature* **320:** 628–631.

98. Kapoun, A. M. and G. M. Shackleford. 1997. Preferential activation of FGF8 by proviral insertion im mammary tumor of Wnt1 transgenic mice. *Oncogene* **14:** 2985–2989.

99. Coleman-Krnacik, S. and J. M. Rosen. 1994. Differential temporal and spatial gene expression of fibroblast growth factor family members during mouse mammary gland development. *Mol. Endocrinol.* **8:** 218–229.

100. Jakobovits, A., G. M. Shackleford, H. E. Varmus, and G. R. Martin. 1986. Two proto-oncogenes implicated in mammary carcinogenesis, int-1 and int-2, are independently regulated during mouse development. *Proc. Natl. Acad. Sci USA* **83:** 7806–7810.

101. Li, S. and G. D. Shipley. 1991. Expression of multiple species of basic fibroblast growth factor mRNA and protein in normal and tumor-derived mammary epithelial cells in culture. *Cell Growth Differ.* **2:** 195–202.

102. Luqmani, Y. A., M. Graham, and R. C. Coombes. 1992. Expression of basic fibroblast growth factor, FGFR1 and FGFR2 in normal and malignant human breast, and comparison with other normal tissues. *Br. J. Cancer* **66:** 273–280.

103. Ke, Y., D. G. Fernig, M. C. Wilkinson, J. H. Winstanley, J. A. Smith, P. S. Rudland, and R. Barraclough. 1993. The expression of basic fibroblast growth factor and its receptor in cell lines derived from normal human mammary gland and a benign mammary lesion. *J. Cell Sci.* **106:** 135–143.

104. Gomm, J. J., P. J. Browne, R. C. Coope, G. S. Bansal, C. Yiangou, C. L. Johnston, R. Mason, and R. C. Coombes. 1997. A paracrine role for myoepithelial cell-derived FGF2 in the normal human breast. *Exp. Cell Res.* **234:** 165–173.

105. Anandappa, S. Y., J. H. Winstanley, S. Leinster, B. Green, P. S. Rudland, and R. Barraclough. 1994. Comparative expression of fibroblast growth factor mRNAs in benign and malignant breast disease. *Br. J. Cancer* **69:** 772–776.

106. El Yazidi, I. and Y. Boilly-Marer. 1995. Production of acidic and basic fibroblast growth factor by the hormone-independent breast cancer cell line MDA-MB-231. *Anticancer Res.* **15:** 783–790.

107. Lee, Y. J., S. S. Galoforo, C. M. Berns, G. Erdos, A. K. Gupta, D. K. Ways, and P. M. Corry. 1995. Effect of ionizing radiation on AP-1 binding activity and basic fibroblast growth factor gene expression in drug-sensitive human breast carcinoma MCF-7 and multidrug-resistant MCF-7/ADR cells. *J. Biol. Chem.* **270:** 28,790–28,796.

108. Bansal, G. S., C. Yiangou, R. C. Coope, J. J. Gomm, Y. A. Luqmani, R. C. Coombes, and C. L. Johnston. 1995. Expression of fibroblast growth factor 1 is lower in breast cancer than in normal human breast. *Br. J. Cancer* **72:** 420–1426.

109. Renaud, F., I. El Yazidi, Y. Boilly-Marer, Y. Courtois, and M. Laurent. 1996. Expression and regulation by serum of multiple FGF1 mRNA in normal transformed, and malignant human mammary epithelial cells. *Biochem. Biophys. Res. Commun.* **219:** 679–685.

110. Payson, R. A., J. Wu, Y. Liu, and I. M. Chiu. 1996. The human FGF-8 gene localizes on chromosome 10q24 and is subjected to induction by androgen in breast cancer cells. *Oncogene* **13:** 47–53.

111. Werner, S., W. K. Roth, B. Bates, M. Goldfarb, and P. H. Hofsneider. 1991. Fibroblast growth factor 5 proto-oncogene is expressed in normal human fibroblasts and induced by serum growth factors. *Oncogene* **6:** 2137–2144.

112. Relf, M., S. LeJeune, P. A. Scott, S. Fox, K. Smith, R. Leek, et al. 1997. Expression of the angiogenic factors vascular endothelial cell growth factor, acidic and basic fibroblast growth factor, tumor growth factor beta-1, platelet-derived endothelial cell growth factor, placenta growth factor, and pleiotrophin in human primary breast cancer and its relation to angiogenesis. *Cancer Res.* **57:** 963–969.

113. Smith, J., A. Yelland, R. Baillie, and R. C. Coombes. 1994. Acidic and basic fibroblast growth factors in human breast tissue. *Eur. J. Cancer* **30A:** 496–503.

114. Yiangou, C., J. J. Gomm, R. C. Coope, M. Law, Y. A. Luqmani, S. Shousha, R. C. Coombes, and C. L. Johnston. 1997. Fibroblast growth factor 2 in breast cancer: occurrence and prognostic significance. *Br. J. Cancer* **75:** 28–33.

115. Yoshiji, H., D. E. Gomez, M. Shibuya, and U. P. Thorgeirsson. 1996. Expression of vascular endothelial growth factor, its receptor, and other angiogenic factors in human breast cancer. *Cancer Res.* **56:** 2013–2016.

116. Koos, R. D., P. K. Banks, S. E. Inkster, W. Yue, and A. M. Brodie. 1993. Detection of aromatase and keratinocyte growth factor expression in breast tumors using reverse transcription-polymerase chain reaction. *J. Steroid Biochem. Mol. Biol.* **45:** 217–225.

117. Gomm, J. J., J. Smith, G. K. Ryall, R. Baillie, L. Turnbull, and R. C. Coombes. 1991. Localization of basic fibroblast growth factor and transforming growth factor beta 1 in the human mammary gland. *Cancer Res.* **51:** 4685–4692.

118. Visscher, D. W., F. De Mattia, S. Ottosen, F. H. Sarkar, and J. D. Crissman. 1995. Biologic and clinical significance of basic fibroblast growth factor immunostaining in breast carcinoma. *Mod. Pathol.* **8:** 665–670.

119. Coope, R. C., P. J. Browne, C. Yiangou, G. S. Bansal, J. Walters, N. Groome, et al. 1997. The location of acidic fibroblast growth factor in the breast is dependent on the activity of proteases present in breast cancer tissue. *Br. J. Cancer* **75:** 1621–1630.

120. Zhang, L., S. Kharbanda, D. Chen, J. Bullocks, D. L. Miller, I. Y. F. Ding, et al. 1997. MCF-7 breast carcinoma cells overexpressing FGF-1 form vascularized, metastatic tumors in ovariectomized or tamoxifen-treated nude mice. *Oncogene* **15:** 2093–2108.

121. Aviezer, D., D. Hecht, M. Safran, M. Eisinger, G. David, and A. Yayon. 1994. Perlecan, basal lamina proteoglycan, promotes basic fibroblast growth factor-receptor binding, mitogenesis, and angiogenesis. *Cell* **79:** 1005–1013.

122. Iozzo, R. V., I. R. Cohen, S. Grassel, and A. D. Murdoch. 1994. The biology of perlecan: the multifaceted heparan sulphate proteoglycan of basement membranes and pericellular matrices. *Biochem. J.* **302:** 625–639.

123. Murdoch, A. D., B. Liu, R. Schwarting, R. S. Tuan, and R. V. Iozzo. 1994. Widespread expression of perlecan proteoglycan in basement membranes and extracellular matrices of human tissues as detected by a novel monoclonal antibody against domain iii and by in situ hybridization. *J. Histochem. Cytochem.* **42:** 239–249.

124. Briozzo, P., J. Badet, F. Capony, I. Pieri, P. Montcourrier, D. Barritault, and H. Rochefort. 1991. MCF7 mammary cancer cells respond to bFGF and internalize it following its release from extracellular matrix: a permissive role of cathepsin D. *Exp. Cell Res.* **194:** 252–259.

125. Peyrat, J. P., H. Hondermark, M. M. Louchez, and B. Boilly. 1991. Demonstration of basic fibroblast growth factor high and low affinity binding sites in human breast cancer cell lines. *Cancer Commun.* **3:** 323–329.

126. Delehedde, M., E. Deudon, B. Boilly, and H. Hondermarck. 1997. Production of sulfated proteoglycans by human breast cancer cell lines: binding to fibroblast growth factor-2. *J. Cell Biochem.* **64:** 605–617.

127. Johnston, C. L., H. C. Cox, J. J. Gomm, and R. C. Coombes. 1995. Fibroblast growth factor receptors (FGFRs) localize in different cellular compartments. a splice variant of FGFR-3 localizes to the nucleus. *J. Biol. Chem.* **270:** 30,643–30,650.

128. Adnane, J., P. Gaudray, C. A. Dionne, G. Crumley, M. Jaye, J. Schlessinger, et al. 1991. BEK and FLG, two receptors to members of the FGF family, are amplified in subsets of human breast cancers. *Oncogene* **6:** 659–663.

129. Jacquemier, J., J. Adelaide, P. Parc, F. Penault-Llorca, J. Planche, O. deLapeyriere, and D. Birnbaum. 1994. Expression of the FGFR1 gene in human breast-carcinoma cells. *Int. J. Cancer* **59:** 373–378.

130. Theillet, C., J. Adelaide, G. Louason, F. Bonnet-Dorion, J. Jacquemier, J. Adnane, et al. 1993. FGFRI and PLAT genes and DNA amplification at 8p12 in breast and ovarian cancers. *Genes Chromosom. Cancer* **7:** 219–226.

131. Lafage, M., F. Pedeutour, S. Marchetto, J. Simonetti, M. T. Prosperi, P. Gaudray, and D. Birnbaum. 1992. Fusion and amplification of two originally non-syntenic chromosomal regions in a mammary carcinoma cell line. *Genes Chromosom. Cancer* **5:** 40–49.

132. Jaakkola, S., P. Salmikangas, S. Nylund, J. Partanen, E. Armstrong, S. Pyrhonen, P. Lehtovirta, and H. Nevanlinna. 1993. Amplification of fgfr4 gene in human breast and gynecological cancers. *Int. J. Cancer* **54:** 378–382.

133. Ron, D., R. Reich, M. Chedid, C. Lengel, O. E. Cohen, A. M. Chan, et al. 1993. Fibroblast growth factor receptor 4 is a high affinity receptor for both acidic and basic fibroblast growth factor but not for keratinocyte growth factor. *J. Biol. Chem.* **268:** 5388–5394.

134. Maher, P. A. 1996. Nuclear translocation of fibroblast growth factor (FGF) receptors in response to FGF-2. *J. Cell Biol.* **134:** 529–536.

135. Wang, F., M. Kan, G. Yan, J. Xu, and W. L. McKeehan. 1995. Alternately spliced NH2-terminal immunoglobulin-like loop I in the ectodomain of the fibroblast growth factor (FGF) receptor 1 lowers affinity for both heparin and FGF-1. *J. Biol. Chem.* **270:** 10,231–10,235.

136. Yamaguchi, F., S. Saya, J. M. Bruner, and R. S. Morrison. 1994. Differential expression of two fibroblast growth factor-receptor genes is associated with malignant progression in human astrocytomas. *Proc. Natl. Acad. Sci. USA* **91:** 484–488.

137. Kobrin, M. S., Y. Yamanaka, H. Friess, M. E. Lopez, and M. Korc. 1993. Aberrant expression of type I fibroblast growth factor receptor in human pancreatic adenocarcinomas. *Cancer Res.* **53:** 4741–4744.

138. Morikawa, Y., Y. Ishihara, K. Tohya, K. Kakudo, M. K. Seo, and N. Matsuura. 1996. Expression of the fibroblast growth factor receptor-1 in human normal tissues and tumors determined by a new monoclonal antibody. *Arch. Pathol. Lab. Med.* **120:** 490–496.

139. Hughes, S. E. and P. A. Hall. 1993. Immunolocalization of fibroblast growth factor receptor 1 and its ligands in human tissues. *Lab. Invest.* **69:** 173–182.

140. Luqmani, Y. A., C. Mortimer, C. Yiangou, C. L. Johnston, G. S. Bansal, D. Sinnett, M. Law, and R. C. Coombes. 1995. Expression of 2 variant forms of fibroblast growth factor receptor 1 in human breast. *Int. J. Cancer* **64:** 274–279.

141. Yiangou, C., H. Cox, G. S. Bansal, R. Coope, J. J. Gomm, R. Barnard, et al. 1997. Down-regulation of a novel form of fibroblast growth factor receptor 1 in human breast cancer. *Br. J. Cancer* **76:** 1419–1427.

142. Miki, T., D. P. Bottaro, T. P. Fleming, C. L. Smith, W. H. Burgess, A. M. Chan, and S. A. Aaronson. 1992. Determination of ligand-binding specificity by alternative splicing: two distinct growth factor receptors encoded by a single gene. *Proc. Natl. Acad. Sci. USA* **89:** 246–250.

143. Yan, G., Y. Fukabori, G. McBride, S. Nikolaropolous, and W. L. McKeehan. 1993. Exon switching and activation of stromal and embryonic fibroblast growth factor (FGF)-FGF receptor genes in prostate epithelial cells accompany stromal independence and malignancy. *Mol. Cell. Biol.* **13:** 4513–4522.

144. Savagner, P., A. M. Valles, J. Jouanneau, K. M. Yamada, and J. P. Thiery. 1994. Alternative splicing in fibroblast growth factor receptor 2 is associated with induced epithelial-mesenchymal transition in rat bladder carcinoma cells. *Mol. Biol. Cell* **5:** 851–862.

145. Feng, S., F. Wang, A. Matsubara, M. Kan, and W. L. McKeehan. 1997. Fibroblast growth factor receptor 2 limits and receptor 1 accelerates tumorigenicity of prostate epithelial cells. *Cancer Res.* **57:** 5369–5378.

146. Carstens, R. P., J. V. Eaton, H. R. Kringman, P. J. Walther, and M. A. Garcia-Blanco. 1997. Alternative splicing of fibroblast growth factor receptor 2 (FGF-R2) in human prostate cancer. *Oncogene* **15:** 3059–3065.

147. Bansal, G. S., H. C. Cox, S. Marsh, J. J. Gomm, C. Yiangou, Y. Luqmani, R. C. Coombes, and C. L. Johnston. 1997. Expression of keratinocyte growth factor and its receptor in human breast cancer. *Br. J. Cancer* **75:** 1567–1574.

148. Finch, P. W., J. S. Rubin, T. Miki, D. Ron, and S. A. Aaronson. 1989. Human KGF is FGF-related with properties of a paracrine effector of epithelial cell growth. *Science* **245:** 752–755.

149. Luqmani, Y. A., G. S. Bansal, C. Mortimer, L. Buluwela, and R. C. Coombes. 1997. Expression of FGFR2 BEK and K-SAM mRNA variants in normal and malignant human breast. *Eur. J. Cancer* **32A:** 518–524.

150. Li, Y., K. Mangasarian, A. Mansukhani, and C. Basilico. 1997. Activation of FGF receptors by mutations in the transmembrane domain. *Oncogene* **14:** 1397–1406.

151. Neilson, K. M. and R. E. Friesel. 1995. Constitutive activation of fibroblast growth factor receptor-2 by a point mutation associated with Crouzon syndrome. *J. Biol. Chem.* **270:** 26,037–26,040.

152. Webster, M. K., P. Y. D'Avis, S. C. Robertson, and D. J. Donoghue. 1996. Profound ligand-independent kinase activation of fibroblast growth factor receptor 3 by the activation loop mutation responsible for a lethal skeletal dysplasia, thanatophoric dysplasia type II. *Mol. Cell. Biol.* **16:** 4081–4087.

153. Webster, M. K. and D. J. Donoghue. 1997. FGFR activation in skeletal disorders: too much of a good thing. *Trends Genet.* **13:** 178–182.

154. Bellus, G. A., I. McIntosh, E. A. Smith, A. S. Aylsworth, I. Kaitila, W. A. Horton, et al. 1995. A recurrent mutation in the tyrosine kinase domain of fibroblast growth factor receptor 3 causes hypochondroplasia. *Nat. Genet.* **10:** 357–359.

155. Tavormina, P. L., R. Shiang, L. M. Thompson, Y. Z. Zhu, D. J. Wilkin, R. S. Lachman, et al. 1995. Thanatophoric dysplasia (types I and II) caused by distinct mutations in fibroblast growth factor receptor 3. *Nat. Genet.* **9:** 321–328.

156. Webster, M. K. and D. J. Donoghue. 1996. Constitutive activation of fibroblast growth factor receptor 3 by the transmembrane domain point mutation found in achondroplasia. *EMBO J.* **15:** 520–527.

157. Deng, C., A. Wynshaw-Boris, F. Zhou, A. Kuo, and P. Leder. 1996. Fibroblast growth factor receptor 3 is a negative regulator of bone growth. *Cell* **84:** 911–921.

158. Thompson, L. M., S. Raffioni, J. J. Wasmuth, and R. A. Bradshaw. 1997. Chimeras of the native form or achondroplasia mutant (G375C) of human fibroblast growth factor receptor 3 induce ligand-dependent differentiation of PC12 cells. *Mol. Cell. Biol.* **17:** 4169–4177.

159. Chesi, M., E. Nardini, L. A. Brents, E. Schrock, T. Ried, W. M. Kuehl, and P. L. Bergsagel. 1997. Frequent translocation t(4;14)(p16.3;q32.3) in multiple myeloma is associated with increased expression and activating mutations of fibroblast growth factor receptor 3. *Nat. Genet.* **16:** 260–264.

160. Webster, M. K. and D. J. Donoghue. 1997. Enhanced signaling and morphological transformation by a membrane-localized derivative of the fibroblast growth factor receptor 3 kinase domain. *Mol. Cell. Biol.* **17:** 5739–5747.

161. Lorenzi, M. V., P. Castagnino, Q. Chen, M. Chedid, and T. Miki. 1997. Ligand-independent activation of fibroblast growth factor receptor-2 by carboxyl terminal alterations. *Oncogene* **15:** 817–826.

162. Doherty, P., E. Williams, and F. S. Walsh. 1994. Activation of the FGF receptor underlies neurite outgrowth stimulated by L1, N-CAM, and N-cadherin. *Neuron* **13:** 583–594.

163. Gao, G. and M. Goldfarb. 1995. Heparin can activate a receptor tyrosine kinase. *EMBO J.* **14:** 2183–2190.

164. Green, P. J., F. S. Walsh, and P. Doherty. 1996. Promiscuity of fibroblast growth factor receptors. *Bioessays* **18:** 639–646.

165. Rudland, P. S., R. C. Hallowes, H. Durbin, and D. Lewis. 1977. Mitogenic activity of pituitary hormones on cell cultures of normal and carcinogen-induced tumor epithelium from rat mammary glands. *J. Cell. Biol.* **73:** 561–577.

166. Smith, J. A., D. P. Winslow, and P. S. Rudland. 1984. Different growth factors stimulate cell division of rat mammary epithelial, myoepithelial, and stromal cell lines in culture. *J. Cell. Physiol.* **119:** 320–326.

167. Imagawa, W., G. R. Cunha, P. Young, and S. Nandi. 1994. Keratinocyte growth factor and acidic fibroblast growth factor are mitogens for primary cultures of mammary epithelium. *Biochem. Biophys. Res. Commun.* **204:** 1165–1169.

168. Ulich, T. R., E. S. Yi, R. Cardiff, S. Yin, N. Bikhazi, R. Biltz, C. F. Morris, and G. F. Pierce. 1994. Keratinocyte growth factor is a growth factor for mammary epithelium in vivo. The mammary epithelium of lactating rats is resistant to the proliferative action of keratinocyte growth factor. *Am. J. Pathol.* **144:** 862–868.

169. Yi, E. S., A. A. Bedoya, H. Lee, S. Kim, R. M. Housley, S. L. Aukerman, et al. 1994. Keratinocyte growth factor causes cystic dilation of the mammary glands of mice. interactions of keratinocyte growth factor, estrogen, and progesterone in vivo. *Am. J. Pathol.* **145:** 1015–1022.

170. Kitsberg, D. I. and P. Leder. 1996. Keratinocyte growth factor induces mammary and prostatic hyperplasia and mammary adenocarcinoma in transgenic mice. *Oncogene* **13:** 2507–2515.

171. Wilkinson, D. G., S. Bhatt, and A. P. McMahon. 1989. Expression pattern of the FGF-related proto-oncogene int-2 suggests multiple roles in fetal development. *Development* **105:** 131–136.

172. Wilkinson, D. G., G. Peters, C. Dickson, and A. P. McMahon. 1988. Expression of the FGF-related proto-oncogene int-2 during gastrulation and neurulation in the mouse. *EMBO J.* **7:** 691–695.

173. Mathieu, M., E. Chatelain, D. Ornitz, J. Bresnick, I. Mason, P. Kiefer, and C. Dickson. 1995. Receptor binding and mitogenic properties of mouse fibroblast growth factor 3. Modulation of response by heparin. *J. Biol. Chem.* **270:** 24,197–24,203.

174. Venesio, T., D. Taverna, N. E. Hynes, R. Deed, D. MacAllan, F. Ciardiello, et al. 1992. The int-2 gene product acts as a growth factor and substitutes for basic fibroblast growth factor in promoting the differentiation of a normal mouse mammary epithelial cell line. *Cell Growth Differ.* **3:** 63–71.

175. Basolo, F., T. Venesio, S. Calvo, L. Fiore, G. Fontanini, F. Ciardello, et al. 1994. The effect of FGF-3/int3 on growth and transformation of MCF-10A normal human mammary epithelial cells is distinct from FGF-1 and FGF-2. *Int. J. Oncol.* **4:** 1365–1370.

176. Levay-Young, B. K., W. Imagawa, D. R. Wallace, and S. Nandi. 1989. Basic fibroblast growth factor stimulates the growth and inhibits casein accumulation in mouse mammary epithelial cells in vitro. *Mol. Cell. Endocrinol.* **62:** 327–336.

177. Souttou, B., R. Hamelin, and M. Crepin. 1994. FGF2 as an autocrine growth factor for immortal human breast epithelial cells. *Cell Growth Differ.* **5:** 615–623.

178. Valverius, E. M., F. Ciardiello, N. E. Heldin, B. Blondel, G. Merlo, G. Smith, et al. 1990. Stromal influences on transformation of human mammary epithelial cells overexpressing c-myc and SV40T. *J. Cell. Physiol.* **145:** 207–216.

179. Johnston, C. L., H. C. Cox, J. J. Gomm, and R. C. Coombes. 1995. bFGF and aFGF induce membrane ruffling in breast cancer cells but not in normal breast epithelial cells: FGFR-4 involvement. *Biochem. J.* **306:** 609–616.

180. Filmus, J., M. N. Pollak, R. Cailleau, and R. N. Buick. 1985. MDA-468, a human breast cancer cell line with a high number of epidermal growth factor (EGF) receptors, has an amplified EGF receptor gene and is growth inhibited by EGF. *Biochem. Biophys. Res. Comm.* **128:** 898–905.

181. Delehedde, M., B. Boilly, and H. Hondermarck. 1995. Differential responsiveness of human breast cancer cells to basic fibroblast growth factor: a cell kinetics study. *Oncol. Res.* **7:** 399–405.

182. Delehedde, M., E. Deudon, B. Boilly, and H. Hondermarck. 1996. Heparan sulfate proteoglycans play a dual role in regulating fibroblast growth factor-2 mitogenic activity in human breast cancer cells. *Exp. Cell Res.* **229:** 398–406.

183. Karey, K. P. and D. A. Sirbasku. 1988. Differential responsiveness of human breast cancer cell lines MCF-7 and T47D to growth factors and 17 beta-estradiol. *Cancer Res.* **48:** 4083–4092.

184. Peyrat, J. P., J. Bonneterre, H. Hondermarck, B. Hecquet, A. Adenis, M. M. Louchez, et al. 1992. Basic fibroblast growth factor (bFGF): mitogenic activity and binding sites in human breast cancer. *J. Steroid Biochem. Mol. Biol.* **43:** 87–94.

185. Stewart, A. J., B. R. Westley, and F. E. B. May. 1992. Modulation of the proliferative response of breast cancer cells to growth factors by oestrogen. *Br. J. Cancer* **66:** 640–648.

186. Fenig, E., R. Wieder, S. Paglin, H. Wang, R. Resaud, A. Haimovitz-Friedman, Z. Fuks, and J. Yahalom. 1997. Basic fibroblast growth factor confers growth inhibition and mitogen-activated protein kinase activation in human breast cancer cells. *Clin. Cancer Res.* **3:** 135–142.

187. Wang, H., M. Rubin, E. Fenig, A. DeBlasio, J. Mendelsohn, J. Yahalom, and R. Wieder. 1997. Basic fibroblast growth factor causes growth arrest in MCF-7 human breast cancer cells while inducing both mitogenic and inhibitory G1 events. *Cancer Res.* **57:** 1750–1757.

188. Souttou, B., C. Gamby, M. Crepin, and R. Hamelin. 1996. Tumoral progression of human breast epithelial cells secreting FGF2 an FGF4. *Int. J. Cancer* **68**: 1–7.
189. McLeskey, S. W., J. Kurebayashi, S. F. Honig, J. Zwiebel, M. E. Lippman, R. B. Dickson, and F. G. Kern. 1993. Fibroblast growth factor 4 transfection of MCF-7 cells produces cell lines that are tumorigenic and metastatic in ovariectomized or tamoxifen-treated athymic nude mice. *Cancer Res.* **53**: 2168–2177.
190. McLeskey, S. W., L. Zhang, D. El-Ashry, B. J. Trock, C. A. Lopez, S. Kharbanda, et al. 1998. Tamoxifen-resistant FGF-transfected MCF-7 cells are cross-resistant in vivo to the antiestrogen, ICI 182,780 and two aromatase inhibitors. *Clin. Cancer Res.* **4**: 697–711.
191. Wakeling, A. E., M. Dukes, and J. Bowler. 1991. A potent specific pure antiestrogen with clinical potential. *Cancer Res.* **51**: 3867–3873.
192. Howell, A., S. Downey, and E. Anderson. 1996. New endocrine therapies for breast cancer. *Eur. J. Cancer* **32A**: 576–588.
193. Howell, A. and J. Robertson. 1995. Response to a specific antioestrogen (ICI 182780) in tamoxifen-resistant breast cancer. *Lancet* **345**: 989–990.
194. Kato, S., H. Endoh, H. Masuhiro, T. Kitamoto, S. Uchiyama, H. Sasaki, et al. 1995. Activation of the estrogen receptor through phosphorylation by mitogen-activated protein kinase. *Science* **270**: 1491–1494.
195. Katzenellenbogen, B. S., M. M. Montano, P. Le Goff, D. J. Schodin, W. L. Kraus, B. Bhardwaj, and N. Fujimoto. 1995. Antiestrogens: mechanisms and actions in target cells. *J. Steroid Biochem. Mol. Biol.* **53**: 387–393.
196. Bunone, G., P.-A. Briand, R. J. Miksicek, and D. Picard. 1996. Activation of the unliganded estrogen receptor by EGF involves the MAP kinase pathway and direct phosphorylation. *EMBO J.* **15**: 2174–2183.
197. Ignar-Trowbridge, D. M., M. Pimentel, M. G. Parker, J. A. Mclachlan, and K. S. Korach. 1996. Peptide growth factor cross-talk with the estrogen receptor requires the A/B domain and occurs independently of protein kinase C or estradiol. *Endocrinology* **137**: 1735–1744.
198. Ignar-Trowbridge, D. M., C. T. Teng, K. A. Ross, M. G. Parker, K. S. Korach, and J. A. Mclachlan. 1993. Peptide growth factors elicit estrogen receptor-dependent transcriptional activation of an estrogen-responsive element. *Mol. Endocrinol.* **7**: 992–998.
199. Pietras, R. J., J. Arboleda, D. M. Reese, N. Wongvipat, M. D. Pegram, L. Ramos, et al. 1995. HER-2 tyrosine kinase pathway targets estrogen receptor and promotes hormone-independent growth in human breast cancer cells. *Oncogene* **10**: 2435–2446.
200. Delli-Bovi, P., A. M. Curatola, K. M. Newman, Y. Sato, D. Moscatelli, R. M. Hewick, D. B. Rifkin, and C. Basilico. 1988. Processing, secretion, and biological properties of a novel growth factor of the fibroblast growth factor family with oncogenic potential. *Mol. Cell. Biol.* **8**: 2933–2941.
201. Thomas, K. A., M. Rios-Candelore, G. Gimenez-Gallego, S. DiSalvo, C. Bennett, J. Rodkey, and S. Fitzpatrick. 1985. Pure brain-derived acidic fibroblast growth factor is a potent angiogenic vascular endothelial cell mitogen with sequence homology to interleukin 1. *Proc. Natl. Acad. Sci. USA* **82**: 6409–6413.
202. Folkman, J. 1990. What is the evidence that tumors are angiogenesis dependent? *J. Natl. Cancer Inst.* **82**: 1–5.
203. Folkman, J., K. Watson, D. Ingber, and D. Hanahan. 1989. Induction of angiogenesis during the transition from hyperplasia to neoplasia. *Nature* **339**: 58–61.
204. Hanahan, D. and J. Folkman. 1996. Patterns and emerging mechanisms of the angiogenic switch during tumorigenesis. *Cell* **86**: 353–364.
205. McLeskey, S. W., L. Zhang, S. Kharbanda, Y. Liu, B. J. Trock, M. M. Gottardis, M. E. Lippman, and F. G. Kern. 1996. Effects of AGM-1470 and pentosan polysulfate on tumorigenicity and metastasis of FGF-transfected MCF-7 cells. *Br. J. Cancer* **73**: 1053–1062.

206. Zhang, L., S. Kharbanda, J. Hanfelt, and F. G. Kern. 1998. Both autocrine and paracrine effects of transfected acidic fibroblast growth factor are involved in the estrogen-independent and antiestrogen-resistant growth of MCF-7 breast cancer cells. *Cancer Res.* **58:** 352–361.

207. Holmgren, L., M. S. O'Reilly, and J. Folkman. 1995. Dormancy of micrometastases: balanced proliferation and apoptosis in the presence of angiogenesis suppression. *Nat. Med.* **1:** 149–153.

208. Lu, C. and N. Tanigawa. 1997. Spontaneous apoptosis is inversely related to intratumoral microvessel density in gastric carcinoma. *Cancer Res.* **57:** 221–224.

209. O'Reilly, M. S., L. Holmgren, C. Chen, and J. Folkman. 1996. Angiostatin induces and sustains dormancy of human primary tumors in mice. *Nat. Med.* **2:** 689–692.

210. Bullocks, J., L. Zhang, I. Y. F. Ding, S. W. McLeskey, C. A. Tobias, D. L. Miller, and F. G. Kern. 1997. Overexpression of vascular endothelial growth factor (VEGF) in MCF-7 breast carcinoma cells facilitates growth in tamoxifen-treated nude mice and tumor cell dissemination. *Proc. Am. Assoc. Cancer Res.* **38:** A3521(Abstract)

211. Macaulay, V. M., S. B. Fox, H. Zhang, R. M. Whitehouse, R. D. Leek, K. C. Gatter, R. Bicknell, and A. L. Harris. 1997. Breast cancer angiogenesis and tamoxifen resistance. *Endocr.-Related Cancer* **2:** 97–103.

212. Fox, S. B., R. D. Leek, M. P. Weekes, R. M. Whitehouse, K. C. Gatter, and A. L. Harris. 1995. Quantitation and prognostic value of breast cancer angiogenesis: comparison of microvessel density, Chalkley count, and computer image analysis. *J. Pathol.* **177:** 275–283.

213. Gasparini, G. and A. L. Harris. 1995. Clinical importance of the determination of tumor angiogenesis in breast carcinoma: much more than a new prognostic tool. *J. Clin. Oncol.* **13:** 765–782.

214. Weidner, N., J. P. Semple, W. R. Welch, and J. Folkman. 1991. Tumor angiogenesis and metastasis: correlation in invasive breast carcinoma. *N. Engl. J. Med.* **324:** 1–8.

215. Murakami, A., H. Tanaka, and A. Matzuzawa. 1990. Association of hst gene expression with metastatic phenotype in mouse mammary tumors. *Cell Growth Differ.* **1:** 225–231.

216. Kern, F. G., S. W. McLeskey, L. Zhang, J. Kurebayashi, Y. Liu, I. Y. F. Ding, et al. 1994. Transfected MCF-7 cells as a model for breast cancer progression. *Breast Cancer Res. Treatment* **31:** 153–165.

217. Kurebayashi, J., S. W. McLeskey, M. D. Johnson, M. E. Lippman, R. B. Dickson, and F. G. Kern. 1993. Quantitative demonstration of spontaneous metastasis by MCF-7 human breast cancer cells cotransfected with fibroblast growth factor 4 and lacZ. *Cancer Res.* **53:** 2178–2187.

218. McLeskey, S. W., L. Zhang, S. Kharbanda, J. Kurebayashi, M. E. Lippman, R. B. Dickson, and F. G. Kern. 1996. Fibroblast growth factor overexpressing breast carcinoma cells as models of angiogenesis and metastasis. *Breast Cancer Res. Treatment* **39:** 103–117.

219. Fox, S. B., R. D. Leek, J. Bliss, J. L. Mansi, B. Gusterson, K. C. Gatter, and A. L. Harris. 1997. Association of tumor angiogenesis with bone marrow micrometastases in breast cancer patients. *J. Natl. Cancer Inst.* **89:** 1044–1049.

220. Chen, C., S. Parangi, M. J. Tolentino, and J. Folkman. 1995. A strategy to discover circulating angiogenesis inhibitors generated by human tumors. *Cancer Res.* **55:** 4230–4233.

221. Folkman, J. 1995. Angiogenesis inhibitors generated by tumors. *Mol. Med.* **1:** 120–122.

222. O'Reilly, M. S., T. Boehm, Y. Shing, N. Fukai, G. Vasios, W. S. Lane, et al. 1997. Endostatin: an endogenous inhibitor of angiogenesis and tumor growth. *Cell* **88:** 277–285.

223. O'Reilly, M. S., L. Holmgren, Y. Shing, C. Chen, R. A. Rosenthal, M. Moses, et al. 1994. Angiostatin: a novel angiogenesis inhibitor that mediates the suppression of metastases by a Lewis lung carcinoma. *Cell* **79**: 315–328.

224. Zhang, L., S. Kharbanda, and F. G. Kern. 1996. Characterization of the metastatic properties of FGF-1 transfected MCF-7 breast cancer cells. *Proc. Am. Assoc. Cancer Res.* **37**: A418(Abstract)

225. Gasparini, G., M. Toi, M. Gion, P. Verderio, R. Dittadi, M. Hanatani, et al. 1997. Prognostic significance of vascular endothelial growth factor protein in node-negative breast carcinoma. *J. Natl. Cancer Inst.* **89**: 139–147.

226. Toi, M., S. Hoshina, T. Takayanagi, and T. Tominaga. 1994. Association of vascular endothelial growth factor expression with tumor angiogenesis and with early relapse in primary breast cancer. *Jpn. J. Cancer Res.* **85**: 1045–1049.

227. Toi, M., K. Inada, H. Suzuki, and T. Tominaga. 1995. Tumor angiogenesis in breast cancer: its importance as a prognostic indicator and the association with vascular endothelial growth factor expression. *Breast Cancer Res. Treatment* **36**: 193–204.

228. Lukas, J., J. Bartkova, and J. Bartek. 1996. Convergence of mitogenic signalling cascades from diverse classes of receptors at the cyclin D-cyclin-dependent kinase-pRB-controlled G1 checkpoint. *Mol. Cell. Biol.* **16**: 6917–6925.

229. Ishii, H., T. Yoshida, H. Oh, S. Yoshida, and M. Terada. 1995. A truncated K-sam product lacking the distal carboxyl-terminal portion provides a reduced level of autophosphorylation and greater resistance against induction of differentiation. *Mol. Cell. Biol.* **15**: 3664–3671.

230. Shaoul, E., R. Reich-Slotky, B. Berman, and D. Ron. 1995. Fibroblast growth factor receptors display both common and distinct signaling pathways. *Oncogene* **10**: 1553–1561.

231. Wang, J.-K., G. Gao, and M. Goldfarb. 1994. Fibroblast growth factor receptors have different signaling and mitogenic potentials. *Mol. Cell. Biol.* **14**: 181–188.

232. Fantl, W. J., D. E. Johnson, and L. T. Williams. 1993. Signalling by receptor tyrosine kinases. *Annu. Rev. Biochem.* **62**: 453–481.

233. Kavanaugh, W. M. and L. T. Williams. 1994. An alternative to SH2 domains for binding tyrosine-phosphorylated proteins. *Science* **266**: 1862–1865.

234. Mohammadi, M., I. Dikic, A. Sorokin, W. H. Burgess, M. Jaye, and J. Schlessinger. 1996. Identification of six novel autophosphorylation sites on fibroblast growth factor receptor 1 and elucidation of their importance in receptor activation and signal transduction. *Mol. Cell. Biol.* **16**: 977–989.

235. Mohammadi, M., C. A. Dionne, W. Li, N. Li, T. Spivak, A. M. Honegger, M. Jaye, and J. Schlessinger. 1992. Point mutation in FGF receptor eliminates phosphatidylinositol hydrolysis without affecting mitogenesis. *Nature* **358**: 681–684.

236. Peters, K. G., J. Marie, E. Wilson, H. E. Ives, J. Escobedo, M. Del Rosario, D. Mirda, and L. T. Williams. 1992. Point mutation of an FGF receptor abolishes phosphatidylinositol turnover and Ca2+ flux but not mitogenesis. *Nature* **358**: 678–681.

237. Ward, C. W., K. H. Gough, M. Rashke, S. S. Wan, G. Tribbick, and J. Wang. 1996. Systematic mapping of potential binding sites for Shc and Grb2 SH2 domains on insulin receptor substrate-1 and the receptors for insulin, epidermal growth factor, platelet-derived growth factor, and fibroblast growth factor. *J. Biol. Chem.* **271**: 5603–5609.

238. Friesel, R. E. and T. Maciag. 1995. Molecular mechanisms of angiogenesis: fibroblast growth factor signal transduction. *FASEB J.* **9**: 919–925.

239. MacNichol, A. M., A. J. Muslin, and L. T. Williams. 1993. Raf-1 kinase is essential for early xenopus development and mediates the induction of mesoderm by FGF. *Cell* **73**: 571–583.

240. Morrison, D. K., D. R. Kaplan, U. Rapp, and T. M. Roberts. 1988. Signal transduction from membrane to cytoplasm: growth factors and membrane-bound oncogene products increase Raf-1 phosphorylation and associated protein kinase activity. *Proc. Natl. Acad. Sci. USA* **85:** 8855–8859.

241. Newberry, E. P., D. Willis, T. Latifi, J. M. Boudreaux, and D. A. Towler. 1997. Fibroblast growth factor receptor signaling activates the human interstitial collagenase promoter via the bipartite Ets-AP1 element. *Mol. Endocrinol.* **11:** 1129–1144.

242. Vainikka, S., V. Joukov, S. Wennstrom, M. Bergman, P. G. Pelicci, and K. Alitalo. 1994. Signal transduction by fibroblast growth factor receptor-4 (FGFR-4). Comparison with FGFR-1. *J. Biol. Chem.* **269:** 18,320–18,326.

243. Wood, K. W., C. Sarnecki, T. M. Roberts, and J. Blenis. 1992. Ras mediates nerve growth factor receptor modulation of three signal-transducing protein kinases: MAP kinase, Raf-1 and RSK. *Cell* **68:** 1041–1050.

244. Klint, P., S. Kanda, and L. Claesson-Welsh. 1995. Shc and a novel 89-kda component couple to the Grb2-Sos complex in fibroblast growth factor-2-stimulated cells. *J. Biol. Chem.* **270:** 23,337–23,344.

245. Kouhara, H., Y. R. Hadari, T. Spivak-Kroizman, J. Schilling, D. Bar-Sagi, and J. Schlessinger. 1997. A lipid-anchored Grb2-binding protein that links FGF-receptor activation to the Ras/MAPK signaling pathway. *Cell* **89:** 693–702.

246. Ong, S. H., K. C. Goh, Y. P. Lim, B. C. Low, P. Klint, L. Claesson-Welsh, et al. 1996. Suc1-associated neurotrophic factor target (SNT) protein is a major FGF-stimulated tyrosine phosphorylated 90-kDa protein which binds to the SH2 domain of GRB2. *Biochem. Biophys. Res. Commun.* **225:** 1021–1026.

247. Wang, J.-K., H. Xu, H.-C. Li, and M. Goldfarb. 1996. Broadly expressed SNT-like proteins link FGF receptor stimulation to activators of Ras. *Oncogene* **13:** 721–729.

248. Oldham, S. M., G. J. Clark, L. M. Gangarosa, R. J. Coffey, Jr., and C. J. Der. 1996. Activation of the Raf-1/MAP kinase cascade is not sufficient for Ras transformation of RIE-1 epithelial cells. *Proc. Natl. Acad. Sci. USA* **93:** 6924–6928.

249. Burgering, B. M. and P. J. Coffer. 1995. Protein kinase B (c-Akt) in phosphatidylinositol-3-OH kinase signal transduction. *Nature* **376:** 599–602.

250. Franke, T. F., D. R. Kaplan, L. C. Cantley, and A. Toker. 1997. Direct regulation of the Akt proto-oncogene product by phosphatidylinositol-3,4-bisphosphate. *Science* **275:** 666–668.

251. Klippel, A., W. M. Kavanaugh, D. Pot, and L. T. Williams. 1997. A specific product of phosphatidylinositol 3-kinase directly activates the protein kinase Akt through its pleckstrin homology domain. *Mol. Cell. Biol.* **17:** 338–344.

252. Dudek, H., S. R. Datta, T. F. Franke, M. J. Birnbaum, R. Yao, G. M. Cooper, et al. 1997. Regulation of neuronal survival by the serine-threonine protein kinase Akt. *Science* **275:** 661–665.

253. Franke, T. F., D. R. Kaplan, and L. C. Cantley. 1997. PI3K: downstream AKTion blocks apoptosis. *Cell* **88:** 435–437.

254. Rodriguez-Viciana, P., P. H. Warne, A. Khwaja, B. M. Marte, D. Pappin, P. Das, M. D. Waterfield, and J. Downward. 1997. Role of phosphoinositide 3-OH kinase in cell transformation and control of the actin cytoskeleton by Ras. *Cell* **89:** 457–467.

255. Khosravi-Far, R., P. A. Solski, G. J. Clark, M. S. Kinch, and C. J. Der. 1995. Activation of Rac1, RhoA, and mitogen-activated protein kinases is required for Ras transformation. *Mol. Cell. Biol.* **15:** 6443–6453.

256. Prendergast, G. C., R. Khosravi-Far, P. A. Solski, H. Kurzawa, P. F. Lebowitz, and C. J. Der. 1995. Critical role of Rho in cell transformation by oncogenic Ras. *Oncogene* **10:** 2289–2296.

257. Qiu, R. G., J. Chen, D. Kirn, F. McCormick, and M. Symons. 1995. An essential role for Rac in Ras transformation. *Nature* **374:** 457–459.

258. Qiu, R. G., J. Chen, F. McCormick, and M. Symons. 1995. A role for Rho in Ras transformation. *Proc. Natl. Acad. Sci. USA* **92:** 11,781–11,785.

259. Logan, A. and S. D. Logan. 1991. Studies on the mechanisms of signalling and inhibition by pertussis toxin of fibroblast growth factor-stimulated mitogenesis in Balb/c 3T3 cells. *Cell Signal.* **3:** 215–223.

260. Jarvis, M. F., G. W. Gessner, G. E. Martin, M. Jaye, M. W. Ravera, and C. A. Dionne. 1992. Characterization of [^{125}I]acidic fibroblast growth factor binding to the cloned human fibroblast growth factor receptor, FGF-flg, on NIH 3T3 cell membranes: inhibitory effects of heparin, pertussis toxin and guanine nucleotides. *J. Pharmacol. Exp. Ther.* **263:** 253–263.

261. Landgren, E., P. Blume-Jensen, S. A. Courtneidge, and L. Claesson-Welsh. 1995. Fibroblast growth factor receptor-1 regulation of src family kinases. *Oncogene* **10:** 2027–2035.

262. Yayon, A., Y. S. Ma, M. Safran, M. Klagsbrun, and R. Halaban. 1997. Suppression of autocrine cell proliferation and tumorigenesis of human melanoma cells and fibroblast growth factor transformed fibroblasts by a kinase-deficient FGF receptor 1: evidence for the involvement of Src-family kinases. *Oncogene* **14:** 2999–3009.

263. Campbell, D. H., A. de Fazio, R. L. Sutherland, and R. J. Daly. 1996. Expression and tyrosine phosphorylation of EMS1 in human breast cancer cell lines. *Int. J. Cancer* **68:** 485–492.

264. Plopper, G. E., H. P. McNamee, L. E. Dike, K. Bojanowski, and D. E. Ingber. 1995. Convergence of integrin and growth factor receptor signaling pathways within the focal adhesion complex. *Mol. Biol. Cell* **6:** 1349–1365.

4

Transforming Growth Factor-β and Breast Cancer

Katri M. Koli and Carlos L. Arteaga

1. INTRODUCTION

Transforming growth factor-βs (TGF-βs) and their receptor proteins are produced by most cell types. Signals generated by TGF-β receptor-ligand interactions are involved in cell-growth regulation, development, morphogenesis, chemotaxis, and connective-tissue and extracellular-matrix production *(1–3)*. TGF-β inhibits the growth of mammary epithelial cells and acts as an autocrine growth regulator. In stepwise tumor progression, the loss of TGF-β responsiveness is thought to be a critical event in breast tumorigenesis. However, several carcinoma cells, although not always growth-inhibited by exogenous TGF-β, may still exhibit modulation of their proteolytic and/or adhesive activities by added ligand. Often during breast cancer progression, tumor cells produce enhanced amount of TGF-βs, which may provide an, albeit indirect, positive growth effect through enhanced angiogenesis, decreased host immune function, increase peritumoral-stroma formation, and cell adhesion. The cumulative data on this field suggest that the net effect of tumor cell TGF-βs on the progression of breast carcinoma depends on the balance between the TGF-βs-mediated autocrine growth inhibition of mammary tumor cells and the effects of the TGF-βs on the host which indirectly foster tumor progression.

2. TGF-β

TGF-βs and receptor proteins are produced ubiquitously by various normal and malignant cells *(4–6)*. The biologically active 25-kDa TGF-β1 is composed of two identical 112 amino-acid polypeptides each containing nine cysteines, of which seven are well-conserved. Eight of these cysteines form a rigid structure known as the cysteine knot, whereas the ninth cysteine forms an interchain disulfide bond with the corresponding residue in the other polypeptide monomer chain. This conserved structure is characteristic to all of the five members of the TGF-β family. Three of them, the mammalian TGF-β1, TGF-β2, and TGF-β3 are found in mammals; TGF-β4 was isolated from chicken *(7)*, and TGF-β5 from Xenopus *(8)*. The three mammalian TGF-β isoforms are products of different genes, but overall exhibit similar biological activity in vitro. Despite a high degree of functional similarity in vitro between the TGF-β isoforms, targeted disruption of the TGF-β1 *(9,10)*, TGF-β2 *(11)*, and TGF-β3 *(12,13)* genes in mice has revealed different phenotypes, suggesting isoform-specific activities in vivo.

From: Breast Cancer: *Molecular Genetics, Pathogenesis, and Therapeutics*
Edited by: *A. M. Bowcock © Humana Press Inc., Totowa, NJ*

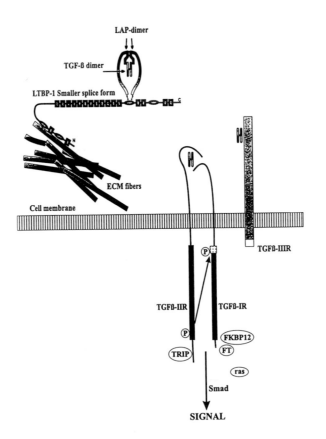

Fig. 1. Structures of large latent TGF-β and the heteromeric TGF-β receptor complexes. TGF-β itself is a 25-kDa dimer held together by a disulfide bond. The latency-associated protein (LAP) is dimerized as well and remains associated with the TGF-β dimer forming the small latent complex. The latent TGF-β binding protein (LTBP) covalently associates with the LAP region of the latent TGF-β complex forming the large latent complex *(15)*. This large latent complex is frequently associated with the ECM and activation of this complex is required to release biologically active TGF-β dimers. The type I and II TGF-β receptors contain serine/threonine kinases in their intracytoplasmic domain. Upon ligand binding, the type-II receptor serine/threonine kinase phosphorylates the type I receptor. The role of TRIP (TGF-β-receptor interacting protein-1), FKBP12, FT (farnesyl transferase) and ras in the transduction of TGF-β mediated signals is still unclear. Smad proteins have recently been identified as intracellular mediators of TGF-β signals. The main function of the type II TGF-β receptor (TGF-IIIR) appears to be in ligand presentation for the signaling receptors *(4,47)*.

2.1. Latent TGF-β Complexes

TGF-βs are usually synthesized and secreted in a latent form (Fig. 1). The TGF-β preproprotein consists of two disulfide-bridged 390–412-amino-acid polypeptide chains, each containing several glycosylation sites and a mannose-6-phosphate receptor-binding site. The precursor structure is shared by members of the TGF-β superfamily and it seems to be essential for the folding and transport of the latent complex. The carboxy-terminal region, representing the mature TGF-β, is cleaved between two arginine residues. The amino-terminal peptide, also called latency-associated protein

(LAP), remains associated with the mature growth factor via noncovalent interactions and is able to render TGF-β latent. The TGF-β protein associated with the LAP is frequently called the small latent complex *(14)*.

Additional proteins are associated with small latent TGF-β to yield large latent complexes (Fig. 1). Latent TGF-β binding protein-1 (LTBP-1), first identified from platelets, binds to LAP covalently by its third 8-cystein repeat *(15)*. The size of LTBP-1 secreted by cultured fibroblasts is 190 kDa, whereas the platelet form appears to be smaller (125–160 kDa), evidently owing to proteolytic processing. LTBP-1 is involved in the secretion of TGF-β and it appears to have a function in the targeting of the latent complexes to extracellular matrix (ECM) *(14,16)*. TGF-β and LTBP-1 are both coregulated in several cell systems; in fibroblasts the assembly and secretion of properly disulfide-bonded TGF-β is dependent on LTBP-1 *(17)*. It has been proposed that LTBP-1 plays a role in the activation process of TGF-β *(18)*. At least two additional LTBPs have been cloned *(19–21)*. These all share a similar domain structure with LTBP-1.

2.2. Activation of TGF-β

Activation of TGF-β comprises a sequence of biochemical events leading to the release of an active TGF-β dimer. In the absence of activation, latent TGF-β forms produced my most cells are not able to interact with cell surface receptors. The interaction between TGF-β and LAP is noncovalent and can be disrupted in vitro by extremes of pH, chaotropic agents, certain glycosidases, or heat treatment *(22)*. The acidic environment in bone tissue and in healing wounds might trigger the release of mature TGF-β, but mechanisms involving proteolysis are more likely to operate in vivo. Several proteases including plasmin, thrombin, and cathepsin D are able to release latent complexes from extracellular matrices and enhance TGF-β activation *(23,24)*. It has also been reported that γ-irradiation specifically generates active TGF-β in the murine mammary gland (Barcellos-Hoff et al., 1994). γ-irradiation generates reactive oxygen species, which were shown to activate latent TGF-β in vitro providing a redox-mediated mechanism of activation *(26)*.

The large latent complex is targeted to the ECM via LTBP *(16)*. LTBP then associates with extracellular fibers morphologically indistinguishable from those of fibronectin-collagen fibers in the pericellular matrix of cultured fibroblasts *(27)*. The amino terminal region of LTBP is involved in this covalent binding *(15)*. Inhibition of LTBP with antibodies or addition of excess free LTBP can inhibit the activation of TGF-β in cocultures of bovine endothelial cells and smooth-muscle cells *(18)*. Evidence for plasmin-mediated activation has been found in many experimental systems *(23,28,29)*. Inhibition of plasmin-mediated proteolysis or transglutaminase prevents the production of active TGF-β *(30)*. Cell-cell contacts and targeting of TGF-β and other factors involved in the activation process seem to be crucial for the production of active TGF-β in the coculture system. The retinoid-induced activation of TGF-β in bovine endothelial cells is also mediated through an increase in plasmin-mediated proteolysis *(31)*. Plasmin, a broad-spectrum serine protease, can cleave LAP and disrupt the interactions between mature TGF-β and LAP *(28)*. The reaction is self-limiting, because TGF-β induces the production of a plasminogen-activator inhibitor (PAI-1), which decreases the formation of active plasmin *(32)*. Vitamin D can also induce the production of active TGF-β in human and murine keratinocytes, but this activation does not seem to be plasmin-mediated because the production and secretion of plasminogen-activator activity decreases rapidly after the addition of vitamin D *(33,34)*. These observations have suggested the use of antibodies against specific regions of the mature protein in conjunction with LAP-specific antibodies to address activation of TGF-β in tissues. Elevated immunoreactivity with mature TGF-β-specific antibodies coupled with loss of LAP immunoreactivity and simultaneous spatial upregulation of a known TGF-β target in those same tissues would serve as reasonable indicators of TGF-β activation *in situ* during physiological and/or pathological processes *(35)*.

Thrombospondin, a platelet α-granule and ECM protein, binds active TGF-β and activates latent TGF-β forms through cell- and protease-independent mechanisms *(36)*. Type-1 repeats of thrombospondin have been found to be the part of the molecule responsible for the binding and activation of TGF-β *(37)*. Despite the general consensus of the importance of post-translational control mechanisms to regulate TGF-β actions *in situ*, little is known about the physiological mechanisms of activation in benign and malignant processes affecting the mammary gland.

2.3. TGF-β Receptor Signaling

Three major cell-surface receptors that bind TGF-β have been identified and named type-I, -II, and -III receptors *(38–40)*. TGFβ-IIIR is a proteoglycan also known as betaglycan, which most likely functions as a storage protein as well as in the presentation of ligand to the signaling type-II and -I receptors *(41)*. TGFβ-IR *(42)* and TGFβ-IIR *(43)* are transmembrane serine/threonine kinases directly involved in signal transduction (Fig. 1). Several different receptor complexes can bind TGF-β *in vitro*, but so far only TGFβ-IR/IIR complexes have been shown to induce TGF-β signals *(44)*. TGFβ-IIR is constitutively phosphorylated in the absence of ligand and this phosphorylation is not altered by exogenous TGF-β binding *(45)*. It is believed that TGF-IIR binds ligand first and determines the ligand specificity of the complex. TGFβ-IR, which alone cannot bind TGF-β, is then recruited to a heteromeric complex, most likely containing several receptor molecules *(46,47)*. A ligand-dependent phosphorylation of the (GS) domain of TGFβ-IR by TGFβ-IIR is required for signal propagation and leads to the activation of downstream signaling *(45,48)*. The effects of TGF-β on growth and ECM production can be uncoupled and the functional contribution to these effects by type-I and -II receptors is under investigation *(49,50)*.

Several proteins that associate with the intracellular domains of the signaling receptors have been identified, but their role in signal propagation is still open. FKBP-12 and farnesyl transferase bind to the cytoplasmic domain of TGFβ-IR *(51,52)*. Chen et al. *(53)* reported a (WD)-domain-containing protein named TRIP-1 (TGF-β-receptor interacting protein-1) that associates with TGFβ-IIR and is phosphorylated by the receptor kinase. A new family of proteins called Mads (Mothers against dpp) has recently been shown to mediate signal transduction by TGF-β receptors *(54)*. Smad2 and Smad3 are closely related and, in association with DPC4, have been implicated as mediators of activin and TGF-β responses *(55–57)*. Smad3 interacts directly with the receptor complex and when overexpressed induces TGF-β-like responses in the absence of ligand *(58)*. Recently, Nakao et al. *(59)* demonstrated that TGF-β induces phosphorylation and nuclear localization of Smad2 protein in mink lung epithelial cells.

TGF-β arrests cell growth in the G_1-phase of the cell cycle and most probably affects multiple signaling pathways *(5,40)*. TGF-β has been shown to retain the retinoblastoma susceptibility gene (pRb) in a hypophosphorylated form, which prevents cells from traversing the G_1/S boundary *(60)*. By regulating the formation of Cdk- cyclin complexes and their inhibitor levels, TGF-β contributes to the accumulation of hypophosphorylated pRb *(61)*. In several cell lines, TGF-β1 also induces rapid downregulation of c-*myc* expression *(62,63)*, suggesting this as an additional mechanism by which these peptides potently suppress epithelial-cell proliferation.

3. TGF-β EXPRESSION IN BREAST EPITHELIAL CELLS

Normal and tumorigenic human-breast epithelial cells in culture express TGF-β1 mRNA and secrete receptor-reactive TGF-β activity into their medium *(64,65,73)*. In one study, steady state levels of TGF-β1 mRNA were grossly similar in a panel of normal and tumor breast epithelial cells *(64)*. We have measured secreted TGF-β activity in conditioned medium from a panel of nontumor and tumor, both estrogen receptor (ER)-positive and ER-negative, human-breast cell lines using a ^{125}I-TGF-β1 radioreceptor assay. In this assay, TGF-β1 and TGF-β2 are equipotent in displacing ^{125}I-TGF-β1 binding *(66)*. In all cell lines examined, TGF-β activity was only detectable by this assay after transient acidification of conditioned medium, suggesting that cultured cells mainly secrete inactive TGF-β and/or that they rapidly internalize it upon activation at the cell surface. In general, the more tumorigenic hormone-independent, ER-negative tumor lines secrete higher levels of TGF-β activity than the estrogen-dependent, ER-positive tumor and nontumorigenic cell lines *(67)*. Baillie et al. *(68)* studied the secretion and content of immunoreactive TGF-β forms in homogeneates from breast tumors and normal peritumoral tissues. By immunological methods, a 50-kDa biologically active TGF-β1 form was more frequently detected in peritumoral tissues compared to tumor homogeneates and in ER-negative vs ER-positive tumors, suggesting that peritumoral tissues are the target for TGF-βs and that these peptides are probably expressed/secreted in excess by the more malignant hormone-independent breast carcinomas than the ER-positive tumors.

Other studies with mammary tumor cell lines suggest changes in expression levels of TGF-βs induced by the presence of ECM and/or culture conditions. TGF-β1 mRNA was readily detectable in MDA-231 breast-cancer cells growing as monolayer. The steady-state mRNA level was not significantly changed by treating the cells with recombinant TGF-β1. In contrast, TGF-β1 mRNA level was much lower in cells growing as tridimensional spheroids and was highly inducible by exogenous TGF-β1 *(69)*. Using mammary epithelial cells, Streuli et al. *(70)* reported marked induction of the TGF-β1 promoter when cells were grown in plastic in the absence of a basement membrane. In contrast, transcription from the TGF-β1 promoter was suppressed when the cells were in contact with endogenously- synthesized or exogenous basement membrane. On the other hand, TGF-β2 mRNA levels were the same in either substratum *(70)*. These reports indicate that TGF-β1 expression can change dramatically depending on intercellular spacial orientation and perhaps tissue architecture, and raise questions about the biological implications derived from TGF-β expression data obtained with cultured cell systems.

Few studies have examined expression of all three TGF-β isoforms systematically in mammary-tumor cell lines or tissues. In one study, coexpression of TGF-β1, -β2, and -β3 mRNA transcripts was not present in all of four breast-cancer cell lines examined *(71)*. This information might be relevant to tumor/host cell paracrine interactions since TGF-β2 binds with a lower affinity to the TGF-βIIR than TGF-β1 and TGF-β3 *(72)*. In a survey by MacCallum et al., most of 50 breast-cancer specimens expressed the mRNA for at least one isoform of TGF-β (90% for TGF-β1, 78% for -β2, and 94% for -β3) but there were different patterns of mRNA expression among individual tumors *(74)*. Barrett-Lee et al. reported TGF-β1 mRNA expression in 69/69 breast carcinomas and 20/20 nonneoplastic mammary tissues but the levels were clearly higher in the tumor specimens *(75)*. Several epidemiological studies have confirmed predominant staining of malignant mammary epithelia with TGF-β1, -β2, and/or -β3 antibodies as well as *in situ* hybridization with RNA probes relative to nontransformed epithelia, myoepithelial cells and stromal elements *(76–80)*. The *in situ* targets of these tumor-associated ligands, as determined by TGF-β receptor studies, have not been addressed and at this time remain unclear.

4. ROLE IN NORMAL MAMMARY EPITHELIUM DEVELOPMENT AND FUNCTION

The growth of ductal structures of the mammary gland is tightly controlled in different stages of breast development. During puberty and sexual maturation, significant elongation and branching of ductal epithelium takes place, and a patterning with typical interductal spaces is formed. During pregnancy, further ductal outgrowth and formation of secretory alveoli generates the lactating phenotype. After weaning, the secretory tissue degenerates and the mammary gland reverts to a state similar to that of a virgin gland. This highly regulated balance between proliferation, differentiation, and regression (apoptosis) requires fine control by hormones and growth factors, as well as cross talk between epithelial cells and stromal fibroblasts of the mammary gland.

TGF-β isoforms are expressed in a developmentally regulated manner in the mammary gland within the epithelium of actively growing mammary end buds during branching morphogenesis *(81)*. By immunohistochemistry, the mature peptides are located in the stroma but not in front of the advancing end buds, thus preventing lateral ductal branching and modulating gland formation (*82* and references therein). A complex epithelium-matrix interaction resulting in TGF-β activation might also be involved in the regulation of ductal outgrowth *(83)*. Exogenous TGF-βs have potent effects in the mouse mammary gland. Slow-release TGF-β1, -β2, and -β3 pellets result in inhibition of mammary-duct elongation, rapid involution of ductal end buds, and localized matrix deposition at the alveolar bud tips *(82)*. TGF-β3 is the only isoform detected in mouse mammary myoepithelial cells. The expression of all three TGF-βs is markedly downregulated during lactation.

Transgenic mice overexpressing constitutively active TGF-β1 in the mammary gland under the control of the (mouse mammary tumor virus [MMTV]/LTR) promoter enhancer exhibit severe ductal epithelial hypoplasia and ductal hypoproliferation *in situ*. For these studies, the cysteine residues in positions 223 and 225 within the proregion of the TGF-β1 precursor were changed to serine codons, thus resulting in production of an active TGF-β1 protein unable to acquire a latent conformation *(84)*. Of note, overexpression of the wild-type and therefore latent TGF-β1 protein resulted in no evident mammary phenotype, underscoring the essential regulatory control of TGF-β actions by activation *in situ*. However, active (mutant) TGF-β1 overexpression did not not inhibit mammary development during pregnancy, and alveolar differentiation and lactation proceeded normally in these transgenic mice *(84)*. If TGF-β1 expression is driven under the whey-acidic protein (WAP)-promoter, which targets transgene expression to the pregnant mammary gland, alveolar development and lactation are both inhibited *(85)*. TGF-β might function to limit the accumulation of milk proteins in pregnancy since the expression of TGF-β2 and -β3 is increased during pregnancy but decreases dramatically at the onset of lactation *(85,86)*. In a subsequent study, transplantation of WAP-TGF-β1 mammary glands from young post-pubertal virgin females into nonpregnant hosts revealed that the transgenic implants had a reduced ability to repopulate epithelium-free mammary fat pads, suggesting that the ectopic expression of TGF-β1 not only impairs lobular progenitors but also promotes early senescence of those stem cells committed to ductal formation *(87)*.

5. ROLE OF THE TGFB AUTOCRINE PATHWAY IN TUMOR INHIBITION AND RESPONSE TO ANTIESTROGENS

5.1. Autocrine Growth Inhibition of Breast Carcinoma Cells by TGF-β

Several studies indicate that breast epithelial cell TGF-βs are autocrine regulators of tumor and nontumor mammary-cell proliferation. Exogenous TGF-β1 and -β2 inhibit the growth of normal human mammary epithelial cells and, to a lesser degree, several breast-carcinoma cell lines in culture *(73,88–92)*. Several reports indicate this growth inhibition follows arrest in G1 mediated by different biochemical signals. In the 184 human mammary cell line derived from reduction mammoplasty tissue, TGF-β1 increases mRNA and protein stability of the Cdk inhibitor p15. p15, in turn, associates with cdk4, disrupts cdk4/cyclin D1 complexes, which are necessary for the G1 to S transition, and induces G1 arrest. In the TGF-β-resistant 184A1L5 subline, although the p15 mRNA was increased, the p15 protein was not stabilized and the cdk4/cyclin E association was not inhibited *(93)*. Iavarone and Masague *(94)* recently reported p15-independent cell-cycle arrest mediated by TGF-β in MCF-10A human mammary epithelial cells. This cell has a normal phenotype but lacks p15 and p16. TGF-β repressed the expression of the Cdk tyrosine phosphatase Cdc25A, thus enhancing the tyrosine phosphorylation of Cdk4 and Cdk6 and inhibiting their kinase activity *(94)*. In MCF-7 human breast-cancer cells, TGF-β1 has been shown to induce cell-cycle arrest in G1, inhibition of Cdk2 kinase activity, and nuclear accumulation of p21[WAF1/CIP1] *(95,96)*.

In some cases the growth-inhibitory effect of TGF-β1 is dominant over the growth-promoting effect of carcinogens or oncogenes as reported by Pierce et al. *(96a)*. In one of these studies, transgenic mice were generated by injecting embryos with a constitutively active mutant TGF-β1 gene under the control of the MMTV promoter/enhancer *(84)*. Tissue-specific expression of the transgene in mouse mammary glands resulted in marked ductal hypoplasia, suppression of ductal branching, and a concordant reduction of bromodeoxyuridine labeling in mammary epithelium. In a subsequent study, MMTV/(mutant) TGF-β1 transgenic mouse were resistant to 7,12-dimethyl benzanthracene (DMBA)-induced breast tumorigenesis. When cross-bred with MMTV/TGFα mice, the double-transgenic animals (MMTV/TGF-β1 and MMTV/TGFα) failed to develop TGFα induced mammary hyperplasia or carcinomas while maintaining the TGF-β1 hypoplastic phenotype *(96a)*. Because the MMTV promoter, driving transcription of the mutant TGF-β1 transgene, was constitutively expressed, this apparent protection from carcinogenesis may mainly reflect the drastically reduced mammary-epithelial population at risk for transformation but may not necessarily address the net effect of TGF-β1 on a fully developed mammary epithelium subjected to the same transforming events.

In addition to a direct inhibitory effect by exogenous TGF-βs, tumor-cell proliferation is temporally associated with lower levels of TGF-β expression and/or secretion. For example, growth stimulation of hormone-dependent breast-cancer cells with either estradiol *(71,97)* or the testosterone-derivative norethindrone *(98)* downregulates TGF-β2 and -β3 mRNAs, whereas TGF-β1 expression is not altered. On the other hand, growth inhibition of these cells with the antiestrogens tamoxifen *(89)* or toremifene *(99)* and the progestin analog gestodene *(100)* is associated with enhanced expression of TGF-β1 mRNA and/or secretion of TGF-β protein. In the latter study, gestodene-mediated growth inhibition was partially blocked with an antiserum that neutralizes TGF-β1 and -β2 *(100)*, suggesting the TGF-βs mediated growth inhibition. Vitamin D_3 and potent growth inhibitory analogs induce TGF-β1 mRNA and protein as well as latent TGF-β binding protein in the vitamin D_3-sensitive BT-20 breast cancer line *(101)*. In another study, anti-TGF-β1 and -β2 neutralizing antisera markedly stimulated the proliferation of ER-negative MDA-231 and HS578T cell lines while upregulating endogenous TGF-β binding sites and decreasing TGF-β1 steady-state mRNA levels *(102)*, supporting at least in cell culture an operative TGF-β-mediated growth-control autocrine pathway. The significance of these in vitro data is questioned by the fact that neutralizing anti-TGFβ antibodies do not enhance MDA-231 tumor growth in nude mice *(103)*. Furthermore, systemic administration of recombinant TGF-β1 to athymic mice bearing MDA-231 tumors, at doses that induced marked toxic effects in host tissues, did not inhibit MDA-231 xenografts *(104)*.

5.2. Mechanisms of Resistance to TGF-β Induced Growth Arrest

Escape from TGF-β autocrine growth control is a common phenomenon in tumor progression. Because TGF-β responsiveness correlates with TGFβ-IIR levels, *(105,106)* attention has been given to mutational changes or deletions of TGFβ-IIR in cancer cells. In colon and gastric cancers with microsatellite instability, TGFβ-IIR mutations in the polyadenine tract are common *(107–109)*. In squamous carcinomas of the head and neck, point mutations in the kinase domain have been reported *(110)*. Futhermore, T-cell malignancies, retinoblastomas, prostate carcinoma, and other neoplasms exhibit mutations in the TGFβ-IIR gene and/or loss of receptor expression, resulting in aberrant TGF-β responsiveness and potentially contributing to tumor progression *(111–114)*.

Loss of autocrine TGF-β-mediated growth regulation has also been proposed as a critical event in breast tumorigenesis. Sun et al., by re-expressing the type-II TGF-β receptor by transfection into MCF-7 cells, reduced the ability of these cells to form tumors in athymic mice *(105)*. Chen et al. *(115)* transfected a tetracycline-repressible type-III TGF-β receptor-expression vector into MCF-7 cells and observed enhanced binding to TGFβ-IR and TGFβ-IIR as well as markedly reduced growth in vitro, suggesting that post-receptor signaling mechanisms had remained intact in these tumor cells. No experiments in mice were reported with this study. Benzopyrene-immortalized nontumorigenic human-breast epithelial cells from reduction mammoplasty tissue can be selected in culture for TGF-β1 resistance . Different to the MCF-7 breast-cancer cells transfected by Sun et al. *(105)*, these resistant sublines still exhibit TGF-β1 binding, suggesting defects in post-binding signal transduction as a mechanim for the lack of TGF-β response and that these defects can occur early before the acquisition of a fully tumorigenic phenotype *(88)*. Younes et al. recently reported the expression of TGF-β type II receptor (IIR) in 111 cases of invasive breast carcinoma as detected by immunohistochemistry *(116)*. Staining for TGFβ-IIR was negative or present in <10% of the tumor cells in 103 of 111 (93%) tissue sections. Only 3% had >50% of tumor cells exhibiting TGFβ-IIR positivity. Unfortunately, most stromal cells and benign adjacent epithelial cells, putative TGF-β targets and potential internal controls for this survey, were also negative or weakly positive for TGFβ-IIR staining thus not allowing for comparisons between tumor and nontumor compartments *(116)*.

Although TGF-β receptor signaling and cell-cycle regulatory molecules are altered in some breast carcinomas *(40)*, some highly tumorigenic breast-cancer cells in culture do retain sensitivity to TGF-βs in vitro. In general estrogen receptor-positive breast carcinoma cell lines lose sensitivity more often owing to inadequate TGFβ-IIR expression, whereas most estrogen receptor-negative cell lines express TGFβ-IIR and retain a low level of sensitivity to added ligand *(117)*. The mutations in the TGFβ-IIR gene reported in other tumor systems have not been found in several human-breast carcinoma cell lines, suggesting other mechanisms to explain TGF-β resistance *(118)*. In MCF-7 cells that lack membrane TGFβ-IIR, a cytosolic pool of receptors has been described *(128)*. The inability of cells to localize a functional receptor to the plasma membrane appears to result in TGF-β insensitivity. Interestingly, exogenous agents that induce differentiation restored the trafficking of TGFβ-IIR to the cell surface as well as TGF-β response *(128)*, suggesting this defect in trafficking is owing to a phenotypic rather than a genetic alteration.

In addition to defects in TGFβ-IR, unresponsiveness to TGF-β can result from aberrant post- receptor intracellular signaling. The recently identified DPC4 protein has been found to be inactive in 48% of pancreatic carcinomas *(119)* as well as in a cohort of breast and ovarian cancers. The human breast carcinoma cell line MDA-MB468 exhibits adequate levels of cell surface TGFβ-IIR and a deletion of the DPC4 gene. Responsiveness to TGF-β is restored by transfection of a functional DPC4 expression vector *(56)*.

More recent data from in vivo experiments suggest an alternative role for breast tumor cell TGF-β receptors: in some scenarios, these molecules may be involved in tumor/host interactions that are deleterious to the host. Guise et al. developed a nude mouse model in which MDA-231 human breast-cancer cells form bone metastases, secrete parathyroid hormone-related protein (PTHrP), and induce hypercalcemia, osteolysis, and early host death *(120)*. TGF-β is abundantly present in bone matrix and enhances PTHrP expression by breast-cancer cells *(121,122)*. These data lead to the hypothesis that metastatic breast tumor cells in bone exhibit functional TGF-β receptors that respond to bone-derived TGF-β by secreting enhanced levels of PTHrP. PTHrP, in turn, increases osteolysis and induces further release of TGF-β from bone matrix. To test this hypothesis, MDA-231 cells were transfected with an expression vector encoding for a dominant negative TGFβ-IIR lacking the receptor's cytoplasmic domain. The transfected cells did not increase PTHrP expression in response to added TGF-β. Animals injected with these cells exhibited less osteolysis, higher body weight, lower serum calcium and PTHrP levels, and statistically longer survival than mice injected with control MDA-231 tumor cells *(123)*. These data suggest additional roles for the type II TGF-β receptor in the net progression of mammary carcinoma cells that may subvert any operational autocrine negative effects.

5.3. Role of Antiestrogen Induced TGF-βs

The role of antiestrogen-induced TGF-βs in breast carcinoma is not well-established. In a small number of breast cancer patients reported by Butta et al., 3 mo of tamoxifen therapy resulted in enhanced TGF-β1 staining around the stromal fibroblasts in breast-tumor biopsies with no effect on the staining of malignant epithelium for TGF-β1, -β2, and -β3 *(124)*. The stromal fibroblasts were ER-negative by immunohistochemistry and the induction of TGF-β1 occurred regardless of the ER status of the tumors, suggesting that the induction of the TGF-βs was independent of ER. The therapeutic significance of this proposed paracrine effect of the TGF-βs is unclear because information on the patients' clinical response to antiestrogen treatment was not provided *(124)*. Consistent with these data, Baillie et al. *(68)* reported the presence of a bioactive 50-kDa TGF-β1 complex in 4/6 breast-tumor extracts from tamoxifen-treated patients but in only 4/34 treatment-free tumor homogeneates. In two other studies, a rise in the circulating level of TGF-β2 *(125)* or in the tumor levels of TGF-β2 mRNA *(126)* correlated directly with a clinical response to tamoxifen, suggesting the potential use of circulating or tumor TGF-β2 as a surrogate marker for effective antiestrogen action. On the other hand, Herman and Katzenellenbogen *(127)* reported that MCF-7 cells, selected for tamoxifen resistance in culture, were also resistant to exogenous TGF-β1 and expressed higher levels of TGF-β1, -β2, and -β3 mRNAs, indicating a circumstantial association between loss of both antiestrogen and TGF-β responsiveness.

Other studies, however, suggest that the growth-inhibitory response of breast cancer cells to antiestrogens is unrelated to autocrine effects of endogenous TGF-βs. Late-passage MCF-7, T47D, and CAMA-1 human breast-cancer cell lines can exhibit resistance to TGF-β1-mediated growth inhibition, despite retaining tamoxifen sensitivity *(92,96,129,130)*. In T47D cells, growth arrest by progestins is not associated with enhanced production of TGF-βs nor is it inhibited by anti-TGF-β neutralizing antibodies *(131)*. In addition, TGF-β-binding sites are low to undetectable in most MCF-7 lines *(90,92,131)* whereas mRNA for the TGFβ-IIR, critical for TGF-βs-mediated signaling, is absent in T47D and CAMA-1 cells *(92,96,128,131)*. Not surprisingly then, expression of a tetracycline-repressible dominant negative TGFβ-IIR lacking its serine/threonine kinase domain into early passage MCF-7 cells blocks TGF-β1 growth inhibition but does not block antiestrogen-induced growth arrest *(96)*. In addition, TGF-β treatment upregulated the Cdk inhibitor p21 and induced its association with Cdk2 in TGF-β sensitive MCF-7 cells, whereas tamoxifen had no effect on p21, indicating alternative biochemical mechanisms for the cytostatic effect of both inhibitors *(96)*.

6. POSITIVE ROLE FOR TUMOR CELL TGFBS
IN TUMOR PROGRESSION: EFFECTS ON THE HOST

Paradoxically, the more tumorigenic hormone-independent, ER-negative breast-cancer cell lines secrete higher levels of TGF-β activity than nontumor and other less tumorigenic breast-cancer cells *(67)*. For example, adriamycin-resistant ER-negative MCF-7 cells secrete >3-fold higher levels of TGF-β activity into conditioned medium compared to parental cells. They exhibit >10-fold higher ^{125}I-TGF-β1 binding as well as type-I, -II, and -III receptors by affinity crosslinking. Despite being more sensitive than parental cells to TGF-β1 in vitro *(128)*, they rapidly form large tumors in ovariectomized nude mice in the absence of estrogen supplementation (CL Arteaga, unpublished data), thus showing that an intact autocrine TGF-β growth circuit is not always associated with reduced tumorigenicity in vivo. Similarly, LCC2 human breast-cancer cells selected for tamoxifen resistance in vitro, overexpress TGF-β2 mRNA and all three TGF-β receptors compared to LCC1 parental cells. Despite exhibiting TGF-β sensitivity in culture, they are highly tumorigenic in nude mice compared to the parental LCC1 antiestrogen-sensitive subline *(132)*.

A positive association between tumor-cell TGF-βs and the progression or maintenance of breast-carcinoma cells has been suggested by many studies. MCF-7 cells transfected with v-Ha-ras escape estrogen dependence and secrete >5-fold higher levels of TGF-β activity than wild-type cells *(133)*. Loss of estrogen dependence in T47D breast-cancer cells is associated with an acquired growth-stimulatory response to exogenous TGF-β1 and a marked increase in TGF-β1 mRNA levels *(134)*. Development of hormone-autonomous proliferation in MCF-7 cells is temporally associated with 3 to 10-fold higher levels of TGF-β1, -β2, and -β3 mRNAs *(127,135)*. TGF-β1 mRNA transcripts are more abundant in highly proliferating tumor than nontumor mammary tissues *(75)*. By Western blot, 78% of ER/PgR-negative but only 13% of the more indolent ER/PgR-positive primary human breast tumors exhibited a high level of TGF-β1 protein *(136)*. In addition, coexpression of all three TGF-β isoforms in breast tumor RNA has been statistically associated with the presence of lymph node metastases whereas tumors expressing only one TGF-β isoform usually exhibited tumor-free axillary lymph nodes at the time of mastectomy *(74)*. Exogenous TGF-β1 can increase the membrane-degrading activity and metastatic ability of mammary tumor cells in the rat *(137)*. TGF-β1 reactivity in breast tumor cells by immunohistochemistry is greater in invasive than in ductal carcinoma *in situ* and is associated with a higher clinical stage *(138)*. An immunohistochemical study in 28 breast-tumor specimens showed more frequent and more intense intra and extracellular staining for TGF-β1 in metastatic sites than in primary tumor tissues *(80)*. The predominant staining for secreted TGF-β1 was detected at advancing tumor edges and lymph-node metastases *(80)*, consistent with a possible role for tumor TGF-βs on invasion. Treatment with exogenous TGF-β1 increased cell-associated urokinase-type plasminogen activator and plasminogen activator inhibitor-1 in medium conditioned by MDA-231 breast-cancer cells *(138)*. These TGF-β1-induced molecules could perhaps facilitate tumor-cell invasion and protect blood-born tumor emboli from host-related fibrinolysis. Consistent with the proposed role for tumor TGF-βs in invasion and stroma formation, a study in 86 invasive breast cancers showed prominent TGF-β1 staining to be associated with the presence of lymph-node metastases, increased stromal fibronectin and tenascin, and altered CD4/CD8 lymphocyte populations *(139)*. In a restropective analysis of 42 breast tumors, intense TGF-β1 staining was associated with a shorter disease-free interval after mastectomy independent of the clinical stage and ER status compared to tumors with low or no TGF-β1 immunoreactivity *(140)*. Thompson et al. *(141)* reported that breast tumors unresponsive to the antiestrogen tamoxifen, when rebiopsied, expressed significantly higher levels of TGF-β1 mRNA than clinically-responsive tumors, further supporting a positive role for tumor TGF-βs in the progression of breast carcinoma. More recently, Relf et al. *(142)* reported statistically higher levels of TGF-β1 mRNA in breast tumors exhibiting a high angiogenic response as measured by microvessel density in tissue section, consistent with the reported angiogenic effect of the TGF-βs *(142a)*. Comparisons between tissue studies examining mRNA expression vs. protein content have not infrequently been at odds. This lack of correlation probably reflects the possibility that most of the regulation of the TGF-βs is post-translational through the activation of the latent complexes. In addition, protein abundance *in situ* may not reflect biological activity if analyzed with antisera that do not discriminate between active and latent protein.

The growth-inhibitory effect of TGF-β1 against breast-cancer cells in vitro was not confirmed in experimental animals. Exogenous TGF-β1 did not inhibit (in vitro-sensitive) MDA-231 tumors in athymic mice. However, TGF-β1 induced marked cachexia and generalized interstitial fibrosis especially in the spleen *(104)*, consistent with the immunosuppressive and stroma-inducing function of TGF-β1. These results and the circumstantial evidence associating high TGF-β1 expression with enhanced tumorigenicity (above) led to other more direct experiments. In one of these studies, MCF-7 estrogen-dependent breast-cancer cells transfected with an expression vector containing a full-length mouse TGF-β1 cDNA encoding for latent TGF-β1 protein were able to form tumors in castrated nude mice in the absence of estrogen supplementation. These tumors were histologically indistinguishable from estrogen-primed parental tumors *(143)*. Administration of 2G7, an IgG2b monoclonal antibody (MAb) that neutralizes all three TGF-β isoforms (antipan TGF-β) inhibited MCF-7$^{TGF-β1}$ tumors, but not wild-type MCF-7 tumor formation in estradiol-supplemented nude mice. Exogenous TGF-β1 had a similar net effect on MCF-7 tumorigenicity: Daily injections of recombinant TGF-β1 supported tumor formation by wild-type MCF-7 cells in castrated nude mice. This result suggested that the TGF-β1-mediated enhanced tumorigenesis of MCF-7 cells was not owing to a direct (autocrine) effect of the transfected gene product on the MCF-7$^{TGF-β1}$ transfectants but rather to an effect on the host which, in turn, favored the establishment and maintenance of MCF-7$^{TGF-β1}$ xenografts.

A possible mechanism for the aforementioned results is suggested by experiments using blocking anti-TGF-β antiboidies against MDA-231 breast xenografts in vivo. These cells express high levels of TGF-β1 and -β2 mRNAs *(71)*. Establishment of intraperitoneal (ip) MDA-231 tumors downregulated mouse-spleen natural killer (NK) function. The 2G7 anti-pan TGF-β antibody suppressed the establishment of ip MDA-231 tumors and lung metastases in athymic mice *(103)*. 2G7 also prevented the inhibition of NK function induced by MDA-231 tumors. These observations strongly suggest that TGF-βs expressed by MDA-231 tumors can immunosuppress the xenograft-bearing host. In addition, they are consistent with the well-established potent immunosuppressive effect of the TGF-βs *(144)*, as well as with clinical observations of altered NK- and T-cell function in patients with glioblastoma whose tumors overexpress TGF-β2 *(145)*. The antibody-mediated effect on NK function appeared to be critical for the observed antitumor effect in that 2G7 did not inhibit MDA-231 tumors in NK-deficient animals. Moreover, anti-TGF-β antibodies do not inhibit but rather stimulate growth of MDA-231 cells in culture *(102,103)*, conditions under which an indirect effect of NK cells would not be expected. The 2G7-treated tumor-free animals exhibited a >4-fold higher spleen NK function than animals treated with a control IgG2. This result supports the notion that the endogenously produced TGF-βs regulate immune function, as indicated by studies in TGF-β1 null mice. These animals exhibit a massive, multiorgan infiltration with lymphocytes and macrophages leading to tissue necrosis, organ failure, and early death *(9,10)*.

To study the role of TGF-β1 on tumor-host immune responses, Park et al. introduced a retroviral vector-encoding antisense TGF-β1 into the EMT6 mouse mammary tumor cell line. Cell medium from the antisense-expressing cells exhibited a reduced capacity to inhibit alloantigen-specific T-cell responses in vitro compared to medium conditioned by cells transfected with backbone vector alone. In addition, antisense-expressing cells exhibited reduced tumorigenicity in BALB/c immunocompetent mice compared to cells transfected with vector alone *(146)*. Reduced tumorigenicity was not observed in *scid* mice compared to EMT6 control tumors, suggesting that the impaired ability to form tumors by the antisense-modified cells was owing to an immunomodulatory effect of the antisense TGF-β1 transgene. These data suggest, first, that tumor cell modified with antisense TGF-β1 could alter afferent immunity against unmodified cancer cells and potentially confer long-term antitumor immunity. In addition, these results also suggest that elimination of tumor cell TGF-β counteracts (tumor-mediated) host immunosuppression and enhances antitumor responses. The practical application of anti-TGF-β strategies as a means of adoptive immunotherapy against against TGF-β overexpressing tumors in currently under active investigation.

7. TGF-β AND DRUG RESISTANCE

Recent data suggest a causal association between TGF-β1 overexpression in tumor cells and resistance to DNA-damaging chemotherapeutic drugs. Intraperitoneal administration of anti-panTGF-β neutralizing antibodies or the TGF-β inhibitor decorin to mice bearing established EMT-6 mammary tumors increased the sensitivity of both sensitive and resistant EMT-6 mammary tumors to cyclophosphamide and cisplatin *(147,148)*. In sensitive tumors, TGF-β1 expression and secretion was highly inducible by DNA-damaging agents whereas the resistant tumors exhibited high constitutive TGF-β1 mRNA levels *(148,149)*. The biological role of this upregulation is unknown but it is tempting to speculate that TGF-β1 induction protects the cell from DNA damage: following drug exposure, TGF-β1 is upregulated with subsequent hypophosphorylation of Rb and induction of other cyclin-dependent kinase inhibitors like $p21^{WAF1/CIP1}$, p27, $p16^{INK4}$, and $p15^{INK4B}$ *(40)*. These cellular responses result in recruitment of tumor cells in the G1 phase of the cell cycle and block progression to apoptosis *(150,151)*. Consistent with this speculation, TGF-β1 has been shown to protect L929 fibroblasts from tumor necrosis factor (TNF) cytotoxicity by inducing G1 arrest *(152)*. Another potential mechanism for the acquisition of drug resistance is gene amplification. Huang et al. *(153)* recently proposed that TGF-β1 promotes gene amplification and drug resistance. 10T^1/2 cells transfected with an inducible TGF-β1 construct encoding for active TGF-β1 exhibited in vitro resistance to N-phos-phonacetyl-L-aspartate (PALA) only under conditions that led to elevated levels of the transgene. All drug-resistant clones exhibited amplification of the CAD gene which encodes for the protein target of PALA. By fluctuation analysis, the increased rate of CAD gene amplification was limited to the TGF-β1 overexpressing clones.

We recently reported TGF-β2 overexpression in the antiestrogen-resistant MCF-7 subline LCC2 *(132)*. Established LCC2 tumors in nude mice treated with tamoxifen and anti-TGF-β neutralizing antibodies failed to grow whereas tumors treated with the antiestrogen and a control IgG2 continued to grow rapidly. These data suggest that the reported overexpression of TGF-βs by breast tumors treated with tamoxifen *(68,126,141)* may in fact contribute to antiestrogen resistance. This observation further challenges the hypothesis that TGF-β signaling mediates the cellular response to antiestrogens.

Demonstration of a causal association between tumor TGF-βs and drug resistance will require additional direct experiments. Conceptually this association may well fit with epidemiological data linking high TGF-β1 expression in mammary tumors with poor prognosis *(80,140,141)* If confirmed further, this association would also raise the possibility that in some breast-tumor cells, an intact TGF-β autocrine system, perhaps via paracrine may indeed serve to protect from either antiestrogens or DNA-damaging anticancer drugs and therefore contribute to tumor progression and poor patient outcome.

8. FUTURE DIRECTIONS (OR CONCLUSIONS)

A large body of experimental data support a role for the TGF-βs in human-breast carcinoma. The once proposed use of TGF-β as an antitumor agent in breast cancer, based on a minor growth attenuation of breast cancer cell lines in culture, has not been documented in in vivo models and at this time would appear unjustified to pursue. Defects in TGF-β receptor(s) expression and signaling have been reported in breast-tumor cell lines but these alterations do not match the mutations observed in other neoplasms. Further epidemiological studies in normal, hyperplastic, preneoplastic, and breast tumor tissues examining expression of TGF-β receptors and cellular substrates would be valuable to infer the prevalence and timing of loss of TGF-β receptor signaling in stepwise mammary carcinogenesis. Although loss of endogenous TGF-β receptor signaling would clearly favor the proliferation of tumor or nontumor mammary cells, maintenance of functional TGF-β receptors by breast cancer cells may mediate paracine tumor/host interactions potentially deleterious to the tumor host. This possibility underscores the severe limitations of cell autonomous models for the study of signaling systems mediating paracrine interactions that are critical for tumor viability and/or progression. It also highlights the need to study the TGF-β receptor system in the context of multicellular experimental cancer systems and/or intact tumor-bearing animals to assess its net contribution to human breast cancer biology.

An excess of TGF-β1 potently inhibits normal breast epithelium. However, a large amount of circumstantial and direct data support a positive effect for the TGF-βs in

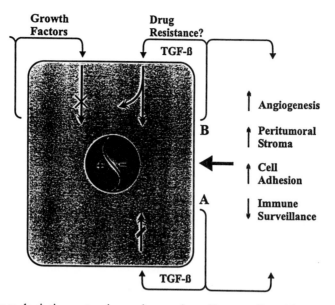

Fig. 2. Diagram depicting autocrine and paracrine effects mediated by tumor-cell TGF-βs. TGF-β-mediated autocrine growth control is operative in nontumor mammary cells. However, some tumor cells lose this autocrine control owing to TGF-β receptor loss and/or defective post-receptor signaling **(A)**. Some breast tumors, with or without loss of TGF-β autocrine signaling, may also overexpress TGF-βs. These ligands via paracrine effects on host cells may then indirectly foster tumor progression **(B)**.

fully transformed mammary cells. It follows then that at some step in stochastic mammary carcinogenesis, the ability of TGF-β to arrest growth (and/or transformation) is lost and/or switches to one in which it accelerates transformation and/or the progression of breast carcinomas by several possible mechanisms, i.e., host immunosuppression, enhanced angiogenesis, deregulation of pericellular proteolysis with increased cell adhesion, increased peritumoral stroma, and possibly drug resistance (Fig. 2). Definition of this TGF-β "switch" may be experimentally approachable in mice temporally-controllable TGF-β transgenes expressed in mammary epithelium. Results from this type of studies may lead us to re-examine the dynamic role of the TGF-β system in mammary transformation and carcinogenesis and, on that basis, to the optimal conception of TGF-β-based chemoprevention strategies. Finally, studies with neutralizing antibodies and stable antisense-expression vectors suggest that perturbation of tumor cell TGF-βs results in a measurable antitumor effect. The therapeutic applicability of these approaches is under study. A marked alteration in the natural history of experimental mammary cancers by elimination of tumor cell-TGF-βs would suggest that these molecules are rational and testable targets for novel antitumor interventions in patients with breast carcinoma.

ACKNOWLEDGMENTS

Supported by NIH grant CA62212, Merit Review and Clinical Investigator grants from the Department of Veteran Affairs, and the T. J. Martell Foundation.

REFERENCES

1. Masague, J. 1990. The transforming growth factor-beta family. *Annu. Rev. Cell Biol.* **6:** 597–641.
2. Moses, H. L. 1990. The biological action of transforming growth factor β, in *Growth Factors from Genes to Clinical Application* (Sara, V., K. Hall, and H. Low, eds.), Raven, New York, pp. 141–155.
3. Roberts, A. B. and M. B. Sporn. 1990. The transforming growth factor-βs, in *Handbook of Experimental Pharmacology*, vol. 95 (Sporn, M. B. and A. B. Roberts, eds.), Springer-Verlag, Heidelberg, **95:** pp. 419–472.
4. Miyazono, K., H. Ichijo, C. H. Heldin. 1993. Transforming growth factor-β: latent forms, binding proteins and receptors. *Growth Factors* **8:** 11–22.
5. Alexandrow M. G. and H. L. Moses. 1995. Transforming growth factor β and cell cycle regulation. *Cancer Res.* **55:** 1452–1457.
6. Koli, K. and J. Keski-Oja. 1996. Transforming growth factor-β system and its regulation by members of the steroid-thyroid hormone superfamily. *Adv. Cancer Res.* **70:** 63–94.
7. Jakowlew, S. B., P. J. Dillard, M. B. Sporn, and A. B. Roberts. 1988. Complementary deoxyribonucleic acid cloning of messenger ribonucleic acid encoding transforming growth factor β4 from chicken embryo chondrocytes. *Mol. Endocrinol.* **2:** 1186–1195.
8. Kondaiah, P., M. J. Sands, J. M. Smith, A. Fields, A. B. Roberts, M. B. Sporn, and D. A. Melton. 1990. Identification of a novel transforming growth factor-β (TGF-β5) mRNA in Xenopus laevis. *J. Biol. Chem.* **265:** 1089–1093.
9. Shull, M. M., I. Ormsby, A. B. Kier, S. Pawlowski, R. J. Diebold, M. Yin, R. Allen, C. Sidman, G. Proetzel, D. Calvin, N. Annunziata, and T. Doetschman. 1993. Targeted disruption of the mouse transforming growth factor-β1 in multifocal inflammatory disease. *Nature* **359:** 693–699.
10. Kulkarni, A. B., C.-G. Huh, D. Becker, A. Geiser, M. Lyght, K. C. Flanders, A. B. Roberts, M. B. Sporn, J. M. Ward, and S. Karlsson. 1993. Transforming growth factor β_1 null mutation in mice causes excessive inflammatory response and early death. *Proc. Natl. Acad. Sci. USA* **90:** 770–774.
11. Sanford, l. . P., I. Ormsby, A. C. Gittenberg-de Groot, H. Sariola, F. Friedman, G. P. Boivin, E. L. Cardell, and T. Doetschman. 1997. TGF2 knockout mice have multiple developmental defects that are non overlapping with other TGF knockout phentypes. *Development* **124:** 2659–2670.
12. Proetzel, G., S. A. Pawlowski, M. V. Wiles, M. Y. Yin, G. P. Boivin, P. N. Howles, J. X. Ding, M. W. J. Ferguson, and T. Doetschman. 1995. Transforming growth factor-β3 is required for secondary palate fusion. *Nature Genet.* **11:** 409–414.
13. Kaartinen, V., J. W. Voncken, C. Shuler, D. Warburton, D. Bu, N. Heisterkamp, and J. Groffen. 1995. Abnormal lung development and cleft palate in mice lacking TGF-β3 indicates defects of epithelial-mesenchymal interaction. *Nature* Genet. **11:** 415–421.
14. Olofsson, A., K. Miyazono, T. Kanzaki, P. Colosetti, U. Engström, and C.-H. Heldin. 1992. Transforming growth factor-β1,-β2, and-β3 secreted by human glioblastoma cell line. Identification of small and different forms of latent complexes. *J. Biol. Chem.* **267:** 19482–19488.
15. Saharinen, J., J. Taipale, and J. Keski-Oja. 1996. Association of the small latent transforming growth factor-β with an eight cysteine repeat of its binding protein LTBP-1. *EMBO J.* **15:** 245- 253.
16. Taipale, J., K. Miyazono, C.-H. Heldin, and J. Keski-Oja. 1994. Latent transforming growth factor-β1 associates to fibroblast extracellular matrix via latent TGF-β binding protein. *J. Cell Biol.* **124:** 171–181.
17. Miyazono, K., A. Olofsson, P. Colosetti, and C.-H. Heldin. 1991. A role of the latent TGF-β-binding protein in the assembly and secretion of TGF-β1. *EMBO J.* **10:** 1091–1101.

18. Flaumenhaft, R., M. Abe, Y. Sato, K. Miyazono, J. G. Harpel, C.-H. Heldin, and D. B. Rifkin. 1993. Role of the latent TGF-β binding protein in the activation of latent TGF-β by cocultures of endothelial and smooth muscle cells. *J. Cell Biol.* **120:** 995–1002.

19. Morén, A., A. Olofsson, G. Stenman, P. Sahlin, T. Kanzaki, L. Claesson-Welsh, P. ten Dijke, K. Miyazono, and C.-H. Heldin. 1994. Identification and characterization of LTBP-2, a novel latent transforming growth factor-β-binding protein. *J. Biol. Chem.* **269:** 32,469–32,478.

20. Li, X., W. Yin, L. Perez-Jurado, J. Bonadio, and U. Francke. 1995. Mapping of human and murine genes for latent TGF-β binding protein–2 (LTBP–2). Mamm. Genome **6:** 42–45.

21. Yin, W., E. Smiley, J. Germiller, R. P. Mecham, J. B. Florer, R. J. Wenstrup, and J. Bonadio. 1995. Isolation of a novel latent transforming growth factor βbinding protein gene (LTBP–3). *J. Biol. Chem.* **270:** 10,147–10,160.

22. Brown, P. D., L. M. Wakefield, A. D. Levinson, and M. B. Sporn. 1990. Physiochemical activation of recombinant latent transforming growth factor-β's 1, 2, 3. *Growth Factors* **3:** 35–43.

23. Lyons, R. M., J. Keski-Oja, H. L. Moses. 1988. Proteolytic activation of latent transforming growth factor-β from fibroblast-conditioned medium. *J. Cell Biol.* **106:** 1659–1665.

24. Taipale, J., K. Koli, and J. Keski-Oja. 1992. Release of transforming growth factor-β1 form the pericellular matrix of cultured fibroblasts and fibrosarcoma cells by plasmin and thrombin. *J. Biol. Chem.* **267:** 25,378–25,384.

25. Barcellos-Hoff, M. H., R. Derynck, M. L.-S. Tsang, and J. A. Wearherbee. 1994. Transforming growth factor-β activation in irradiated murine mammary galnd. *J. Clin. Invest.* **93:** 892–899.

26. Barcellos-Hoff M. H. and T. A. Dix. 1996. Redox-mediated activation of latent transforming growth factor-β1. *Mol. Endocrinol.* **10:** 1077–1083.

27. Taipale, J., J. Saharinen, K. Hedman, and J. Keski-Oja. 1996. Latent transforming growth factor-β1 and its binding protein are components of extracellular matrix microfibrils. *J. Histochem. Cytochem.* **44:** 875–889.

28. Lyons, R. M., L. E. Gentry, A. F. Purchio, and H. L. Moses. 1990. Mechanism of activation of latent recombinant transforming growth factor-β1 by plasmin. *J. Cell Biol.* **110:** 1361–1367.

29. Nunes, I., J. S. Munger, J. G. Harpel, Y. Nagano, R. L. Shapiro, P.-E. Gleizes, and D. B. Rifkin. 1996. Structure and activation of the large latent transforming growth factor-β complex. *Int. J. Obesity* **20:** S4-S8.

30. Kojima, S., K. Nara, and D. B. Rifkin. 1993. Requirement for transglutaminase in the activation of latent transforming growth factor-β in bovine endothelial cells. *J. Cell Biol.* **121:** 439–448.

31. Kojima, S. and D. B. Rifkin. 1993. Mechanism of retinoid-induced activation of latent transforming growth factor-β in bovine endothelial cells. *J. Cell Physiol.* **155:** 323–332.

32. Laiho, M., O. Saksela, P. A. Andreasen, and J. Keski-Oja. 1986. Enhanced production and extracellular deposition of the endothelial-type plasminogen activator inhibitor in cultured human lung fibroblasts by transforming growth factor-β. *J. Cell Biol.* **103:** 2403–2410.

33. Koli, K. and J. Keski-Oja. 1993a. Vitamin D$_3$ and calcipotriol enhance the secretion of transforming growth factor-β1 and -β2 in cultured murine keratinocytes. Growth Factors **8:** 153–163.

34. Koli, K. and J. Keski-Oja. 1993b. Vitamin D$_3$ and calcipotriol decrease extracellular plaminogen activator activity in cultured keratinocytes. *J. Invest. Dermatol.* **101:** 706–712.

35. Barcellos-Hoff, M. H. 1996a. Latency and activation in the control of TGF-β. *J. Mammary Gland Biol. Neopl.* **1:** 353–363.

36. Schultz-Cherry, S., S. Ribeiro, L. Gentry, and J. E. Murphy-Ullrich. 1994. Thrombospondin binds and activates the small and large forms of latent transforming growth factor-β in a chemically defined system. *J. Biol. Chem.* **268:** 26,775–26,782.

37. Schultz-Cherry, S., H. Chen, D. F. Mosher, T. M. Misenheimer, H. C. Krutzsch, D. D. Roberts, and J. E. Murphy-Ullrich. 1995. Regulation of transforming growth factor-beta activation by discrete sequences of thrombospondin 1. *J. Biol. Chem.* **270:** 7304–7310.

38. Massagué, J., L. Attisano, J. L. Wrana. 1994. The TGF-β family and its composite receptors. *Trends Cell Biol.* **4:** 172–178.

39. Derynck, R. 1994. TGF-β-receptor-mediated signaling. *Trends Biochem. Sci.* **19:** 548–553.

40. Yingling, J. M., X.-F. Wang, and C. H. Bassing. 1995. Signaling by transforming growth factor-β receptors. *Biochem. Biophys. Acta* **1242:** 115–136.

41. Wang, X.-F., H. Y. Lin, E. Ng-Eaton, J. Downward, H. F. Lodish, and R. A. Weinberg. 1991. Expression cloning and characterization of the TGF-β type III receptor. *Cell* **67:** 797–805.

42. Franzén, P., P. ten Dijke, H. Ichijo, H. Yamashita, P. Schultz, C.-H. Heldin, and K. Miyazono. 1993. Cloning of the TGF-β type I receptor that forms a heteromeric complex with the TGF-β type II receptor. *Cell* **75:** 681–692.

43. Lin, H. Y., X.-F. Wang, E. Ng-Eaton, R. A. Weinberg, and H. F. Lodish. 1992. Expression cloning of the TGF-β type II receptor, a functional transmembrane serine/threonine kinase. *Cell* **68:** 775–758.

44. ten Dijke, P., H. Yamashita, H. Ichijo, P. Franzén, M. Laiho, K. Miyazono, and C.-H. Heldin. 1994. Characterization of type I receptors for transforming growth factor-β and activin. *Science* (Washington DC) **264:** 101–104.

45. Wrana, J. L., L. Attisano, J. Cárcamo, A. Zentella, J. Doody, M. Laiho, X.-F. Wang, and J. Massagué. 1992. TGF-β signals through a heteromeric protein kinase receptor complex. *Cell* **71:** 1003–1014.

46. Weis-Garcia, F. and J. Massagué. 1996. Complementation between kinase-defective and activation-defective TGF-β receptors reveals a novel form of receptor cooperativity essential for signaling. *EMBO J.* **15:** 276–289.

47. Wrana, J. L., L. Attisano, R. Wiser, F. Ventura, and J. Massagué. 1994. Mechanism of activation of the TGF-β receptor. *Nature* (Lond.) **370:** 341–347.

48. Chen, F. and R. A. Weinberg. 1995. Biochemical evidence for the autophosphorylation and transphosphorylation of transforming growth factor β receptor kinases. *Proc. Natl. Acad. Sci. USA* **92:** 1565–1569.

49. Chen, R.-H., R. Ebner, and R. Derynck. 1993. Inactivation of the type II receptor reveals two receptor pathways for the diverse TGF-β activities. Science (Washington DC) **260:** 1335–1338.

50. Saitoh, M., H. Nishitoh, T. Amagasa, K. Miyazono, M. Takagi, and H. Ichijo. 1996. Identification of important regions in the cytoplasmic juxtamembrane domain of type I receptor that separate signaling pathways of transforming growth factor-β. *J. Biol. Chem.* **271:** 2769–2775.

51. Wang, T., P. K. Donahoe, and A. S. Servos. 1994. Specific interaction of type I receptors of the TGF-β family with the immunophilin FKBP-12. *Science* (Washington, DC) **265:** 674–676.

52. Kawabata, M., T. Imamura, K. Miyazono, M. Engel, and H. L. Moses. 1995. Interaction of the transforming growth factor-β type I receptor with farnesyl-protein transferase-alpha. *J. Biol. Chem.* **270:** 29,628–29,631.

53. Chen, R.-H., P. J. Miettinen, E. M. Maruoka, L. Choy, and R. Derynck. 1995. A WD-domain protein that is associated and phosphorylated by the type II TGF-β receptor. *Nature* (Lond.) **377:** 548–552.

54. Massagué, J. 1996. TGF-β signaling: receptors, transducers, and Mad proteins. *Cell* **85**: 947–950.

55. Macias-Silva, M., S. Abdollad, P. A. Hoodless, R. Pirone, L. Attisano, and J. L. Wrana. 1996. MADR2 is a substrate of the TGF-β receptor and its phosphorylation is required for nuclear accumulation and signaling. *Cell* **87**: 1215–1224.

56. Lagna, G., A. Hata, A. Hemmati-Brivanlou, and J. Massagué. 1996. Partnership between DPC4 and SMAD proteins in TGF-β signaling pathways. *Nature* **383**: 832–836.

57. Wu, R.-Y., Y. Zhang, X.-H. Feng, R. Derynck. 1997. Heteromeric and homomeric interactions correlate with signaling activity and functional cooperativity of Smad3 and Smad4/DPC4. *Mol. Cell. Biol.* **17**: 2521–2528.

58. Zhang, Y., X.-H. Feng, R.-Y. Wu, and R. Derynck. 1996. Receptor-associated Mad homologues synergize as effectors of the TGF-β-beta response. *Nature* **383**: 168–172.

59. Nakao, A., E. Röijer, T. Imamura, S. Souchelnytskyi, G. Stenman, C.-H. Heldin, and P. ten Dijke. 1997. Identification of Smad2, a human Mad-related protein in the transforming growth factor β signaling pathway. *J. Biol. Chem.* **272**: 2896–2900.

60. Laiho, M., J. A. DeCaprio, J. W. Ludlow, D. M. Livingstone, and J. Massagué. 1990. Growth inhibition by TGF-β linked to suppression of retinoblatoma protein phosphorylation. *Cell* **62**: 175–185.

61. Hunter, T. 1993. Braking the cycle. *Cell* **75**: 839–841.

62. Pietenpol, J. A., J. T. Holt, R. W. Stein, and H. L. Moses. 1990. Transforming growth factor-β 1 suppression of c-myc gene transcription: role in inhibition of keratinocyte proliferation. *Proc. Natl. Acad. Sci. USA* **87**: 3758–3762.

63. Chen, A. R. and L. R. Rohrschneider. 1993. Mechanism of differential inhibition of factor-β dependent cell proliferation by transforming growth factor-β1: selective uncoupling of FMS form MYC. *Blood* **81**: 2539–2546.

64. Zajchowski, D., V. Band, N. Pauzie, A. Tager, M. Stampfer, and R. Sager. 1988. Expression of growth factors and oncogenes in normal and tumor-derived human mammary epithelial cells. *Cancer Res.* **48**: 7041–7047.

65. Dickson, R. B., S. E. Bates, M. E. McManaway, and M. E. Lippman. 1986a. Characterization of estrogen responsive transforming activity in human breast-cancer cell lines. *Cancer Res.* **48**: 1707–1713.

66. Lyons, R. M., D. A. Miller, J. L. Graycar, H. L. Moses, and R. Derynck. 1991. Differential binding of transforming growth factor-β1,-β2, and -β3 by fibroblasts and epithelial cells measured by affinity cross-linking of cell surface receptors. *Mol. Endocrinol.* **5**: 1887–1896.

67. Koli, K. M. and C. L. Arteaga. 1996. Complex role of tumor cell transforming growth factor (TGF)-βs on breast carcinoma progression. *J. Mammary Gland Biol. Neopl.* **1**: 373–380.

68. Baillie, R., R. C. Coombes, and J. Smith. 1996. Multiple forms of TGF-β in breast tissue: a biologically active form of the small latent complex of TGF-β1. *Eur. J. Cancer* **32A**: 1566–1573.

69. Theodorescu, D., C. Sheehan, and R. S. Kerbel. 1993. TGF-β gene expression depends on tissue architecture. *In Vitro Cell Devel. Biol.* **28A**: 105–108.

70. Streuli, C. H., Schmidhauser, M. Kobrin, M. J. Bissell, and R. Derynck. 1993. Extracellular matrix regulates expression of the TGF-β1 gene. *J. Cell Biol.* **120**: 253–260.

71. Arrick, B. A., M. Korc, and R. Derynck. 1990. Differential regulation of expression of three transforming growth factor β species in human breast-cancer cell lines by estradiol. *Cancer Res.* **50**: 299–303.

72. Moustakas, A., T. Takumi, H. Y. Lin, and H. F. Lodish. 1995. GH3 pituitary tumor cells contain heteromeric type I and type II receptor complexes for transforming growth factor β and activin –A. *J. Biol Chem.* **270**: 765–769.

73. Valverius, E. M., D. Walker-Jones, S. E. Bates, M. R. Stampfer, R. Clark, F. McCormick, R. B. Dickson and M. E. Lippman. 1989. Production of and responsiveness to transforming growth factor-β in normal and oncogene-transformed human mammary epithelial cells. *Cancer Res.* **49:** 6269–6274.

74. MacCallum, J., J. M. S. Bartlett, A. M. Thompson, J. C. Keen, J. M. Dixon, and W. R. Miller. 1994. Expression of transforming growth factor beta mRNA isoforms in human breast cancer. *Br. J. Cancer* **69:** 1006–1009.

75. Barrett-Lee, P., M. Travers, Y. Luqmani, and R. C. Coombes. 1990. Transcripts for transforming growth factors in human breast cancer: clinical correlates. *Br. J. Cancer* **61:** 612–617.

76. McCune, B. K., B. R. Mullin, K. C. Flanders, W. J. Jaffurs, L. T. Mullen, and M. B. Sporn. 1992. Localization of transforming growth factor-β isotypes in lesions of the human breast. *Human Pathol.* **20:** 13–20.

77. Dublin, E. A., D. M. Barnes, D. Y. Wang, R. J. B. King, and D. A. Levison. 1993. TGF alpha and TGF beta expression in mammary carcinomas. *J. Pathol.* **170:** 15–22.

78. Mitzukami, Y., A. Nonomura, T. Yamada, H. Kurumaya, M. Hayashi, N. Koyasaki, T. Taniya, M. Noguchi, S. Nakamura, and F. Matsubara. 1990. Immunohistochemical demonstration of growth factors, TGF-β, TGF-β, IGF-I, and neu oncogene product in benign and malignat human breast tissue. *Anticancer Res.* **10:** 1115–1126.

79. Walker, R. A., and B. Gallagher. 1995. Determination of transforming growth factor βeta₁ mRNA expression in breast carcinomas by *in situ* hybridization. *J. Pathol.* **177:** 123–127.

80. Dalal, B. I., P. A. Keown, and A. H. Greenberg. 1993. Immunocytochemical localization of secreted transforming growth factor-β1 to the advancing edges of primary tumors and to lymph-node metastasis of human mammary carcinoma. *Am. J. Pathol.* **43:** 381–389.

81. Robinson, S. D., G. B. Silberstein, A. B. Roberts, K. C. Flanders, and C. W. Daniel. 1991. Regulated expression and growth inhibitory effects of transforming growth factor-β isoforms in mouse mammary gland development. *Development* **113:** 867–878.

82. Daniel, C. W., S. Robinson, and G. B. Silberstein. 1996. The role of TGF-β in patterning and growth of the mammary ductal tree. *J. Mammary Gland Biol. Neopl.* **1:** 331–341.

83. Howlett, A. R. and M. J. Bissell. 1993. The influence of tissue microenvironment (stroma and extracellular matrix) on the development and function of mammary epithelium. *Epithelial Cell Biol.* **2:** 79–89.

84. Pierce, D. F., M. D. Johnson, Y. Matsui, S. D. Robinson, L. I. Gold, A. F. Purchio, C. W. Daniel, B. L. M. Hogan, and H. L. Moses. 1993. Inhibition of mammary duct development but not alveolar outgrowth during pregnancy in transgenic mice expressing active TGF-β1. *Genes Devel.* **7:** 2308–2317.

85. Jhappan, C., A. G. Geiser, E. C. Kordon, D. Bagheri, L. Henninghausen, A. B. Roberts, G. H. Smith, and G. Merlino. 1993. Targeting expression of a transforming growth factor beta 1 transgene to the pregnant mammary gland inhibits alveolar development and lactation. *EMBO J.* **12:** 1835–1845.

86. Robinson, S. D., A. B. Roberts, and C. W. Daniel. 1993. TGF beta suppresses casein synthesis in mouse mammary explants and may play a role in controlling milk levels during pregnancy. *J. Cell Biol.* **120:** 245–251.

87. Kordon, E. C., R. A. McKnight, C. Jhappan, L. Henninghausen, G. Merlino, and G. H. Smith. 1995. Ectopic TGFβ1 expression in the secretory mammary epithelium induces early senescence of the epithelial stem cell populaiton. *Dev. Biol.* **168:** 47–61.

88. Stampfer, M. R., P. Yaswen, M. Alhadeff, and J. Hosoda. 1993. TGF-β induction of matrix associated proteins in normal and transformed human mammary epithelial cells in culture is dependent of growth effects. *J. Cell Physiol.* **155:** 210–221.

89. Knabbe, C., M. E. Lippman, L. M. Wakefield, K. C. Flanders, A. Kasid, R. Derynck, and R. B. Dickson. 1987. Evidence that transforming growth factor-β is a hormonally regulated negative growth factor βin human breast-cancer cells. *Cell* **48:** 417–428.

90. Arteaga, C. L., A. K. Tandon, D. D. Von Hoff, and C. K. Osborne. 1988. Transforming growth factor β: a potential autocrine growth inhibitor of estrogen receptor-negative human breast-cancer cells. *Cancer Res.* **48:** 3898–3904.

91. Zugmaier, G., B. W. Ennis, B. Deschauer, D. Katz, C. Knabbe, G. Wilding, P. Daly, M. E. Lippman, and R. B. Dickson. 1989. Transforming growth factors type β1 and β2 are equipotent growth inhibitors of human breast-cancer cell lines. *J. Cell Physiol.* **141:** 353–361.

92. Kalkhoven, E., B. A. J. Roelen, J. P. de Winter, C. L. Mummery, A. J. M. van den Eijnden-van Raaij, P. T. van der Saag, and B. van der Burg. 1995. Resistance to transforming growth factor β and activin due to reduced receptor expression in human breast tumor cell lines. *Cell Growth Diff.* **6:** 1151–1161.

93. Sandhu, C., J. Garbe, N. Bhattacharya, J. Daksis, C.-H. Pan, P. Yaswen, J. Koh, J. M. Slingerland, and M. R. Stampfer. 1997. Transforming growth factor β stabilizes p15*INK4B* protein, increases p15*INK4B*-cdk4 complexes, and inhibits cyclin D1-cdk4 association in human mammary epithelial cells. *Mol Cell. Biol.* **17:** 2458–2467.

94. Iavarone, A. and J. Masague. (1997) Repression of the CDK activator Cdc25A and cell-cycle arrest by cytokine TGF-β in cells lacking the CDK inhibitor p15. *Nature* **387:** 417–422.

95. Mazars, P., N. Barboule, V. Baldin, S. Vidal, B. Ducommun, and N. Valetta. 1995. Effects of TGF-β1 (transforming growth factor-β1) on the cell cycle regulation of human breast adenocarcinoma (MCF-7) cells. *FEBS Lett.* **362:** 295–300.

96. Koli, K. M., T. T. Ramsey, Y. Ko, T. C. Dugger, M. G. Brattain, and C. L. Arteaga. 1997. Blockade of TGF-β signaling does not abrogate antiestrogen-induced growth inhibition of human breast carcinoma cells. *J. Biol. Chem.* **272:** 8296–8302.

96a. Pierce D. F., A. E. Gorska, A. Chytil, K. S. Meise, D. L. Page, R. J. Coffey, H. L. Moses. 1995. Mammary tumor suppression by transforming growth factor β1 transgene expression. *Proc. Natl. Acad. Sci. USA* **92:** 4254–4258.

97. Jeng M.-H., P. ten Dijke, K. K. Iwata, and V. C. Jordan. 1993. Regulation of the levels of three transforming growth factor β mRNAs by estrogen and their effects on the proliferation of human breast-cancer cells. *Mol. Cell Endocrinol.* **97:** 115–123.

98. Jeng M.-H., and V. C. Jordan. 1991. Growth stimulation and differential regulation of transforming growth factor-β1 (TGF-β1), TGF-β2, and TGF-β3 messenger RNA levels by norethindrone in MCF-7 human breastcancer cells. *Mol. Endocrinol.* **5:** 1120–1128.

99. Warri A. M., R. L. Huovinen, A. M. Laine, P. M. Martikainen, and P. L. Härkonen. 1993. Apoptosis in toremifene-induced growth inhibition of human breast-cancer cells in vitro and in vivo. *J. Natl. Cancer Inst.* **85:** 1412–1418.

100. Colletta A. A , L. M. Wakefield, F. V. Howell, D. Danielpour, M. Baum, M. B. Sporn MB. 1991. The growth inhibition of human breast cancer cells by a novel synthetic progestin involves the induction of transforming growth factor β. *J. Clin. Invest.* **87:** 277–283.

101. Koli, K. and J. Keski-Oja. 1995. 1,25-dihydroxyvitamin D_3 enhances the expression of transforming growth factor β1 and its latent form binding protein in cultured breast carcinoma cells. *Cancer Res.* **55:** 1540–1546.

102. Arteaga, C. L., R. J. Coffey, T. C. Dugger, C. M. McCutchen, H. L. Moses, and R. M. Lyons. 1990. Growth stimulation of breast-cancer cells with anti-transforming growth factor β antibodies: Evidence for negative autocrine growth regulation by transforming growth factor β. *Cell Growth Diff.* **1:** 367–374.

103. Arteaga, C. L., S. D. Hurd, A. R. Winnier, M. D. Johnson, B. M. Fendly, and J. T. Forbes. 1993a. Anti-transforming growth factor (TGF)-β antibodies inhibit breast-cancer cell tumorigenicity and increase mouse spleen natural killer cell activity: implications for a possible role of tumor cell/host TGF-β interactions in human breast cancer progression. *J. Clin. Invest.* **92:** 2569–2576.

104. Zugmaier, G., S. Paik, G. Wilding, C. Knabbe, M. Bano, R. Lupu, B. Deschauer, S. Simpson, R. B. Dickson, and M. E. Lippman. 1991. Transforming growth factor β_1 induces cachexia and systemic fibrosis without an antitumor effect in nude mice. *Cancer Res.* **51:** 3590- 3594.

105. Sun, L., G. Wu, J. K. V. Willson, E. Zborowska, J. Yang, I. Rajkarunanayake, J. Wang, L. E. Gentry, X.-F. Wang, and M. G. Brattain. 1994. Expression of transforming growth factor β type II receptor leads to reduced malignancy in human breast cancer MCF-7 cells. *J. Biol. Chem.* **268:** 26,449–26,455.

106. Nørgaard, P., L. Damstrup, K. Rygaard, M. Spang-Thomsen, and H. S. Poulsen. 1994. Growth suppression by transforming growth factor-β1 of human small-cell lung cancer cell lines is associated with expression of the type II receptor. *Br. J. Cancer* **69:** 802–808.

107. Markowitz, S., J. Wang, L. Myeroff, R. Parsons, L. Sun, J. Lutterbaugh, R. S. Fan, E. Zborowska, K. W. Kinzler, B. Vogelstein, M. Brattain, and J. K. V. Willson. 1995. Inactivation of the type II TGF-β receptor in colon cancer cells with microsatellite instability. *Science* (Washington, DC) **268:** 1336–1338.

108. Parsons, R., L. L. Myeroff, B. Liu, J. K. V. Willson, S. D. Markowitz, K. W. Kinzler, and B. Vogelstein. 1995. Microsatellite instability and mutations of the transforming growth factor β type II receptor gene in colorectal cancer. *Cancer Res.* **55:** 5548–5550.

109. Park, K., S.-J. Kim, Y.-J. Bang, J.-G. Park, N. K. Kim, A. B. Roberts, and M. B. Sporn. 1994. Genetic changes in the transforming growth factor β (TGF-β) type II receptor gene in human gastric cancer cells: correlation with sensitivity to growth inhibition by TGF-β. *Proc. Natl. Acad. Sci. USA* **91:** 8772–8776.

110. Garrigue-Antar, L., T. Munos-Antonia, S. J. Antonia, J. Gesmonde, V. F. Vellucci, and M. Reiss. 1995. Missense mutations of the transforming growth factor β type II receptor in human head and neck squamous carcinoma cells. *Cancer Res.* **55:** 3982–3987.

111. Kadin, M. E., M. W. Cavaille-Coll, R. Gertz, J. Massagué, S. Cheifetz, and D. George. 1994. Loss of receptors for transforming growth factor β in human T-cell malignancies. *Proc. Natl. Acad. Sci. USA* **91:** 6002–6006.

112. Nørgaard, P., S. Hougaard, H. S. Poulsen, and M. Spang-Thomsen. 1995. Transforming growth factor β and cancer. *Cancer Treat. Rev.* **21:** 367–403.

113. Kim, I. Y., H.-J. Ahn, D. J. Zelner, J. W. Shaw, S. Lang, M. Kato, M. G. Oefelin, K. Miyazono, J. A. Nemeth, J. M. Kozlowski, and C. Lee. 1996. Loss of expression of transforming growth factor β type I and II receptors correlates with tumor grade in human prostate cancer tissues. *Clin. Cancer Res.* **2:** 1255–1261.

114. Knaus, P. I., D. Lindemann, J. F. DeCoteau, R. Perlman, H. Yankelev, M. Hille, M. E. Kadin, and H. F. Lodish. 1996. A dominant inhibitory mutant of the type II transforming growth factor β receptor in the malignant progression of a cutaneous T-cell lymphoma. *Mol. Cell. Biol.* **16:** 3480–3489.

115. Chen, C., X.-F. Wang, and L. Sun. 1997. Expression of transforming growth factor β type III receptor restores autocrine TGF_1 activity in human breast cancer MCF–7 cells. *J. Biol. Chem.* **272:** 12,862–12,867.

116. Younes, M., L. Fernandez, and R. Laucirica. 1996. Transforming growth factor-β type II receptor is infrequently expressed in human breast cancer. *Breast J.* **2:** 150–153.

117. Brattain, M. G., Y. Ko, S. S. Banerji, G. Wu, and J. K. V. Willson. 1996. Defects of TGF-β receptor signaling in mammary cell tumorigenesis. *J. Mammary Gland Biol. Neopl.* **1:** 364–372.

118. Vincent, F., M. Nagashima, S. Takenoshita, M. A. Khan, A. Gemma, K. Hagiwara, and W. P. Bennett. 1997. Mutation analysis of the transforming growth factor-β type II receptor in human cell lines resistant to growth inhibition by transforming growth factor-β. *Oncogene* **15:** 117–122.

119. Schutte, M., R. H. Hruban, L. Hedrick, K. R. Cho, G. M. Nadasdy, C. L. Weinstein, G. S. Bova, W. B. Isaacs, P. Cairns, H. Nawroz, D. Sidransky, R. A. Casero, Jr., P. S. Meltzer, S. A. Hahn, and S. E. Kern. 1996. DPC4 gene in various tumor types. *Cancer Res.* **56:** 2527–2530.

120. Guise, T. A., J. J. Yin, S. D. Taylor, Y. Kumagai, M. Dallas, B. F. Joyce, T. Yoneda, and G. R. Mundy. 1996. Evidence for a causal role of parathyroid hormone-related protein in the pathogenesis of human breast cancer-mediated osteolysis. *J. Clin. Invest.* **98:** 1544–1549.

121. Hauschka, P. V., A. E. Mavrakos, M. D. Iafrati, S. E. Doleman, and M. Klagsburn. 1986. Growth factors in bone matrix. *J. Biol. Chem.* **261:** 12665–12674.

122. Kiriyama, T., M. T. Gillespie, J. A. Glatz, S. Fukumoto, J. M. Moseley, and T. J. Martin. 1992. Transforming growth factor β stimulation of parathyroid hormone-related protein (PTHrP): a paracrine regulator? *Mol. Cell. Endocrinol.* **92:** 55–62.

123. Yin, J. J., J. M. Chrigwin, S. D. Taylor, M. Dallas, J. Masague, G. R. Mundy, and T. A. Guise. 1996. Dominant negative blockade of the transforming growth factor β (TGFβ) type II receptor decreases breast cancer-mediated osteolysis. *Breast Cancer Res. Treat.* **41:** 220A.

124. Butta, A., K. MacLennan, K. C. Flanders, N. P. M. Sacs, I. Smith, A. McKinna, M. Dowsett, L. M. Wakefield, M. B. Sporn, M. Baum, and A. A. Colletta. 1992. Induction of transforming growth factor β$_1$ in human breast cancer in vivo following tamoxifen treatment. *Cancer Res.* **52:** 4261–4264.

125. Kopp A., W. Jonat, M. Schmahl, and C. Knabbe. 1995. Transforming growth factor β2 (TGF-β2) levels in plasma of patients with metastatic breast cancer treated with tamoxifen. *Cancer Res.* **55:** 4512–4515.

126. MacCallum, J., J. C. Keen, J. M. S. Barlett, A. M. Thompson, J. M. Dixon, and W. R. Miller. 1996. Changes in expression of transforming growth factor beta mRNA isoforms in patients undergoing tamoxifen therapy. *Br. J. Cancer* **74:** 474–478.

127. Herman, M. E., and B. S. Katzenellenbogen. 1994. Alterations in transforming growth factor-α and -β production and cell responsiveness during the progression of MCF-7 human breast-cancer cells to estrogen-autonomous growth. *Cancer Res.* **54:** 5867–5874.

128. Koli, K. M. and C. L. Arteaga. 1997. Predominant cytosolic localization of type II transforming growth factor β receptors in human breast carcinoma cells. *Cancer Res.* **57:** 970–977.

129. Arteaga, C. L. and C. K. Osborne. 1991. Growth factors as mediators of estrogen/antiestrogen action in human breast-cancer cells, in *Regulatory Mechanisms in Breast Cancer* (Lippman, M. and R. Dickson, eds.), Kluwer, Boston, pp. 289–304.

130. Ji, H., L. E. Stout, Q. Zhang, R. Zhang, H. T. Leung, and B. S. Leung. 1994. Absence of transforming growth factor-β responsiveness in the tamoxifen growth-inhibited human breast cancer cell line CAMA-1. *J. Cell Biochem.* **54:** 332–342.

131. Kalkhoven, E., L. Kwakkenbos-Isbrucker, C. L. Mummery, S. W. de Laat, A. J. M. van den Eijnden-van Raaij, P. T. van der Saag, and B. van der Burg. 1995. The role of TGF-β production in growth inhibition of breast-tumor cell by progestins. *Int. J. Cancer* **61:** 80–86.

132. Arteaga, C. L., K. M. Koli, T. C. Dugger, and R. Clarke. 1998. Reversal of tamoxifen resistance of human breast carcinomas in vivo with anti-transforming growth factor-β antibodies involves paracrine mechanisms. *J. Natl. Cancer Inst.*, in press.

133. Dickson, R. B., A. Kasid, K. K. Huff, S. E. Bates, C. Knabbe, D. Bronzert, E. P. Gelmann, and M. E. Lippman. 1986b. Activation of growth factor βsecretion in tumorigenic states of breast cancer by 17β-estradiol or v-Ha-ras oncogene. *Proc. Natl. Acad. Sci. USA* **84:** 837–841.

134. Daly, R. J., R. J. B. King, and P. D. Darbre. 1990. Interaction of growth factors during progression towards steroid independence in T47D human breast cancer cells. *J. Cell Biochem.* **43:** 199–211.

135. Herman, M. E. and B. S. Katzenellenbogen. 1996. Response-specific antiestrogen resistance in a newly characterized MCF-7 human breast-cancer cell line resulting form long-term exposure to *trans*-hybroxytamoxifen. *J. Steroid Biochem. Biol.* **59:** 121–134.

136. King, R. J. B., D. Y. Wang, R. J. Daly, and P. D. Darbre. 1989. Approaches to studying the role of growth factors in the progression of breast tumors from steroid sensitive to insensitive state. *J. Steroid Biochem.* **34:** 133–138.

138. Walker, R. A. and S. J. Dearing. 1992. Transforming growth factor β1 in ductal carcinoma in situ and invasive carcinomas of the breast. *Eur. J. Cancer* **28:** 641–644.

137. Welch, D. R., A. Fabra, and M. Nakajima. 1990. Transforming growth factor β stimulates mammary adenocarcinoma cell invasion and metastatic potential. *Proc. Natl. Acad. Sci. USA* **87:** 7678–7682.

138. Arnoletti, J. P., D. Albo, M. S. Granick, M. P. Solomon, A. Castiglioni, V. L. Rothman, and G. P. Tuszynski. 1995. Thrombospondin and transforming growth factor-β1 increase expression of urokinase-type plasminogen activator and plasminogen activator inhibitor-1 in human MDA-231 breast-cancer cells. *Cancer* **76:** 998–1005.

139. Walker, R. J., S. J. Dearing, and B. Gallagher. 1994. Relationship of transforming growth factor β_1 to extracellular matrix and stromal infiltrates in invasive breast carcinoma. *Br. J. Cancer* **69:** 1160–1165.

140. Gorsch, S. M., V. A. Menoli, T. A. Stukel, L. I. Gold, and B. A. Arrick. 1992. Immuno-histochemical staining for transforming growth factor β_1 associates with disease progression in human breast cancer. *Cancer Res.* **52:** 6949–6952.

141. Thompson, A. M., D. J. Kerr, and C. M. Steel. 1991. Transforming growth factor β_1 is implicated in the failure of tamoxifen therapy in human breast cancer. *Br. J. Cancer* **63:** 609–614.

142. Relf, M., S. LeJeune, P. A. E. Scott, et al. 1997. Expression of the angiogenic factors vascular endothelial cell growth factor, acidic and basic fibroblast growth factor, tumor growth factor β-1, platelet-derived endothelial cell growth factor, placenta growth factor, and pleiotrophin in human primary breast cancer and its relationship to angiogenesis. *Cancer Res.* **57:** 963–969.

142a. Pepper, M. S. 1997. Transforming growth factor-beta: Vasculogenesis, angiogenesis, and vessel wall integrity. *Cytokine & Growth Factors Rev.* **8:** 21–43.

143. Arteaga, C. L., T. Carty-Dugger, H. L. Moses, S. D. Hurd, and J. A. Pietenpol. 1993. Transforming growth factor β_1 can induce estrogen-independent tumorigenicity of human breast-cancer cells in athymic mice. *Cell Growth Diff.* **4:** 193–201.

144. Letterio, J. J. and A. B. Roberts. 1998. Regulation of immune responses by TGF-β. *Annu. Rev. Immunol.* **16:** 137–161.

145. de Martin, R., B. Haendler, R. Wofer-Harbinek, H. Gaugitsch, M. Wrann, H. Schlusener, J. M. Seifert, S. Bodmer, A. Fontana, and E. Hofer. 1987. Complementary DNA for human glioblastoma-derived T-cell suppressor factor, a novel member of the transforming growth factor gene family. *EMBO J.* **6:** 3673–3677.

146. Park, J. A., E. Wang, R. A. Kurt, S. F. Schluter, E. M. Hersh, and E. T. Akporiaye. 1997. Expression of an antisense transforming growth factor-β1 transgene reduces tumorigenicity of EMT6 mammary tumor cells. *Cancer Gene Ther.* **4:** 42–50.

147. Teicher, B. A., S. A. Holden, G. Ara, and G. Chen. 1996. Transforming growth factor-β in *in vivo* resistance. *Cancer Chemother. Pharmacol.* **37:** 601–609.

148. Teicher, B. A., Y. Maehara, Y. Kakeji, G. Ara, S. R. Keyes, J. Wong, and R. Herbst. 1997. Reversal of *in vivo* drug resistance by the transforming growth factor-β inhibitor decorin. *Int. J. Cancer* **71**: 49–58.

149. Kakeji, Y., Y. Maehara, M. Ikebe, B. A. Teicher. 1997. Dynamics of tumor oxygenation, CD31 staining, and transforming growth factor-β levels after treatment with radiation or cyclophosphamide in the rat 13762 mammary carcinoma. *Int. J. Radiation Oncol. Biol. Phys.* **37**: 1115–1123.

150. Lowe, S. W., H. E. Ruley, T. Jacks, and D. E. Housman. 1993. p53-dependent apoptosis modulates the cytotoxicity of anticancer agents. *Cell* **74**: 957–967.

151. Li, J. J. and R. J. Deshaies. 1993. Exercising self-restraint: discouraging illicit acts of S and M in eukaryotes. *Cell* **74**: 223–226.

152. Belizario, J. E. and C. A. Dinarello. 1991. Interleukin 1, interleukin 6, tumor necrosis factor, and transforming growth factor β increase cell resistance to tumor necrosis factor cytotoxicity by growth arrest in the G_1 of the cell cycle. *Cancer Res.* **51**: 2379–2385.

153. Huang, A., H. Jin, and J. A. Wright. 1995. Drug resistance and gene amplification potential regulated by transforming growth factor $β_1$ gene expression. *Cancer Res.* **55**: 1758–1762.

5

The Insulin-Like Growth Factor Network and Breast Cancer

Matthew J. Ellis

1. INTRODUCTION

The insulin-like growth factors, IGF1 and IGF2, are an increasingly important focus for breast cancer research. Expressed in most organs, IGF1 and IGF2 are circulating peptide hormones and locally acting growth factors with paracrine/autocrine functions. Both IGFs signal through a common tyrosine kinase receptor, the insulin-like growth factor 1 receptor (IGF1R), and have mitogenic, antiapoptotic, and insulin-like actions that are essential for embryogenesis and postnatal growth physiology. IGF1 and IGF2 also interact with a family of seven soluble IGF-binding proteins (IGFBP1–7) that tightly regulate free IGF1 and IGF2 concentrations. Release of active IGF1 and IGF2 from IGFBP complexes is mediated by IGFBP proteinases synthesized by target cells. Additionally, IGF2 activity is regulated by the mannose 6-phosphate/IGF2 receptor (M6P/IGF2R), a protein transporter that targets IGF2 for lysosomal degradation. This complex network of ligands, receptors, and binding proteins is disturbed in breast cancer, leading to excess IGF1R activation and tyrosine kinase signaling. Evidence for this conclusion includes the following observations: IGF2 is strongly and aberrantly expressed by stromal cells within breast cancers; M6P/IGF2R is mutated in breast cancer epithelial cells, leading to loss of IGF2 degradation; IGF1R is overexpressed by malignant breast epithelial cells; and complex changes in IGFBP expression occur during breast cancer progression. Further, synergistic interaction between IGF1R and estrogen signaling implies that IGF network changes play an important role in pathogenesis of hormone-dependent breast cancer. Abnormal levels of IGF1R signaling could, therefore, alter the response to antiestrogen therapy by modifying estrogen receptor (ER) function. Additionally, it has been shown that IGF1R activation, by generating a cell survival signal, may inhibit the effectiveness of radiotherapy and chemotherapy. Since IGF signaling potentially impacts on all three nonsurgical modalities of breast cancer therapy, IGF network proteins are being evaluated as therapeutic response markers. Furthermore, the link between IGF and therapy has raised the intriguing possibility that inhibitors of IGF1R activation could prove to be logical and effective approaches to improve the efficacy of multimodality breast cancer treatment.

From: Breast Cancer: *Molecular Genetics, Pathogenesis, and Therapeutics*
Edited by: A. M. Bowcock © Humana Press Inc., Totowa, NJ

2. THE IGF NETWORK

2.1. Introduction

The IGF network is composed of ligands, receptors, and binding proteins that determine the overall level of signaling through the tyrosine kinase receptor, IGF1R. A summary of the functions of each IGF network component is a necessary prerequisite for a discussion of the role of IGF signaling in breast cancer pathogenesis. IGF network components can be classified as IGF activators, modulators, and inhibitors (Fig. 1). IGF activators are composed of the peptide ligands, IGF1 and IGF2, and their common receptor, IGF1R *(1)*. The insulin receptor (IR) is also an IGF activator, since IGF2 can activate IR *(2)*, and IGF1R and IR form signaling-competent heterodimers *(3)*. IGFBPs can be classified as IGF network modulators. When IGF1 and IGF2 are in a complex with IGFBPs, they are inactive. However, through the action of IGFBP proteinases, IGF1 and IGF2 are released from IGFBPs in the vicinity of a target cell. IGFBPs, therefore, tightly regulate IGF concentrations within tissues, and have both stimulatory and inhibitory roles *(4)*. The M6P/IGF2R is an IGF network inhibitor that selectively targets IGF2 for lysosomal degradation *(5)*. The recent recognition that the M6P/IGF2R is subject to loss of function mutations in breast cancer cells provides one of the most direct links between aberrant IGF signaling and human breast cancer pathogenesis *(6)*.

2.2. Insulin-like Growth Factors 1 and 2

Mature IGF1 (somatomedin) and IGF2 are 7.5 kDa polypeptide growth factors that arise from proteolytic cleavage of prohormones, in a manner analogous to insulin. IGF1 is the principal mediator of the effects of growth hormone (GH) on postnatal growth. IGF2 has an important growth-promoting action during embryogenesis; however, the role of IGF2 in postnatal physiology is ill-defined, since IGF2 is not GH-regulated, and no human IGF2 deficiency syndromes have been described. Both IGF1 and IGF2 circulate at high levels in the peripheral blood, bound to IGFBPs. In the case of IGF1, the principal source of circulating protein is the liver. IGF2, on the other hand, has a widespread pattern of expression, and the circulating pool presumably has multiple sources *(7,8)*. Synthesis of both IGFs has been shown to be under the control of estrogen *(9,10)*. This observation may be important therapeutically, since IGF1 levels (but not IGF2 levels) are suppressed in patients receiving the antiestrogen tamoxifen *(11)*. Additional controls on IGF synthesis exist; for example, IGF2 promotes its own translation via a growth factor-activated, S6-kinase-regulated positive feedback loop *(12)*. Furthermore, transcriptional control of IGF2 is highly complex, with four promoters differentially driving six exons that encode four alternative 5' untranslated regions *(12)*. Each IGF2 promoter has a distinct pattern of tissue-specific and embryonic expression *(13)*, and transcription is restricted to the paternal allele as a result of genomic imprinting. IGF2 imprinting is relaxed in some human tumors, leading to abnormal biallelic expression *(14)*.

2.3. IGF1 Receptor and the Insulin Receptor

IGF1 and IGF2 signal through the IGF1R, a ligand-activated tyrosine kinase *(1)*. IGF1R is highly homologous to the IR (85% amino acid homology). IGF1R and IR

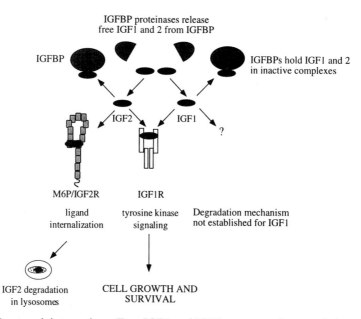

IGFBP proteinases release
free IGF1 and 2 from IGFBP

IGFBP

IGFBPs hold IGF1 and 2
in inactive complexes

IGF2   IGF1

?

M6P/IGF2R   IGF1R

ligand   tyrosine kinase   Degradation mechanism
internalization   signaling   not established for IGF1

IGF2 degradation   CELL GROWTH AND
in lysosomes   SURVIVAL

Fig. 1. IGF network interactions. Free IGF1 and IGF2 concentrations, and, therefore, IGF1R tyrosine kinase activity, are tightly regulated by a complex network of binding proteins, binding protein proteinases, and a lysosomal transport receptor.

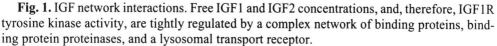

form heterodimeric receptor structures consisting of disulfide-linked α- and β-chain dimers, which serve ligand binding and signal transduction, respectively *(15)*. IGF1R and IR have traditionally been considered to have distinct physiological roles. IGF1R was thought to predominantly regulate cellular proliferation, and IR, to regulate cellular metabolism. This proposed division of labor was based on the observation that IGF1 promotes growth hormone-dependent postnatal growth exclusively through the IGF1R *(16,17)*. Conversely, studies of insulin action focused mainly on cellular metabolism, rather than on proliferation. In keeping with these distinct roles, insulin and IGF1 exhibit highly selective affinity for IR and IGF1R. However, recent studies of insulin and IGF action at the molecular level have revealed several receptor crosstalk mechanisms that reduce specificity (Fig. 2). Specifically, heterodimers form between the IR and the IGF1R, consisting of an α and β chain of each receptor type, generating a hybrid receptor *(3)*. The exact signaling properties, tissue distribution, and physiological role of IR/IGF1R hybrids are unclear, although the presence of hybrid receptors in the breast cancer cell line MCF7 implies a potential role in breast cancer pathophysiology *(18)*. Furthermore, IGF2 binds and activates both IR and IGF1R homodimers, as well as (presumably) hybrid receptors *(2)*. This insulin-like action of IGF2 leads to hypoglycemia in patients with IGF2-overexpressing malignancies *(19,20)*. Intracellularly, a myriad of postreceptor crosstalk mechanisms must also exist, since IR and IGF1R activate related, and, in many instances, identical signal transduction molecules. A comprehensive review of IGF1R and IR signal transduction is inappropriate here; however, a number of excellent reviews are available *(21–23)*.

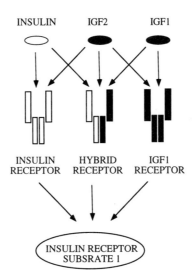

Fig. 2. Crosstalk between insulin receptor and IGF1 receptor. Crosstalk occurs at three levels: a) at the ligand level, since IGF2 can activate both insulin receptor and the IGF1 receptor; b) at the receptor level, since insulin receptor and insulin-like growth factor form hybrid receptors; and c) at the signal transduction level, since insulin receptors and IGF1 receptor signal tranduction pathways utilize common signal transduction molecules, for example, insulin receptor substrate 1.

2.4. IGF-Binding Proteins and Proteinases

IGFBPs consist of a family of six proteins that has recently been joined by a seventh *(24)*. The functions of the IGFBPs 1–7 are complex and have been reviewed recently *(4)*. The affinity of IGFBPs for IGF1 and IGF2 exceeds the affinity of these ligands for IGF1R *(25)*. The IGFBPs show tissue-specific expression patterns, and IGFBP synthesis is regulated by hormonal signals that include sex steroids, retinoids, cyclic AMP, cytokines, and gonadotrophins. Controversy concerning IGFBP action has arisen because IGFBPs have been shown to both stimulate and inhibit IGF action. Clearly, binding to an IGFBP will temporarily inactivate IGF1 and IGF2; however, this interaction also stabilizes IGF ligands and protects them from degradation. In response to physiologic or pathophysiologic stimuli, target cells can trigger the release of IGF1 and IGF2 from binding protein complexes by expressing IGFBP proteinases *(26)*. IGFBP proteinases can be IGFBP-specific, such as the IGFBP3 serine proteinase *(27)*, or have a more general IGFBP proteinase effect, such as the metalloproteinases, MMP1 and MMP2 *(28)*. Prostate-specific antigen (PSA) is another recently defined IGFBP proteinase *(29)* expressed by breast cancer cells *(30)*. Adding further biological complexities, IGFBPs have additional growth-regulatory actions that are independent of their activity as IGF network modulators. For example, overexpression of IGFBP3 unexpectedly inhibits the growth of IGF1R-deficient fibroblasts. Theoretically, IGFBP3 could directly generate an inhibitory growth signal, because a pool of IGFBP3 molecules are associated with the cell membrane. Alternatively, IGFBP3 could somehow modulate the activity of other growth factor receptors *(31)*.

2.5. Ligand Degradation

Ligand degradation is a critical aspect of IGF network regulation. In the case of IGF2, a dedicated degradation pathway is provided by the M6P/IGF2R, a lysosomal trafficking protein that transports IGF2 to lysosomes *(5)*. M6P/IGF2R also binds mannose 6-phosphorylated lysosomal enzymes and transports nascent lysosomal proteins from the Golgi to the endosomal compartment *(32)*. A 275–300 kD integral membrane protein, M6P/IGF2R has a large extracellular domain composed of 15 cysteine-rich repeats, each an average of 147 amino acids in length. The C-terminal 300 amino acids include a transmembrane domain and a short cytoplasmic domain that is believed to be devoid of enzymatic activities associated with signal transduction *(33)*. IGF2 binds within repeat 11 *(34–36)* and mannose 6-phosphorylated proteins bind to a bipartite domain composed of amino acids in both repeats 3 and 9 *(37)*. Despite the lack of a tyrosine kinase domain or other signaling motifs, investigators have proposed an active signaling role for the M6P/IGF2R cytoplasmic domain, possibly through a G-protein-linked mechanism *(38)*. However, interactions between M6P/IGF2R and G proteins have proved difficult to confirm *(39)*, and recent evidence supports the notion that the only role of the M6P/IGF2R in IGF signaling is to degrade IGF2, thereby downregulating IGF1R activity *(40-42)*. M6P/IGF2R expression is increased by IGF2 *(43)*, indicating that regulation of IGF2 by M6P/IGF2R is part of a negative-feedback mechanism. In this model, IGF2 activates IGF1R, stimulating M6P/IGF2R synthesis, which, in turn, reduces extracellular IGF2 by targeted degradation, thereby reducing IGF1R activation *(41)*. IGF1 and insulin are not regulated by M6P/IGF2R, and insulin is routed for degradation in the endosomal compartment directly, via its interaction with IR. Liganded IR is internalized from coated pits, and traffics to the endosomal compartment. Insulin is then degraded in lysosomes, and intact IR recycles to the cell surface *(44)*. It is not known if analogous IGF1 degradation occurs via the IGF1R or even via a receptor-independent mechanism.

3. THE IGF NETWORK AND REPRODUCTIVE ORGAN PHYSIOLOGY

3.1. Animal Studies

What role does the IGF network play in reproductive organ physiology, and, more specifically, the physiology of the mammary gland? In rodents, IGF signaling is critical for reproductive organ development, since *Igf-1* gene knock-out mice exhibit testicular, uterine, ovarian, and mammary hypoplasia *(45)*. Since female ER knock-out mice are also sterile *(46)*, dual signals from both IGF1R and ER must be considered obligatory requirements for reproductive organ development in rodents. Evidence for a critical interplay between ER and IGF1R signaling is supported by a number of additional animal studies; for example: estrogen stimulates IGF1R phosphorylation in uterine tissue *(47)*; IGF1 is an estrogen-regulated gene in the ovary and uterus *(48,49)*; transgenic expression of IGFBP1 inhibits estrogen-dependent uterine growth *(50)*; estrogen treatment enhances the stimulatory effect of IGF1 on mammary gland development *(51,52)*; and transgenic overexpression of IGF1 in the mouse and rat mammary gland is associated with incomplete mammary involution, ductal hypertrophy, loss of secretory lobules, and increased deposition of collagen *(53,54)*.

3.2. *Human Studies*

Examination of human individuals with defects in IGF signaling provides an opportunity to compare IGF physiology between rodents and humans. A human male with short stature and a homozygous deletion in the *IGF1* gene has recently been described *(16)*. This patient had begun puberty, but at the time of the report it was unclear whether full sexual maturation would occur. In male IGF1-deficient mice, testicular hypoplasia and low testosterone levels have been observed *(45)*. However, it is possible that the consequences of IGF1 deficiency in humans may be attenuated by IGF2, which is present at higher levels in adult humans than in adult mice *(55,56)*. No females with deletions in *IGF1* have been described to date. The Efi Pygmies of Northern Zaire provide another interesting example of the consequences of reduced IGF signaling. Immortalized lymphocytes from Efi Pygmies exhibit a defect in IGF1R tyrosine kinase activation, even though high affinity binding takes place *(57)*. Interestingly, although Efi Pygmies are short, they are fertile, despite defective IGF1R signaling. A possible explanation for the "short but fertile" Efi phenotype is IGF2-dependent IR activation (2). Perhaps the IGF2/IR pathway provides sufficient stimulus for reproductive organs to mature. While this hypothesis is difficult to confirm, IGF2 is expressed in the human ovary *(58)* and breast *(59,60)*, implying that IGF2 may have a role in human reproductive organ function. Determination of the role IGF2 plays in adult human physiology awaits the identification of IGF2-deficient individuals.

4. IGF SIGNALING AND PROLIFERATION

IGF1 and IGF2 promote cellular proliferation through the IGF1R tyrosine kinase. A requirement for IGF1R activation for cell-cycle progression has been noted in studies on the growth of primary cells in response to various growth factor combinations. These data lead to the proposition that IGF1R activation is a restriction point in the cell cycle *(61)*. A critical aspect of the action of IGF1 and IGF2 on breast tissue is the well-established synergistic effect of combined estrogen and IGF exposure on breast epithelial growth (Fig. 3). This interaction is obvious both in vitro *(41,62)* and in vivo *(51,52)*. At least part of the interaction between estrogen and IGF signaling occurs at the level of the ER, since IGF1 and IGF2 activate transcription from estrogen response elements in the presence of liganded ER *(63–65)*. ER is, therefore, a nuclear target for IGF1R signaling. Activation of transcription by ER is complex and requires not only estrogen, but ER phosphorylation and the action of coactivator proteins that connect ER to the basal transcriptional machinery. By activating the mitogen-activated protein (MAP) kinase cascade, IGF1R increases ER protein phosphorylation and elevates transcriptional activity *(66)*. In addition, both IGF1R and ER activation increase the expression of a recently-described ER coactivator, cyclin D1 *(67,68)*. Cyclin D1 has been shown to form a complex with ER that promotes transcription from an estrogen response element *(69)*. Genetic manipulation of IGF1R expression levels in breast cells in vitro provides further evidence for a role for IGF1R in hormone-dependent breast cancer proliferation: overexpression of IGF1R by gene transfection sensitizes cells to IGF1, reduces the requirement for estrogen, and increases cell adhesion *(70)*, and antisense-mediated reduction of IGF1R expression inhibits MCF7 cell growth in the presence of IGF1 *(71)*. Furthermore steroidal antiestrogens inhibit the IGF1-dependent growth of ER-positive breast cancers and downregulate IGF1R expression *(72)*. These data, the

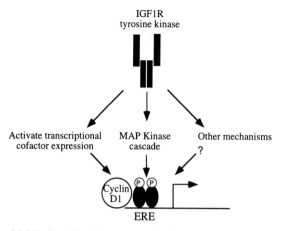

Fig. 3. Estrogen and IGF signaling interact at the level of the estrogen receptor. Activation of the IGF1 receptor induces MAP kinase phosphorylation of the estrogen receptor. In addition, IGF1R stimulates the expression of transcriptional co-activators such as cyclin D. These events lead to an increase in the ability of liganded ER to drive transcription through estrogen response elements (ERE).

observation that ER-negative cell lines are frequently insensitive to the growth-promoting actions of IGF1 *(73,74)*, and the consequences of *Igf-I* gene knock-out on the development of estrogen-regulated tissue in mice *(45)*, all support the conclusion that ER is an obligatory component for IGF-induced mitogenesis in breast cancer cells. However, other important consequences of IGF1R activation, for example, inhibition of apoptosis, could be ER-independent, since distinct signal transduction pathways are likely to be involved.

5. IGF SIGNALING AND APOPTOSIS

It is well established that genetic lesions that transform cells may, paradoxically, also increase the rate of cell death. One of the best examples of this phenomenon comes from studies of the *c-myc* oncogene, which induces apoptosis as well as cellular proliferation when constitutively expressed in nontransformed fibroblasts *(75)*. Intriguingly, IGF1 and IGF2 suppress c-*myc*-induced apoptosis *(76)*. Epithelial cell lines from MMTV c-*myc*-induced mammary tumors, like their fibroblast counterparts, also undergo apoptosis that can be reversed with EGF or IGF1 *(77)*. By increasing the survival of transformed cells with aberrant oncogene expression, the IGFs could have profound effects on the rate of malignant progression and tumor growth. IGF1R activation appears to be a prerequisite for transformation, since mouse embryonic fibroblasts from IGFIR-deficient transgenic mice cannot be transformed by SV40 T-antigen, or *SRC*, by signal transduction components such as *RAS* and *RAF*, or by other tyrosine kinase-linked receptors such as the epidermal growth factor receptor (EGFR). IGF-IR therefore generates a critical signal for cellular transformation *(78)*. Based on these observations, it can be argued that genetic or epigenetic events that lead to an increase in IGF1R activity are a critical early event in cellular transformation that allows a cell to tolerate otherwise lethal mutations.

6. IGF SIGNALING AND TRANSFORMATION

Transgenic technology has provided a further opportunity to examine the relationship between IGF signaling and cancer. A key example of such studies is a pancreatic cancer model generated by the introduction into the mouse germline of a rat insulin promoter-driven oncogene SV40 large T-antigen (RIP TAg). Formation of vascular tumors in animals harboring the RIP TAg construct is associated with a marked increase in tumor IGF2 expression. This increase in IGF2 expression is critical for tumor formation, because the number and size of the pancreatic tumors were markedly reduced when RIP TAg mice were crossed into an IGF2-deficient knock-out background *(79)*. Generation of transgenic mice with IGF2 constructs that drive IGF2 overexpression has also confirmed that increased IGF2 expression directly promotes malignant transformation. Mice bearing a major urinary protein promoter-IGF2 transgene, which targets IGF2 expression to the liver, develop diverse tumors, with a preponderance of hepatocellular carcinomas *(80)*. Similarly, when IGF2 is placed under the control of the sheep β-lactoglobin promoter, mice develop an excess of mammary tumors *(81)*. On the basis of these transgenic experiments, IGF2 can be considered an oncogene, since IGF2 is the genetic cause of malignancy in these transgenic experiments *(82)*.

7. IGF SIGNALING AND P53

p53 is a transcription factor that activates genes responsible for cell-cycle arrest, DNA repair, and apoptosis in response to DNA damage *(83)*. IGFBP3 has recently been identified in a screen for p53-regulated genes. In keeping with a role in p53-mediated tumor suppression, IGFBP3 is induced by exposure to chemotherapy *(84)*. p53 also suppresses transcription from the IGF2 P3 promoter *(85)* and the IR promoter *(86)*. Inhibition of IGF signaling is, therefore, an integral aspect of the p53-mediated cellular response. Presumably, this is because an IGF1R-dependent cell survival signal suppresses apoptosis and opposes the ability of p53 to guard the genome *(87)*. Further evidence linking IGF1R activity to resistance to genotoxic stress can be found in studies linking IGF1R and resistance to chemotherapy and radiation; for example, etoposide-induced apoptosis, a p53-dependent process, is suppressed by IGF-I *(88)*; IGF1R activity is associated with radiation resistance in vitro, and elevated IGF1R expression by breast cancer cells has been associated with in-breast cancer recurrence after breast irradiation *(89)*.

8. EXPRESSION OF IGF NETWORK PROTEINS IN BREAST CANCER

Correlation between IGF network components and responses to breast cancer therapies have provided fresh impetus for studies of IGF network proteins in breast cancer specimens. New reagents, particularly monoclonal antibodies, will be essential in future attempts to determine the value of IGF network proteins as prognostic or therapeutic markers. Currently available data, summarized in this section, support the hypothesis that aberrant IGF1R activation is associated with hormone-dependent breast cancer and, therefore, the early stages of breast cancer evolution. In late-stage breast cancer, IGF1R signaling may contribute to radiotherapy and chemotherapy resistance through mechanisms that may be ER-independent.

8.1. Insulin-like Growth Factor 2

Both *in situ* mRNA analysis and immunohistochemistry have demonstrated that IGF2 is the dominant IGF ligand expressed in breast cancer. However, unlike in sarcoma and colon cancer, IGF2 in breast cancer is predominantly produced by the tumoral stroma, rather than malignant epithelial cells *(60,90)*. In mesenchymal and endodermal tumors, IGF2 expression has been proposed to reflect recapitulation of a "fetal" pattern of gene expression *(91)*. In contrast, stromal IGF2 expression in breast cancer reflects the complex stromal–epithelial interactions that occur during breast cancer evolution *(92)*. Malignant breast epithelial cells presumably secrete factor(s) that promote IGF2 expression in surrounding stromal cells. Stromal IGF2, in turn, acts on ductal epithelial cells to increase cell growth and survival. Activation of stromal IGF2 expression may be the result of inward migration of IGF2-expressing fibroblasts. However, in vitro coculture experiments with breast cancer cells (MCF7) and fibroblasts derived from normal breast tissue suggest that soluble tumor factor(s) promote localized proliferation of IGF2-expressing fibroblasts *(93)*. In addition to paracrine interactions, IGF-mediated stromal–epithelial interactions are strongly modulated by endocrine signals. IGF2 expression is markedly increased in biopsies from pregnant women *(94)*, and, in animal breast cancer models, stromal IGF2 expression decreases after ovariectomy *(95)*. Since the influence of stromal signals is thought to decline with disease progression, the significance of stromal IGF2 expression may be limited to the early phase of breast cancer evolution. This conclusion is supported by a report of an association between IGF2 expression and low tumor grade *(96)*, and observations of prominent stromal IGF2 expression around preinvasive intraductal breast cancers (Ellis et al., manuscript in preparation). However, the literature is not completely consistent on this issue. For example, one report noted a negative correlation between ER and the IGF2 content of tumor cytosols, suggesting that IGF2 expression drives ER-independent growth *(97)*. Inconsistent results may reflect differences in the assays employed to estimate tumor IGF2 content in these studies. Biochemical assays for IGF2 on tumor extracts are prone to inaccuracies caused by inadequate separation of IGF2 from IGFBPs *(98)*. On the other hand, the stromal staining pattern renders immunohistochemical assays for IGF2 difficult to quantify. Theoretically, immunohistochemistry could also be affected by IGFBPs, although this has not been investigated.

8.2. Insulin-like Growth Factor 1 Receptor

Robust positive correlation between IGF1R and ER expression in breast cancer specimens is further strong evidence that IGF1R signaling promotes hormone-dependent breast cancer growth *(99–102)*. In addition, in these studies IGF1R levels also correlated with markers of favorable prognosis and an indolent clinical phenotype (diploid, low S-phase tumors). The association of ER and IGF1R is probably a consequence of ER activity, since IGF1R expression has been shown to be regulated by estrogen in breast tissue *(103)*. IGF1R overexpression in breast cancer may also be a consequence of gene amplification in 15q26, but, unlike another major growth factor receptor implicated in breast cancer pathogenesis, *ERBB2, IGF1R* gene amplification is uncommon (2–3% of unselected breast cancers) *(104)*. In early studies, IGF1R was measured by radioimmunoassay or radioreceptor assay of tumor cytosols, a technique not suitable for analysis of paraffin-embedded, formalin-fixed material. Recently, IGF1R estimation by immunohistochemistry has confirmed a strong positive correlation with ER expression *(105)*. A reliable immunohistochemical assay for IGF1R would open the way for a reexamination of the prognostic and therapeutic value of IGF1R analysis. A study by Railo et al. observed that IGF1R was an adverse prognostic marker in an ER-negative group, but a favorable prognostic marker in an ER-positive subgroup *(106)*. The converse consequences of IGF1R expression in this report seem consistent with the multiple roles IGF1R plays in ER-mediated signal transduction, chemotherapy resistance, and radiation resistance. Given these data, the emphasis for IGF1R analysis in breast cancer is beginning to shift from prognostic to therapeutic marker studies. Analysis of the *ERBB2* oncogene went through a similar transition after an interaction between ErbB2 signaling and resistance to hormone therapy and chemotherapy was defined *(107)*.

8.3. Insulin Receptor

Like IGF1R, IRs are also overexpressed in breast cancer. Upregulation of IRs may be a direct consequence of p53 mutation, as wild-type p53 suppresses IR gene transcription *(86)*. IR overexpression may have an impact on breast cancer growth as breast cancer cells proliferate in vitro in response to insulin *(108,109)*. Although the role of IR in breast cancer is less well defined than that of IGF1R, insulin action could underlie the important epidemiological connection between high animal-fat intake, obesity, and breast cancer. Excess dietary fat leads to insulin resistance, with high levels of circulating insulin. Excessive insulin, together with increased estrogen levels that result from aromatase activity in adipose tissue, could conceivably contribute to abnormal breast epithelial proliferation and, ultimately, breast cancer *(110)*.

8.4. Mannose 6-Phosphate/Insulin-like Growth Factor 2 Receptor

Gene mutation screens have recently established that the mannose 6-phosphate/insulin-like growth factor 2 receptor *(M6P/IGF2R)* is a candidate tumor suppressor gene in a broad spectrum of malignancies, including breast cancer. Loss of heterozygosity (LOH) at the *M6P/IGF2R* locus is present in approx 30% of both invasive and *in situ* breast carcinomas, suggesting that mutations in this gene occur early in breast cancer evolution *(6)*. Consistent with the genetic fingerprint of a tumor-suppressor gene (TSG), loss-of-function mutations in the remaining allele in breast cancer cases exhibiting LOH have been identified *(6)*. Somatic mutations in *M6P/IGF2R* have also been described in hepatoma *(111)* and gastrointestinal and endometrial cancers with the replication error positive phenotype *(112,113)*. Loss of M6P/IGF2R will result in defective IGF2 degradation, leading to aberrant IGF1R activation. In addition, defective Golgi-to-endosome transfer will lead to extracellular release of destructive lysosomal enzymes. Other growth factor pathways may also be affected; for example, proteolytic activation of the negative-growth regulator, latent transforming growth factor-β (TGF-β), may be reduced in M6P/IGF2R-deficient cells. Loss of M6P/IGF2R may, therefore, contribute to several aspects of the malignant phenotype, including deregulated cell growth and tissue invasion *(5)*. The relationship between M6P/IGF2R expression/mutation status and breast cancer phenotype is unknown. One might predict that loss of M6P/IGF2R, by deregulating IGF2 activity, could be a feature of hormone-dependent breast cancer evolution. In addition, M6P/IGF2R mutant tumors could be resistant to both radiotherapy and chemotherapy as a consequence of excessive IGF1R signaling.

8.5. Insulin-like Growth Factor Binding Proteins

Most of the IGFBPs have been found to be expressed in breast cancer cell lines or in clinical specimens. Ligand-blotting studies on breast cancer samples (a technique that detects the IGFBP expression profile) and immunoassay techniques have revealed that IGFBP3 is one of the most prominently expressed IGFBPs, and is particularly elevated in ER-negative, high S-phase, aneuploid tumors with a poor prognosis *(114,115)*. The elevation of IGFBP3 in ER-negative breast cancer, together with the observations that IGFBP3 is both induced by antiestrogens and opposes estrogen-stimulated growth *(116,117)*, implies that IGFBP3 expression may be a marker for hormone resistance. These observations are not restricted to IGFBP3. For example, IGFBP5 is also upregulated in cells exposed to antiestrogens *(118)*, and IGFBP1 both suppresses the estrogen-dependent growth of MCF7 cells *(119)* and is elevated in the serum of patients on antiestrogen therapy *(120)*. Overexpression of IGFBP3 by breast cancer cells with aggressive biological features is a paradox, since IGFBP3 is a breast cancer growth inhibitor that mediates cell-cycle arrest in response to retinoids, TGFβ, p53 and antiestrogens *(84,118,121)*. Perhaps, as a consequence of the transition to hormone-independence, breast cancer cells become resistant to the growth-inhibitory effects of IGFBP3.

8.6. Insulin-like Growth Factor Binding Protein Proteinases

Very little systematic research has been conducted on the role of IGFBP proteinases in breast cancer. The exception has been PSA, since highly specific antibodies are readily available. Breast cancer patients with elevated PSA in tumor extracts have a better prognosis in a multivariate analysis *(122)*, and PSA levels fall in the transition from benign to malignant breast tissue *(123)*. It is not clear how these observations relate to the IGFBP3 proteinase action of PSA. However, release of IGF1 and IGF2 from IGFBPs will increase IGF1R activity, which is, as discussed earlier, a feature of early breast cancer. A glimpse of further complexities in the interaction between IGFs, IGFBPs, and proteinases has recently been provided by evidence that breast cancer cells secrete an IGF-induced IGFBP proteinase-inhibitor *(124)*. A family of IGFBP proteinase inhibitors would add a further tier of complexity to our already elaborate model of interactions within the IGF network.

9. IGF AND BREAST CANCER TREATMENT

9.1. The IGF Network as a Target for Therapy

Given the central role of the IGFs and receptors in breast cancer pathophysiology, these molecules represent excellent therapeutic targets for antibody-based approaches, small-molecule inhibitors, and gene therapy. In addition, it can be envisioned that recombinant formulations of IGF network modulators and antagonists could be used directly to inhibit IGF1R activity.

9.2. Ligand and Receptor Antagonists

A number of groups have looked at developing IGFIR antagonists based on antireceptor antibodies. A monoclonal antibody directed against the IGFIR (αIR-3) has been shown to inhibit the growth of IGF2-overexpressing malignancies (125,126). αIR-3 is also effective against breast cancer cell lines growing in nude mice (127). Ligand–antibody fusions have also been developed. These molecules are designed to bind to the IGF1R on target cells and activate complement-mediated cell lysis (128). Clearly, as our understanding of IGF ligand receptor interaction grows, peptide or peptide mimetic IGF-IR antagonists will become realistic alternatives to antireceptor antibodies. An alternative to directly interrupting the interaction between IGF1R and IGF1 or IGF2 is to use IGFBP or ligand-binding receptor fragments as ligand decoys. IGFBPs are effective breast cancer inhibitors in vitro, and clinical trials with recombinant IGFBPs can be anticipated (119).

9.3. Endocrine Cancer Therapy and IGF1 Expression

Systemic IGF1 levels fall during tamoxifen therapy for breast cancer (11). Suppression of IGF1 expression may, therefore, contribute to the therapeutic action of ER antagonists. Recently, there has been interest in enhancing tamoxifen-induced IGF1 suppression with somatostatin analogs. By inhibiting GH secretion by the anterior pituitary, somatostatin analogs suppress GH-driven IGF1 expression by the liver. Unfortunately, somatostatin analogs have not proved to be effective treatments for metastatic breast cancer (129,130), and did not add to the antitumor activity of tamoxifen in one reasonably sized randomized trial (131). A potential reason for the lack of efficacy of somatostatin analogs in breast cancer is the failure to target IGF2, which is unaffected by tamoxifen or somatostatin analog therapy. These data not withstanding, an adjuvant trial of tamoxifen, plus or minus monthly sustained release somatostatin injections, has been opened by the National Surgical Adjuvant Breast and Bowel Project (NSABP) (NSABP B-29), in the hope that increased activity for the combination can be detected in the minimal disease setting. B-29 is a groundbreaking trial as the first randomized study that tests the logic of combining anti-IGF therapy and hormone therapy in the adjuvant setting. This trial may set the scene for future randomized trials of growth factor inhibitor/antiestrogen combinations.

9.4. Drugs that Modulate IGF Network Protein Levels or Function

The mechanism of a number of anticancer agents may involve modulating IGF or IGF receptor expression in tumor cells. Both estrogen and tamoxifen have been shown to induce growth arrest and regression of T61 human breast cancer xenografts, accompanied by downregulation of IGF2 mRNA expression (132). Other noncytotoxic breast cancer therapies are also linked to inhibition of IGF network activity. For example, monoterpenes have antineoplastic activities in a variety of animal systems (133), and induce an increase in expression of the IGF2 antagonist receptor, m6p/igf2r (134); activation of IGF1R blunts the antiproliferative effect of retinoids on breast cancer cells in vitro (135); and fenretinide, like tamoxifen, is associated with a fall in circulating IGF1 (136). Based on these data, a combined somatostatin analog/retinoid trial is a logical thing to consider.

9.5. Genetic Approaches

IGF1, IGF2, and IGF1R expression or function could be suppressed by antisense approaches, or by dominant negative-receptor molecules. The IGF antagonist genes (IGFBP and M6P/IGF2R), or engineered constructs based on IGFBP or M6P/IGF2R ligand-binding domains, could be used to inhibit IGF signaling by gene transfer. However, genetic therapies for cancer are limited by inefficient tumor-targeting strategies, unless there is a significant bystander effect (i.e., nongenetically-transduced cells are inhibited by cells successfully targeted). This may be the case for IGF1R antisense therapy, because IGF1R antisense-treated C6 rat glioblastoma cells inhibit the growth of a contralateral injection of C6 control cells *(137)*. Immune-system activation has been proposed as the mechanism underlying this observation, and similar results have been obtained in rodent breast cancer models *(138)*. Clinical trials employing IGF1R antisense gene therapy have been initiated.

10. CONCLUSION

Rather than attempt an exhaustive review of the relationship between the IGF network and breast cancer, this chapter has tried to create a framework for the reader to consider new data in this rapidly evolving area of breast cancer research. As must be abundantly clear from the discussion, the IGF network represents a complex, yet exciting area for clinical exploitation. Clinical trials of anti-IGF therapies will be the ultimate test of the integrity of data linking IGF1R activity and breast cancer pathophysiology, and preclinical data dictates that novel anti-IGF therapies should not only be tested alone, but in combination with chemotherapy, radiotherapy, and antiestrogens.

ACKNOWLEDGMENTS

This work was supported by NIH grant CA67302.

REFERENCES

1. Ellis, M., F. Garmroudi, and K. Cullen. 1997. Insulin receptors (IGF1 and IGF2), in *Encyclopedia of Cancer*, vol. 2 (Bertino, J., ed.) San Diego Academic Press, San Diego, CA, pp. 927–939.
2. Morrione, A., B. Valentinis, X. Shi-Qiong, G. Yumaet, A. Louvi, A. Efstratiadis, and R. Baserga. 1997. Insulin-like growth factor II stimulates cell proliferation through the insulin receptor. *Proc. Natl. Acad. Sci. USA* **94:** 3777–3782.
3. Moxham, C. and S. Jabobs. 1992. Insulin/IGF-I receptor hybrids: a mechanism for increasing receptor diversity. *J. Cell. Biochem.* **48:** 136–140.
4. Clemmons, R. 1997. Insulin-like growth factor binding proteins and their role in controlling IGF actions. *Cytokine Growth Factor Rev.* **8:** 45–62.
5. Oates, A., L. Schumaker, S. Jenkins, A. Pearce, S. DaCosta, B. Arun, and M. Ellis. 1998. The mannose 6-phosphate/insulin-like growth factor 2 receptor (*M6P/IGF2R*), a putative breast tumor suppressor gene. *Br. Cancer Res. Treat.* **47:** 269–281.
6. Hankins, G. R., A. T. De Sousa, R. C. Bentley, M. R. Patel, J. R. Marks, J. D. Iglehart, and R. L. Jirtle. 1996. M6P/IGF2 receptor: a candidate breast tumor suppressor gene. *Oncogene* **12:** 2003–2009.
7. Cohick, W. S. and D. R. Clemmons. 1993. Insulin-like growth factors. *Annu. Rev. Physiol.* **55:** 131–153.

8. Humbel, R. E. 1990. Insulin-like growth factors I and II. *Eur. J. Biochem.* **190:** 445–462.

9. Yee, D., K. J. Cullen, S. Paik, J. F. Perdue, B. Hampton, A. Schwartz, M. E. Lippman, and N. Rosen. 1988. Insulin-like growth factor II mRNA expression in human breast cancer. *Cancer Res.* **48:** 6691–6696.

10. Huynh, H. T. and M. Pollak. 1993. Insulin-like growth factor I gene expression in the uterus is stimulated by tamoxifen and inhibited by the pure antiestrogen ICI 182780. *Cancer Res.* **53:** 5585–5588.

11. Pollak, M. 1993. Effects of adjuvent tamoxifen therapy on growth hormone and insulin-like growth factor I (IGF-I) physiology, in *Adjuvant Therapy of Cancer* VII edition (Salmon, S., ed.), Lippincott-Raven, Philadelphia, PA, pp. 43–54.

12. Neilson, F. C., L. Ostergaard, J. Nielson, and J. Christiansen. 1995. Growth-dependent translation of IGF-II mRNA by a rapamycin-sensitive pathway. *Nature* **377:** 358–362.

13. Hu, J., T. Vu, and A. Hoffman. 1995. Differential biallelic activation of three insulin-like growth factor II promoters in the mouse central nervous system. *Mol. Endocrinol.* **9:** 628–636.

14. Rainier, S., L. A. Johnson, C. J. Dobry, A. J. Ping, P. E. Grundy, and A. P. Feinberg. 1993. Relaxation of imprinted genes in human cancer. *Nature* **362:** 747–749.

15. Siddle, K. 1992. The insulin receptor and type I IGF receptor: comparison of structure and function. *Prog. Growth Factor Res.* **4:** 301–320.

16. Woods, K., C. Camacho-Hubner, M. Savage, and A. Clark. 1996. Intrauterine growth retardation and postnatal growth failure associated with deletion of the insulin-like growth factor 1 gene. *N. Engl. J. Med.* **335:** 1363–1367.

17. Lui, J., J. Baker, A. Perkins, E. Robertson, and A. Efstratidis. 1993. Mice carrying null mutations of the the the genes encoding insulin-like growth factor I (*igf-I*) and type I IGF receptor (*igf-Ir*). *Cell* **75:** 59–72.

18. Milazzo, G., C. C. Yip, B. A. Maddux, R. Vigneri, and I. D. Goldfine. 1992. High affinity Insulin binding to an atypical insulin-like growth factor-I receptor in human breast cancer cells. *J. Clin. Invest.* **89:** 899–908.

19. Baxter, R. and W. Daughaday. 1991. Impared formation of the ternary insulin-like growth factor-binding protein complex in patients with hypoglycemia due to nonislet cell tumors. *J. Clin. Endocrinol. Metab.* **73:** 696–702.

20. Daughaday, W. H., B. Trivedi, and R. C. Baxter. 1993. Serum "big insulin-like growth factor II" from patients with tumor hypoglycemia lacks normal E-domain O-linked glycosylation, a possible determinant of normal propeptide processing. *Proc. Natl. Acad. Sci. USA* **90:** 5823–5827.

21. Yenush, L. and M. White. 1997. The IRS-signaling system during insulin and cytokine action. *BioEssays* **19:** 491–500.

22. White, M. and C. Kahn. 1994. The insulin signalling system. *J. Biol. Chem.* **269:** 1–4.

23. Cheatham, B. and C. Kahn. 1995. Insulin action and the insulin signalling network. *Endocr. Rev.* **16:** 117–142.

24. Oh, Y., S. Nagalla, Y. Yamanaka, H. Kim, E. Wilson, and R. Rosenfeld. 1996. Synthesis and characterization of insulin-like growth factor-binding protein (IGFBP)-7. Recombinant human mac25 protein specifically binds IGF-I and -II. *J. Biol. Chem.* **271:** 30,322–30,325.

25. Bach, L. A., S. Hsieh, K. Sakano, H. Fujiwara, J. F. Perdue, and M. M. Rechler. 1993. Binding of mutants of human insulin-like growth factor-II to insulin-like growth factor binding proteins 1 to 6. *J. Biol. Chem.* **268:** 9246–9254.

26. Rajah, R., L. Katz, S. Nunn, P. Solberg, T. Beers, and P. Cohen. 1995. Insulin-like growth factor binding protein (IGFBP) proteinases: functional regulators of cell growth. *Prog. Growth Factor Res.* **6:** 273–284.

27. Lee, C. and M. Rechler. 1995. Proteolysis of insulin-like growth factor binding protein 3 in 150 kilodalton IGFBP complexes by a cation dependent protein activity in adult rat serum promotes the release of IGF1. *Endocrinology* **136:** 4982–4989.
28. Fowlkes, J., K. Thrailkill, D. Serra, K. Suzuki, and H. Nagase. 1995. Matrix metalloproteinases as insulin-like growth factor binding protein-degrading proteinases. *Prog. Growth Factor Res.* **6:** 255–263.
29. Cohen, P., D. Peehl, H. Graves, and R. Rosenfeld. 1994. Biological effects of prostate specific antigen as an insulin-like growth factor binding protein-3 protease. *J. Endocrinol.* **142:** 407–415.
30. Bodey, B., S. Siegel, and H. Kaiser. 1997. Immmunocytochemical detection of prostate specific antigen (PSA) in breast carcinomas. *Proc. AACR.* **38:** 205(Abstract).
31. Valentinis, B., A. Bhala, T. De Angelis, R. Baserga, and P. Cohen. 1995. The human insulin-like growth factor (IGF) binding protein-3 inhibits the growth of fibroblasts with a targeted disruption of the IGF-I receptor gene. *Mol. Endocrinol.* **9:** 361–367.
32. Lobel, P., K. Fujimoto, R. D. Ye, G. Griffiths, and S. Kornfeld. 1989. Mutations in the cytoplasmic domain of the 275 kd mannose 6-phosphate receptor differentially alter lysosomal enzyme sorting and endocytosis. *Cell* **57:** 787–796.
33. Kornfeld, S. 1992. Structure and function of the mannose 6-phosphate /insulin-like growth factor II receptors. *Annu. Rev. Biochem.* **61:** 307–330.
34. Dahms, N. M., D. A. Wick, and M. A. Brzychi-Wessell. 1994. The bovine mannose 6-phosphate/insulin-like growth factor II receptor: localization of the insulin-like growth factor II binding site to domains 5-11. *J. Biol. Chem.* **269:** 3802–3809.
35. Garmroudi, F., G. Devi, D. H. Slentz, B. Schaffer, and R. G. MacDonald. 1996. Truncated forms of the insulin-like growth factor II (IGF-II)/mannose 6-phosphate receptor encompassing the IGF-II binding site: characterization of a point mutation that abolishes IGF-II binding. *Mol. Endocrinol.* **10:** 642–651.
36. Garmroudi, F. and R. G. MacDonald. 1994. Localization of the insulin-like growth factor II (IGF-II) binding/cross-linking site of the IGF-II/mannose 6-phosphate receptor to extracellular repeats 10-11. *J. Biol. Chem.* **269:** 26,944–26,952.
37. Dahms, N. M., P. A. Rose, J. D. Molkentin, Y. Zhang, and M. A. Brzycki. 1993. The bovine mannose 6-phosphate/insulin-like growth factor II receptor: the role of arginine residues in mannose 6-phosphate binding. *J. Biol. Chem.* **268:** 5457–5463.
38. Okamoto, T., T. Katata, Y. Murayama, M. Ui, E. Ogata, and I. Nishimoto. 1990. A simple structure encodes G protein-activating function of the IGF-II/mannose 6-phosphate receptor. *Cell* **62:** 709–717.
39. Korner, C., B. Nurnberg, M. Uhde, and T. Braulke. 1995. Mannose 6-phosphate/insulin-like growth factor II receptor fails to interact with G-proteins. *J. Biol. Chem.* **270:** 287–295.
40. Wang, Z.-Q., M. R. Fung, D. P. Barlow, and E. F. Wagner. 1994. Regulation of embryonic growth and lysosomal targeting by the imprinted *Igf2/Mpr* gene. *Nature* **372:** 464–467.
41. Ellis, M. J. C., B. A. Leav, Z. Yang, A. Rasmussen, A. Pearce, J. A. Zweibel, M. E. Lippman, and K. J. Cullen. 1996. Affinity for the insulin-like growth factor-II (IGF-II) receptor inhibits autocrine IGF-II activity in MCF-7 breast cancer cells. *Mol. Endocrinol.* **10:** 286–297.
42. Lau, M. M. H., C. E. H. Stewart, Z. Liu, H. Bhatt, P. Rotwein, and C. L. Stewart. 1994. Loss of the imprinted IGF2/cation-independent mannose 6-phosphate receptor results in fetal overgrowth and perinatal lethality. *Genes Dev.* **8:** 2953–2963.
43. Claussen, M., D. Buergisser, A. G. P. Schuller, U. Matzner, and T. Braulke. 1995. Regulation of insulin-like growth factor (IGF)-binding protein-6 and mannose 6-phosphate/IGF-II receptor expression in IGF-II-overexpressing NIH 3T3 cells. *Mol. Endocrinol.* **9:** 902–912.

44. Formisano, P., S. Najjar, C. Gross, N. Philippe, F. Oriente, C. Kern-Buell, D. Accili, and P. Gorden. 1995. Receptor-mediated internalization of insulin. Potential role of pp120/HA4, a substrate of the insulin receptor kinase. *J. Biol. Chem.* **270:** 24,073–24,077.

45. Baker, J., M. P. Hardy, J. Zhou, C. Bondy, F. Lupu, A. R. Bellve, and A. Efstratiadis. 1996. Effects of an *Igf1* gene null mutation on mouse reproduction. *Mol. Endocrinol.* **10:** 903–918.

46. Korach, K., J. Couse, S. Curtis, T. Washburn, J. Lindzey, K. Kimbro, et al. 1996. Estrogen receptor gene disruption: molecular characterization and experimental and clinical phenotypes. *Recent Prog. Horm. Res.* **51:** 159–186.

47. Richards, R., R. Di Augustine, P. Petrusz, G. Clark, and J. Sebastian. 1996. Estradiol stimulates tyrosine phosphorylation of the insulin-like growth factor receptor and insulin receptor substrate-1 in the uterus. *Proc. Natl. Acad. Sci. USA* **93:** 12,002–12,007.

48. Adesanya, O., J. Zhou, and C. Bondy. 1996. Sex steroid regulation of insulin-like growth factor system gene expression and proliferation in primate myometrium. *J. Clin. Endocrinol. Metab.* **81:** 1967–1974.

49. Hernandez, E. 1995. Regulation of the genes for insulin-like growth factor (IGF) 1 and 2 and their receptors by steroids and gonadotrphins in the ovary. *J. Steroid Biochem. Mol. Biol.* **53:** 219–221.

50. Rajkumar, K., T. Dheen, M. Krsek, and L. Murphy. 1996. Impared estrogen action in the uterus of insulin-like growth factor binding protein-1 transgenic mice. *Endocrinology* **137:** 1258–1264.

51. Ruan, W., C. Newman, and D. Kleinberg. 1992. Intact and amino-terminally shortened forms of insulin-like growth factor I induce mammary gland differentiation and development. *Proc. Natl. Acad. Sci. USA* **89:** 10,872–10,876.

52. Ruan, W., V. Catanese, R. Wieczorek, M. Feldman, and D. Kleinberg. 1995. Estradiol enhances the stimulatory effect of insulin-like growth factor-1 (IGF1) on mammary development and growth hormone-induced IGF1 meseenger ribonucleic acid. *Endocrinology* **136:** 1296–1302.

53. Neuenschwander, S., A. Schwartz, T. Wood, C. J. Roberts, L. Henninghausen, and D. Le Roith. 1996. Involution of the lactating mammary gland is inhibited by the IGF system in a transgenic mouse model. *J. Clin. Invest.* **97:** 2225–2232.

54. Hadsell, D. L., N. M. Greenberg, J. M. Fligger, C. R. Baumrucker, and J. M. Rosen. 1996. Targeted expression of des(1-3) human insulin-like growth factor I in transgenic mice influences mammary gland development and IGF-binding protein expression. *Endocrinology* **137:** 321–330.

55. Nissley, S. P. and M. M. Rechler. 1986. Insulin-like growth factors: biosynthesis, receptors, and carrier proteins. *Hormones Proteins Peptides* **12:** 127–203.

56. Unterman, T., R. Simmons, R. Glick, and E. Ogata. 1993. Circulating levels of insulin, insulin-like growth factor-I (IGF-I), IGF-II, and IGF-binding proteins in the small for gestational age fetal rat. *Endocrinology* **132:** 327–336.

57. Hattori, Y., J. Vera, C. Rivas, N. Bersch, R. Bailey, M. Geffner, and D. Golde. 1996. Decreased insulin-like growth factor I receptor expression and function in immortalized African Pygmy T cells. *J. Clin. Endocrinol. Metab.* **81:** 2257–2263.

58. el-Roeiy, A., X. Chen, V. Roberts, S. Shimasakai, N. Ling, D. Le Roith, C. J. Roberts, and S. Yen. 1994. Expression of the genes encoding the insulin-like growth factors (IGF-I and II), the IGF and insulin receptors, and IGF-binding proteins-1-6 and the localization of their gene products in normal and polycystic ovary syndrome ovaries. *J. Clin. Endocrinol. Metab.* **78:** 1488–1496.

59. Yee, D., S. Paik, G. S. Lebovic, R. R.Marcus, R. E. Favoni, K. J. Cullen, M. E. Lippman, and N. Rosen. 1989. Analysis of insulin-like growth factor I gene expression in malignancy: evidence for a paracrine role in human breast cancer. *Mol. Endocrinol.* **3:** 509–517.

60. Giani, C., K. J. Cullen, D. Campani, and A. Rasmussen. 1996. IGF-II mRNA and protein are expressed in the stroma of invasive breast cancers: an *in situ* hybridization and immunohistochemical study. *Br. Cancer Res. Treatment* **41**: 43–50.

61. Baserga, R. 1992. IGF-I receptor as the restriction point of the cell cycle. *Ann. NY Acad. Sci.* **663**: 154–157.

62. Stewart, A., M. Johnson, F. May, and B. Westley. 1990. Role of insulin-like growth factors and type I insulin-like growth factor receptor in the estrogen stimulated proliferation of human breast cancer cells. *J. Biol. Chem.* **265**: 31,172–21,178.

63. Lee, A., C. Weng, J. Jackson, and D. Yee. 1997. Activation of estrogen receptor-mediated gene transcription by IGF1 in human breast cancer cells. *J. Endocrinol.* **152**: 39–47.

64. el-Tanani, M. and C. Green. 1996. Insulin/IGF-1 modulation of the expression of two estrogen-induced genes in MCF-7 cells. *Mol. Cell. Endocrinol.* **121**: 29–35.

65. Hafner, F., E. Holler, and E. von Angerer. 1996. Effect of growth factors of estrogen mediated gene expression. *J. Steroid Biochem. Mol. Biol.* **58**: 385–393.

66. Kato, S., H. Endoh, Y. Masuhiro, T. Kitamoto, S. Uchiyama, H. Sasaki, et al. 1995. Activation of the estrogen receptor through phosphorylation by mitogen-activated protein kinase. *Science* **270**: 1491–1494.

67. Sweeney, K., E. Musgrove, C. Watts, and R. Sutherland. 1996. Cyclins and breast cancer. *Br. Cancer Res. Treatment* **83**: 141–170.

68. Furlanetto, R., S. Harwell, and K. Frick. 1994. Insulin-like growth factor-I induces cyclin-D1 expression in MG63 human osteosarcoma cells *in vitro*. *Mol. Endocrinol.* **8**: 510–517.

69. Zwijsen, R., E. Wientjens, R. Klompmaker, J. van der Sman, R. Bernards, and R. Michalides. 1997. CDK-independent activation of estrogen receptor by cyclin D1. *Cell* **88**: 405–415.

70. Guvakova, M. and E. Surmacz. 1997. Overexpressed IGF-I receptors reduce estrogen growth requirements, enhance survival, and promote E-cadherin-mediated cell–cell adhesion in human breast cancer cells. *Exp. Cell Res.* **231**: 149–162.

71. Neuenschwander, S., C. J. Roberts, and D. Le Roith. 1995. Growth inhibition of MCF-7 breast cancer cells by stable expression of an insulin-like growth factor I receptor antisense ribonucleic acid. *Endocrinology* **136**: 4298–4303.

72. de Cupis, A., D. Noonan, P. Pirani, A. Ferrera, L. Clerico, and R. Favoni. 1995. Comparison between novel steroid-like and conventional nonsteroidal antioestrogens in inhibiting oestradiol- and IGF-I-induced proliferation of human breast cancer-derived cells. *Br. J. Pharmacol.* **116**: 2391–2400.

73. Kawamura, I., E. Lacey, T. Mizota, S. Tsujimoto, F. Nishigaki, T. Manda, and K. Shimomura. 1994. The effect of droloxifene on the insulin-like growth factor-I-stimulated growth of breast cancer cells. *Anticancer Res.* **14**: 427–431.

74. Sepp-Lorenzino, L., N. Rosen, and D. Lebwohl. 1994. Insulin and insulin-like growth factor signaling are defective in the MDA MB-468 human breast cancer cell line. *Cell Growth Differ.* **5**: 1077–1083.

75. Evan, G. I., A. H. Wyllie, C. S. Gilbert, T. D. Littlewood, H. Land, M. Brooks, et al. 1992. Induction of apoptosis in fibroblasts by c-myc protein. *Cell* **69**: 119–128.

76. Harrington, E. A., M. R. Bennett, A. Fanidi, and G. I. Evan. 1994. c-Myc-induced apoptosis in fibroblasts is inhibited by specific cytokines. *EMBO J.* **13**: 3286–3295.

77. Amundadottir, L. T., M. D. Johnson, G. Merlino, G. H. Smith, and R. B. Dickson. 1995. Synergistic interaction of transforming growth factor _ and c-*myc* in mouse mammary and salivary gland tumorigenesis. *Cell Growth Differ.* **6**: 737–748.

78. Baserga, R. 1995. The insulin-like growth factor I receptor: a key to tumor growth? *Cancer Res.* **55**: 249–252.

79. Christofori, G., P. Naik, and D. Hanahan. 1994. A second signal supplied by insulin-like growth factor II in oncogene-induced tumorigenesis. *Nature* **369**: 414–418.

80. Rogler, C. E., D. Yang, L. Rossetti, J. Donohoe, E. Alt, C. J. Chang, et al. 1994. Altered body composition and increased frequency of diverse malignancies in insulin-like growth factor-II transgenic mice. *J. Biol. Chem.* **269:** 13,779–13,784.

81. Bates, P., R. Fisher, A. Ward, L. Richardson, D. J. Hill, and C. F. Graham. 1995. Mammary cancer in transgenic mice expressing insulin-like growth factor II (IGF-II). *Br. J. Cancer* **72:** 1189–1193.

82. Westley, B. and F. May. 1995. Insulin-like growth factors: the unrecognised oncogenes. *Br. J. Cancer* **72:** 1065–1066.

83. Cox, L. and D. Lane. 1995. Tumour suppressors, kinases and clamps: how p53 regulates the cell cycle in response to DNA damage. *Bioessays* (England) **17:** 501–508.

84. Buckbinder, L., R. Talbott, S. Velasco-Miguel, I. Takenaka, B. Faha, B. R. Seizinger, and N. Kley. 1995. Induction of the growth inhibitor IGF-binding protein 3 by p53. *Nature* **377:** 646–649.

85. Zhang, L., F. Kashanchi, Q. Zhan, S. Zhan, J. Brady, A. Fornace, P. Seth, and L. Helman. 1996. Regulation of insulin-like growth factor II P3 promotor by p53: a potential mechanism for tumorigenesis. *Cancer Res.* **56:** 1367–1373.

86. Webster, N., J. Resnik, D. Reichart, B. Strauss, M. Haas, and B. Seely. 1996. Repression of the insulin receptor promoter by the tumor suppressor gene product p53: a possible mechanism for receptor overexpression in breast cancer. *Cancer Res.* **56:** 2781–2788.

87. Lane, D. 1994. The regulation of p53 function: Steiner Award Lecture. *Int. J. Cancer* **57:** 623–627.

88. Sell, C., R. Baserga, and R. Rubin. 1995. Insulin-like growth factor I (IGF-I) and the IGF-1 receptor prevent etoposide-induced apoptosis. *Cancer Res.* **55:** 303–306.

89. Turner, B., B. Haffty, L. Narayanan, J. Yuan, P. Havre, A. Gumbs, et al. 1997. Insulin-like growth factor-I receptor overexpression mediates cellular radioresistance and local breast cancer recurrence after lumpectomy and radiation. *Cancer Res.* **57:** 3079–3083.

90. Cullen, K. J., H. S. Smith, S. Hill, N. Rosen, and M. E. Lippman. 1991. Growth factor messenger RNA expression by human breast fibroblasts from benign and malignant lesions. *Cancer Res.* **51:** 4978.

91. Singer, C., A. Rasmussen, M. Lippman, and K. Cullen. 1997. Coexpression of Stromelysin-3 and insulin-like growth factor II in tumors of ectodermal, mesodermal and endodermal origin: indicator of a fetal cell phenotype. *J. Clin. Endocr. Metab.* **82:** 1917–1927.

92. Ellis, M. J. C., C. Singer, A. Hornby, A. Rasmussen, and K. J. Cullen. 1994. Insulin-like growth factor mediated stromal-epithelial interactions in human breast cancer. *Br. Cancer Res. Treatment* **31:** 249–261.

93. Singer, C., A. Rassmussen, H. Smith, M. Lippman, H. Lynch, and K. Cullen. 1995. Malignant breast epithelium selects for IGF-II expression in breast stroma. Evidence for paracrine function. *Cancer Res.* **55:** 2448–2454.

94. Huynh, H., L. Alpert, and M. Pollak. 1996. Pregnancy-dependent growth of mammary tumors is associated with overexpression of insulin-like growth factor II. *Cancer Res.* **56:** 3651–3654.

95. Manni, A., B. Badger, L. Wei, A. Zaenglein, R. Grove, S. Khin, et al. 1994. Hormonal regulation of insulin-like growth factor-II and insulin-like growth factor-binding protein expression by breast cancer cells *in vivo*. evidence for stromal epithelial interactions. *Cancer Res.* **54:** 2934–2942.

96. Torapainen, E., P. Lipponen, and K. Syrjanen. 1995. Expression of insulin-like growth factor II in female breast cancer as related to established prognostic factors and long term prognosis. *Anticancer Res.* **15:** 2669–2674.

97. Yu, H., M. Levesque, M. Khosravi, A. Papanastasiou-Diamandi, G. Clark, and E. Diamandis. 1996. Associations between insulin-like growth factors and their binding proteins and other prognostic indicators in breast cancer. *Br. J. Cancer* **74:** 1242–1247.

98. Rivero, F., L. Goya, and A. M. Pascual-Leone. 1994. Comparison of extraction methods for insulin-like growth factor-binding proteins prior to measurement of insulin-like growth factor-1 in undernourished neonatal and adult rat serum. *J. Endocrinol.* **140:** 257–263.

99. Papa, V., G. Biancamaria, G. Clark, W. McGuire, D. Moore, Y. Fujita-Yamaguchi, et al. 1993. Insulin-like growth factor receptors are overexpressed and predict a low risk in human breast cancer. *Cancer Res.* **53:** 3736–3740.

100. Foekens, J., H. Portengen, W. van Putten, A. Trapman, J. Reubi, J. Alexieva-Figusch, and J. Klijn. 1989. Prognostic value of receptors for insulin-like growth factor 1, somatostatin, and epidermal growth factor in human breast cancer. *Cancer Res.* **49:** 7002–7009.

101. Peyrat, J., J. Bonneterre, P. Vennin, H. Jammes, R. Beuscart, B. Hecquet, et al. 1990. Insulin-like growth factor 1 receptors (IGF1-R) and IGF1 in human breast tumors. *J. Steroid Biochem. Mol. Biol.* **37:** 823–827.

102. Bonneterre, J., J. Peyrat, R. Beuscart, and A. Demaille. 1990. Prognostic significance of insulin-like growth factor 1 receptors in human breast cancer. *Cancer Res.* **50:** 6931–6935.

103. Clarke, R., A. Howell, and E. Anderson. 1997. Type I insulin-like growth factor receptor gene expression in normal human breast tissue treated with oestrogen and progesterone. *Br. J. Cancer* **75:** 251–257.

104. Almeida, A., M. Muleris, B. Dutrillaux, and B. Malfoy. 1994. The insulin-like growth factor I receptor gene is the target for the 15q26 amplicon in breast cancer. *Genes Chromosomes Cancer* **11:** 63–65.

105. Happerfield, L., D. Miles, D. Barnes, L. Thompsen, and A. M. Hanby. 1997. The localization of the insulin-like growth factor receptor 1 (IGFR1) in benign and malignant breast tissue. *Proc. AACR* **38:** 374(Abstract).

106. Railo, M., K. von Smitten, and F. Pekonen. 1994. The prognostic value of insulin-like growth factor-I receptor in breast cancer patients. Results of a follow-up study on 126 patients. *Eur. J. Cancer* **30A:** 307–311.

107. Ellis, M.J. and D. Hayes. 1997. Improving hormonal therapy for breast cancer. *Breast* **3(Suppl.):** 57–68.

108. Belfiore, A., L. Frittitta, A. Costantino, F. Frasco, G. Pandina, L. Sciacca, I. Goldfine, and R. Vigneri. 1996. Insulin receptors and breast cancer. *Ann. NY Acad. Sci.* **784:** 173–188.

109. Papa, V. and A. Belfiore. 1996. Insulin receptors in breast cancer: biological and clinical role. *J. Endocrinol. Invest.* **19:** 324–333.

110. Stoll, B. 1996. Nutrition and breast cancer risk: can an effect via insulin resistance be demonstrated? *Br. Cancer Res. Treatment* **38:** 239–246.

111. De Souza, A. T., G. R. Hankins, M. K. Washington, T. C. Orton, and R. L. Jirtle. 1995. M6P/IGF2R gene is mutated in human hepatocellular carcinomas with loss of heterozygosity. *Nat. Genet.* **11:** 447–449.

112. Ouyang, H., H. O. Shiwaku, H. Hagiwara, K. Miura, T. Abe, Y. Kato, et al. 1997. The *insulin-like growth factor II receptor* gene is mutated in genetically unstable cancers of the endometrium, stomach and colorectum. *Cancer Res.* **57:** 1851–1854.

113. Souza, R., R. Appel, J. Yin, S. Wang, K. Smolinski, J. Abraham, et al. 1996. Microsatellite instability in the insulin-like growth factor II receptor gene in gastrointestinal tumours. *Nat. Genet.* **14:** 255–257.

114. Rocha, R., S. Hilsenbeck, J. Jackson, C. VanDenBerg, C. Wend, A. Lee, and D. Yee. 1997. Insulin-like Growth Factor Binding Protein-3 and Insulin Receptor substrate-1 in breast cancer: correlation with clinical parameters and disease free survival. *Clin. Cancer Res.* **3:** 103–109.

115. Rocha, R., S. Hilsenbeck, J. Jackson, A. Lee, J. Figueroa, and D. Yee. 1996. Correlation of insulin-like growth factor-binding protein-3 messenger RNA with protein expression in primary breast cancer tissues: detection of higher levels in tumors with poor prognostic features. *J. Natl. Cancer. Inst.* **88:** 601–606.

116. Pratt, S. and M. Pollak. 1994. Insulin-like growth factor binding protein 3 (IGF-BP3) inhibits estrogen-stimulated breast cancer cell proliferation. *Biochem. Biophys. Res. Commun.* **198:** 292–297.

117. Pratt, S. and M. Pollak. 1993. Estrogen and antiestrogen modulation of MCF7 human breast cancer cell proliferation is associated with specific alterations in accumulation of insulin-like growth factor-binding proteins in conditioned media. *Cancer Res.* **53:** 5193–5198.

118. Huynh, H., X. Yang, and M. Pollak. 1996. A role for insulin-like growth factor binding protein 5 in the antiproliferative action of the antiestrogen ICI 182780. *Cell Growth Differ.* **7:** 1501–1506.

119. Yee, D., J. Jackson, T. Kozelsky, and J. Figueroa. 1994. Insulin-like growth factor binding protein 1 expression inhibits insulin-like growth factor I action in MCF-7 breast cancer cells. *Cell Growth Differ.* **5:** 73–77.

120. Lahti, E., M. Knip, and T. Laatikainen. 1994. Plasma insulin-like growth factor I and its binding proteins 1 and 3 in postmenopausal patients with breast cancer receiving long term tamoxifen. *Cancer* **74:** 618–624.

121. Gucev, Z., Y. Oh, K. Kelley, and R. Rosenfeld. 1996. Insulin-like growth factor binding protein 3 mediates retinoic acid- and transforming growth factor beta2-induced growth inhibition in human breast cancer cells. *Cancer Res.* **56:** 1545–1550.

122. Yu, H., M. Levesque, G. Clark, and E. Diamandis. 1997. Prognostic value of PSA in Breast Cancer: a large US cohort study. *Proc. Am. Assoc. Cancer Res.* **38:** 2924(Abstract).

123. Yu, H., E. Diamandis, M. Levesque, M. Giai, and R. Roagna. 1996. Prostate specific antigen in breast cancer, benign breast disease and normal breast tissue. *Br. Cancer Res. Treatment* **40:** 171–178.

124. Salahifar, H., R. Baxter, and J. Martin. 1997. Insulin-like growth factor binding protein (IGFBP)-3 protease activity secreted by MCF-7 breast cancer cells: inhibition by IGFs does not require IGF-IGFBP interaction. *Endocrinology* **138:** 1683–1690.

125. Gansler, T., R. Furlanetto, T. S. Gramling, K. A. Robinson, N. Blocker, M. Buse, D. A. Sens, and A. J. Garvin. 1986. Antibody to Type I insulin-like growth factor receptor inhibits the growth of Wilm's tumor in culture and in athymic nude mice. *Am. J. Pathol.* **135:** 961–966.

126. Kalebic, T., M. Tsokos, and L. Helman. 1994. In vivo treatment with antibody against IGF-1 receptor suppresses growth of human rhabdomyosarcoma and down-regulates p34cdc2. *Cancer Res.* **54:** 5531–5534.

127. Arteaga, C. L. 1992. Interference with the IGF system as a strategy to inhibit breast cancer growth. *Br. Cancer Res. Treatment* **22:** 101–106.

128. Shin, S., P. Friden, M. Moran, and S. Morrison. 1994. Functional properties of antibody insulin-like growth factor fusion proteins. *J. Biol. Chem.* **269:** 4979–4985.

129. Ingle, J., C. Kardinal, V. Suman, J. Krook, and A. Hatfield. 1996. Octreotide as first-line treatment for women with metastatic breast cancer. *Invest. New Drugs* **14:** 235–237.

130. Di Leo, A., L. Ferrari, E. Bajetta, C. Bartoli, G. Vicario, D. Moglia, et al. 1995. Biological and clinical evaluation of lanreotide (BIM 23014), a somatostatin analogue, in the treatment of advanced breast cancer. A pilot study by the I.T.M.O. Group. Italian Trials in Medical Oncology. *Br. Cancer Res. Treatment* **34:** 237–244.

131. Ingle, J., C. Kardinal, V. Suman, M. Krook, and M. Pollak. 1997. Randomized trial of tamoxifen (Tam) alone or combined with octreotide (Oct) in women with metastatic breast cancer. *Proc. ASCO* **16:** 526(Abstract).

132. Brunner, N., C. Moser, R. Clarke, and K. Cullen. 1992. IGF-I and IGF-II expression in human breast cancer xenografts: relationship to hormone independence. *Br. Cancer Res. Treatment* **22**: 39–45.

133. Gould, M. N. 1995. Prevention and therapy of mammary cancer by monoterpenes. *J. Cell. Biochem.* **22(Suppl.):** 139–144.

134. Jirtle, R. L., G. R. Hankins, H. Reisenbichler, and I. J. Boyer. 1994. Regulation of mannose 6-phosphate/insulin-like growth factor-II receptors and transforming growth factor beta during liver tumor promotion with phenobarbital. *Carcinogenesis* **15**: 1473–1478.

135. Bentel, J., D. Lebwohl, K. Cullen, M. Rubin, N. Rosen, J. Mendelsohn, and W. J. Miller. 1995. Insulin-like growth factors modulate the growth inhibitory effects of retinoic acid on MCF-7 breast cancer cells. *J. Cell. Physiol.* **165**: 212–221.

136. Formelli, F., L. Cleris, E. Cavadini, T. Camerini, M. Di Mauro, T. Campa, et al. 1996. Analysis of fenretinide (4-HPR) effects on plasma IGF1 levels in relation with age and chemopreventive efficacy in breast cancer patients. *Proc. AACR* **37**: 1263(Abstract).

137. Resnicoff, M., C. Sell, M. Rubini, D. Coppola, D. Ambrose, R. Baserga, and R. Rubin. 1994. Rat glioblastoma cells expressing an antisense RNA to the insulin-like growth factor-1 (IGF-1) receptor are nontumorigenic and induce regression of wild-type tumors. *Cancer Res.* **54**: 2218–2222.

138. Wallenfriedman, M., J. Conrad, L. Chiang, L. DeLaBarre, W. Jean, M. Garwood, et al. 1997. Peripheral vaccine for breast cancer: Insulin-like grwoth factor receptor (IGF1-R) antisense oligonucleotide (AON) modified tumor cells protect against peripheral disease and brain metastases. *Proc. AACR* **38**: 4143(Abstract).

6

Molecular Alterations in Breast Cancer

Ivan Bergstein

1. INTRODUCTION

Although not obligatory, many breast cancers appear to develop through a series of premalignant stages histologically defined as atypical hyperplasia and carcinoma *in situ* leading to invasive cancer *(1,2)*. Accompanying this histologic progression are numerous molecular alterations that result in oncogene activation and/or tumor suppressor inactivation *(2–4)*. These genetic changes accumulate in a notoriously variable fashion, some maintained throughout different stages of tumorigenesis, others specific to particular stages, while still others have no obvious linkage to progression *(4–8)*. Amid this considerable heterogeneity is a general trend toward increasing mutational load, with tumor evolution comprised in part by recognizable cycles of mutational diversification followed by clonal selection *(7,8)*. Accordingly, it has been suggested that mutations are causally responsible for driving mammary tumorigenesis but that significant modifications to the simple linear progression model are warranted to wholly account for this complex evolutionary cascade *(7–9)*.

The most common molecular alterations known in breast cancer involve large scale gains and/or losses of genetic material resulting in allelic imbalances *(4)*. The great majority of invasive breast cancers contain multiple examples of such imbalances— most commonly losses of chromosomes 17p, 16q, 8p as well as 6q, 7q, 9p, 11q, 13q, 17q, 18q, in addition to gains of chromosomes 1q, 8q as well as 3q, 6p,17q22–24, 20q13 *(2–11)*. Additionally, several monosomies (chromosomes 6, 8, 11, 13, 16, 17, 22, X) as well as trisomies (chromosomes 7,18) have also been documented in breast cancer *(4)*. A number of genes, some of which are amid these mentioned loci, have been implicated in breast tumorigenesis. These include the proto-oncogene products c-myc, cyclins, c-erbB2, bcl-2 and the tumor suppressor gene products Rb, cyclin-dependent kinase inhibitors (CDIs), p53, and DNA-mismatch repair proteins *(2–4)*.

Interestingly, while the number of molecular alterations increases with breast tumor evolution *(5,9–12)*, there is evidence that the most common changes can occur at the earliest stages of tumorigenesis *(5–8,13,14)*. For example, loss of 16q and 17p have been detected in atypical ductal hyperplasia (ADH) *(14)*, and losses of these as well as other commonly lost loci in invasive cancer (i.e., 6q, 7q, 8p, 9p, 11q, 13q, 17q) have also been reported in ductal carcinoma *in situ* (DCIS) *(8,10)*. There are also data implying that many of these as well as other early alterations can be maintained throughout

From: Breast Cancer: *Molecular Genetics, Pathogenesis, and Therapeutics*
Edited by: A. M. Bowcock © Humana Press Inc., Totowa, NJ

progression to more advanced stages *(5–7,11)*. For example, amplification of c-myc has been detected in DCIS and adjacent invasive ductal carcinoma (IDC) *(15)*, and overexpression of c-erbB2 and cyclin D1 as well as TP53 mutations have all been detected in DCIS, adjoining IDC, and corresponding metastatic lesions *(3,5,9,16)*. In a related manner, while certain TP53 mutations are conserved throughout breast tumor evolution *(17)*, the prevalence of TP53 mutant cells increases with tumor invasiveness and bcl-2 expression decreases *(18)*. Stage-specific alterations have also been noted. For example, losses of 3p, 11p, 18p have been preferentially found in IDC versus DCIS *(1–4)*, loss of 11p in IDC (but not adjacent DCIS) *(1)*, loss of 18q at nodal sites (more so than in corresponding primary tumor) *(5)*, and gains in 11q, Xq12–22, and possibly 7q in metastatic versus primary lesions *(5,7)*. Moreover, cyclin D1 is overexpressed at the ADH-DCIS boundary indicating a possible causal role in this particular stage of mammary tumorigenesis *(16)*.

As mentioned, breast tumor evolution does not seem to follow a simple linear progression model but rather appears to involve a more complex process characterized by periods of expansion followed by contraction concomitant with simultaneous evolution of multiple independent tumor regions—a scenario likely responsible for the great mutational heterogeneity witnessed in this disease *(5–8,19)*. It has been noted by several investigators that tumor heterogeneity (i.e., expansion) is greatest at transition phases (i.e., DCIS-IDC, or IDC-metastatic boundaries) and less so following these phases (i.e., contraction) presumably owing to alternating periods of mutational diversity followed by clonal selection *(6,7,11,19)*. However, it is not clear that all breast tumor-related evolution proceeds in this manner. That is, there are a number of enigmatic examples wherein certain molecular alterations are present in less advanced lesions but seemingly "lost" during tumor progression to more invasive lesions *(5,7,8,20)*. For example, some investigators have found a lack of correspondence between the mutational spectrum (in terms of allelic imbalances) among adjoining DCIS and IDC *(11,21)*, as well as between primary breast tumors and their corresponding metastases *(7)*. Moreover, individual allelic changes such as gain of Xq as well as overexpression of cyclin D1 and c-erbB2 have been shown to occur preferentially in DCIS versus later stages *(8,9,15,20)*, and loss of 11q23-qter as well as c-myc amplification have been detected in primary tumors but surprisingly not their metastases *(5,20)*. Whether these enigmatic findings reflect progression of an undetected subset of cells (from DCIS to IDC, or from primary tumor to metastasis), or rather independent evolution of DCIS, IDC, and metastatic lesions remains to be determined.

Despite this heterogeneity, it is clear that certain molecular alterations are important for the evolution of mammary epithelial cells to frank malignancy. As mentioned, a number of these changes involve known proto-oncogenes and/or tumor suppressor genes. That additional breast cancer-related genes await identification is suggested by 1) significant frequency of altered loci in breast cancer without a known culprit gene (i.e., 16q), and 2) even at loci harboring known genes, many contain multiple breakpoint regions (i.e., two regions within 17p and 8p, three regions within 17q, and likely multiple within 13q) indicating that more than one gene may be involved in these cases *(2–4,12)*.

Thus far, investigators have sought to determine the function of certain breast cancer-related genes by analyzing their relation to well-studied clinicopathological features of tumors. Moreover, it has been a major goal of the oncologist to be able to discern prognostic information as well as predictive data (in reference to treatment response) from molecular aberrations. This information could afford clinicians with the maneuverability to tailor types and/or aggressiveness of therapy. In addition, some have undertaken preliminary studies which target some of the more common breast cancer-related mutant gene products with novel forms of cancer treatment including immunotherapy and gene therapy.

2. PROTO-ONCOGENES IN BREAST CANCER

2.1. c-myc

c-myc is a transcription factor involved in the regulation of a host of cellular activities including proliferation, differentiation, as well as apoptosis *(2,22)*. The MYC gene, located on chromosome 8q24, is amplified in approx 20–30% of breast cancers but this poorly correlates with c-myc expression at either the mRNA or protein levels *(12)*. MYC amplification has been detected in DCIS, however, in contrast to cyclin D1 and c-cerbB2 that are amplified at higher frequencies in DCIS than IDC, amplified MYC is slightly more prevalent in IDC versus DCIS *(15)*. Although some have argued that MYC amplification is an early event in mammary tumorigenesis *(12)*, others have suggested a role in tumor promotion by virtue of demonstrated associations between MYC amplification and certain aggressive features (i.e., large tumor size, high tumor grade) *(2,23)*, as well as poor short-term outcome in some small studies *(23,24)*. Interestingly, c-myc alterations, while present in certain primary breast cancers, are not always detectable in corresponding lymph node metastases, thereby indicating a potential role in initiation and promotion prior to invasion but not a prerequisite for subsequent metastasis *(20)*.

2.2. Cyclin D1

The CCND1/BCL1/PRAD1 gene, located on chromosome 11q13, encodes cyclin D1 protein which when complexed to certain cyclin-dependent complexes (CDKs) controls cell cycle progression through G1/S via phosphorylation of pRB *(12)*. The 11q13 locus is amplified in 15–20% breast cancers (2,25) and has been associated in some reports with estrogen receptor (ER) positivity and poor prognosis *(2,4,25–27)*. Cyclin D1 overexpression, more common in breast cancer (35–50% of cases) than amplification *(12,25)*, has also been associated with ER-positivity but not significantly with prognosis *(28–30)*.

Borg et al. and Schuuring et al. found an association between 11q13 amplification and unfavorable clinical course but in different subgroups, i.e., node-negative and node-positive patients, respectively *(26,27)*. Several other studies report similar findings *(31,32)*, however Lonn et al. failed to find prognostic value for this amplicon *(33)*. With regard to cyclin D1 overexpression, although there is a general consensus of an association with ER-positivity *(12,28,34)*, there is less so with prognosis *(12,28–30,35)*. Gillett et al. and van Diest et al. noted an association between cyclin D1 expression and low histologic grade, but neither could demonstrate prognostic value in 345 and 148 tumors examined, respectively *(30,34)*. Data from Nielsen et al, like Gillett et al, even suggest a seemingly paradoxical direct relationship between cyclin D1 expression and favorable outcome *(30,35)*. In a related manner, Michalides et al. reviewed 248 early (stage I, II) tumors and found no prognostic value for cyclin D1 over-expression after a median follow-up of 8.5 yr *(28)*, and McIntosh et al. found no corre-lation between cyclin D1 overexpression and survival in 93 cases with mean follow-up of 6 yr *(29)*. It has been suggested that the discrepancy in potential prognostic value for cyclin D1 at the DNA versus protein levels could be due to contribution of another oncogene on the 11q13 amplicon, to irrelevant protein staining from epigenetic effects (i.e., hormone induced up-regulation), or rather to absence of cyclin D1 protein stain-ing in Rb-negative cells (i.e., when p16 becomes up-regulated, following pRb inactiva-tion and sequesters CDKs, leading to cyclin D1 destabilization) *(35)*.

It has been suggested that alterations in cyclin D1 may represent a relatively early event in breast tumor development *(3,36)*. Indeed, both amplification of 11q13 as well as cyclin D1 overexpression have been detected in some premalignant breast lesions *(15,16)*. Moreover, Weinstat-Saslow et al. have demonstrated by *in situ* hybridization that cyclin D1 overexpression may represent a boundary between premalignancy and cancer as they report elevated mRNA in only 18% of cases of atypical ductal hyperpla-sia (ADH), but in 76–87% of cases of ductal carcinoma *in situ* (DCIS) and 83% of infiltrating ductal carcinomas (IDCs) *(16)*. 11q13 amplification rates also, like those of overexpression, appear to be relatively constant from DCIS to IDC *(15)*. There is also evidence that cyclin D1 overexpression is conserved during metastasis *(36)*, indicating that while it acts at the ADH-DCIS boundary *(16)*, it may also function in the later stages of breast tumorigenesis. Moreover, increased cyclin D1 amplification has been reported to continue during the later stages of tumor progression in patients with late stage disease treated with second-line hormonal therapy *(37)*.

2.3. Cyclin E

Cyclin E is a late G1 cyclin that complexes with CDK2 to control progression through G1S via phosphorylation of pRB *(25)*. During cell cycle progression, the cyclin D1-complex phosphorylates pRB thereby releasing E2F that can then activate cyclin E expression *(38)*. Mechanistically, there is some recent evidence that pRB normally cooperates with a histone deacetylase (HDAC1) to repress cyclin E by impairing access by E2F to the cyclin E promoter via stabilization of its nucleosomal structure *(38a)*. With phosphorylation of pRB, Cyclin E becomes involved in a positive autoregulatory loop wherein, upon complexing with CDK2 and phosphorylation of pRB, E2F contin-ues to be released and cyclin E expression is maintained thereby ensuring pRB inacti-vation and cell cycle progression into S-phase *(25,38)*.

Altered cyclin E expression has been detected in a variety of malignancies including breast *(25)*. For example, quantitative as well as qualitative changes in cyclin E protein have been found in a number of breast cancer cell lines *(25)*. Moreover, cyclin E overexpression has been shown to correlate with tumor aggressiveness as determined by stage and grade *(38)*. Nielsen et al. examined 114 breast tumors by Western blotting and found cyclin E overexpression in 25% of cases that associated with ER-negativity and increased death in patients without evidence of metastatic disease at the time of diagnosis *(25)*. Further study of these patients revealed that, when combined with low cyclin D1 expression, cyclin E expression correlated with inactive pRB and was even more predictive of poor outcome *(38)*. Whether cyclin E overexpression leading to inactivation (via inappropriate phosphorylation) of pRB is a more significant pathway than the reverse (i.e., primarily inactivated pRB causing cyclin E upregulation) remains to be determined. Porter et al. have also shown that high cyclin E expression (especially when combined with low p27 expression) correlated with increased mortality in a study of 278 young women with a median follow-up of 5.2 yr *(39)*.

2.4. c-erbB2

The c-erbB2 (HER2/neu) proto-oncogene is located on chromosome 17q21 and encodes a transmembrane tyrosine kinase receptor which shares extensive homology with epidermal growth factor receptor (EGFR) *(2,4)* (*see* Chapter 2). Amplification of c-erbB2 has been detected in 20–30% of invasive breast tumors *(2,4,12,40)*, a finding that parallels its frequency of tumor-related overexpression *(41,42)*. Interestingly, c-erbB2 alterations have been reported in as many as 40–60% of cases of DCIS, and are more prevalent in comedo than cribriform subtypes indicating a role in the progression of premalignant lesions *(4,12,15)*. Whether diminished presence of c-erbB2 alterations in IDC (compared with DCIS) indicates a down-regulation event, that evolution of DCIS is independent of IDC, or that alternative c-erbB2-independent pathways are possible in early breast tumorigenesis remains to be determined *(12)*. It should be noted that c-erbB2 alterations present in primary IDCs can be maintained during progression to metastatic disease suggesting a potential role in the later stages of breast tumor evolution as well *(43)*. This variability in early versus late effects of c-erbB2 on breast tumorigenesis may account for some of the heterogeneity reported with regard to associations between c-erbB2 alterations and markers of tumor aggressiveness (i.e., high nuclear grade, increased size, ER-negativity) *(12,44,45)*.

Slamon et al. were the first to report prognostic significance for c-erbB2 alterations *(46,47)*. Namely, these investigators examined 187 and then 526 patients and found an independent correlation between c-erbB2 amplification and both disease-free survival (DFS) as well as overall survival (OS) in the node-positive subgroups *(46,47)*. Subsequent studies have been conflicting as some have corroborated these results *(48,49)*, while others have not *(50–52)*. A host of reports concerning the prognostic significance of c-erbB2 overexpression have similarly left this question unresolved—the majority reporting no value, while some showing trends toward worse OS *(41,42)*. Recently, however, Sjögren et al. reported a positive study wherein c-erbB2 overexpression was found to have prognostic value in 315 cases with follow-up of 5–10 yr, and was independent of other parameters *(53)*. It has been suggested that lack of consensus in these studies may be due in part to lack of standardization of antibodies and methods of analyses used, as well as the relatively small size and short follow-up of most studies *(43,54)*. In an attempt to increase the numbers of patients analyzed, when Gullick et al. combined the results of three studies these investigators were able to show a correlation between c-erbB2 overexpression and both DFS as well as OS irrespective of nodal status *(44)*. These results await prospective studies.

The data concerning c-erbB2 in the node-negative subgroup are similarly without consensus. While Slamon et al. originally did not find prognostic value for c-erbB2 amplification in node-negative patients *(46,47)*, a later study did report an association with decreased DFS but only by univariate analysis *(55)*. While some subsequent studies were able to show independent prognostic value in the node-negative subgroup

(49), others have not *(50,52,56,57)*. In expression studies, the large majority have not been able to demonstrate prognostic value for c-erbB2 in node-negative patients (41,42). Similarly, a more recent study by Carlomagno et al. of 145 node-negative patients followed for a median of 12 yr reported that although c-erbB2 overexpression did correlate with unfavorable features (i.e., large tumor size and steroid receptor-negativity), it was not prognostic *(45)*. It has been suggested that some of these conflicting data may be owing, not only to previously mentioned variability in staining techniques and interpretation thereof, but also to the significant heterogeneity in management of node-negative patients (i.e., no treatment versus various adjuvant regimens) *(45,54)*. In an attempt to limit some of these sources of variability, Press et al. analyzed by fluorescence *in situ* hybridization (FISH) only tumors from node-negative patients who did not receive any adjuvant therapy. They reported that c-erbB2 amplification was an independent predictor of poor clinical outcome *(54)*. This technique awaits independent confirmation and prospective randomized analyses.

As pointed out by Press et al. *(54)*, and suggested previously by others *(41)*, some of the discrepancies concerning the potential prognostic value of c-erbB2 for both node-negative as well as -positive patients may result from an interaction between c-erbB2 status and certain therapies. With regard to systemic chemotherapy, however, this concept remains unresolved. Namely, several studies report an association between c-erbB2 and chemoresistance (i.e., in response to cyclophosphamide, methotrexate, fluorouracil—CMF regimens) in the adjuvant setting *(56–58)*, but not in metastatic disease *(59)*. Gusterson et al. reported that c-erbB2-negativity was more predictive of better DFS and OS in node-positive patients treated with multiple (rather than 1 or 2) cycles of a CMF-based regimen, while there was no difference in the c-erbB2-positive group. These investigators also found value in c-erbB2 for predicting CMF-based treatment response (i.e., OS) in a node-negative subgroup *(59)*. Similarly, Allred et al. demonstrated an association between c-erbB2-negativity and improved survival in high risk (tumor size >3 cm, ER-negative) node-negative patients treated with a CMF-based regimen, while there was no survival difference between the treated and untreated c-erbB2-positive group *(60)*. On the other hand, Klijn et al. found that c-erbB2 overexpression was a predictor of good response to CMF in patients with metastatic disease *(61)*.

Consensus is also lacking with regard to the predictive power of c-erbB2 in anthracycline-containing regimens. Namely, in a large randomized adjuvant chemotherapy trial by the Cancer and Leukemia Group B (CALGB), c-erbB2 overexpression was associated with better DFS and OS following higher dose therapy with cyclophosphamide, doxorubicin, fluorouracil (CAF), while it was not predictive of outcome in patients treated with lower dose therapy *(62)*. However, in a small study of 68 patients with metastatic disease, Wright et al. reported marginally poorer outcome in c-erbB2-positive patients treated with mitoxantrone *(63)*. In order to account for some of these inconsistent data, it has been suggested that c-erbB2 might preferentially potentiate adriamycin activity (i.e., via effects on multi-drug resistance proteins), and that the effects of CMF-based regimens on c-erbB2-positive patients may have been somewhat confounded by concomitant use of endocrine therapy (to which some c-erbB2-positive cells may have resistance) *(45)*.

With regard to endocrine therapy, two small studies have found negative prognostic value for c-erbB2 in hormonally-treated patients with advanced disease *(64,65)*. In the adjuvant setting, Borg et al. showed that c-erbB2-positivity associated with tamoxifen-resistance in node-positive patients *(66)*, and Tetu et al. found a correlation between c-erbB2 and decreased DFS as well as OS in 888 node-positive patients treated with adjuvant hormonal therapy (and/or CMF-based chemotherapy) *(58)*. Similarly, Sjögren et al. have recently reported a relation between c-erbB2 and poor outcome in node-positive patients treated with adjuvant tamoxifen, although this subgroup was small in number *(53)*. With regard to node-negative patients, Carlomagno et al. found c-erbB2-negativity to be associated with prolonged DFS and OS (median follow-up 12 yr) in that subgroup (99 patients) of 145 patients randomized to receive adjuvant tamoxifen *(45)*. In a related manner, Lonn et al. found that c-erbB2 amplification increased with progression of disease on second-line hormonal therapy *(67)*. However, Archer et al. did not find c-erbB2 overexpression to predict resistance to hormonal therapy in 92 patients with either locally advanced or metastatic breast cancer *(68)*. Similarly, in a recent report from the Southwest Oncology Group (SWOG), Elledge et al. analyzed metastatic ER-positive tumors from 205 previously untreated patients and did not find c-erbB2 expression to associate with poor outcome following tamoxifen therapy after a median follow-up of 9 yr *(69)*. These investigators argued that their rigorous exclusion of ER-negative tumors (a parameter often correlated with c-erbB2-positivity), not routinely excluded in other studies, might explain adequate responses to tamoxifen by their c-erbB2-positive cases *(69)*. Considering the relatively small size of this study, larger studies with longer follow-up are required to resolve the issue of tamoxifen-resistance in c-erbB2-positive tumors.

2.5. Bcl-2

BCL2 encodes an inner mitochondrial protein involved in suppression of programmed cell death (apoptosis) *(3)*. bcl-2 is expressed in normal breast tissue (>95% of cells) and is found in decreasing frequency as tumors progress from DCIS (79–91%), higher in noncomedo (82%) versus comedo (67%) subtypes, to IDC (45–79%) *(18,70)*. As might be expected from these data, bcl-2 expression has also been found to correlate with certain favorable features, most notably hormone receptor-positivity *(3,18,70–73)*, as well as small size and/or low tumor grade (18,74,75). It has been suggested that paradoxical loss of expression of an apoptosis-suppressing factor (bcl-2) with tumor progression, coupled with its association with less aggressive clinicopathological parameters, might be owing to a relation of bcl-2 with differentiation (rather than apoptosis) whereby certain tumors assume alternative (i.e., bcl-2-independent) mechanisms of survival as they progress *(70,72,74)*. Along these lines, some but not all studies have found that bcl-2 expression relates to good prognosis. Namely, Joensuu et al. analyzed 174 cases and reported an association between bcl-2 and certain favorable features as well as with better prognosis (but not independently of other factors), after a long-term median follow-up of 31 yr *(76)*. Similarly, Hurlimann et al. demonstrated prognostic value for bcl-2 in terms of increased DFS in 190 patients *(77)*, and Hellemans et al. analyzed 251 invasive ductal carcinomas and found that absence of bcl-2 expression was independently correlated with decreased DFS and OS in node-positive (but not node-negative) patients after median follow-up of 91 mo *(78)*. However, like Joensuu et al. *(76)*, Silvestrini et al. were unable to attribute independent prognostic value to bcl-2 in 283 (node-negative) patients after 6 yr *(79)*, and Barbareschi et al. found no value for bcl-2 as a prognosticator in 178 node-negative cases after a median follow-up of 60 mo *(75)*.

There are also some preliminary data, although no consensus, that bcl-2 might predict good treatment response. For example, Silvestrini et al. found bcl-2 to be of only weak predictive value and not independent of other factors, as previously demonstrated by this group *(79)*, after a 5 yr follow-up of 240 postmenopausal ER-positive node-positive patients treated with tamoxifen *(80)*. On the other hand, in a similar group of ER-positive metastatic cases treated with tamoxifen, Elledge et al. demonstrated that bcl-2 expression was an independent predictor of decreased time to treatment failure but not OS in 205 patients followed for up to 8 yr *(81)*. Similarly, Gasparini et al. evaluated 180 node-positive (largely hormone receptor-positive) cases and found bcl-2 to independently correlate with improved DFS but not OS following adjuvant hormonal therapy *(72)*. This same group also showed that bcl-2 independently associated with improved OS (but not DFS) in patients treated with adjuvant chemotherapy (cyclophosphamide, methotrexate, fluorouracil) after median follow-up of 63 mo *(72)*. There are also some indirect preliminary data that decreased bcl-2 expression might unexpectedly afford a benefit in terms of local relapse in patients treated with chest wall radiation, although this study needs to be confirmed by larger randomized ones *(82)*.

3. TUMOR SUPPRESSOR GENES IN BREAST CANCER

3.1. Rb

The RB gene, located on chromosome 13q14, encodes a nuclear protein (pRB) that when phosphorylated by cyclin-CDK complexes releases E2F thereby allowing cell cycle progression into S-phase *(12,25)*. LOH of 13q14 has been found in approx 25% of breast cancers, the significance of which remains to be determined *(25)*. For example, while some studies have cited an association between loss of the RB locus and aggressive features (i.e., aneuploidy, high S-phase fraction, high tumor grade) *(83,84)*, others have either failed to find a correlation between RB deletion and clinicopathological parameters *(85)*, or else have noted an association between RB gene alterations and favorable features (tumor size <2 cm, node-negativity) *(86)*. One possible explanation for these conflicting data is that a tumor suppressor at or close to 13q14 (e.g., BRCA2, Brush-1) is lost in some breast tumors *(12,86)*.

Another potential confounder of these genetic data is the inconsistent correlation between alterations in pRB expression (detected in 10–45% of breast cancers) and loss of the RB locus *(2,4,25)*. Similar to Varley et al. *(84)*, Trudel et al. report an association between RB alterations (in this case abnormal pRB expression) and poor tumor differentiation *(87)*. However, Sawan et al. examined pRB protein expression in 197 tumors and found, in contrast to Berns et al. who analyzed the Rb gene *(86)*, an association between abnormalities and node-positivity *(88)*. Some have suggested that the discrepancies between genetic and protein alteration may be due to the wide range (10–45%) of detected pRB alteration frequencies (i.e., presumably over-detecting) when using different immunostaining techniques, or else that epigenetic pRB inactivation (i.e., without concomitant genetic change at the RB locus) occurs to a significant degree as a consequence of deregulated cyclin or CDK action *(25)*. One preliminary consensus that has been reached thus far, however, is an apparent lack of prognostic value for RB in breast cancer at either the gene or protein level *(25,86,88)*.

3.2. Cyclin-Dependent Kinase Inhibitors (CDIs)

Alterations in the G1-S cell cycle checkpoint have been implicated in human breast cancer *(25)*. In the native state, CDKs complex with various sequentially activated cyclins to initiate progression into S-phase via phosphorylation of pRB and release of the E2F transcription factor that activates genes responsible for DNA replication *(2,25)*. In addition, a variety of CDK inhibitors (CDIs) compete with cyclins for binding of CDKs to prevent progression of G1-S *(25)*. In this manner, certain CDIs could have tumor suppressor function.

One family of CDIs includes the Ink4 proteins (p15, p16, p18, p19) that share four ankyrin repeats and complex with CDK4 and CDK6 as well as with D-type cyclins to halt progression *(25)*. Another group is the Cip/Kip proteins which include p21, p27, p57 and have a wide range of specificity and spectrum of inhibitory activities *(25)*. Some of these CDIs have been preliminarily implicated in breast cancer, these include an Ink4 protein (p16), and two Cip/Kip proteins (p21, p27).

3.2.1. p16

p16 (MTS1/INK4A/CDKN2) inhibits cell cycle progression at G1-S by interfering with action of the cyclin D/CDK4 complex (25). Both homozygous as well as hemizygous deletions of the p16 locus at 9p21–22 (the latter with accompanying point mutations in the remaining allele) have been detected in numerous cancer cell lines (50–60% of breast cancer cell lines) thereby strongly implicating p16 with tumor suppressor function *(89,90)*. However, in general, primary tumors have only been found to harbor genetic alterations at this locus at low frequency *(91)*. There is some evidence, however, that p16 may be epigenetically inactivated in certain tumors including breast *(92)*.

In breast cancer, most studies report LOH at 9p to be a rare finding, with some exceptions *(93,94)*, despite high frequency of homozygous allelic deletion in breast cancer cell lines *(91)*. Moreover, several studies have failed to detect any significant level of point mutations in the p16 gene in primary breast tumors *(89,91,94,95)*. For example, Quesnel et al. found no evidence of allelic deletion by Southern blotting and only a single point mutation after screening 35 breast cancers *(91)*, and Berns et al. reviewed 164 primary breast cancers and detected only two point-mutations in the p16 gene (89). Of note, Geradts et al. demonstrated complete or focal loss of p16 expression by IHC in 49% of 104 breast tumors examined without correlation with other parameters *(92)*. Others claim similar results using Western blotting *(25)*. Mechanistically, Herman et al. have shown that 31% of breast cancers displayed de novo methylation of a 5' CpG island *(96)*. Whether aberrant methylation is a common means by which p16 contributes to breast cancer remains to be investigated.

3.2.2. p21

p21 (WAF1/CIP1) can inhibit a variety of CDKs in both G1-S or G2-M and cause cell cycle arrest in the setting of differentiation or in response to DNA damage *(97)*. Induction of p21 can proceed via both p53-dependent as well as p53-independent pathways, and there is preliminary evidence that p21 may also be transactivated by BRCA1 in some instances *(98–100)*. Although these actions suggest a possible tumor suppressor role for p21, the data thus far in this regard are conflicting.

In line with a classical tumor suppressor function for p21, Wakasugi et al. reported correlation between p21 expression (by IHC, >10% staining) and favorable parameters (i.e., low histologic grade, ER-positivity, node-negativity), as well as an independent association between low expression with worse outcome (i.e., shorter DFS) for 104 patients with mean follow-up 3 yr *(101)*. Similarly, Jiang et al, upon analysis of tumors from 106 patients with mean follow-up of 4.3 yr, found a relation between p21 expression (by IHC, >25% staining) and well-differentiated tumors as well as independent prognostic value for low p21 expression and shortened survival *(102)*. The results of these studies are consistent with several concerning colon cancer wherein p21 expression related to differentiation, decreased proliferation, and early stage *(102)*. In contradistinction, however, Barbareschi et al. examined 91 tumors for p21 expression by IHC (>10% cells staining) and found an association between expression and high histologic grade and poor outcome (i.e., shortened DFS) *(97)*. In the same vein, Johnson et al. described a correlation between p21 expression in node-negative patients and relapse *(103)*. Caffo et al. also reported a relation between p21 overexpression and decreased DFS, particularly in the node-negative group *(104)*. In order to account for these conflicting results, it has been proposed that, in certain instances, IHC-positive p21 might reflect mutant protein with prolonged half-life and possible dominant-negative function (i.e., analogous to p53) rather than wild type with growth-suppressing function *(102)*. It should be noted, however, that preliminary analyses have not yet revealed evidence of p21 mutations in breast cancers *(105)*.

3.2.3. p27

p27 (KIP1) mediates G1-S arrest through inhibition of cyclin D/CDK4 and to a lesser extent cyclin E/CDK2 complexes *(106)*. Analyses of numerous tumor types have revealed that genetic alteration of p27 is a rare event in cancer *(106)*. In breast cancers, Spirin et al. failed to find evidence of homozygous p27 deletion by Southern blotting, and reported only one somatic point mutation in 36 primary tumors examined. Moreover, although these investigators did detect five cases of LOH of p27, four were accompanied by a remaining allele which was wild type *(107)*. Ferrando et al. examined 30 primary breast cancers and found no p27 mutations (108). There is experimental evidence, however, that p27 expression can be regulated post-transcriptionally at the level of protein translation and/or degradation *(106,109)*.

Expression level alterations in p27 have been detected in breast cancers and, in general, appear to correlate with tumor aggressiveness. Fredersdorf et al. analyzed 84 breast and 80 colon cancer specimens and found a statistically significant inverse relationship between p27 expression and malignant features (histologic grade, depth of invasion) *(106)*. Catzavelos et al. demonstrated, in breast tumors derived from 168 patients, that low p27 expression (as measured by IHC and Western blotting) correlated with high tumor grade (in both DCIS and invasive cancer) and was also an independent prognostic marker for poor DFS after a short median follow-up of 2 yr *(109)*. Tan et al. also reported a statistically significant correlation between decreased p27 protein and poor outcome in 202 patients with small tumors (<1 cm) *(110)*. Similarly, Porter et al. examined tumors from 278 patients (<45 yr old) and found that low p27 expression was an independent prognostic marker for increased mortality with a median follow-up of 5.2 yr. In this study, the prognostic value to p27 was significantly improved when used in combination with cyclin E overexpression *(111)*. In contrast, Sgamboto et al. upon analysis of 52 primary breast cancers were unable to demonstrate prognostic value for low p27 expression, and also found cases wherein p27 expression was actually higher in tumor than adjacent normal tissue *(111a)*.

It should also be noted that in the study of Fredersdorf et al, there was surprisingly no association between p27 expression and proliferation rates in 5 of 12 breast cancer cell lines *(106)*. In a number of those highly proliferative cell lines with paradoxical elevated p27 expression there was concomitant elevated cyclin D1 expression suggesting that, in certain cases, it may be the balance between oppositely-acting cell cycle proteins which ultimately determines the phenotype of the cancer cell *(106)*.

3.3. p53

The TP53 gene is located on human chromosome 17p13 and encodes a 393-amino acid nuclear phosphoprotein that functions in cell cycle control as a mediator of differentiation, DNA repair, and apoptosis *(112,113)*. As such, TP53 is a tumor suppressor that is the most common somatically mutated gene in sporadic cancers and, when mutant in the germline, forms the inherited cancer susceptibility locus responsible for the Li-Fraumeni Syndrome *(2,3,112,113)*. In human breast cancer, alterations in p53 at the protein or DNA levels have been detected in 25–50% or 15–35% of cases, respectively *(2–4,112,113)*. There is evidence that such aberrations cause either loss of function or dominant-negative action which disrupts the native growth-regulatory role of p53 thereby contributing to tumorigenesis *(2–4)*. More specifically, there are data indicating that aberrant p53 function can lead to derangements in differentiation and cell cycle control including disruption of the G1-S checkpoint resulting loss of the apoptotic response to DNA damage and untoward DNA replication of an unrepaired genome (i.e., increasing genomic instability) *(112,113)*.

Alterations at the TP53 locus have been detected at the earliest stages of breast tumorigenesis. Using microdissection and polymerase chain reaction (PCR) techniques, Lakhani et al. were able to demonstrate loss of heterozygosity (LOH) of 17p in 2/8 informative cases of atypical ductal hyperplasia (ADH), an early premalignant breast lesion *(14)*. Interestingly, there is even some preliminary evidence that LOH of TP53 can occur in histologically "normal" lobules adjacent to invasive cancer *(114)*. In a slightly more advanced lesion, ductal carcinoma *in situ* (DCIS), Radford et al. describe LOH of 17p in 8/28 specimens examined *(13)*, and in a follow-up paper report an association between LOH at 17p with DCIS preferentially of the comedo and high nuclear grade subtypes *(10)*. In a related manner, altered p53 protein (presumed to occur subsequent to allelic loss) has been reported in 15–24% of cases of DCIS *(4,18,115)*, and there is preliminary evidence that p53 expression (like LOH of 17p) may be slightly more pronounced in comedo vs noncomedo subtypes *(18)*.

It appears that early p53 alterations can be maintained during progression to more advanced breast lesions. For example, allelic loss at 17p has been found in synchronous lesions containing DCIS and invasive cancer, as well as in primary tumors and their corresponding lymph node metastases, although not always in either case *(11,17)*.

Moreover, there is preliminary evidence that the frequency of p53 alterations may potentially correlate with tumor progression *(18)*, which suggests that not only are p53 derangements maintained during evolution but also may be causally involved in the advancement to more invasive forms, possibly by promoting further genomic instability and resistance to therapy *(112,113)*. This idea is consistent with the well-documented association of p53 alterations with a variety of aggressive features of invasive cancers including high proliferative index, S-phase fraction, poorly differentiated grade, as well as ER-negativity *(4,12,25)*. From a clinical standpoint, maintenance of altered p53 during tumor evolution coupled with its association with aggressive features hints that p53 may possess prognostic value. That p53 alterations are often not associated with the most common prognostic variables (i.e., tumor size and nodal status) indicates that p53, if found to be prognostic, could represent an independent variable potentially useful in risk stratification and subsequent clinical management of node-negative disease *(116)*. However, at this point in time there are conflicting data with regard to the prognostic value of p53 in breast cancer.

The majority of studies investigating whether p53 is prognostic in breast cancer have utilized immunohistochemistry (IHC) as an indirect measure of TP53 mutation *(42,117,118)*. This technique can be used because the majority of TP53 mutant alleles are missense and encode a mutant protein with prolonged half-life that accumulates intracellularly and can be detected by IHC *(117,118)*. IHC has some benefit over DNA sequencing when employed in large studies because it is considerably less labor-intensive and can be used on archival paraffin-embedded material *(117,118)*. As reviewed by Bosari, approx one-third of large studies have found p53 to be of prognostic value, while the majority have not *(118)*. Interestingly, many of these positive studies concern node-negative patients but as previously noted these are fraught with experimental variability *(42,118)*. Namely, Thor et al. reported an independent association between p53 and poor outcome (after a mean follow-up of 7 yr) most significantly in the node-negative subgroup of the 295 tumors examined, when IHC positivity was defined as any cell staining *(119)*. Silvestrini et al. analyzed 256 patients with predominantly small node-negative tumors and demonstrated independent prognostic value for p53 staining (>5% positive cells) with regard to both OS and DFS after a mean follow-up of 72 mo *(120)*. Similarly, Gasparini et al. reported an independent correlation between p53(+) IHC and DFS for 203 node-negative patients after a median follow-up of 62 mo *(121)*. Allred et al, also found an independent association between p53 staining (but with two monoclonal antibodies [MAb]) and poor outcome upon examination of 316 node-negative cases *(122)*. Using both a different (polyclonal) antibody and a higher threshold for IHC positivity (>20% cells staining), Isola et al. demonstrated prognostic value for p53, but not independent of S-phase fraction in 289 node-negative tumors with an average follow-up of 8.5 yr *(123)*.

On the other hand, Pietilainen et al, upon examination of 392 node-negative tumors, showed that p53 staining did not correlate with outcome *(124)*. In addition, Lipponen et al. were unable to find an association between p53 staining and outcome in a mixture of 193 node-negative and -positive patients after >13 yr *(125)*. Moreover, Rosen et al, upon analysis of 440 specimens from node-negative patients, could not demonstrate independent prognostic value for p53 staining (>10% positive cells) after a median follow-up of 10 yr *(116)*. Similarly, Barbareschi et al. showed that p53 staining lacked independent prognostic value for 178 node-negative patients with median follow-up of 60 mo *(75)*. More recently, Seshadri et al, looked prospectively at >900 patients and although showing prognostic significance for p53 staining (>10% positive cells), did not find it to be independent of other parameters although median follow-up was only 66 mo *(126)*. In addition, Sjögren et al. did not report p53 staining to be prognostic in 316 tumors examined (when IHC threshold was set for any cell staining), but prognostic value was attributed to p53 staining in a secondary analysis when the threshold for IHC positivity was raised *(127)*. Accordingly, it has been suggested that these conflicting results with regard to p53 and prognosis in node-negative patients (as well as in node-positive ones, as previously mentioned) might be due in part to the significant variability of methods used (i.e., antibodies, staining thresholds), which to rectify would require more stringent standardization of techniques *(42,117,118)*.

Some have proposed that evaluation of TP53 at the DNA level, rather than at the protein level, might provide a less variable and more accurate assessment of p53 action in breast cancer *(128)*. For one, a number of investigators have shown discordance between IHC and mutation in certain settings *(118,127)*. It has been proposed that IHC might fail to detect certain mutant TP53 null alleles, or alternatively over-detect irrelevant instances of wild type protein stabilization (i.e., owing to transient cellular response to DNA damage, intercellular signals, or interaction with proteins such as MDM-2) *(112,113,117,118)*. Most reports seeking to determine the prognostic significance of TP53 mutations in breast cancer have concentrated on the most highly conserved regions of TP53 (i.e., exons 5–8) and have utilized a combination of direct sequencing with PCR coupled to DNA mobility shift assays such as single strand conformation polymorphism (SSCP), constant denaturant gel electrophoresis (CDGE), and denaturing gradient gel electrophoresis (DGGE) *(117,118,128)*. Elledge et al. reported an independent association between DFS (mean of 71 mo follow-up) and TP53 mutations in exons 5–9 as detected by SSCP upon analysis of 200 node-negative specimens *(129)*. Similarly, in two smaller studies comprised of a mixture of node-negative and -positive patients, both Anderson et al. and Thoraclius et al. showed a relation between TP53 mutations and poor outcome by CDGE (130,131). However, while Caleffi et al. were able to detect a trend toward prognostic value, these investigators were unable to demonstrate a statistically significant association between TP53 mutations and outcome, having evaluated 192 specimens by DGGE in exons 5-9 for a median follow-up of 48 mo *(132)*. Moreover, while Seshadri et al. demonstrated a significant association between outcome and TP53 mutation (in exons 5 and 6 by SSCP), this result was not subjected to complete multivariate analysis *(126)*. Accordingly, as in the case of IHC, there is as yet no consensus regarding the prognostic worth of genetic analysis of TP53 in breast cancer and this awaits larger studies with longer follow-ups.

Some investigators have used very sensitive techniques in an attempt to more accurately assess the prognostic value, if any, of TP53. Namely, in a small study by Kovach et al, all TP53 coding exons in tumors from 90 patients were screened by dideoxy-fingerprinting (ddF) of touch preparation specimens (i.e., an extremely sensitive technique) *(128,133)*. Whereas in most positive studies tumors harboring TP53 mutations were found to carry relative risks of poor outcome between 2.3-3.3, this study reported relative risks as high as 4.7 and 23.2 for recurrence and death, respectively for TP53 mutation *(128,133)*. Multivariate analyses revealed that TP53 mutation was independent of steroid receptor and nodal status *(133)*. In a related manner, Bergh et al. have also shown that extensive sequence analysis can not only improve prognostic value but can identify specific mutations which are particularly prognostic. Namely, these investigators, upon sequencing the entire coding region of TP53 cDNA in tumors from 316 patients, found that TP53 mutations had a statistically significant association with short survival, which was independent of other factors in node-positive patients *(134)*. In addition, mutations in two highly conserved regions of the TP53 gene correlated with a worse OS than did mutations outside this region, although this aspect of the study was quite small *(134)*. These findings are similar to a previous report of an association between the another highly conserved region of TP53 (i.e., the zinc-binding domain) and poor prognosis *(135)*.

It has been suggested that some of the discrepancies with regard to p53 and prognosis may be owing to effects of p53, not on inherent tumor behavior, but on certain therapeutic regimens which vary considerably from study to study *(136)*. There is some preliminary support for this idea. For example, although Bergh et al. found p53 status to predict outcome of node-positive patients treated with adjuvant therapy, it was not predictive of outcome in untreated node-negative patients *(134)*. Similarly, although Clahsen et al. and Elledge et al. reported a relation between p53 and outcome of node-negative patients treated with adjuvant chemotherapy, prognosis was similar in the untreated groups regardless of p53 status *(136,137)*. In these studies, Clahsen et al. have shown that while 441 node-negative patients randomized to receive chemotherapy (one cycle of CAF) fared better if without p53 alteration, those patients not receiving adjuvant therapy had equivalent outcomes whether p53-negative or -positive *(136)*. Elledge et al. also found a trend between p53 and outcome in 564 patients receiving adjuvant chemotherapy (six cycles of CMF and prednisone) but not in those randomized to receive no systemic treatment *(137)*. Similarly, Bergh et al. reported a trend between TP53 mutations and resistance to adjuvant CMF *(134)*, and in a related manner Aas et al. showed that TP53 mutations (in the highly conserved DNA-binding domain) were associated with resistance to adriamycin in metastatic breast cancer *(138)*. However, two other smaller studies failed to find a correlation between p53 status and various chemotherapeutic regimens *(139,140)*.

Two large studies investigating the predictive value of p53 with respect to tamoxifen-treated patients have yielded conflicting results. Namely, Elledge et al. in their analysis of 205 patients with metastatic disease not did show a correlation between p53 and response to tamoxifen *(141)*, while in the adjuvant setting Silvestrini et al. found p53 to independently predict poor response to tamoxifen in 240 node-positive ER-positive patients with resectable disease *(142)*. Berns et al. recently reported that p53 associated with decreased response to tamoxifen but mostly in that subset of 401 relapsed patients with low steroid receptor levels after a median follow-up of 69 mo *(142a)*. Bergh et al. have also shown, although in a small study, that p53 mutations (especially in conserved regions) can correlate with tamoxifen-resistance in node-positive patients in the adjuvant setting *(134)*. Interestingly, two reports have suggested that p53 alterations might predict a beneficial response to local radiation therapy *(143,144)*.

3.4. DNA Mismatch Repair Proteins

Expansion or contraction of nucleotide repeat elements (i.e., microsatellite instability, MI) was first reported in cancers of the colon and rectum *(145–147)*. Subsequently, hereditary nonpolyposis colorectal carcinoma (HNPCC) was shown to be caused by inheritance of a mutant DNA mismatch repair gene leading to a MI phenotype in colorectal tumors derived from these patients *(148,149)*. In breast cancers, MI has been detected in 10–40% tumors *(2,150)*. Unlike its relatively favorable associations in colorectal cancer, breast cancer-related MI has been found to correlate with unfavorable parameters such as large tumor size and node-positivity *(40,150)*, as well as with decreased DFS and OS in a relatively small study that needs to be confirmed *(150)*. Interestingly, MI has been detected in hyperplastic as well as DCIS specimens *(12,150a)*, and there is some evidence that it may act at an earlier stage of mammary tumorigenesis than other types of alterations (i.e., LOH) *(151)*.

3.5. Inherited Breast Cancer Genes

There are conflicting data as to the role, in sporadic mammary tumors, of genes associated with inherited breast cancer syndromes. The 2 most common inherited breast cancer predispostion genes are BRCA1 (at 17q) and BRCA2 (at 13q) *(3,40)* (*see* Chapters 9 and 10). The PTEN/MMAC1 gene, located at 10q23, encodes a tyrosine phosphatase (with homology to tensin, a cytoskeletal protein) and when inherited in a mutant form is responsible for Cowden's disease—a syndrome marked by mucocutaneous lesions, multiple benign hamartomas, and an increased incidence of malignancy (including breast cancer) *(3,40,152–154)*. The findings that the corresponding wild type allele is deleted in breast tumors derived from patients with germline mutations in BRCA1, BRCA2, and PTEN/MMAC1 indicates a tumor suppressor function by these genes in inherited breast cancers *(3,40,152–154)*. In support of similar role in noninherited cases is the frequent detection of LOH at 17q, 13q, and less commonly 10q in some sporadic tumors *(3,40,152–154)*. Additionally, decreased BRCA1 mRNA has been detected in sporadic breast cancers, a finding consistent with a tumor suppressor function in these cases *(155)*. However, only a paucity of mutations have been found in the corresponding remaining alleles of BRCA1, BRCA2, and PTEN/MMAC1 (in sporadic cases) thereby calling into question the mechanism by which, if any, these genes contribute to noninherited breast cancers *(3,12,40,152–154)*. It remains to be determined whether these or other genes associated with even rarer syndromes that predispose to an elevated breast cancer risk (i.e., STK11 at 19p13.3 for Peutz-Jeghers syndrome, ATM at 11q22 for ataxia telangiectasia) play a role in the pathogenesis of sporadic breast cancers *(3,40,156)*.

4. CONCLUSION

As described, a host of oncogenes and tumor suppressor genes have been implicated in the development of human breast cancer *(2–4)*. The most common alterations affecting these genes include amplification events of oncogenic loci and allelic deletions of tumor suppressor loci *(2–4,12)*. These genetic changes have been detected at different stages of breast tumorigenesis, some correlating with clinicopathological features, and a subset possessing prognostic and/or treatment-related predictive value *(2–4,12,40–*

42). It should also be noted that other less well characterized loci are likely to harbor additional breast cancer-related genes as evidenced by their nonrandom loss or gain in sporadic tumors (i.e., three deleted regions within 1p, 16q, 17q, two within 8p, 11q, 17p, at least one at 6q, 7q, 9p, 18q, and gained regions at 1q, 3q, 6p,2 0q) *(2–4)*. At present there are some candidate genes which map to these regions (i.e., ATM at 11q, p16 at 9p; DCC at 11q; E-cadherin at 16q; BRCA1, nm23 at 17q) *(2–4,15)*.

As mentioned, the most common mechanisms leading to gene deregulation in breast cancer are amplification and deletion (with or without accompanying point mutation) of oncogenes and tumor suppressors, respectively *(2–4)*. It should be noted, however, that although such genetic changes are often accompanied by corresponding expression changes (and vice versa) there are exceptions to this rule. For example, amplification correlates well with overexpression of c-erbB2 but slightly less so with cyclin D1, and appears to be unrelated to c-myc expression *(12,25,41,42)*. Similarly, down-regulation of tumor suppressor products p53, pRb, and certain CDI's are only variably associated with concomitant alterations at their respective genetic loci *(25,91,92,105,106,127,128)*. Several potential explanations have been offered to account for those instances wherein expression change occurs without obvious genetic change: 1) mutations affecting expression are not readily detectable (i.e., are within regulatory regions or splice sites), or 2) overexpression results not from mutation but as an epigenetic consequence of aberrant expression of upstream gene products (i.e., altered expression of a cell cycle product such as cyclin, p53, pRb, and CDI's may influence expression of the others) *(35,106,155)*. On the other hand, in order to explain instances wherein genetic alteration occurs without expression change, some have implicated the action of linked breast cancer-related genes within an amplicon (i.e., 11q13) or within a deleted region (i.e., 17p or 13q) *(2–4,25,35)*.

The major molecular alterations affecting breast cancer-related genes are present at some or all stages of tumorigenesis (*see* Fig. 1), and associate at times with known clinicopathological features *(2–4,12,15)*. In ductal hyperplasia, several alterations including LOH at 16q and 17p have been detected *(14)*. Subsequent to this stage, there is evidence that breast tumors evolve through the oncogenic action of cyclin D1 from ADH to DCIS, c-erbB2 in DCIS, and c-myc from DCIS to primary IDC (prior to metastasis) *(12,15,16,20)*. Cyclin D1 and c-erbB2, as well as acting in premalignancy, have also been found in more advanced primary as well as metastatic lesions *(15,36,43)*, and correlate with either favorable or in some reports aggressive features, respectively *(12,25–27,44,45)*. Alterations in MYC, more consistently so than c-erbB2, have been associated with certain unfavorable parameters *(2,23)*. BCL2 is unique in that, unlike other breast cancer-related oncogenes, its expression does not appear to be affected by large scale genetic events and is paradoxically both down-regulated as breast tumors advance as well as associated with several favorable features *(18,70–75)*. With regard to tumor suppressor genes, altered p53 expression has been detected in early premalignant lesions (subsequent to LOH of 17p) but with increasing frequency as tumors progress to more invasive forms *(18,115)*, and correlates with a number of aggressive clinicopathological features *(4,12,25)*. LOH at 13q is found in both DCIS and invasive cancer *(8,10,25)*, but there are conflicting data concerning associations between Rb deregulation and other tumor-related parameters *(25,83–86)*.

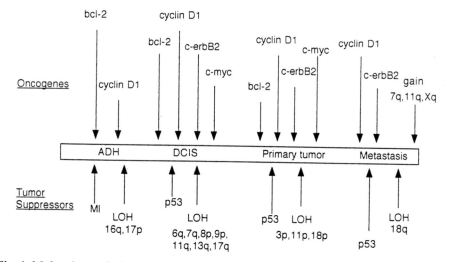

Fig. 1. Molecular evolution of breast cancer. Temporal relationships between breast cancer-related oncogenes and tumor suppressors at various stages of tumorigenesis. Arrow length of a given gene, which represents its relative expression level, is not drawn to scale and not intended for inter-gene comparisons.

There are numerous reports investigating the potential prognostic and predictive value of breast cancer-related molecular alterations. Several small studies have reported preliminary associations between amplification of MYC and cyclin D1 (but not overexpression of cyclin D1) with poor prognosis, while alterations affecting bcl-2 and Rb have been of more questionable prognostic value *(23–27,75–79,86,88)*. The bulk of reported studies, however, have examined c-erbB2 and p53 and have found suggestions (although by no means a consensus) that their deregulation may serve as indicators of poor prognosis in some node-positive and -negative patients, respectively *(41,42)*. With regard to possible predictive value to treatment response, there are some data indicating that c-erbB2 may correlate with tamoxifen-resistance and p53 with poor response to chemotherapy *(41,42)*. It should be noted, however, that the former idea has recently been challenged *(69)*, and the latter is not always statistically significant in larger studies *(134,136,137)*. Accordingly, it appears that the issue of prognostic or predictive value for c-erbB2 and p53 remains to be defined by larger prospective randomized trials with longer follow-up *(41,42)*. There are some existing reports, however, that prognostic value may be appreciated for 1) c-erbB2 (in node-negative patients) only following rigorous standardization of techniques and use of strict inclusion/exclusion criteria *(54)*, and 2) p53, only when techniques with significantly improved sensitivity for mutation detection are employed *(128,133)*. These studies await independent confirmation.

Aberrantly functional gene products involved in the development of breast cancer may also potentially serve as targets for novel methods of therapeutic intervention. Recent studies have revealed some efficacy when c-erbB2 is used as a target for immunotherapy. Namely, a humanized monoclonal antibody has been shown in phase II trials to be relatively well tolerated and capable of inducing tumor response

(157,158). Moreover, tumor suppressors p53 and BRCA1 have been used in preliminary gene therapy experiments. Adenovirally-introduced p53 has been shown capable of potentiating chemotherapy-induced apoptosis in breast cancer cell lines as well as growth inhibition of human breast cancer cell line xenografts in nude mice *(159,160).* Similarly, retrovirally-introduced BRCA1 inhibits the growth of MCF-7 cells when xenografted into nude mice *(161).* In ovarian cancer, a phase I study using BRCA1-containing retrovirus in 12 patients with advanced stage disease resulted in vector stability and minimal antibody response, as well as eight cases of relatively stable disease and three with tumor reduction, albeit after a short follow-up time *(162).* Clinical studies using gene therapy for breast cancer are eagerly anticipated.

ACKNOWLEDGMENTS

I would like to thank Dr. Anthony Brown for helpful comments on the manuscript, and Dr. Michael Osborne for encouragement and support to study human breast cancer. I would also like to thank Dr. Anne Bowcock for the opportunity to prepare this chapter.

REFERENCES

1. Radford, D. M., N. J. Phillips, K. L. Fair, J. H. Ritter, M. S. Holt, and H. Donis-Keller. 1995. Allelic loss and the progression of breast cancer. *Cancer Res.* **55:** 5180–5183.
2. Brenner, A. J. and C. M. Aldaz. 1997. The genetics of sporadic breast cancer, in *Etiology of Breast and Gynecological Cancers* (Aldaz, C. M., M. N. Gould, J. McLauchlan, and T. J. Slaga, eds.),Wiley-Liss, New York, NY, pp. 63–82.
3. Couch, F. J. and B. L. Weber. 1998. Breast cancer, in *The Genetic Basis of Human Cancer* (Vogelstein, B. and K. W. Kinzler, eds.), McGraw Hill, New York, NY, pp. 537–563.
4. Devilee, P. and C. J. Cornelisse. 1994. Somatic genetic changes in human breast cancer. *Biochim. Biophys. ACTA* **1198:** 113–130.
5. Nishizaki, T., S. DeVries, K. Chew, W. H. Goodson, III, B.-M. Ljung , A. Thor, and F. M. Waldman. 1997. Genetic alterations in primary breast cancers and their metastases: direct comparison using modified comparative genomic hybridization. *Genes Chrom. Cancer* **19:** 267–272.
6. Bonsing, B. A., P. Devilee, A.-M. Cleton-Jansen, N. Kuipers-Dijkshoorn, G. Jan Fleuren, and C. J. Cornelisse. 1993. Evidence for limited molecular genetic heterogeneity as defined by allelotyping and clonal analysis in nine metastatic breast carcinomas. *Cancer Res.* **53:** 3804–3811.
7. Kuukasjarvi, T., R. Karhu, M. Tanner, M. Kahkonen, A. Schaffer, N. Nupponen, S. Pennanen, A. Kallionemi, O.-P. Kallionemi, and J. Isola. 1997. Genetic heterogeneity and clonal evolution underlying development of asynchronous metastasis in human breast cancer. *Cancer Res.* **57:** 1597–1604.
8. Kuukasjarvi, T., M. Tanner, S. Pennanen, R. Karhu, O.-P. Kallionemi , and J. Isola. 1997. Genetic changes in intraductal breast cancer detected by comparative genomic hybridization. *Am. J. Path.* **150:** 1465–1471.
9. Tsuda, H., T. Fukutomi, and S. Hirohashi. 1995. Pattern of gene alterations in intraductal breast neoplasms associated with histological type and grade. *Clin. Cancer Res.* **1:** 261–267.
10. Radford, D. M., K. L. Fair, N. J. Phillips, J. H. Ritter, T. Steinbrueck, M. S. Holt, and H. Donis-Keller. 1995. Allelotyping of ductal carcinoma in situ of the breast: deletion of loci on 8p, 13q, 16q, 17p, and 17q. *Cancer Res.* **55:** 3399–3405.

11. Fujii, H., C. Marsh, P. Cairns, D. Sidransky, and E. Gabrielson. 1996. Genetic divergence in the clonal evolution of breast dancer. *Cancer Res.* **56:** 1493–1497.

12. Walker, R. A., J. L. Jones, S. Chappell, T. Walsh, and J. A. Shaw. 1997. Molecular pathology of breast cancer and its application to cllinical management. *Cancer Metast. Rev.* **16:** 5–27.

13. Radford, D. M., K. L. Fair, A. M. Thompson, J. H. Ritter, M. S. Holt, T. Steinbrueck, M. Wallace, S. A. Wells Jr., and H. R. Donis-Keller. 1993. Allelic loss on chromosome 17 in ductal carcinoma in situ of the breast. *Cancer Res.* **53:** 2947–2950.

14. Lakhani, S. R., N. Collins, M. R. Stratton, and J. P. Sloane. 1995. Atypical ductal hyperplasia of the breast: clonal proliferation with loss of heterozygosity on chromosomes 16q and 17p. *J. Clin. Pathol.* **48:** 611–615.

15. Beckmann, M. W., D. Niederacher, H.-G. Schnurch, B. A. Gusterson, and H. G. Bender. 1997. Multistep carcinogenesis of breast cancer and tumor heterogeneity. *J. Mol. Med.* **75:** 429–439.

16. Weinstat-Saslow, D., M. J. Merino, R. E. Manrow, J. A. Lawrence, R. F. Bluth, K. D. Wittenbel, J. F. Simpson, D. L Page, and P. S. Steeg. 1995. Overexpression of cyclin D mRNA distinguishes invasive and in situ breast carcinomas from non-malignant lesions. *Nature Med.* **1:** 1257–1260.

17. Davidoff, A. M., B.-J. M. Kerns, J. D. Iglehart, and J. R. Marks. 1991. Maintenance of p53 alterations throughout breast cancer progression. *Cancer Res.* **51:** 2605–2610.

18. Zhang, G.-J., I. Kimijima, R. Abe, M. Kanno, N. Katagata, K. Hara, T. Watanabe, and A. Tsuchiya. 1997. Correlation between the Expression of apoptosis-related bcl-2 and p53 oncoproteins and the carcinogenesis and progression of breast carcinomas. *Clin. Cancer Res.* **3:** 2329–2335.

19. Teixera, M. R., G. Bardi, J. A. Anderson, and S. Heim. 1996. Karyotypic comparisons of multiple tumorous and macroscopically normal surrounding tissue samples from patients with breast cancer. *Cancer Res.* **56:** 855–859.

20. Watson, P. H., J. R. Safneck, K. Lee, D. Dubik, and R. P. C. Shiu. 1993. Relationship of c-myc amplification to progression of breast cancer from in situ to invasive tumor and lymph node metastasis. *J. Natl. Cancer Inst.* **85:** 902–907.

21. O'Connell, P., V. Pekkel, S. Fuqua, C. K. Osborne, and D. C. Allred. 1994. Molecular genetic studies of early breast cancer evolution. *Breast Cancer Res. Treat.* **32:** 5–12.

22. Escot, C., C. Theillet, R. Lidereau, F. Spyratos, M.-H. Champeme, J. Gest, and R. Callahan. 1986. Genetic alterations of the c-myc oncogene (MYC) in human breast carcinomas. *Proc. Natl. Acad. Sci. USA* **83:** 4834–4838.

23. Berns, P. M. J. J., J. G. M. Klijn, W. L. J. Van Putten, I. L. Van Steveren, H. Portengen, and J. A. Foekens. 1992. C-myc amplification is a better prognostic factor than HER2/neu amplification in primary breast cancer. *Cancer Res.* **52:** 1107–1113.

24. Varley, J. M., J. E. Swallow, W. J. Brammar, J. L. Whittaker, and R. A. Walker. 1987. Alterations to either C-ERBB-2 (NEU) or C-MYC proto-oncogenes in breast carcinomas correlate with poor short term prognosis. *Oncogene* **1:** 423–430.

25. Landberg, G., G. Roos. 1997. The cell cycle in breast cancer. *APMIS* **105:** 575–589.

26. Borg, A., H. Sigurdsson, G. M. Clark, M. Freno, S. A. W. Fuqua, J. Olsson, D. Killander, and W. L. McQuire. 1991. Association of INT1/HST1 coamplification in primary breast cancer with hormone-dependent phenotype and poor prognosis. *Br. J. Cancer* **63:** 136–142.

27. Schuuring, E., E. Verhoeven, H. van Tinteren, J. L. Peterse, B. Nunnink, F. B. J. M. Thunnissen, P. Devilee, C. J. Cornelisse, M. J. van de Vijver, W. J. Mooi, and R. J. A. M. Michalides. 1992. Amplification of genes within the chromosome 11q13 region is indicative of poor prognosis in patients with operable breast cancer. *Cancer Res.* **52:** 5229–5234.

28. Michalides, R., P. Hageman, H. van Tinteren, L. Houben, E. Wientjens, R. Klompmaker, and J. Peterse. 1996. A clinicopathological study on overexpression of cyclin D1 and of p53 in a series of 248 patients wiht operable breast cancer. *Br. J. Cancer* **73:** 728–734.

29. McIntosh, G. G., J. J. Anderson, I. Milton, M. Steward, A. H. Parr, M. D. Thomas, J. A. Henry, B. Angus, T. W. J. Lennard, and C. H. W. Horne. 1995. *Oncogene* **11:** 885–891.

30. Gillett, C., P. Smith, W. Gregory, M. Richards, R. Millis, G. Peters, and D. Barnes. 1996. Cyclin D1 And prognosis in human breast cancer. *Int. J. Cancer* **69:** 92–99.

31. Adnane, J., P. Gaudray, M. Simon, J. Simony-Lafontaine, P. Jeanteur, and C. Theillet. 1989. Proto-oncogene amplification and human tumor phenotype. *Oncogene* **4:** 1389–1395.

32. Tsuda, H., S. Hirohashi, Y. Shimosato, T. Hirota, S. Tsugane, H. Yamamoto, N. Miyajima, K. Toyoshima, T. Yamamoto, J. Yokota, T. Yoshida, H. Sakamoto, M. Terada, and T. Sugimura. 1989. Correlation between long-term survival in breast cancer patients and amplification of two putative oncogene-coamplification units: hst–1/int–2 and c-erbB2/ear–1. *Cancer Res.* **49:** 3104–3108.

33. Lonn, U., S. Lonn, B. Nilsson, and B. Stenvist. 1994. Breast cancer: prognostic significance of c-erbB2 and int–2 amplification compared with DNA ploidy, S-phase fraction, and conventional clinicopathological features. *Breast Cancer Res. Treat.* **29:** 237–254.

34. van Diest, P. J., R. J. A. M. Michalides, I. Jannick, P. van der Valk, H. L. Peterse, J. S. de Jong, C. J. L. M. Meijer, and J. P. A. Baak. 1997. Cyclin D1 expression in invasive breast cancer. *Am. J. Pathol.* **150:** 705–711.

35. Nielsen, N. H., S. O. Emdin, J. Cajander, and G. Landberg. 1997. Deregulation of cyclin E and D1 in breast cancer is associated with inactivation of the retinoblastoma protein. *Oncogene* **14:** 295–304.

36. Bartkova, J., J. Lucas, H. Muller, D. Lutzhoft, M. Strauss, and J. Bartek. 1994. Cyclin D1 protein expression and function in human breast cancer. *Int. J. Cancer* **57:** 353–361.

37. Lonn, U., S. Lonn, H. Ingelman-Sundberg, B. Nilsson, and B. Stenkvist. C-ERB2/INT–2 amplification appears faster in breast-cancer patients receiving second-line endocrine treatment. 1996. *Int. J. Cancer* **69:** 273–277.

38. Nielsen, N. H., S. O. Emdin, J. Cajander, and G. Landberg. 1997. Deregulation of cyclin E and D1 in breast cancer is associated with inactivation of the retinoblastoma protein. *Oncogene* **14:** 295–304.

38a. Brehm, A., E. A. Miska, D. J. McCance, J. L. Reid, A. J. Bannister, and T. Kouzarides. 1998. Retinoblastoma protein recruits histone deacetylase to repress transcription. *Nature* **391:** 597–601.

39. Porter, P. L., K. E. Malone, P. J. Heagerty, G. M. Alexander, L. A. Gatti, E. J. Firpo, J. R. Daling, and J. M. Roberts. 1996. Expression of cell-cycle regulators p27Kip and Cyclin E, alone and in combination, correlate with survival in young breast cancer patients. *Nature Med.* **3:** 222–225.

40. Radice, P. and M. A. Pierotti. 1997. Molecular genetics of breast cancer. *Q. J. Nucl. Med.* **41:** 189–199.

41. Ravdin, P. M. and G. C. Chamness. 1995. The c-erbB-2 proto-oncogene as a prognostic and predictive marker in breast cancer: a paradigm for the development of other macromolecular markers- a review. *Gene* **159:** 19–27.

42. American Society of Clinical Oncology (ASCO). 1996. Clinical practice guidelines for the use of tumor markers in breast and colorectal cancer. *J. Clin. Oncol.* **14:** 2843–2877.

43. Iglehart, J. D., M. H. Kraus, B. C. Langton, G. Huper, B. J. Kerns, and J. R. Marks. 1990. Increased erbB-2 gene copies and expression in multiple stages of breast cancer. *Cancer Res.* 6701–6707.

44. Gullick, W. J., S. B. Love, C. Wright, D. M. Barnes, B. Gusterson, A. L. Harris, and D. G. Altman. 1991. c-erbB-2 protein overexpression in breast cancer is a risk factor in patients with involved and uninvolved lymph nodes. *Br. J. Cancer* **63:** 434–438.

45. Carlomagno, C., F. Perrone, C. Gallo, M. De Laurentis, R. Lauria, A. Morabito, G. Pettinato, L. Panico, A. D'Antonio, A. R. Bianco, and S. De Placido. 1996. c-erbB2 Overexpression decreases the benefit of adjuvant tamoxifen in early-stage breast cancer without axillary lymph node metastases. *J. Clin. Oncol.* **10**: 2702–2708.

46. Slamon, D. J., G. M. Clark, S. G. Wong, W. J. Levin, A. Ullrich, and W. L. McGuire. 1987. Human breast cancer: correlation of felapse and xurvival with amplification of the HER-2/neu oncogene. *Science* **235**: 177–182.

47. Slamon, D. J., W. Godolphin, L. A. Jones, J. A. Holt, S. G. Wong, D. E. Keith, W. J. Levin, S. G. Stuart, J. Udove, A. Ullrich, and M. F. Press. 1989. Studies of the HER-2/neu Proto-ncogene in Human Breast and Ovarian Cancer. *Science* **244**: 707–712.

48. Winstanley, J., T. Cooke, G. D. Murray, A. Platt-Higgins, W. D. George, S. Holt, M. Myskov, A. Spedding, B. R. Barraclough, and P. S. Rudland. 1991. The long term prognostic significance of c-erbB2 in primary breast cancer. *Br. J. Cancer* **63**: 447–450.

49. Paterson, M. C., K. D. Dietrich, J. Danyluk, A. H. Paterson, A. W. Lees, N. Jamil, J. Hanson, H. Jenkins, B. E. Krause, W. A. McBlain, D. J. Slamon, and R. M. Fourney. 1991. *Cancer Res.* **51**: 556–567.

50. Borg, A., A. K. Tandon, H. Sigurdsson, G. M. Clark, M. Ferno, S. A. Fuqua, D. Killander, and W. L. McGuire. 1990. HER-2/neu amplification predicts poor survival in node-positive breast cancer. *Cancer Res.* **50**: 4332–4337.

51. Berns, E. M., J. G. Klijn, W. L. van Putten, I. L. van Staveren, H. Portengen, and J. A. Foekens. 1992. c-myc amplification is a better prognostic factor than HER2/neu in primary breast cancer. *Cancer Res.* **52**: 1107–1113.

52. Clark, G. M. and W. L. McGuire. 1991. Follow-up study of HER-2/neu amplification in primary breast cancer. *Cancer Res.* **51**: 944–948.

53. Sjögren, S., M. Inganas, A. Lindgren, L. Holmberg, and J. Bergh. 1998. Prognostic and predictive value of c-erbB-2 overexpression in primary breast cancer, alone and in combination with other prognostic markers. *J. Clin. Oncol.* **16**: 462–469.

54. Press, M. F., L. Bernstein, P. A. Thomas, L. F. Meisner, J.-Y. Zhou, Y. Ma, G. Hung, R. A. Robinson, C. Harris, A. El-Naggar, D. J. Slamon, R. N. Phillips, J. S. Ross, S. R. Wolman, and K. J. Flom. 1997. HER-2/neu gene amplification characterized by fluorescence in situ hybridization: poor prognosis in node-negative breast carcinomas. *J. Clin. Oncol.* **15**: 2894–2904.

55. Press, M. F., M. C. Pike, V. R. Chazin, G. Hung, J. A. Udove, M. Markowicz, J. Danyluk, W. Godolphin, M. Sliwkowski, R. Akita, M. C. Patterson, and D. J. Slamon. 1993. Her-2/neu expression in node-negative breast cancer: direct tissue quantitation by computerized image analysis and association of overexpression with increased risk of recurrent disease. *Cancer Res.* **53**: 4960–4970.

56. Ali, I. U., G. Campbell, R. Lidereau, and R. Callahan. 1988. Lack of evidence for the prognostic significance of c-erbB-2 amplification. *Oncogene Res.* **3**: 139–146.

57. Tsuda, H., S. Hirohashi, Y. Shimosato, T. Tanaka, T. Hirota, S. Tsugane, M. Shiraishi, K. Toyoshima, T. Yamamoto, and M. Terada. 1990. Immunohistochemical study on overexpression of c-erbB-2 protein in human breast cancer: its correlation with gene amplification and long-term survival of patients. *Jpn. J. Cancer Res.* **81**: 327–332.

58. Tetu, B. and J. Brisson. 1994. Prognostic significance of HER-2/neu oncoprotein expression in node-positive breast cancer. The influence of the pattern of immunostaining and adjuvant therapy. *Cancer* **73**: 2359–2365.

59. Gusterson, B. A., R. D. Gelber, A. Goldhirsch, K. N. Price, J. Save-Soderborgh, R. Anbazhagan, J. Styles, C.-M. Rudenstam, R. Golouh, R. Reed, F. Martinez-Tello, A. Tiltman, J. Torhorst, P. Grigolato, R. Bettelheim, A. M. Neville, K. Burki, M. Catiglione, J. Collins, J. Lindtner, and H.-J. Senn. 1992. Prognostic importance of c-erbB-2 expression in breast cancer. *J. Clin. Oncol.* **10**: 1049–1056.

60. Allred, D. C., G. M. Clark, A. K. Tandon, R. Molina, D. C. Tormey, C. K. Osborne, K. W. Gilchrist, E. G. Mansour, M. Abeloff, L. Eudey, and W. L. McGuire. 1992. HER-2/neu in node-negative breast cancer: prognostic significance of overexpression influenced by the presence of in situ carcinoma. *J. Clin. Oncol.* **10:** 599–605.

61. Klijn, J. G., E. M. Berns, M. Bontenbal, and J. Foekens. 1993. Cell biological factors associated with the response of breast cancer to systemic treatment. *Cancer Treat. Rev.* **19(Suppl. B):** 45–63.

63. Muss, H. B., A. D. Thor, D. A. Berry, T. Kute, E. T. Liu, F. Koerner, C. T. Cirrincione, D. R. Budman, W. C. Wood, M. Barcos, and I. C. Henderson. 1994. c-erbB-2 expression and response to adjuvant therapy in women with node-positive breast cancer. *N. Engl. J. Med.* **330:** 1260–1266.

63. Wright, C., J. Cairns, B. J. Cantwell, A. R. Cattan, A. G. Hall, A. L. Harris, and C. H. Horne. 1992. Response to mitoxantrone in advanced breast cancer: correlation with expression of c-erbB2 protein and glutathione S-transferases. *Br. J. Cancer* **65:** 271–274.

64. Wright, C., S. Nicholson, B. Angus, J. R. C. Sainsbury, J. Farndon, J. Cairns, A. L. Harris, and C. H. Horne. 1992. Relationship between c-erbB2 protein product expression and response to endocrine therapy in advanced breast cancer. *Br. J. Cancer* **65:** 118–121.

65. Berns, M. J. J., J. A. Foekens, I. L. van Staveren, W. L. J. van Putten, H. Y. W. C. M. de Koning, H. Portenegen, and J. G. M. Klijn. 1995. *Oncogene* amplification and prognosis in breast cancer: relationship with systemic treatment. *Gene* **159:** 11–18.

66. Borg, A., B. Baldetorp, M. Ferno, D. Killander, H. Olsson, S. Ryden, and H. Sigurdsson. 1994. ERBB2 amplification is associated with tamoxifen resistance in steroid-receptor positive breast cancer. *Cancer Lett.* **8:** 137–144.

67. Lonn, U., S. Lonn, H. Ingelman-Sundberg, B. Nilsson, and B. Stenkvist. C-ERB2/INT–2 amplification appears faster in breast-cancer patients receiving second-line endocrine treatment. 1996. *Int. J. Cancer* **69:** 273–277.

68. Archer, S. G., A. Eliopoulos, D. Spandidos, D. Barnes, I. O. Ellis, R. W. Blamey, R. I. Nicholson, and J. F. Robertson. 1995. Expression of ras p21, p53, and c-erbB-2 in advanced breast cancer and response to first line hormonal therapy. *Br. J. Cancer* **72:** 1259–1266.

69. Elledge, R. M., S. Green, D. Ciocca, R. Pugh, D. C. Allred, G. M. Clark, J. Hill, P. Ravdin, J. O'Sullivan, S. Martino, and C. K. Osborne. 1998. HER-2 expression and response to tamoxifen in estrogen receptor-positive breast cancer: a southwest oncology group study. Clin *Cancer Res.* **4:** 7–12.

70. Leek, R. D., L. Kaklamanis, F. Pezzella, K. C. Gatter, and A. L. Harris. 1994. Bcl-2 in normal human breast and carcinoma, association with oestrogen receptor-positive, epidermal growth factor receptor-negative tumours and in situ cancer. *Br. J. Cancer* **69:** 135–139.

71. Gee, J. M. W., J. F. R. Robertson, I. O. Ellis, P. Willsher, R. A. McClelland, H. B. Hoyle, S. R. Kyme, P. Finlay, R. W. Blamey, and R. I. Nicholson. 1994. Immunocytochemical localization of bcl-2 protein in human breast cancers and its relationship to a series of prognostic markers and response to endocrine therapy. *Int. J. Cancer* **59:** 619–628.

72. Gasparini, G., M. Barbareschi, C. Doglioni, P. D. Palma, F. A. Mauri, P. Borrachi, P. Bevilacqua, O. Caffo, L. Morelli, P. Verderio, F. Pezzella, and A. L. Harris. 1995. Expression of bcl-2 protein predicts efficacy of adjuvant treatments in operable node-positive breast cancer. *Clin. Cancer Res.* **1:** 189–198.

73. Elledge, R. M., S. Green, L. Howes, G. M. Clark, M. Berardo, D. C. Allred, R. Pugh, D. Ciocca, P. Ravdin, J. O'Sullivan, S. Rivkin, S. Martino, and C. K. Osborne. 1997. bcl-2, p53, and response to tamoxifen in estrogen receptor-positive metastatic breast cancer: a southwest oncology group study. *J. Clin. Oncol.* **15:** 1916–1922.

74. Silvestrini R., S. Veneroni, M. G. Daidone, E. Benini, P. Borrachi, M. Mezzetti, G. Di Fronzo, F. Rilke, and U. Veronesi. 1994. The Bcl-2 protein: A prognostic indicator strongly related to p53 protein in lymph node-negative breast cancer patients *J. Natl. Cancer Inst.* **86:** 499–504.

75. Barbareschi, M., O. Caffo, S. Veronese, L. D. Leek, P. Fina, S. Fox, M. Bonzanini, S. Girlando, L. Morelli, C. Eccher, F. Pezzella, C. Doglioni, P. D. Plama, and A. Harris. 1996. Bcl-2 and p53 expression in node-negative breast carcinoma. *Hum. Pathol.* **27:** 1149–1155.

76. Joensuu, H., L. Pylkkanen, and S. Toikkanen. 1994. Bcl-2 protein expression and long-term survival in breast cancer. *Am. J. Pathol.* **145:** 1191–1198.

77. Hurlimann, J., B. Larrinaga, and D. L. M. Vala. 1995. bcl-2 protein in invasive ductal breast carcinomas. *Virchows Archiv.* **426:** 163–168.

78. Hellemans, P., P. A. van Dam, J. Weyler, A. T. van Oosterom, P. Buytaert, and E. Van Marck. 1995. Prognostic value of bcl-2 expression in invasive breast cancer. *Br. J. Cancer* **72:** 354–360.

79. Silvestrini R., S. Veneroni, M. G. Daidone, E. Benini, P. Borrachi, M. Mezzetti, G. Di Fronzo, F. Rilke, and U. Veronesi. 1994. The Bcl-2 protein: A prognostic indicator strongly related to p53 protein in lymph node-negative breast cancer patients *J. Natl. Cancer Inst.* **86:** 499–504.

80. Silvestrini, R., E. Benini, S. Veneroni, M. G. Daidone, G. Tomasic, P. Squicciarini, and B. Salvadori. 1996. p53 and bcl-2 Expression correlates with xlinical outcome in a series of node-positive breast cancer patients. *J. Clin. Oncol.* **14:** 1604–1610.

81. Elledge, R. M., S. Green, L. Howes, G. M. Clark, M. Berardo, D. C. Allred, R. Pugh, D. Ciocca, P. Ravdin, J. O'Sullivan, S. Rivkin, S. Martino, and C. K. Osborne. 1997. bcl-2, p53, and response to tamoxifen in estrogen receptor-positive metastatic breast cancer: a southwest oncology group study. *J. Clin. Oncol.* **15:** 1916–1922.

82. Silvestrini, R., S. Veneroni, E. Benini, M. G. Daidone, A. Luisi, M. Leutner, A. Maucione, R. Kenda, R. Zucali, U. Veronesi. 1997. Expression of p53, glutathione S-transferase, and Bcl-2 proteins and benefit from adjuvant radiotherapy in breast cancer. *J. Natl. Cancer Inst.* **89:** 639–645.

83. Borg, A., Q.-X. Zhang, P. Alm, H. Olsson, and,G. Sellberg. 1992. The retinoblastoma gene in breast cancer: allele loss is not correlated with loss of gene protein expression. *Cancer Res.* **52:** 2991–2994.

84. Varley, J. M., J. Armour, J. E. Swallow, A. J. Jeffreys, B. A. J. Ponder, A. T'Ang, Y.-K. Fung, W. J. Brammar, and R. A. Walker. 1989. The retinoblastoma gene is frequently altered leading to loss of expression in primary breast tumours. *Oncogene* **4:** 725–729.

85. Thoraclius, S., O. Jonasdottir, and J. E. Eyfjord. 1991. Loss of heterozygosity at selective sites on chromosomes 13 and 17 in human breast carcinoma. *Anticancer Res.* **11:** 1501–1508.

86. Berns, E. M. J. J., A. De Klein, W. L. J. van Putten, I. L. van Staveren, A. Bootsma, J. G. M. Klign, and J. A. Foekens. 1995. Association between RB–1 gene alterations and factors of favorable prognosis in human breast cancer, without effect on survival. *Int. J. Cancer* **64:** 140–145.

87. Trudel, M., L. Mulligan, W. Cavenee, R. Margolese, J. Cote, and G. Gariepy. 1992. Retinoblastoma and p53 gene product expression in breast carcinoma: immunohistochemical analysis and clinicopathologic correlation. *Hum. Pathol.* **23:** 1388–1394.

88. Sawan, A., B. Randall, B. Angus, C. Wright, J. A. Henry, J. Ostrowski, C. Hennessy, T. W. Lennard, I. Corbett, and C. H. Horne. 1992. Retinoblastoma and p53 gene expression related to relapse and survival in human breast cancer: an immunohistochemical study. *J. Pathol.* **168:** 23–28.

89. Berns, E. M. J. J., J. G. M. Klijn, M. Smid, I. L. vsn Staveren, N. A. Gruis, and J. A. Foekens. 1995. Infrequent CDKN2 (MTS/p16) gene alterations in human primary breast cancer. *Br. J. Cancer* **72:** 964–967.

90. An, H. X., D. Niederacher, F. Picard, C. Vanroeyen, H. G. Bender, and M. W. Beckmann. 1996. Frequent allele loss on 9P21–22 defines a smallest common region in the vicinity of the CDKN2 gene in sporadic breast cancer. *Genes Chrom. Cancer* **17**: 14–20.

91. Quesnel, B., P. Fenaux, N. Phillipe, J. Fournier, J. Bonneterre, C. Preudhomme, and J. P. Peyrat. 1995. *Oncogene* **10**: 351–353.

92. Geradts, J. and P. A. Wilson. 1996. High frequency of aberrant p16INK4A expression in human breast cancer. *Am. J. Pathol.* **149**: 15–20.

93. Cairns, P., T. J. Polascik, Y. Eby, K. Tokino, J. Califano, A. Merlo, L. Mao, J. Herath, R. Jenkins, W. Westra, J. L. Rutter, A. Buckler, E. Gabrielson, M. Tockman, K. R. Cho, L. Hedrick, G. S. Bova, W. Isaacs, W. Koch, D. Schwab, and D. Sidransky. 1995. Frequency of homozygous deletion at p16/CDKN2 in primary human tumors. *Nature Genet.* **11**: 210–212.

94. Brenner, A. J. and C. M. Aldaz. 1995. Chromosome 9p allelic loss and p16/CDKN2 in breast cancer and evidence of p16 inactivation in immortal breast epithelial cells. *Cancer Res.* **55**: 2892–2895.

95. Musgrove, E. A., R. Lilischkis, A. L. Cornish, C. S. L. Lee, V. Setlur, R. Seshadri, and R. L. Sutherland. 1995. Expression of the cyclin-dependent kinase inhibitors p16INK4, p15INK4B, and p21WAF1/CIP1 in human breast cancer. *Int. J. Cancer* **63**: 584–591.

96. Herman, J. G., A. Merlo, L. Mao, R. G. Lapidus, J.-P. J. Issa, N. E. Davidson, D. Sidransky, and S. B. Baylin. 1995. Inactivation of the CDKN2/p16/MTS1 gene is frequently associated wtih aberrant DNS methylation in all common human cancers. *Cancer Res.* **55**: 4525–4530.

97. Barbareschi, M., O. Caffo, C. Doglioni, P. Fina, A. Marchetti, F. Buttitta, R. Leek, L. Morelli, E. Leonardi, G. Bevilacqua, P. Dalla Palma, A. L. Harris. 1996. p21WAF1 immunohistochemical expression in breast carcinoma: correlations with clinicopathological data, oestrogen receptor status, MIB1 expression, p53 gene and protein alterations and relapse-free survival. *Br. J. Cancer* **74**: 208–215.

98. Xiong, Y., G. J. Hannon, H. Zhang, D. Casso, R. Kobayashi, and D. Beach. 1993. p21 is a universal inhibitor of cyclin kinases. *Nature* **366**: 701–704.

99. Hunter, T. and J. Pines. 1994. Cyclins and cancer II: cyclin D and CDK inhibitors come of age. *Cell* **79**: 573–582.

100. Somasundaram, K., H. Zhang, Y.-I. Zeng, Y. Houvras, Y. Peng, H. Zhang, G. S. Wu, J. D. Licht, B. L. Weber, and W. S. El-Deiry. 1997. Arrest of the cell cycle by the tumor-suppressor BRCA–1 requires the CDK-inhibitor p21WAF1/CIP1. *Nature* **389**: 187–188.

101. Wakasugi, E., T. Kobayashi, Y. Tamaki, Y. Ito, I. Miyashiro, Y. Komoike, T. Takeda, E. Shin, Y. Takatsuka, N. Kikkawa, T. Monden, and M. Monden. 1997. p21 (Waf1/Cip1) and p53 protein expression in breast cancer. *Am. J. Clin. Pathol.* **107**: 684–691.

102. Jiang, M., Z.-M. Shao, J. Wu, J.-S. Lu, L.-M. Yu, J.-D. Yuan, Q.-X. Han, Z.-Z. Shen, and J. A. Fontana. 1997. p21/waf1/cip1 and mdm–2 expression in breast carcinoma patients as related to prognosis. *Int. J. Cancer* **74**: 529–534.

103. Johnson, E. A., A. G. Davidson, R. B. Hostetter, L. L. Cook, E. M. Thomas, and D. C. Quinlan. 1996. The expression of WAF–1 in node negative infiltrating ductal breast carcinoma. *Proc. Amer. Ass. Cancer Res.* **37**: 569a.

104. Caffo, O., C. Doglioni, S. Veronese, M. Bonzanini, A. Marchetti, F. Buttitta, P. Fina, R. Leek, L. Morelli, P. Dalla Palma, A. L. Harris, and M. Barbareschi. 1996. Prognostic value of p21 WAF1 and p53 expression in breast carcinoma: An immunohistochemical study in 261 patients with long-term followup. *Clin. Cancer Res.* **2**: 1591–1599.

105. Marchetti, A., F. Buttitta, S. Pellegrini, A. Lori, G. Bertacca, and G. Bevilacqua. 1995. Absence of somatic mutations in the coding region of the WAF1/CIP1 gene in

human breast, lung, and ovarian carcinomas: a polymorphism at codon 31. *Int. J. Oncol.* **6:** 187–189.

106. Fredersdorf, S., J. Burns, A. M. Milne, G. Packham, L. Fallis, C. E. Gillett, J. A. Royds, D. Peston, P. A. Hall, A. M. Hanby, D. M. Barnes, S. Shoush, M. J. O'Hare, and X. Lu. 1997. High level expression of p27kip and cyclin D1 in some human breast cancer cells: Inverse correlation between the expression of p27kip and degreee of malignancy in human breast and colorectal cancers. *Proc. Natl. Acad. Sci. USA* **94:** 6380–6385.

107. Spirin, K. S., J. F. Simpson, S. Takeuchi, N. Kawamata, C. W. Miller, and H. P. Koeffler. 1996. p27/Kip1 mutation found in breast cancer. *Cancer Res.* **56:** 2400–2404.

108. Ferrando, A. A., M. Balbin, A. M. Pendas, F. Vizoso, G. Velasco, and C. Lopez-Otin. 1996. Mutational Analysis of the human cyclin dependent kinase inhibitor p27Kip1 in primary breast carcinomas. *Hum. Genet.* **97:** 91–94.

109. Catzavelos, C., N. Bhattacharya, Y. C. Ung, J. A. Wilson, L. Roncari, C. Sandhu, P. Shaw, H. Yeger, I. Morava-Protzner, L. Kapusta, E. Franssen, K. I. Pritchard, and J. M. Slingerland. 1996. Decreased levels of the cell-cycle inhibitor p27Kip protein: prognostic implications in primary breast cancer. *Nature Med.* **3:** 227–230.

110. Tan, P., B. Cady, M. Wanner, P. Worland, B. Cukor, C. Magi-Galluzzi, P. Lavin, G. Draetta, M. Pagano, and M. Loda. 1997. The cell cycle inhibitor p27 is an independent prognostic marker in small (T1a,b) invasive breast carcinomas. *Cancer Res.* **57:** 1259–1263.

111. Porter, P. L., K. E. Malone, P. J. Heagerty, G. M. Alexander, L. A. Gatti, E. J. Firpo, J. R. Daling, and J. M. Roberts. 1996. Expression of cell-cycle regulators p27Kip and Cyclin E, alone and in combination, correlate with survival in young breast cancer patients. *Nature Med.* **3:** 222–225.

111a. Sgambato, A., Y.-J. Zhang, N. Arber, H. Hibshoosh, Y. Doki, M. Ciaparrone, R. M. Santella, A. Cittadini, and I. B. Weinstein. 1997. Deregulated expression of p27Kip1 in human breast cancers. *Clin. Cancer Res.* **3:** 1879–1887.

112. Greenblatt, M. S., W. P Bennett, M. Hollstein, and C. C Harris. 1994. Mutations in the p53 tumor suppressor gene: Clues to cancer etiology and molecular pathogenesis. *Cancer Res.* **54:** 4855–4878.

113. Chang, F., S. Syrjanen, and K. Syrjanen. 1995. Implications of the p53 tumor-suppressor gene in clinical oncology. *J. Clin. Oncol.* **13:** 1009–1022.

114. Deng, G., Y. Lu, G. Zlotnikov, A. D. Thor, and H. S. Smith. 1996. Loss of heterozygosity in normal tissue adjacent to breast carcinomas. *Science* **274:** 2057–2059.

115. Poller, D. N., E. C. Roberts, J. A. Bell, C. W. Elston, R. W. Blamey, and I. O. Ellis. 1993. p53 protein expression in mammary ductal carcinoma in situ: relationship to immunohistochemical expression of estrogen receptor and c-erbB-2 protein. *Hum. Pathol.* **24:** 463–468.

116. Rosen, P. P., M. L. Lesser, C. D. Arroyo, M. Cranor, P. Borgen, and L. Norton. 1995. p53 in node-negative breast carcinoma: an immunohistochemical study of epidemiologic risk factors, histologic features, and prognosis. *J. Clin. Oncol.* **13:** 821–830.

117. Dowell, S. P. and P. A. Hall. 1995. The p53 tumour suppressor gene and tumour prognosis: Is there a relationship? *J. Pathol.* **177:** 221–224.

118. Bosari, S., and G. Viale. 1995. The clinical significance of p53 aberrations in human tumors. *Virchows Arch.* **427:** 229–241, 1995.

119. Thor, A. D., D. H. Moore, S. M. Edgerton, E. S. Kawasaki, E. Reihsaus, H. T. Lynch, J. N. Marcus, L. Schwartz, L.-C. Chen, B. H. Mayall, and H. S. Smith. 1992. Accumulation of p53 tumor suppressor gene protein: An independent marker of prognosis in breast cancers. *J. Natl. Cancer Inst.* **84:** 845–855.

120. Silvestrini, R., E. Benini, M. G. Daidone, S. Veneroni, P. Borrachi, V. Cappelletti, G. Di Fronzo, and U. Veronesi. 1993. p53 as an independent prognostic marker in lymph node-negative breast cancer patients. *J. Natl. Cancer Inst.* **85:** 965–970.

121. Gasparini, G., N. Weidner, P. Bevilacqua, S. Maluta, P. Dalla Palma, O. Caffo, M. Barbareschi, P. Borrachi, E. Marubini, and F. Pozza. 1994. Tumor microvessel density, p53 expression, tumor size, and peritumoral vessel invasion are relevant prognostic markers in node-negative breast carcinoma. *J. Clin. Oncol.* **12**: 454–466.

122. Allred, D. C., G. M. Clark, R. Elledge, S. A. W. Fuqua, R. W. Brown, G. C. Chamness, and C. K. Osborne. 1993. Association of p53 protein expression with tumor cell proliferation rate and clinical outcome in node-negative breast cancer. *J. Natl. Cancer Inst.* **85**: 200–206.

123. Isola, I., T. Visakorpi, K. Holli, and O.-P. Kallionemi. 1992. Association of overexpression of tumor suppressor protein p53 with rapid cell proliferation and poor prognosis in node-negative breast cancer patients. *J. Natl. Cancer Inst.* **84**: 1109–1114.

124. Pietilainen, T., P. Lipponen, S. Aaltomaa, M. Eskelinen, V.-M. Kosma, and K. Syrjanen. 1995. Expression of p53 protein has no independent prognostic value in breast cancer. *J. Pathol.* **177**: 225–232.

125. Lipponen, P., S. Aaltomaa, S. Syrjanen, and K. Syrjanen. 1993. p53 protein expression in breast cancer as related to histopathological characteristics and prognosis. *Int. J. Cancer* **55**: 51–56.

126. Seshadri, R., A. S.-Y. Leong, K. McCaul, F. A. Firgaira, V. Setlur, and D. J. Horsfall. 1996. Relationship between p53 gene abnormalities and other tumour characteristics in breast-cancer prognosis. *Int. J. Cancer* **69**: 135–141.

127. Sjögren, S., M. Inganas, T. Norberg, A. Lindgren, H. Nordgren, L. Holmberg, and J. Bergh. 1996. The p53 gene in breast cancer: prognostic value of complementary DNA sequencing versus immunohistochemistry. *J. Natl. Cancer Inst.* **88**: 173–182.

128. Hartmann, A., H. Blaszyk, J. S. Kovach, and S. S. Sommer. 1997. The molecular epidemiology of P53 gene mutations in human breast cancer. *Trends Genet.* **13**: 27–33.

129. Elledge, R. M., S. A. W. Fuqua, G. M. Clark, P. Pujol, and D. C. Allred. 1993. Prognostic significance of p53 alteration in node-negative breast cancer. *Breast Cancer Res. Treat.* **26**: 225–235.

130. Anderson, T. I., R. Holm, J. M. Nesland, K. R. Keimdal, L. Ottestad, and A. L. Borreson. 1993. Prognostic significance of TP53 in breast carcinoma. *Br. J. Cancer* **68**: 540–548.

131. Thoraclius, S., A.-L. Borresen, and J. E. Eyfjord. 1993. Somatic p53 mutations in human breast carcinomas in an Icelandic population: a prognostic factor. *Cancer Res.* **53**: 1637–1641.

132. Caleffi, M., M. W. Teague, R. A. Jensen, C. L. Vnencak-Jones, W. D. Dupont, and F. F. Parl. 1994. p53 mutations and steroid receptor status in breast cancer. *Cancer* **73**: 2147–2156.

133. Kovach, J. S, A. Hartmann, H. Blaszyk, J. Cunningham, D. Schaid, and S. S. Sommer. 1996. Mutation detection by highly sensitive methods indicates that p53 gene mutations in breast cancer can have important prognostic value. *Proc. Natl. Acad. Sci. USA* **93**: 1093–1096.

134. Bergh, J., T. Norberg, S. Sjögren, A. Lindgren, and L. Holmberg. 1995. Complete sequencing of the p53 gene provides prognostic information in breast cancer patients, particularly in relation to adjuvant systemic therapy and radiotherapy. *Nature Med.* **1**: 1029–1034.

135. Borresen, A.-L., T. I. Andersen, J. E. Eyfjord, R. S. Cornelis, S. Thorlacius, A. Borg, U. Johansson, C. Theillet, S. Scherneck, S. Hartman, C. J. Cornelisse, E. Hovig, and P. Devilee. 1995. TP53 mutations and breast cancer prognosis: particularly poor survival rates for cases with mutations in the zinc-binding domains. *Genes Chromosom. Cancer* **14**: 71–75.

136. Clahsen, P. C., C. J. H. van de Velde, C. Duval, C. Pallud, A.-M. Mandard, A. Delobelle-Deroide, L. van den Broek, T. M. Sahmoud, and M. J. van de Vijver. 1998. p53 protein

accumulation and response to adjuvant chemotherapy in premenopausal women with node-negative early breast cancer. *J. Clin. Oncol.* **16:** 470–479.

137. Elledge, R. M., R. Gray, E. Mansour, Y. Yu, G. M. Clark, P. Ravdin, C. K. Osborne, K. Gilchrist, N. E. Davidson, N. Robert, D. C. Tormey, and D. C. Allred. 1995. Accumulation of p53 protein as a possible predictor of response to adjuvant combination chemotherapy with cyclophosphamide, methotrexate, fluorouracil, and prednisone for breast cancer. *J. Natl. Cancer Inst.* **87:** 1254–1256.

138. Aas, T., A.-L. Borresen, S. Geisler, B. Smith-Sorensen, H. Johnsen, J. E. Varhaug, L. A. Akslen, and P. E. Lonning. 1996. Specific P53 mutations are associated with de novo resistance to doxorubicin in breast cancer patients. *Nature Med.* **2:** 811–814.

139. Makris, A., T. J. Powles, M. Dowsett, and D. C. Allred. 1995. p53 protein overexpression and chemosensitivity in breast cancer (letter). *Lancet* **345:** 1181–1182.

140. Mathieu, M.-C., S. Koscielny, M.-L. Le Bihan, M. Spielmann, and R. Arriagada. 1995. p53 protein overexpression and chemosensitivity in breast cancer (letter). *Lancet* **345:** 1182.

141. Elledge, R. M., S. Green, L. Howes, G. M. Clark, M. Berardo, D. C. Allred, R. Pugh, D. Ciocca, P. Ravdin, J. O'Sullivan, S. Rivkin, S. Martino, and C. K. Osborne. 1997. bcl-2, p53, and response to tamoxifen in estrogen receptor-positive metastatic breast cancer: A Southwest Oncology Group study. *J. Clin. Oncol.* **15:** 1916–1922.

142. Silvestrini, R., E. Benini, S. Veneroni, M. G. Daidone, G. Tomasic, P. Squicciarini, and B. Salvadori. 1996. p53 and bcl-2 Expression correlates with clinical outcome in a series of node-positive breast cancer patients. *J. Clin. Oncol.* **14:** 1604–1610.

142a. Berns, E. M. J. J., J. G. M. Klijn, W. L. J. van Putten, H. H. de Witte, M. P. Look, M. E. Meijer-van Gelder, K. Wilman, H. Portengen, T. J. Benraad, and J. A. Foelkens. 1998. p53 protein accumulation predicts poor response to tamoxifen therapy of patients with recurrent breast cancer. *J. Clin. Oncol.* **16:** 121–127.

143. Jansson, T., M. Inganas, S. Sjögren, T. Norberg, A. Lindgren, L. Holmberg, and J. Bergh. 1995. p53 status predicts survival in breast cancer patients treated with or without postoperative radiotherapy: a novel hypothesis based on clinical findings. *J. Clin. Oncol.* **13:** 2745–2751.

144. Silvestrini, R., S. Veneroni, E. Benini, M. G. Daidone, A. Luisi, M. Leutner, A. Maucione, R. Kenda, R. Zucali, and U. Veronesi. 1997. Expression of p53, glutathione S-transferase, and Bcl-2 proteins and benefit from adjuvant radiotherapy in breast cancer. *JNCI* **89:** 639–645.

145. Aaltonen, L. A., P. Peltomaki, F. S. Leach, P. Sistonen, L. Pylkkanen, J. P. Mecklin, H. Jarvinen, S. M. Powell, J. Jen, S. R. Hamilton, G. M. Petersen, K. W. Kinsler, B. Vogelstein, and A. de la Chapelle. 1993. Clues to the pathogenesis of familial colorectal cancer. *Science* **260:** 812–816.

146. Thibodeau, S. N., G. Bren, D. Schaid. 1993. Microsatellite instability in cancer of the proximal colon. *Science* **269:** 816–819.

147. Ionov, Y., M. A. Peinado, S. Malkhosyan, D. Shibata, and M. Perucho. 1993. Ubiquitous somatic mutations in simple repeated sequences reveal a new mechanism for colonic carcinogenesis. *Nature* **363:** 558–561.

148. Fishel, R., M. K. Lescoe, M. R. S. Rao, N. G. Copeland, N. A. Jenkins, J. Garber, M. Kane, and R. Kolodner. 1993. The human mutator homolog MSH2 and its association with hereditary nonpolyposis colon cancer. *Cell* **75:** 1027–1038.

149. Leach, F. S., N. C. Nicolaides, N. Papadopoulos, B. Liu, J. Jen, R. Parsons, P. Peltomaki, P. Sistonen, L. A. Aaltonen, M. Nystrom-Lahti, X. Y. Guan, J. Zhang, P. S. Meltzer, J. W. Yu, F. T. Kao, D. J. Chen, K. M. Cerosaletti, R. E. K. Fournier, S. Todd, T. Lewis, R. J. Leach, S. L. Naylor, J. Weissenbach, J. P. Mecklin, H. Jarvinen, G. M. Petersen, S. R. Hamilton, J. Green, J. Jass, P. Watson, H. T. Lynch, J. M. Trent, A. de la Chapelle, K. W.

Kinsler, and B. Vogelstein. 1993. Mutations in a MutS homolog in hereditary non-polyposis colorectal cancer. *Cell* **75**: 1215–1225.

150. Paulson, T. G., F. A. Wright, B. A. Parker, V. Russack, and G. M. Wahl. 1996. Microsatellite instability correlates with reduced survival and poor disease prognosis in breast cancer. *Cancer Res.* **56**: 4021–4026.

150a. Kasami, M., C. L. Vnencak-Jones, S. Manning, W. D. Dupont, and D. L. Page. 1997. Loss of heterozygosity and microsatellite instability in breast hyperplasia. No obligate correlation of these genetic alterations with subsequent malignancy. *Am. J. Pathol.* **150**: 1925–1932.

151. Yee, C. J., N. Roodi, C. S. Verrier, and F. F. Parl. 1994. Microsatellite instability and loss of heterozygosity in breast cancer. *Cancer Res.* **54**: 1641–1644.

152. Sakurada, A., A. Suzuki, M. Sato, H. Yamakawa, K. Orikasa, S. Uyeno, T. Ono, N. Ohuchi, S. Fujimura, and A. Horii. 1997. Infrequent genetic alterations of the PTEN/MMAC1 gene in Japanese patients with primary cancers of the breast, lung, pancreas, kidney, and ovary. *Jpn. J. Cancer Res.* **88**: 1025–1028.

153. Rhei, E., L. Kang, F. Bogomolniy, M. G. Federici, P. I. Borgen, and J. Boyd. 1997. Mutation analysis of the putative tumor suppressor gene PTEN/MMAC1 in primary breast carcinomas. *Cancer Res.* **57**: 3657–3659.

154. Steck, P. A., M. A. Pershouse, S. A. Jasser, W. K. A. Yung, H. Lin, A. H. Ligon, L. A. Langford, M. L. Baumgard, T. Hattier, T. Davis, C. Frye, R. Hu, B. Swedlund, D. H. F. Teng, and S. V. Tavtigian. 1997. Identification of a candidate tumour suppressor gene, MMAC1, at chromosome 10q23. 3 that is mutated in multiple advanced cancers. *Nature Genet.* **5**: 356–362.

155. Thompson, M. E., R. A. Jensen, P. S. Obermiller, D. L. Page, and J. T. Holt. 1995. Decreased expression of BRCA–1 accelerates growth and is often present during sporadic breast cancer progression. *Nature Genet.* **9**: 444–450.

156. Jenne, D. E., H. Reimann, J. Nezu, W. Friedel, S. Loff, R. Jeschke, O. Muller, W. Back, and M. Zimmer. 1998. Peutz-Jeghers syndrome is caused by mutations in a novel serine threonine kinase. *Nature Genet.* **18**: 38–43.

157. Baselga, J., D. Tripathy, J. Mendelsohn, S. Baughman, C. C. Benz, L. Dantis, N. T. Sklarin, A. D. Seidman, C. A. Hudis, J. Moore, P. P. Rosen, T. Twaddell, I. C. Henderson, and L. Norton. 1996. Phase II study of weekly intravenous recombinant humanized anti-p185HER2 monoclonal antibody in patients with HER2/neu-overexpressing metastatic breast cancer. *J. Clin. Oncol.* **14**: 737–744.

158. Pegram, M. A., A. Lipton, R. Pietras, D. Hayes, B. Weber, J. Baselga, D. Tripathy, T. Twaddell, J. Glaspy, and D. Slamon. 1995. Phase II study of intravenous recombinant humanized anti-p185HER-2 monoclonal antibody (rhuMAb HER-2) plus cisplatinum in patients with HER-2/neu overexpressing metastatic breast cancer. Proc. Am. Soc. Clin. Oncol. **14**: 106 (Abstract #124).

159. Seth, P., D. Katayose, Z. Lim, M. Kim, R. Wersto, C. Craig, N. Shanmugam, E. Ohri, B. Mudahar, A. N. Rakkar, P. Kodali, and K. Cowan. 1997. A recombinant adenovirus expressing wild type p53 induces apoptosis in drug-resistant human breast cancer cells: a gene therapy approach for drug-resistant cancers. *Cancer Gene Ther.* **4**: 383–390.

160. Nielsen, L. L., J. Dell, E. Maxwell, L. Armstrong, D. Maneval, and J. J. Catino. 1997. Efficacy of p53 adenovirus-mediated gene therapy against human breast cancer xenografts. *Cancer Gene Ther.* **4**: 129–138.

161. Holt, J. T., M. E. Thompson, C. Szabo, C. Robinson-Benion, C.-L. Arteaga, M.-C. King, and R. A. Jensen. 1996. Growth retardation and tumor inhibition by BRCA1. *Nat. Genet.* **12**: 298–302.

162. Tait, D. L., P. S. Obermiller, S. Redlin-Frazier, R. A. Jensen, P. Welcsh, J. Dann, M.-C. King, D. H. Johnson, and J. T. Holt. 1997. A phase I trial of retroviral BRCA1sv gene therapy in ovarian cancer. *Clin. Cancer Res.* **3**: 1959–1968.

7

Apoptosis and the Development of Breast Cancer

Priscilla A. Furth

1. INTRODUCTION

Each year there are more than 180,000 new cases of breast cancer diagnosed in the United States alone. One out of eight American women will experience breast cancer during their lifetime. These numbers alone compel society towards developing a scientific understanding of the pathophysiology of this disease. Research efforts over several decades have determined that both hormonal influences and specific genetic events cooperate in the development of breast cancer. This chapter will focus on the hormonal and genetic factors that regulate apoptosis in the normal mammary gland and in breast cancers.

1.1. Apoptosis and Cell Death

Apoptosis is a genetically regulated process of cell death (1). It was originally recognized as a defined cellular morphology found in regressing tissues such as the mammary gland during involution, the uterus during menses, or the prostate after withdrawal of male hormones (2). Cells which are undergoing apoptosis in these tissues can exhibit shrunken pyknotic nuclei as well as other characteristic changes (3). Molecular analyses of these regressing tissues can demonstrate characteristic nucleosome-sized cleavage patterns of cellular DNA and activation of specific 'death-inducing' cellular genes and their protein products (4). Activation of the cell cycle plays a significant role in the regulation of apoptosis (5). In some cell types and under certain conditions, apoptosis can be shown to occur only at specific stages in the cell cycle (6). Apoptosis is not the only type of cell death. For example, cells can also die through necrosis (9). However, for those persons developing new approaches for the treatment of breast cancer, apoptosis is a particularly attractive target for intervention (8). Because it is a genetically regulated process, it is theoretically possible to specifically activate it in breast-cancer cells, given a sufficient understanding of the molecular processes that control its execution.

1.2. Genetic and Hormonal Factors Regulating Apoptosis
of Mammary Epithelial Cells

Apoptosis is an integral part of the development of all organisms (3). As each organ develops, it is modeled into a finished product through a coordinated process of cellular

From: Breast Cancer: Molecular Genetics, Pathogenesis, and Therapeutics
Edited by: A. M. Bowcock © Humana Press Inc., Totowa, NJ

proliferation, migration, and death. For many tissues, this procedure is primarily embryonic; in other words, it is essentially finished by the time the organism is ready to live in an outside environment. However, the mammary gland is one of the few organs that undergoes most of its development in the mature organism. Even more importantly for students of apoptosis, the mammary gland undergoes sequential waves of apoptosis during development and involution beginning with each pregnancy and ending with each weaning.

Apoptosis features in the development of breast cancer *(9,10)*. The degree of apoptosis can be an important factor in both progression of breast cancer and its response to treatment *(11–13)*.

Researchers have looked to both the normal mammary gland and breast tumors to identify specific hormonal and molecular factors controlling apoptosis of mammary epithelial cells. Animal models have been used to monitor expression patterns of specific gene products and to make dominant-gain experiments and gene-deletion experiments to define the contributions of specific gene products on induction of apoptosis. These models have also been used to examine the effect of chemotherapeutic agents on apoptosis frequency and its activation. Studies of human breast-cancer samples have been used to define the expression patterns of apoptotic-pathway genes in different tumor types. Cell lines generated from human tumors have been used to define the specific apoptotic pathways utilized.

For the most part, breast-cancer researchers have looked to see how known apoptotic-pathway genes play out their roles under the different physiological conditions in which normal or malignant mammary epithelial cells are found. A few studies have focused on using apoptotic mammary epithelial cells to try to identify novel genes that contribute to induction of apoptosis *(11)*.

2. APOPTOSIS DURING NORMAL BREAST DEVELOPMENT AND PHYSIOLOGY

2.1. Hormones, Signaling Molecules, and Genes Regulating Apoptosis in the Normal Mammary Gland

There are both hormonal and nonhormonal factors which regulate apoptosis of mammary epithelial cells. Hormonal regulation of apoptosis of normal mammary epithelial cells has been well-recognized for decades. Mammary-gland involution following weaning results from withdrawal of lactogenic hormones and apoptosis of mammary epithelial cells is an inherent part of this involution *(14)*. However, more recent studies have determined that apoptosis of mammary epithelial cells can also be regulated by hormone-independent mechanisms. Some of the same downstream gene products participate in the regulation of both hormonally and nonhormonally induced apoptosis.

Hormonal factors and signaling molecules that have been implicated in the control of apoptosis in the mammary gland include the developmentally important hormones estrogen and progesterone as well as the lactogenic hormones glucocorticoid and prolactin *(15–17)*. Signaling molecules which appear to play a role in vivo include insulin-like growth factor (IGF)-1 and the IGF-related binding protein *(18)* (reviewed in Chapter 5). Fas and Fas ligand are expressed in both normal and malignant mammary epithelial cells in culture but their role in vivo has not been well established *(19,20)*.

Several members of the bcl-2 gene family such as bcl-2, bax, bcl-x, bad, and bak are expressed in the mammary gland and exhibit distinct changes in their expression pattern through development, lactation, and involution *(21–24)*. Up-regulation of bax expression is temporally correlated with induction of apoptosis at several different timepoints *(21–23,25)*. Developmental studies have demonstrated that p53 is not required for apoptosis of mammary epithelial cells during normal development or involution *(22,23)*.

2.2. Development of the Mammary Gland

Development of the mammary gland has been well-studied in rodent models. These studies serve as general models for development in other species including humans. In the mouse, a rudimentary ductal structure develops within the mammary-gland fat pad as the virgin mouse becomes sexually mature. This remodeling process includes both cell proliferation and apoptosis. Ductal development proceeds through a coordinated process of proliferation at the end bud and cellular apoptosis within the duct to create a lumen. Apoptosis within the duct follows up-regulation of bax expression and does not require the presence of p53 *(22)*.

Maturation of the ductal structure during early pregnancy is associated with expression of the survival inducer bcl-2 in ductal epithelial cells *(26)*. However, bcl-2 expression is down-regulated in the latter half of pregnancy as ductal development is completed. Development of lobulo-alveolar structures dominates the second half of pregnancy. Bcl-2 is not expressed but bcl-x_{long}, bcl-x_{short}, and bax are present *(25)*. The apoptotic index is low, averaging .2%. Even fewer apoptotic cells are found during lactation *(21)*.

2.3. Mammary-Gland Involution

Withdrawal of suckling leads to mammary-gland involution and the induction of apoptosis in mammary epithelial cells *(14)*. Local factors induce apoptosis during the first stage of involution *(16)*. This first stage of involution is reversible when suckling is restored. There is little tissue remodeling. Alveolar structures are maintained even as individual cells undergo apoptosis. It is independent from changes in systemic hormone levels and does not require the presence of p53 *(23)*. Apoptotic cells begin to appear within 24–48 h of the end of suckling as cells enter into the cell cycle *(27,28)*. Increased levels of bax RNA and protein can be found coincident with the appearance of apoptosis. There is a relative increase in expression of the death inducing gene bcl-x_{short} as compared to bcl-x_{long} *(16,21,23,25)*. Changes in the activation patterns of Stat signaling proteins are seen during the first stage of involution *(16,27)*.

The second stage of involution is very different. It is under hormonal control and the entire gland is remodeled as proteinases are activated by withdrawal of the lactogenic hormones glucocorticoid and prolactin *(17,30)*. Apoptotic cells continue to appear as the connective tissue and basement membrane is disrupted. Apoptosis during this stage appears to be primarily regulated by loss of contact with the extracellular matrix *(31)*.

2.4. Estrous Cycle

In the mature organism, mammary epithelial cells also exhibit a cyclical pattern of proliferation and apoptosis with each estrous cycle *(32)*. Apoptotic cell death follows each estrus. Although the downstream genes regulating induction of apoptosis on hormone withdrawal at the end of estrus have not yet been defined, it is likely that at least some of the genes regulating apoptosis during development and involution are involved.

3. APOPTOSIS AND BREAST CANCER

3.1. Apoptosis, Proliferation, and the Extracellular Matrix

Apoptosis can regulate both progression of human breast cancer *(33)* and its response to treatment. However, the effect of changing apoptotic frequency in any individual tumor must be measured against the proliferative capacity of the cells within the tumor. Tumors that have a high apoptotic index but are also highly proliferative can still progress rapidly *(11)*. The most effective treatment regimens for breast cancers will try to both induce apoptosis and reduce proliferation.

From this point of view, it is useful to look at mammary gland involution as a model for understanding what an effective breast-cancer treatment must do. During mammary-gland involution, not only do cells undergo apoptosis but the proliferative capacity of the gland is destroyed by the tissue remodeling process. Individual cells lose the extracellular matrix that they require for survival. The question to determine is how to apply such a combined approach to breast cancers. Critical questions include understanding how apoptosis is controlled in tumor cells, how to effect dissolution of the extracellular matrix in a tumor, and to determine how loss of the cell matrix affects survival of a breast-cancer cell *(24)*.

3.2. Regulation of Apoptosis in Breast-Cancer Cell Lines

One approach to understanding how apoptosis is regulated in breast cancers is to examine specific mechanisms in tissue-culture cell lines prepared from breast cancers *(8)*. Studies in such cell lines have revealed a number of potential mechanisms for regulating apoptosis in breast-cancer cells.

A few common themes have emerged from this research. One is that withdrawal or administration of hormones and specific growth factors can induce apoptosis in certain cell types dependent upon the presence or absence of specific receptors for these growth receptors on the cell membrane *(35–38)*.

A second theme revolves around bcl-2 and $bcl-x_{long}$, inducers of cell survival, and their associated family members bax and $bcl-x_{short}$, cell death inducers. Both bcl-2 and $bcl-x_{long}$ can form heterodimers with bax. Although the specific molecular action of these specific proteins in apoptosis remains ill-defined *(38)*, it has been postulated that relative levels of the survival inducers as compared to death inducers regulate the propensity of a cell to undergo apoptosis *(40)*. Breast cancer cell lines have been used to demonstrate experimentally that increased levels of bax protein are associated with increased apoptosis *(41–43)* and a delay in tumor progression *(44)*. Increasing levels of $bcl-x_{short}$ can sensitize cells to chemotherapy *(45)*. Similarly, increased levels of apoptosis are also found when expression levels of bcl-2 are reduced *(46–49)*. Increased levels of either bcl-2 or $bcl-x_{long}$ can protect cells from apoptosis *(50)*.

One of the experimental approaches is to use specific chemical inducers of apoptosis to identify molecular pathways that induce apoptosis in breast-cancer cell lines *(51–54)*. Regulation of protein phosphorylation has emerged as a possible mediator of apoptosis *(52,53)*.

Fourth, breast-cancer cell lines have been used to investigate the potential of specific chemotherapeutic agents for inducing apoptosis *(55,56)*. Effects of individual growth factors on response to chemotherapy can be tested; for example, IGF-1 can alter the response to chemotherapy by inhibiting the apoptotic response to specific chemotherapeutics *(57)*.

Finally, the different effects of p53 mutation have been investigated in tissue-culture cell lines *(58,59)*. Mutation of the p53 gene is seen in a proportion of human breast cancers *(60,61)*. In tissue-culture cell lines, p53 deficiency is associated with resistance to apoptosis *(62)*; however, p53 is not required for apoptosis in normal mammary epithelial cells *(23)* and absence of p53 in animal models does not accelerate progression of breast cancer by altering the percentage of apoptotic cells *(12,63,64,)*.

3.3. The Role of Apoptosis During Progression of Breast Cancer in Animal Models

Animal models have been used to investigate specific contributions of apoptosis to breast-cancer progression. The relative role of apoptosis as compared to proliferation was examined in myc- and ras-induced tumors in transgenic mice *(11)*. These studies clearly demonstrate that tumor progression is dependent on both apoptosis and proliferation. Neither factor alone can be used to predict tumor growth. In our laboratory we have examined the power of bcl-2-induced apoptosis resistance to accelerate breast-tumor progression. Inhibition of apoptosis by 50% shortened tumor latency by 25% *(73)*.

The contribution of p53 deficiency to apoptosis during breast-cancer progression has been tested in transgenic mouse models *(12,63,64)*. The absence of p53 did not reduce the incidence of apoptosis during tumor progression although it did appear to increase genomic instability. Accelerated tumor progression was observed in Wnt-1 transgenic mice in the absence of p53 even though the apoptotic index was unchanged. p53 deficiency accelerated the appearance of salivary-gland tumors and T-cell lymphomas in MMTV-*ras* *(17)* and MMTV-myc transgenic mice *(64)*, respectively. Expression of a mutant p53 can also accelerate tumorigenesis *(65,66)* but, at least in one model, did so without decreasing apoptotic incidence *(66)*. These results are consistent with the observation that p53-independent, rather than p53-dependent, apoptosis plays the major role in the breast, both in normal development and in malignancy. Deficiency or mutation of p53 can contribute to tumor progression but may not do so through modifying the apoptotic response.

3.4. Human Breast Cancers and Expression of Apoptosis Pathway Genes

Human breast cancer specimens have been used to investigate the relative expression levels of bcl-2, and bax, and to investigate the incidence of mutations in other cellular genes including the p53 gene. A number of studies have found bcl-2 overexpression and associated it with a good prognosis *(67,68)*. In contrast, low levels of bax expression have been associated with a poor clinical outcome *(44,69)*. Further investigation will be required to determine if the associated clinical out comes are directly related to the amount of apoptosis or some other property of these multifunctional proteins *(39)*. Mutation of the p53 gene is found in a subset of human breast cancers *(60,70)*. However, because it also can direct a diverse number of cellular functions *(61,71)*, it is not clear if p53 mutations promote tumor progression through changes in apoptotic frequency *(72)* or some other pathway. As previously outlined, animal studies suggests that p53 mutation leads to genomic instability but does not directly affect the degree of apoptosis.

4. CONCLUDING REMARKS

Apoptosis plays an essential role in normal development and physiology in the breast. Breast-cancer progression is accelerated by reducing the level of apoptosis. Treatment of breast cancer is improved by increasing the percentage of cells undergoing apoptosis. Research into the mechanisms that regulate apoptosis during mammary-gland involution may provide insight for improving current approaches to breast-cancer treatment. Studies in human tissue-culture cell lines and tumors are used to define specific molecular lesions that impact on the propensity of a cell to undergo apoptosis. These molecular lesions are introduced into animal models and their effect on apoptosis during cancer development and treatment tested. Finally, conversion of these results into new treatment regimens for clinical practice will determine how well an improved understanding of apoptotic mechanisms translates into more effective therapies for breast cancer.

ACKNOWLEDGMENTS

This work was supported in part by NIH grants CA70545 and CA68033.

REFERENCES

1. Bellamy, C. O., R. D. Malcolmsom, D. J. Harrison, and A. H. Wyllie. 1995. Cell death in health and disease: the biology and regulation of apoptosis. *Semin. Cancer Biol.* **6:** 3–16.
2. Tenniswood, M. P., R. S. Guenette, J. Lakins, M. Mooibroek, P. Wong, and J.-E. Welsh. 1992. Active cell death in hormone-dependent tissues. *Cancer Metastasis Rev.* **11:** 197–220.
3. Jacobson, M. D., M. Weil, and M. C. Raff. 1997. Programmed cell death in animal development. *Cell* **88:** 347–354.
4. Nagata, S. 1997. Apoptosis by death factor. *Cell* **88:** 355–365.
5. Hunter, T. 1997. Oncoprotein Networks. *Cell* **88:** 333–346.
6. Levine, A. 1997. p53, the cellular gatekeeper for growth and division. *Cell* **88:** 323–331.
7. Columbano, A. 1995. Cell death: current difficulties in discriminating apoptosis from necrosis in the context of pathological processes in vivo. *J. Cell. Biochem.* **58:** 181–190.
8. McCloskey, D. E., D. K. Armstrong, C. Jackisch, and N. E. Davidson. 1996. Programmed cell death in human breast-cancer cells. *Recent Prog. Horm. Res.* **51:** 493–508.
9. Schedin, P. J., L. B. Thackray, P. Malone, S. C. Fontaine, R. R. Friis, and R. Strange. 1996. Programmed cell death and mammary neoplasia. *Cancer Treat. Res.* **83:** 3–22.
10. Wu, J. 1996. Apoptosis and angiogenesis: two promising tumor markers in breast cancer. *Anticancer Res.* **16:** 2233–2239.
11. Hundley, J. E., S. K. Koester, D. A. Troyer, S. G. Hilsenbeck, R. E. Barrington, and J. J. Windle. 1997. Differential regulation of cell cycle characteristics and apoptosis in MMTV-myc and MMTV-ras mouse mammary tumors. *Cancer Res.* **57:** 600–603.
12. Hundley, J. E., S. K. Kotster, D. A. Troyer, S. G. Hilsenbeck, M. A. Subler, and J. J. Windle. 1997. Increased tumor proliferation and genomic instability without decreased apoptosis in MMTV-*ras* mice deficient in p53. *Mol. Cell. Biol.* **17:** 723–731.

13. Muschel, R. J. and W. G. McKenna. 1996. Alterations in cell cycle control during tumor progression: effects on apoptosis and the response to therapeutic agents. *Curr. Topics Microbiol. Immunol.* **213**: 197–213.
14. Furth, P. A., U. Bar-Peled, and M. Li. 1997. *Apoptosis* and mammary gland involution: reviewing the process. *Apoptosis* **2**: 19–24.
15. Feng, Z., A. Marti, B. Jehn, H. J. Altermatt, G. Chicaiza, and R. Jaggi. 1995. Glucocorticoid and progesterone inhibit involution and programmed cell death in the mouse mammary gland. *J. Cell Biol.* **131**: 1095–1103.
16. Li, M., X. Liu, G. Robinson, U. Bar-Peled, K. -U. Wagner, W. S. Young, E. Ginns, L. Hennighausen, and P. A. Furth. 1997. Mammary derived signals activate programmed cell death during the first stage of mammary gland involution. *Proc. Natl. Acad. Sci. USA* **94**: 3425–3430.
17. Lund, L. R., J. Romer, N. Dohy-Thomasset, H. Solberg, C. Pyke, M. J. Bissell, K. Dano, and Z. Werb. 1996. Two distinct phases of apoptosis in mammary gland involution: proteinase-independent and -dependent pathways. *Development* **122**: 181–193.
18. Neuenschwander, S., A. Schwartz, T. L. Wood, C. T. Jr. Roberts, L. Hennighausen, and D. LeRoith. 1996. Involution of the lactating mammary gland is inhibited by the IGF system in a transgenic mouse model. *J. Clin. Invest.* **97**: 2225–2232.
19. Jaattela, M., M. Benedict, M. Tewarui, J. A. Shayman, and V. M. Dixit. 1995. Bcl-x and bcl-2 inhibit TNF and Fas-induced apoptosis and activation of phospholipase A2 in breast carcinoma cells. *Oncogene* **10**: 2297–2305.
20. Keane, M. M., S. A. Ettenberg, G. A. Lowrey, E. K. Russell, and S. Lipkowitz. 1996. Fas expression and function in normal and malignant breast cell lines. *Cancer Res.* **56**: 4791–4798.
21. Heermeier, K., M. Benedict, M. Li, G. Nunez, P. A. Furth, and L. Hennighausen. 1996. Bax and bcl-x$_s$ are induced at the onset of mammary gland involution. *Mech. Devel.* **56**: 197–207.
22. Humphreys, R. C., M. Krajewska, S. Krnacik, R. Jaeger, H. Weiher, S. Krajewski, J. C. Reed, and J. M. Rosen. 1996. Apoptosis in the terminal endbud of the murine mammary gland: a mechanism of ductal morphogenesis. *Development* **122**: 4013–4022.
23. Li, M., J. Hu, K. Heermeier, L. Hennighausen, and P. A. Furth. 1996. *Apoptosis* and remodeling of mammary gland tissue during involution proceeds through p53 independent pathways. *Cell Growth Diff.* **7**: 13–20.
24. Reed, J. C. 1996. Balancing cell life and death: bax, apoptosis, and breast *Cancer. J. Clin. Invest.* **97**: 2403–2404.
25. Li, M., J. Hu, K. Heermeier, L. Hennighausen, and P. A. Furth. 1996. Expression of a viral oncoprotein during development of the mammary gland alters cell fate and function: induction of p53 independent apoptosis is followed by impairment of milk protein production in surviving cells. *Cell Growth Diff.* **7**: 3–11.
26. Pullan, S., J. Wilson, A. Metcalfe, G. Edwards, N. Goberdhan, J. Tilly, J. A. Hickman, C. Dive, and C. H. Streuli. 1996. Requirement of basement membrane for the suppression of programmed cell death in mammary epithelium. *J. Cell Science* **109**: 631–642.
27. Marti, A., Z. Feng, B. Jehn, V. Djonov, G. Chicaiza, H. J. Altermatt, and R. Jaggi. 1995. Expression and activity of cell cycle regulators during proliferation and programmed cell death in the mammary gland. *Cell Death Diff.* **2**: 277–283.
28. Marti, A., B. Jehn, E. Costello, N. Keon, G. Ke, F. Martin, and R. Jaggi. 1994. Protein kinase A and AP-1 (c-Fos/JunD) are induced during apoptosis of mouse mammary epithelial cells. *Oncogene* **9**: 1213–1223.
29. Philp, J. A., T. G. Burdon, and C. J. Watson. 1996. Differential activation of Stats 3 and 5 during mammary gland development. *FEBS Lett.* **396**: 77–80.
30. Travers, M. T., M. C. Barber, E. Tonner, L. Quarrie, C. J. Wilde, and D. J. Flint. 1996. The role of prolactin and growth hormone in the regulation of casein gene expression and

mammary cell survival: relationships to milk synthesis and secretion. *Endocrinology* **137:** 1530–1539.

31. Boudreau, N., C. J. Sympson, Z. Werb, and M. J. Bissell. 1995. Suppression of ICE and apoptosis in mammary epithelial cells by extracellular matrix. *Science* **267:** 891–893.

32. Ferguson, D. J. and T. J. Anderson. 1981. Morphological evaluation of cell turnover in relation to the menstrual cycle in the resting human breast. *Br. J. Cancer* **44:** 177–181.

33. Bodis, S., K. P. Siziopikou, S. J. Schnitt, J. R. Harris, and D. E. Fisher. 1996. Extensive apoptosis in ductal carcinoma in situ of the breast. *Cancer* **77:** 1831–1835.

34. Howlett, A. R., N. Bailey, C. Damsky, O. W. Petersen, and M. Bissell. 1995. Cellular growth and survival are mediated by beta 1 integrins in normal human breast epithelium but not in breast carcinoma. *J. Cell Science* **108:** 1945–1947.

35. Armstrong, D. K., S. H. Kaufmann, Y. L. Ottaviano, Y. Furuya, J. A. Buckley, J. T. Isaacs, and N. E. Davidson. 1994. Epidermal growth factor-mediated apoptosis of MDA-MB-468 human breast cancer cells. *Cancer Res.* **54:** 5280–5283.

36. Simboli-Campbell, M., C. J. Narvaez, M. Tenniswood, and J. Welsh. 1996. 1,25-Dihydroxyvitamin D3 induces morphological and biochemical markers of apoptosis in MCF-7 breast-cancer cells. *J. Steroid Biochem. Mol. Biol.* **58:** 367–376.

37. Wilson, J. W., A. E. Wakeling, I. D. Morris, J. A. Hickman, and C. Dive. 1995. MCF-7 human mammary adenocarcinoma cell death in vitro in response to hormone-withdrawal and DNA damage. *Intl. J. Cancer* **61:** 502–508.

38. Zhang, X. 1996. Retinoic acid receptor beta mediates the growth-inhibitory effect of retinoic acid by promoting apoptosis in human breast cancer cells. *Mol. Cell. Biol.* **16:** 1138–1149.

39. Reed, J. 1997. Double identity for proteins of the bcl-2 family. *Nature* **387:** 773–776.

40. Korsmeyer, S. J., J. R. Shutter, D. J. Veis, D. E. Merry, and Z. N. Oltvai. 1993. Bcl-2/Bax: a rheostat that regulates an antioxidant pathway and cell death. *Semin. Cancer Biol.* **4:** 327–332.

41. Sakakura, C., E. A. Sweeney, T. Shirahama, Y. Igarashi, S. Hakomori, T. Mishi, M. Ohgaki, T. Ohyama, J. Yamazaki, A. Hagiwara, T. Yamaguchi, K. Sawai, and T. Takahashi. 1996. Overexpression of bax sensitizes human breast cancer MCF-7 cells to radiation-induced apoptosis. *Intl. J. Cancer* **67:** 101–105.

42. Sheikh, M. S., M. Garcia, Q. Zhan, Y. Liu, and A. J. Fornace, Jr. 1996. Cell cycle-independent regulation of p21WAF1/Cip1 and retinoblastoma protein during okadaic acid-induced apoptosis is coupled with induction of Bax protein in human breast carcinoma cells. *Cell Growth Diff.* **7:** 1599–1607.

43. Wagener, C., R. C. Bargou, P. T. Daniel, K. Bommert, M. Y. Mapara, H. D. Royer, and B. Dorken. 1996. Induction of the death-promoting gene bax-α sensitizes cultured breast-cancer cells to drug induced apoptosis. *Intl. J. Cancer* **67:** 138–141.

44. Bargour, R. C., C. Wageneer, K. Bommert, M. Y. Mapara, P. T. Daniel, W. Arnold, M. Dietel, H. Guski, A. Feller, H. D. Royer, and B. Dyrken. 1996. Overexpression of the death-promoting gene bax-α which is downregulated in breast cancer restores sensitivity to different apoptotic stimuli and reduces tumor growth in SCID mice. *J. Clin. Invest.* **97:** 2651–2670.

45. Sumantran, V. N., M. W. Ealovega, G. Nunez, M. F. Clarke, and M. S. Wicha. 1995. Overexpression of Bcl-xS sensitizes MCF-7 cells to chemotherapy-induced apoptosis. *Cancer Res.* **55:** 2507–2510.

46. Adam, L., M. Crepin, and L. Israel. 1997. Tumor growth inhibition, apoptosis, and bcl-2 down-regulation of MCF-7*ras* tumors by sodium phenylacetate and tamoxifen combination. *Cancer Res.* **57:** 1023–1029.

47. Huang, Y., S. Ray, J. C. Reed, A. M. Ibrado, C. Tang, A. Nawabi, and K. Bhalla. 1997. Estrogen increases intracellular p26Bcl-2 to p21Bax ratios and inhibits taxol-induced apoptosis of human breast cancer MCF-7 cells. Breast *Cancer Res. Treatment* **42:** 73–81.

48. Mandal, M. and R. Kumar. 1996. Bcl-2 expression regulates sodium butyrate-induced apoptosis in human MCF-7 breast-cancer cells. *Cell Growth Diff.* **7**: 311–318.

49. Teixeira, C., J. C. Reed, and M. A. Pratt. 1995. Estrogen promotes chemotherapeutic drug resistance by a mechanism involving Bcl-2 proto-oncogene expression in human breast-cancer cells. *Cancer Res.* **55**: 3902–3907.

50. Schott, A. F., I. J. Apel, G. Nunez, and M. F. Clarke. 1995. Bcl-xL protects cancer cells from p53-mediated apoptosis. *Oncogene* **11**: 1389–1394.

51. Boe, R., B. T. Gjertsen, S. O. Doskeland, and O. K. Vintermyr. 1995. 8-Chloro-cAMP induces apoptotic cell death in a human mammary carcinoma cell (MCF-7) line. *Br. J. Cancer* **72**: 1151–1159.

52. de Vente, J. E., C. A. Kukoly, W. O. Bryant, K. J. Posekany, J. Chen, D. J. Fletcher, P. J. Parker, G. J. Pettit, G. Lozano, and P. P. Cook. 1995. Phorbolesters induce death in MCF-7 breast-cancer cells with altered expression of protein kinase isoforms. Role for p53-independent induction of gadd–45 in initiating death. *J. Clin. Invest.* **96**: 1874–1886.

53. Kiguchi, K., D. Glesne, C. H. Chubb, H. Fujiki, and E. Huberman. 1994. Differential induction of apoptosis in human breast tumor cells by okadaic acid and related inhibitors of protein phosphatases 1 and 2A. *Cell Growth Diff.* **5**: 995–1004.

54. Lowe, S. W., H. E. Ruley, T. Jacks, and D. Housman. 1993. p53-dependent apoptosis modulates the cytotoxicity of anticancer agents. *Cell* **74**: 957–967.

55. Frankfurt, O. S., E. V. Sugarbaker, J. A. Robb, and L. Villa. 1995. Synergistic induction of apoptosis in breast-cancer cells by tamoxifen and calmodulin inhibitors. *Cancer Lett.* **97**: 149–154.

56. Wosikowski, K., J. T. Regis, R. W. Robey, M. Alvarez, J. T. Buters, J. M. Gudas, and S. E. Bates. 1995. Normal p53 status and function despite the development of drug resistance in human breast cancer cells. *Cell Growth Diff.* **6**: 1395–1403.

57. Dunn, S. E., R. A. Hardman, F. W. Kari, and J. C. Barrett. 1997. Insulin-like growth factor 1 (IGF-1) alters drug sensitivity of HBL100 breast cancer cells by inhibition of apoptosis induced by diverse anticancer drugs. *Cancer Res.* **57**: 2687–2693.

58. Runnebaum, I. B., J. -K. Yee, D. G. Kieback, S. Sukumar, and T. Friedmann. 1994. Wild-type p53 suppresses the malignant phenotype in breast-cancer cells containing mutant p53 alleles. *Anticancer Res.* **14**: 1137–1144.

59. Ryan, J. J., E. Prochownik, C. A. Gottlieb, I. J. Apel, R. Merino, G. Nuñez, and M. F. Clarke. 1994. c-*myc* and *bcl-2* modulate p53 function by altering p53 subcellular trafficking during the cell cycle. *Proc. Natl. Acad. Sci. USA* **91**: 5878–5882.

60. Hartmann, A., H. Blaszyk, J. S. Kovach, and S. S. Sommer. 1997. The molecular epidemiology of p53 gene mutations in human breast cancer. *Trends Genet.* **13**: 27–33.

61. Ozbun, M. A. and J. S. Butel. 1995. Tumor suppressor p53 mutations and breast cancer: a critical analysis. Advances in *Cancer Res.* **66**: 71–141.

62. Haldar, S., M. Negrini, M. Monne, S. Sabbioni, and C. M. Croce. 1994. Down-regulation of bcl-2 by p53 in breast-cancer cells. *Cancer Res.* **54**: 2095–2097s.

63. Donehower, L. A., L. A. Godley, C. M. Aldaz, R. Pyle, Y. P. Shi, D. Pinkel, J. Gray, A. Bradley, D. Medina, and H. E. Varmus. 1995. Deficiency of p53 accelerates mammary tumorigenesis in Wnt-1 transgenic mice and promotes chromosomal instability . *Genes Dev.* **9**: 882–895.

64. Elson, A., C. Deng, J. Campos-Torres, L. A. Donehower, and P. Leder. 1995. The MMTV/c-myc transgene and p53 alleles collaborate to induce T-cell lymphomas, but not mammary carcinomas in transgenic mice. Oncogene **11**: 181–190.

65. Harvey, M., H. Vogel, D. Morris, A. Bradley, A. Bernstein, and L. A. Donehower. 1995. A mutant p53 transgene accelerates tumour development in heterozygous but not nullizygous p53-deficient mice. *Nature Genet.* **9**: 305–311.

66. Li, B., J. M. Rosen, J. McMenamin-Balano, W. J. Muller, and A. S. Perkins. 1997. *neu*/ERRB2 cooperates with *p53–172H* during mammary tumorigenesis in transgenic mice. *Mol. Cell. Biol.* **17**: 3155–3163.

67. Lipponen, P., T. Pietilainen, V. M. Kosma, S. Aaltomaa, M. Eskelinen, and K. Syrjanen. 1995. *Apoptosis* suppressing protein bcl-2 is expressed in well-differentiated breast carcinomas with favourable prognosis. *J. Pathol.* **177:** 49–55.

68. Siziopikou, K. P., J. E. Prileau, J. R. Harris, and S. J. Schnitt. 1996. bcl-2 expression in the spectrum of preinvasive breast lesions. *Cancer* **77:** 499–506.

69. Krajewski, S., C. Blomquist, K. Franssila, M. Krajewska, V. M. Wasenius, E. Niskanen, S. Nordling, and J. C. Reed. 1995. Reduced expression of the proapoptotic gene BAX is associated with poor response rates to combination chemotherapy and shorter survival in women with metastatic breast adenocarcinoma. *Cancer Res.* **55:** 4471–4478.

70. Cunningham, J. M., J. N. Ingle, S. H. Jung, S. S. Cha, L. E. Wold, G. Farr, T. E. Witzig, J. E. Krook, H. S. Wieand, and J. S. Kovach. 1994. p53 gene expression in node-positive breast cancer: relationship to DNA ploidy and prognosis. *JNCI* **86:** 1871–1873.

71. Marx, J. 1994. New link found between *p53* and DNA repair. *Science* **266:** 1321–1322.

72. Lane, D. P., X. Lu, T. Hupp, and P. A. Hall. 1994. The role of the p53 protein in the apoptotic response. *Philos. Trans. R. Soc. Lond. [Biol.]* **345:** 277–280.

73. Bar-Peled, U., M. Li, R. Jaeger, L. Hennighausen, H. Weiher, and P. A. Furth. 1997. Bcl-2 mediated block of bax induced apoptosis accelerates breast tumorigenesis in vivo. Unpublished results.

8

WNT Genes and Breast Cancer

Ivan Bergstein and Anthony M.C. Brown

1. INTRODUCTION

The *Wnt* gene family is a large group of related genes encoding secreted proteins that function as extracellular signaling factors. At least 18 distinct *Wnt* genes have so far been described in mammals, and homologs have been isolated from a broad range of metazoan species from nematodes to humans. Both genetic analysis and experimental studies have shown that *Wnt* genes function in a variety of critical developmental processes and these data imply that Wnt signals have the potential to regulate several aspects of cell behavior, including cell proliferation, cell fate determination, and cell-cell adhesion (for reviews, *see* refs. *1* and *2*). While there has been enormous interest in *Wnt* genes because of their multiple roles in embryonic development, the original *Wnt* gene, mouse *Wnt1*, was discovered as an oncogene activated in mouse mammary carcinomas, and other members of the *Wnt* gene family are also strongly implicated in the genesis of such tumors *(3–5)*. There is now compelling evidence that Wnt proteins serve to regulate mammary development in the mouse, and it is likely that they fulfill a similar role in humans. Ever since the initial identification of *Wnt* genes as mammary oncogenes in the mouse, it has been a reasonable possibility that aberrant expression of *WNT* genes could contribute to human breast cancer. This idea has been strengthened by evidence that several human *WNT* genes are over-expressed in breast cancers, and by recent revelations that downstream components of the Wnt signaling pathway are activated in other forms of human cancer *(6,7)*. It is therefore timely to review the evidence linking *Wnt* genes to breast cancer, both in mouse model systems and in the human disease.

2. WNT PROTEINS AND THEIR SIGNALING PATHWAY

All the vertebrate Wnt proteins so far characterized have a remarkably similar overall structure. Each is 350–400 amino acids in length and has an amino-terminal secretory signal peptide and one or more N-linked glycosylation sites. The sequence identity between different Wnt proteins typically ranges from 35–95% and extends over approximately 300 amino acids, within which there are at least 22 cysteine residues whose relative spacing is highly conserved *(2)*. Sixteen different *Wnt* genes have so far been characterized from the mouse and 13 from humans *(1,8)*.

From: Breast Cancer: Molecular Genetics, Pathogenesis, and Therapeutics
Edited by: A. M. Bowcock © Humana Press Inc., Totowa, NJ

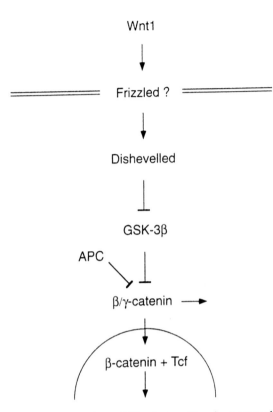

Fig. 1. Diagrammatic representation of Wnt1 signaling in mammalian cells. Outline of a composite pathway derived from studies of Wnt signaling in Drosophila, Xenopus, and mammalian cells. Seven-transmembrane proteins of the Frizzled family are candidate receptors for Wnt proteins. Signals transduced via Dishevelled result in inactivation of the kinase GSK-3 and consequent stabilization of β-catenin or γ-catenin. β-catenin can enter the nucleus and form complexes with Tcf DNA binding proteins that then regulate transcription. Note that stability of β-catenin is also regulated by the tumor suppressor gene product APC. Since catenins also function in adherens junctions, Wnt signals may also modulate cell-cell adhesion. *See text* and refs. *1* and *12* for details.

   Wnt proteins are secreted but have a propensity to associate with cell surfaces and extracellular matrix *(8a,8b)*. Soluble forms are present in low abundance, at least in cell culture, but the biological activity of these forms has demonstrated that Wnt proteins function as extracellular signals *(9–11)*. Information about intracellular Wnt signaling pathways has been derived from a wide variety of genetic and experimental systems, including *Drosophila, Xenopus, C. elegans,* and mammalian cells *(1)*. The apparent conservation of these pathways in evolution has allowed a generic Wnt1 pathway to be outlined that serves as a working model for current research in several systems (Fig. 1). The Frizzled family of seven-transmembrane proteins are the leading candidates for Wnt receptors. These are thought to transduce Wnt signals via one or more members of the Dishevelled protein family, resulting in inactivation of the protein kinase GSK-3β and subsequent stabilization of cytoplasmic β-catenin and/or the related protein plakoglobin. Stabilization of β-catenin appears to be a key step. In addition to its function in cell-cell adhesive junctions, β-catenin can enter the nucleus where it forms complexes with members of the Tcf/LEF-1 family of DNA binding proteins. In response to Wnt signals, these complexes are thought to regulate the transcription of downstream target genes (*see* refs. *1* and *12* for reviews). Besides the role of Wnt proteins themselves in mammary tumorigenesis, there is relatively little information about the involvement of the above intracellular signaling components. However, activation of the distal portion of this pathway through β-catenin stabilization is implicated in the majority of human colorectal cancers and is likely to be of widespread relevance in other epithelial tissues (*6,7,13,14*). In addition, mice bearing homozygous mutations that prevent expression of LEF-1 lack mammary glands, consistent with a crucial role in mammary development for this potential effector of Wnt signaling (*15*).

3. *WNT* GENES IN MOUSE MAMMARY CANCER AND CELL TRANSFORMATION

Studies of mammary tumorigenesis in mice have provided a powerful model system for the identification of oncogenes that contribute to multi-step neoplasia in mammary epithelium. Certain inbred strains of mice, such as C3H, BR6, GR, and RIII, show a high incidence of mammary tumor development as a consequence of chronic infection by the mouse mammary tumor virus (MMTV), a retrovirus which acts by insertional activation of host cell proto-oncogenes (*4*). At least eight candidate proto-oncogenes have been identified as frequent sites of proviral integration in MMTV-induced tumors. These genes were originally named "int," for retroviral "integration," but have since been renamed according to their membership of individual gene families, as determined by sequence comparisons. The genes thus far identified as frequent sites of MMTV integration in tumors are the *Wnt* genes *Wnt1* (formerly *int*-1), *Wnt3*, and *Wnt10b* (*2,16,17*); three members of the *Fgf* family, *Fgf3*, *Fgf4*, and *Fgf8* (*18,19*); the *Notch* family gene, *Notch*-4 (*20*); and *Int6*, which encodes a translation initiation factor subunit (*21*). The *int* nomenclature has also been applied to *Int5*, a gene encoding the P450 enzyme Aromatase, which is a site of MMTV insertion in certain mammary hyperplasias (*22*).

In evaluating the significance of the data associating members of the *Wnt* gene family with mouse mammary tumorigenesis, it is useful to consider *Wnt1* as a paradigm. Approximately 70% of the mammary carcinomas in C3H mice contain MMTV proviral insertions at the *Wnt1* locus and most of these tumors are clonal in origin (*5*). Since there is a huge number of potential MMTV integration sites throughout the mouse genome, the recurrent detection of insertions at the *Wnt1* locus in tumor samples strongly implies a selective growth advantage for cells bearing insertions at this site. MMTV can thus be viewed as a retrotransposon acting as a random insertional mutagen and the resulting tumors as the products of selection for oncogenic mutations. MMTV insertions at the *Wnt1* locus result in expression of *Wnt1* RNA, which is not detectably expressed in normal mammary tissue, and in each case the resulting Wnt1 protein produced is predicted to be wild-type since the insertions lie outside the coding sequence (*4,23*). Similar data pertain to *Wnt3* and *Wnt10b*, the principal differences being that these genes were identified as tumor-associated MMTV insertion sites in different strains of MMTV-infected mice, and insertions at these sites are found in a smaller proportion of the tumors (*3,16,17*). In both cases, the proteins produced from the activated locus are again predicted to be wild-type. Thus it is overproduction or deregulated expression of Wnt proteins which is associated with tumorigenesis. A fourth *Wnt* gene, *Wnt2*, has been found overexpressed in a mouse mammary carcinoma, although in this case the underlying mechanism is gene amplification rather than proviral insertion (24).

The biological consequences of excessive Wnt expression in mammary cells have now been studied for several *Wnt* genes, and again *Wnt1* serves as a paradigm. In order to recapitulate the activation of *Wnt1* experimentally in mammary tissues, Tsukamoto et al. (25) introduced an MMTV-activated *Wnt1* allele into the germline of transgenic mice. These animals expressed *Wnt1* ectopically in their mammary glands and, as a consequence, developed extensive mammary hyperplasia within 8 wk of birth. Subsequently, some of these hyperplasias gave rise to focal carcinomas after several months (25). Besides confirming the otherwise circumstantial evidence that *Wnt1* contributes to tumorigenesis, these results demonstrated that *Wnt1* activation per se is not sufficient for full neoplasia but appears to mediate an early step in the pathway of tumorigenesis. Comparable effects of *Wnt10b* on mammary gland growth and tumorigenesis in transgenic mice have also been reported recently (26).

In addition to the mammary growth-promoting effects of *Wnt* genes in vivo, transforming and mitogenic effects of Wnt proteins are evident in certain mouse mammary epithelial cell lines in culture. These effects were first demonstrated for *Wnt1* in the mammary epithelial line C57MG, and many other *Wnt* genes have since been evaluated in this assay. Expression of *Wnt1* in C57MG cells causes morphological transformation, characterized by an elongated and refractile cell phenotype, and also results in continued cell proliferation in confluent cultures (27). A similar phenotype has been observed in the mammary epithelial line RAC311, with the additional consequence that RAC311/*Wnt1* cells become tumorigenic in nude mice (28,29). Despite this formal evidence of oncogenic potential in a cell line, the transforming effects of *Wnt1* are somewhat limited in comparison with certain other oncogenes. For example, the morphological and mitogenic effects of *Wnt1* seen in C57MG and RAC311 cells appear to be limited to a subset of cell lines as no obvious phenotypic changes are observed when the gene is expressed in other mammary epithelial lines such as MOMMA or MMEC (unpublished observations). Similarly, *Wnt1* expression is thought to have little effect on several fibroblastic cell lines, although there are exceptions in which changes in morphology and growth parameters have been observed (30,31).

Although many questions remain about the transformed phenotype induced by *Wnt1* in the C57MG cell line, these cells have provided a useful experimental system for studying the mechanism of action of *Wnt1* and its protein products. For example, coculture experiments demonstrated that cells expressing Wnt1 could induce transformation of C57MG via a paracrine mechanism (32). Subsequently it was shown that conditioned culture medium containing soluble Wnt1 protein caused morphological transformation and continuing DNA replication in quiescent C57MG cells (10). These results demonstrated that mammalian Wnt proteins can act as extracellular signaling factors with mitogenic effects on mammary cells.

The C57MG cell line has also provided a convenient system for assaying the biological activities of other *Wnt* family members besides *Wnt1* (33–35). In a recent study of this sort, Shimizu et al. (36) used retroviral vectors to express ten different epitope-tagged mouse Wnt proteins in C57MG cells and assessed their ability to cause transformation. The genes were divisible into three functional classes. *Wnt1*, *Wnt2*, *Wnt3*, and *Wnt3a* induced strong transformation, *Wnt6* and *Wnt7a* produced weak phenotypes, and *Wnt4*, *Wnt5a*, *Wnt5b*, and *Wnt7b* had no effect on cell morphology *(36)*. Although it is possible that this differential response to different Wnts depends on which particular Wnt receptors are expressed in these cells, there is a striking concordance between the strongly transforming *Wnt* genes and those family members implicated in mouse mammary tumorigenesis. As mentioned above, *Wnt1* and *Wnt3* are found insertionally activated by MMTV in tumors *(5,17)*, *Wnt2* is implicated by gene amplification *(24)*, and *Wnt3a* encodes a protein that is likely to be functionally redundant with Wnt3 since it is 90% identical *(37)*. The remaining *Wnt* gene activated by MMTV, *Wnt10b*, has not yet been evaluated in the C57MG assay and it will be interesting to test the prediction that it will cause transformation.

Although C57MG has been a useful cell line for assaying the transformation potential of *Wnt* family members, its selective responsiveness to certain *Wnt* genes may not mirror the responsiveness of the many cell types in the mammary gland in vivo. Thus the *Wnt* genes which cause transformation of C57MG cells may represent only a subset of those with oncogenic potential in vivo. In addition, Wnt proteins may contribute to tumorigenesis via phenotypic changes that do not necessarily result in morphological transformation of mammary cell lines. This is illustrated by a recent analysis of the effects of ectopic *Wnt7b* expression in the mammary epithelial cell line HC11 *(38)*. Although there was no major change in the morphology of these cells in culture, when implanted in the mammary fat pads of recipient mice the cells generated adenocarcinomas within 12 wk *(38)*.

4. *WNT* GENES IN MOUSE MAMMARY DEVELOPMENT

At least seven different members of the *Wnt* gene family are expressed during normal development of the mouse mammary gland. These are *Wnt2*, *Wnt4*, *Wnt5a*, *Wnt5b*, *Wnt6*, *Wnt7b*, and *Wnt10b (26,39,40)*. In contrast, *Wnt1* and *Wnt3*, the two family members first identified as mammary oncogenes, are not detectably expressed in adult mammary tissues. Although initially intriguing, the apparent correlation between tumorigenic potential and lack of endogenous expression does not hold true for *Wnt10b*, which is expressed in normal mammary tissue but is oncogenic when activated by MMTV *(26)*.

Northern analysis of mammary RNA at different stages of postnatal development has shown differential temporal expression patterns for each of the expressed *Wnt* genes during ductal proliferation, pregnancy, and lactation. Although there are inconsistencies in the data obtained for *Wnt2* in different studies, these may be attributable to differences in mouse strains. In concise terms, the data thus far indicate that *Wnt2*, *Wnt5a*, *Wnt7b*, *Wnt10b*, and possibly *Wnt4*, are expressed in the ductal phase of development in adolescent mice *(26,39,40)*. At the onset of pregnancy, there is a sharp increase in expression of *Wnt4*, *Wnt5b*, and *Wnt6*, while expression of *Wnt7b* and *Wnt10b* rapidly declines. Once differentiation of the glandular tissue is complete at lactation, most of the *Wnt* transcripts are no longer detectable. This may be due to down-regulation of transcription, although an alternative explanation might be a fall in the relative abundance of *Wnt* transcripts due to the dramatically increased levels of milk protein RNAs *(26)*. During the regression or involution phase after lactation, sev-

Table 1
Mouse *Wnt* Genes Implicated
in Mammary Development and Tumorigenesis

Mouse *Wnt* gene	Expression in mammary gland[a]		Tumorigenic in vivo[b]	Transformation of C57MG cells[c]
Wnt1	−		+	+
Wnt2	+	S	+	+
Wnt3	−		+	+
Wnt3a	−			+
Wnt4	+			−
Wnt5a	+	S		−
Wnt5b	+	E		−
Wnt6	+	E,S		+/−
Wnt7a	−			+/−
Wnt7b	+	E	+	−
Wnt10b	+		+	
Wnt11				+

[a]Expression data in developing mammary glands is summarized from references *(26,39,40,50)*. E, epithelium; S, stroma.

[b]Tumorigenicity is inferred from MMTV insertions (*Wnt1*, *Wnt3*, *Wnt10b*), gene amplification in tumors (*Wnt2*), transgenic mice (*Wnt1* and *Wnt10b*), and mammary outgrowths from transfected cells (*Wnt7b*). *(5,17,24–26, 38)*.

[c]Data are from *(36)*, except for *Wnt11 (72)*. Slightly different results were reported for *Wnt5b* and *Wnt7b* in ref. *35*.

eral *Wnt* mRNAs are once again detectable. Relatively little is known about the localization of *Wnt* transcripts in the mouse mammary gland. However, *in situ* hybridization data are available for *Wnt2* and *Wnt5b (40,50)*, and efforts to distinguish epithelial from stromal expression by separation of primary cells have been described for other mouse *Wnt* genes *(40)*. These data are summarized in Table 1.

One implication from the fluctuating levels of *Wnt* RNAs during development is that certain *Wnt* genes may be regulated by hormonal signals. In support of this notion, Weber-Hall et al. found reduced levels of *Wnt2*, *Wnt4*, and *Wnt5b* RNAs in the mammary glands of ovariectomized mice *(40)*. Although this is consistent with gene regulation by ovarian hormones, it is also possible that it is an indirect consequence of arrested mammary development. Currently there is no evidence of direct transcriptional control of *Wnt* genes by hormonal signals. However, the study of *Wnt* gene promoters and their regulation is still in its infancy.

The temporal patterns of *Wnt* gene expression in the developing mammary gland suggest that Wnt proteins may themselves function in regulating mammary gland growth and differentiation, and that they may be local mediators of more distant hormonal signals. Ectopic expression experiments provide strong support for this model. Apart from the ability of *Wnt1*, *Wnt3*, and *Wnt10b* to act as mammary oncogenes when activated by MMTV insertions, transgenic mice expressing either *Wnt1* or *Wnt10b* from an MMTV promoter develop extensive mammary hyperplasia *(25,26)*. Two aspects of this phenotype are worthy of further consideration here. One is that the hyperplastic glandular tissues display lobulo-alveolar differentiation similar to that normally seen during pregnancy. The other is that male transgenic animals develop mammary hyperplasia as well as females. It therefore appears that deregulated expression of certain *Wnt* genes is sufficient to bypass the need for pregnancy-related hormones in stimulating mammary differentiation, and thus can establish hyperplastic growth of this sort even in a male hormonal context. Since *Wnt10b* is one of the *Wnt* genes normally expressed during mammary development, the in vivo consequences of its deregulated expression are particularly germane and highlight this *Wnt* family member as a positive regulator of mammary gland development *(26)*. One interpretation of the available data would be that *Wnt1* and *Wnt3*, when ectopically expressed in the mammary gland, activate the same receptor pathway as *Wnt10b* and hence have comparable effects in tumorigenesis.

Evidence of ability to induce mammary hyperplasia has also been reported for *Wnt4*, a gene endogenously expressed during early pregnancy *(41)*. In this case the data are from experiments in which primary mammary epithelial cells were infected with a retroviral vector expressing *Wnt4* and transplanted into cleared mammary fat pads. The resulting epithelial outgrowths showed hyperplasia with increased epithelial branching, and were similar to those derived from expression of *Wnt1* in the same system *(41,42)*. Since *Wnt4* does not cause transformation of C57MG mammary cells in culture, although *Wnt1* does *(25,35,36)*, the similar consequences of expressing these two genes in transplanted epithelium suggests that the functional grouping of *Wnt* genes based on C57MG transformation assays may not reflect their potential for functional redundancy in vivo. Consequently, a major question remains as to whether the other members of the *Wnt* gene family expressed endogenously during mouse mammary development have similar mitogenic and morphogenic potential when overexpressed, or whether these effects are limited to a subset of *Wnt* genes. The construction of additional transgenic mice will be one approach towards answering this question and establishing how many different *Wnt* genes have oncogenic potential in the mammary gland.

5. WNT EXPRESSION IN HUMAN BREAST TISSUES

As in the mouse mammary gland, several members of the *WNT* gene family are expressed in the human breast and it is therefore likely that they also function in regulating development and proliferation of the tissue. Of the 13 *WNT* family members thus far isolated from human DNA, transcripts of nine different *WNT* sequences have been reported in normal human breast tissue. These are *WNTs* 2, 3, 4, 5A, 7B, 10B, 13, 14, and 15 *(8,43–46; see* Table 2*)*. A variety of different techniques have been used to generate these data, and it is appropriate to review the limited number of studies in more detail.

Among the more abundant *WNT* transcripts is *WNT5A* RNA, which has been detected in normal breast tissue specimens, both by Northern blotting and by RNase protection *(45,46)*. In a separate study of normal breast tissue specimens, Huguet et al. *(44)* detected transcripts of *WNTs* 2, 3, 4, and 7B by RNase protection assay. By comparable methods of RNase protection, transcripts of *WNT3A* and *WNT7A* were undetectable in either the normal breast specimens or in human mammary cell lines *(44)*. In addition, *WNT1* mRNA has not been detected in human mammary tissue *(47,48)*.

To the extent that data are available for both species, the above findings in human breast mirror the expression data for mouse mammary gland, wherein *Wnts* 2, 4, 5A, and

Table 2
Human *WNT* Genes and Their Expression in Breast Tissues

Human WNT Gene	Normal Breast	Benign Tumor	Breast Cancer	Map Location	References
WNT1	–		–	12q13	*(47,48,73)*
WNT2	+	++	++	7q31	*(44,49,74)*
WNT3	+	+	+	17q21	*(44,75)*
WNT3A	–	–	–		*(44)*
WNT4	+	++	++		*(44)*
WNT5A	+	++	++	3p14–p21	*(45,46,76)*
WNT7A	–	–	–	3p25	*(44,77)*
WNT7B	+	+	++	22q13	*(44,78)*
WNT10B	+	+	++	12q13.1	*(43,79)*
WNT13*	+	+	++	1p13	*(8,80; Fig. 2)*
WNT14	+/–	+/–	+/–	chrom. 1	*(8)*
WNT15	+/–	+/–	+/–	17q21	*(8)*

++ Indicates a report of overexpression, relative to normal tissue, in any proportion of samples analyzed.
+/– Indicates very low levels of RNA. No expression data are currently available for *WNT5B*, *WNT6*, *WNT8B*, or *WNT11*.
*Note that *WNT13* may be renamed *WNT2B* on account of its similarity to WNT2.

7B are also expressed *(39,40,44)*. One exception is *Wnt3*, which was not detected in normal mouse mammary tissue (by Northern blotting) but was detectable by RNase protection in human breast *(39,44)*. This difference may reflect the different sensitivity of the assays used. Also, while there are no data to address changes in *WNT* expression during pregnancy, comparisons of pre- vs postmenopausal breast tissue have not yet revealed differential *WNT* expression with respect to hormonal status in humans *(44,46)*.

For two human *WNT* genes, the expression data for human breast tissue have been refined by *in situ* hybridization. *WNT5A* transcripts were seen in epithelial cells of lobules and ducts, and in some larger ducts the RNA appeared to be within the luminal cells but not the myoepithelial component *(46)*. In contrast, *WNT2* transcripts have been localized exclusively within the stroma of normal breast tissue *(49)*, a finding consistent with the detection of *WNT2* RNA in fibroblasts isolated from mammoplasty specimens but not in mammary cell lines of epithelial derivation *(44)*. These data are comparable to the localization data for *Wnt2* in the stroma of mouse mammary glands *(40,50)*.

Transcripts of a further set of human *WNT* genes have been detected in breast tissue using sensitive RT-PCR techniques without independent confirmation by other methods. For example, *WNT10B* transcripts were not detected in normal breast tissue by RNase protection, but Southern blot analysis of RT-PCR products revealed low levels of *WNT10B* mRNA in normal breast tissue specimens *(43)*. In addition, Bergstein et al. *(8)* detected a spliced transcript of *WNT13* by RT-PCR analysis of three mammoplasty specimens, as well as very low levels of *WNT14* and *WNT15* RNA. Semiquantitative competitive RT-PCR assays of normal breast RNA indicated that *WNT5A* transcript levels were 5–10-fold higher than *WNT13* RNA, and that the latter was at least 10-fold more abundant than either *WNT14* or *WNT15* *(8)* (I.B., unpublished data). Although control reactions confirmed that the PCR products detected with *WNT14* and *WNT15* primers were RNA-dependent, it remains to be determined whether these low abundance transcripts represent significant expression in a small subpopulation of cells, or a low-level background of unprocessed nuclear RNA which may have no functional consequences.

6. ABERRANT WNT EXPRESSION IN HUMAN BREAST CANCER

Following the initial discovery of *Wnt1* as a novel mammary oncogene in the mouse, the first questions about the role of *WNT* genes in human breast cancer were restricted to analysis of human *WNT1*, whose lack of expression in human breast tumors seemed discouraging *(48)*. However, it is now known that there are at least 18 different vertebrate *Wnt* genes, that many of these display functional redundancy with *Wnt1* in experimental assays, and that other *Wnt*s besides *Wnt1* are implicated in mouse mammary tumorigenesis. As the analysis of aberrant *WNT* expression in human breast cancer has broadened to include other family members, evidence of overexpression of certain *WNT* genes has been obtained which is consistent with a role for these genes in abnormal growth of human mammary tissues. Specifically, aberrant expression of *WNT2*, *WNT4*, *WNT5A*, *WNT7B*, and *WNT10B*, has been reported in neoplastic breast biopsies (Table 2).

Two studies have examined *WNT2* RNA levels by RNase protection assay and both found evidence of overexpression of this gene in tumors relative to normal breast tissue *(44,49)*. For example, Huguet et al. *(44)* found 10- to 20-fold overexpression in four out of five benign fibroadenomas analyzed. In addition, Dale et al. *(49)* reported elevated expression of *WNT2* in five out of 11 malignant carcinomas. Since *WNT2* is normally expressed in stromal tissue *(see above)*, its overexpression in fibroadenomas might be predictable because of their large stromal content. Surprisingly, however, Dale et al. detected *WNT2* RNA in both the stromal and epithelial components of the fibroadenomas and carcinomas that displayed elevated expression *(49)*. These authors suggest that WNT2 protein may normally provide a paracrine signal from mammary stroma to epithelium, and that its activation in epithelial cells leads to the creation of an autocrine loop *(49)*. Since *Wnt2* is able to cause transformation of mouse mammary epithelial cells, and the gene is amplified in certain mouse mammary tumors *(24,33,36)*, the above data are consistent with a functional contribution of *WNT2* to the abnormal growth of human breast lesions.

In addition to *WNT2*, Huguet et al. *(44)* also reported overexpression of *WNT4* in four out of five fibroadenomas, the increase being approx 10-fold relative to normal tissue. It is not yet known whether *Wnt4* is expressed in the mammary stroma or epithelium, in either mouse or human, so the expression detected in these benign lesions could be derived from an excess of stromal fibroblasts. The detection of *WNT4* RNA in only one out of 12 human breast epithelial cell lines supports this view *(44)*. Nevertheless, the ability of mouse *Wnt4* to generate hyperplasia in transplanted mammary tissues raises the possibility that expression of this gene may contribute to growth of human fibroadenomas *(41)*.

In the same study, *WNT7B* RNA was not overexpressed in benign breast lesions, but was found up-regulated (by approx 30-fold) in two out of 20 carcinomas examined *(44)*. There is evidence from mouse studies that *Wnt7b* is normally expressed in mammary epithelium rather than stroma *(40)*, and the abundance of *WNT7B* transcripts in 12 human mammary epithelial cell lines supports this *(44)*. By the same arguments applied above to *WNT2* and *WNT4* in stromal tissues, it is possible that the overabundance of *WNT7B* reflects an excess of epithelial cells in the carcinomas relative to normal breast biopsies. However, the overexpression in only 10% of the samples seems to argue against this. Moreover, oncogenic effects of *Wnt7b* have been described in cells implanted into mouse mammary glands *(38)*. More data are now required to clarify the potential role of *WNT7B* in breast cancer, both in terms of sample numbers and the localization of *Wnt7b* expression in mammary tissues.

Two groups have reported *WNT5A* overexpression in human breast tumors. By RNase protection, Lejeune et al. *(46)* found *WNT5A* expressed in five fibroadenomas at 10-fold higher levels on average than in normal breast tissue. This study also demonstrated *WNT5A* overexpression in 10 out of 28 carcinomas, but with an average increase of only fourfold compared with normal breast. Similar results were reported by Iozzo et al. *(45)*, who detected *WNT5A* expression in breast, lung, prostate, and other cancers. Quantitative slot blot analysis showed that *WNT5A* RNA was approx fourfold more abundant in 4 breast carcinomas relative to normal breast tissue *(45)*. *WNT5A* overexpression in tumors could not be attributed to gene amplification or DNA rearrangements and did not appear to correlate with known prognostic parameters, such as estrogen receptor, or nodal status *(45,46)*. Although *WNT5A* was only rarely detected in mammary epithelial cell lines, Lejune et al. *(46)* localized *WNT5A* transcripts to the epithelial component of both benign and malignant tissues by *in situ* hybridization. The evidence of *WNT5A* overexpression in fibroadenomas is thus particularly impressive since the epithelial component of these lesions is likely to be underrepresented. However, in the murine system, *Wnt5a* expression has not been linked to tumorigenesis and instead there is evidence of an inverse correlation between *Wnt5a* RNA levels and mammary cell transformation *(51)*. Although the phenotypic consequences of WNT5A signaling may vary depending on which receptors are expressed in the target cells *(52)*, there is no strong case at present that *WNT5A* contributes to the deregulated growth of mammary tissues. Instead, it may represent a marker for a particular stage of mammary cell differentiation found in tumors, as suggested by Lejeune et al.*(46)*.

As mentioned earlier, results in the murine system strongly implicate Wnt10B protein as a positive regulator of mammary cell proliferation. It is therefore of particular interest to examine the expression of this gene in human breast cancer. There are technical difficulties with this since the expression levels are very low. However, by RNase protection assay, Bui et al. *(43)* were able to detect overexpression of *WNT10B* in three out of 50 carcinomas analyzed. The magnitude of this effect was not quantified since expression in the other samples was hard to detect, but the oncogenic effects of *Wnt10b* in the mouse mammary gland increase the potential significance of these findings *(16,26)*. As with *WNT7B*, the frequency with which overexpression of *WNT10B* is detected is low in the limited sample sizes analyzed. Given the likely redundancy among different WNT proteins, however, it is possible that the proportion of breast tumors with at least one oncogenic *WNT* gene overexpressed is considerably greater.

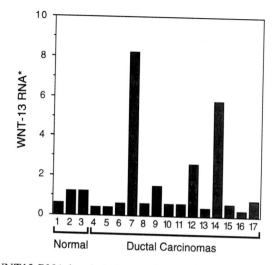

Fig. 2. Relative WNT13 RNA levels in human breast tissue. Levels of *WNT13* RNA in 17 breast tissue specimens were measured by competitive RT-PCR assay and expressed relative to GAPDH levels. GAPDH RNA was first quantified in reactions containing serial dilutions of a GADPH competitor template. *WNT13* RNA levels in the same cDNA samples were then assayed in reactions containing serial dilutions of a *WNT13* competitor template using primers described by Bergstein et al. *(8)*. Relative amounts of *WNT13* RNA in each specimen were determined by normalizing the absolute amounts of *WNT13* RNA to GAPDH transcript levels. Specimens 1–3 were from normal mammoplasty tissue, and 4–17 from infiltrating ductal carcinoma biopsies. Relative *WNT13* RNA levels showed a twofold range in mammoplasty tissue and were within 2.5-fold of that mean value in 12 out of 14 ductal carcinomas. The two remaining tumors showed 5–8-fold higher levels of *WNT13* RNA. *Note that *WNT13* may be renamed *WNT2B* on account of its similarity to *WNT2*.

Our own studies of recent additions to the *WNT* gene family revealed potential evidence of overexpression of *WNT13* in a small number of breast tumors. *WNT13* RNA was detected by RT-PCR analysis using primers that span an intron, and was quantified by comparison with a competitor template of known concentration. In two out of 14 carcinomas, the *WNT13* RNA was 5–8-fold more abundant than in normal breast tissue samples (Fig. 2). At present, however, nothing is known of the spatial expression pattern of *WNT13* in breast tissue, nor of its ability to cause transformation of mammary cells in vitro or in vivo. Similar studies of *WNT14* and *WNT15* showed no evidence of overexpression in the breast tumor samples analyzed (unpublished data).

In summary, the evidence for involvement of *WNT* genes in human breast cancer rests on a growing amount of circumstantial evidence of overexpression, combined with knowledge of the mitogenic and oncogenic potential of certain *Wnt* genes in mouse mammary cells in vivo and in vitro. The genes most strongly implicated so far are *WNT2*, *WNT7B*, and *WNT10B*. To date, there are no reports of DNA rearrangements or mutations in *WNT* genes in human breast cancer, which would otherwise provide much greater evidence of cause and effect in relation to tumorigenesis. In the absence of such data, it is difficult to exclude the alternative possibility that deregulation of *WNT* expression is an indirect consequence of tumorigenesis, or that expression in tumors results from the clonal expansion of a subpopulation of cells that normally express the relevant gene. However, whether or not aberrant expression of WNT proteins in breast cancer is an initiating factor in the disease, the evidence that these proteins regulate mammary cell growth and differentiation suggests that breast cancer cells may be in part dependent on WNT signals, and thus that the proliferation of tumor cells could be influenced by interfering with WNT signaling therapeutically. In this regard it is notable that a family of secreted Frizzled-related proteins, called Frps or Frzbs, has recently been identified. These have been reported to bind Wnt proteins and may act as natural antagonists of Wnt signaling *(53,54)*.

7. WNT SIGNALING COMPONENTS IN BREAST CANCER

Most of the studies of Wnt signaling in breast cancer thus far have focused on expression of *WNT* genes themselves, as described above. However, as the molecular pathways of intracellular Wnt signal transduction become understood in more detail, it will become increasingly possible to assay for mutations in other proteins which may result in ligand-independent activation of the pathway. For example, when the Frizzled proteins or other receptors that transduce Wnt signals at the surface of mammary cells are more clearly defined, there will be good reasons to screen for oncogenic mutations in the relevant genes.

One protein that is already established as a key component of intracellular Wnt signaling is β-catenin (*see* Fig. 1). There have been several studies of the status of this protein in breast tumors and cell lines, but most have focused on β-catenin as a component of cell-cell adhesive junctions. Other components of such junctions include E-cadherin, α-catenin, and plakoglobin *(55)*. In many cases, the expression or function of one or more of these proteins is deficient in breast cancer cells and the resulting loss of adhesion may facilitate invasion and metastasis *(56–62)*. Consistent with this, several studies describe loss of β-catenin staining in breast tumors *(62–64)*. These data therefore appear incompatible with activation of Wnt signaling, which would be expected to increase β-catenin levels. However, the predominant β-catenin staining visible in normal tissues is at the plasma membrane, while the catenin fraction associated with Wnt signaling would be in the cytosol or nucleus. Nuclear staining of β-catenin in mammary tissues may be difficult to detect by standard histochemical techniques and more specific detection methods may be required to assay this fraction. It therefore remains a possibility that the reduced number of cadherin–catenin complexes at the membrane in tumor cells might leave more β-catenin available for Wnt signaling in the nucleus.

High levels of β-catenin protein have been found in other cancers, most notably in colorectal cancer, and in most cases this is a result of mutations in the tumor suppressor gene APC *(13)*. Wild-type APC protein normally participates in destabilization of β-catenin, but the majority of colorectal tumors express only truncated mutant forms of APC that have lost this property *(13,65)*. In some cases, nuclear staining of β-catenin has been reported in such tumors *(66)*. Although there have been reports of LOH at or near the APC locus in human breast cancer, and APC mutations in mice can promote mammary carcinoma in addition to intestinal tumors, there have so far been no reports of APC truncation mutations in human breast cancer *(67–70)*. Another class of mutations that can result in increased β-catenin levels are mutations within the β-catenin gene itself, as recently described in both colon cancer and melanoma cells *(6,7)*. These mutations specifically affect a group of phosphorylation sites near the N-terminus of β-catenin, which govern the protein's stability. Although a previous study of 11 breast carcinomas (9 lobular and 2 ductal) failed to detect mutations in the β-catenin gene by SSCP analysis *(71)*, a question that should now be addressed more specifically is whether breast tumors contain β-catenin mutations that result in more stable protein products. In breast cancer cell lines it should also be possible to screen for transcriptionally active β-catenin/Tcf complexes *(14)*, whose presence might be indicative of any alteration in the Wnt pathway that results in constitutive signal transduction to the nucleus.

8. SUMMARY

Many years of research on mouse mammary carcinomas have led to the identification of *Wnt* genes as oncogenes whose activation is frequently responsible for the genesis of tumors induced by the mouse mammary tumor virus. Although there is apparently no comparable viral etiology for human breast cancer, members of the same gene family have been found overexpressed in a proportion of human tumors. In view of the functions of Wnt proteins in regulating proliferation and differentiation in mammary tissues, it is likely that breast cancer cells are responsive to Wnt signals and possible that they will be sensitive to therapeutic intervention aimed at these signals. Mutations in *WNT* genes themselves have not been described in breast cancer, but precedents from other growth factor signaling pathways would suggest that oncogenic mutations may be more likely in genes encoding intracellular components of the signaling pathway. The framework of a Wnt signaling pathway has recently been elucidated and the stage is therefore set for renewed investigation of the role of WNT proteins and their signal transduction pathway in human breast cancer.

ACKNOWLEDGMENTS

We thank Louise Howe and Stephen Byers for comments on the manuscript, and Dr. Michael Osborne for encouragement to study *WNT* genes in human breast cancer. Work on *WNT* genes in our laboratory was supported by NIH grant CA47207 and by the Iris Cantor Clinical Research Unit at Strang Cancer Prevention Center. I.B. was supported by a Jerome A. Urban Research Fellowship and A.M.C.B. is the recipient of an Irma T. Hirschl Career Scientist award.

REFERENCES

1. Cadigan, K. M. and R. Nusse. 1997. Wnt signaling: a common theme in animal development. *Genes Dev.* **11:** 3286–3305.
2. Nusse, R. and H. E. Varmus. 1992. Wnt genes. *Cell* **69:** 1073–1087.
3. Callahan, R. 1996. MMTV-induced mutations in mouse mammary tumors: their potential relevance to human breast cancer. *Br. Ca. Res. Treat.* **39(1):** 33–44.
4. Nusse, R. 1991. Insertional mutagenesis in mouse mammary tumorigenesis. *Curr. Topics Microbiol Immunol.* **171:** 43–66.
5. Nusse, R. and H. E. Varmus. 1982. Many tumors induced by the mouse mammary tumor virus contain a provirus integrated in the same region of the host genome. *Cell* **31:** 99–109.
6. Morin, P. J., A. B. Sparks, B. Korinek, N. Barker, H. Clevers, B. Vogelstein, and K. W. Kinzler. 1997. Activation of β-catenin-Tcf signaling in colon cancer by mutations in β-catenin or APC. *Science* **275:** 1787.

7. Rubinfeld, B., P. Robbins, M. El-Gamil, I. Albert, E. Porfiri, and P. Polakis. 1997. Stablization of β-catenin by genetic defects in melanoma cell lines. *Science* **275:** 1790

8. Bergstein, I., L. M. Eisenberg, J. Bhalerao, N. A. Jenkins, N. G. Copeland, M. P. Osborne, A. M. Bowcock, and A. M. C. Brown. 1997. Isolation of two novel WNT genes, WNT14 and WNT15, one of which (WNT15) is closely linked to WNT3 on human chromosome 17q21. *Genomics* **46:** 450–458.

8a. Bradley, R. S. and A. M. C. Brown. 1990. The proto-oncogene *int*–1 encodes a secreted protein associated with the extracellular matrix. *EMBO J.* **9:** 1569–1575.

8b. Smolich, B. D., J. A. McMahon, A. P. McMahon, and J. Papkoff. 1993. Wnt family proteins are secreted and associated with the cell surface. *Mol. Biol. Cell.* **4:** 1267–1275.

9. Austin, T. W., G. P. Solar, F. C. Ziegler, L. Liem, and W. Matthews. 1997. A role for the Wnt gene family in hematopoiesis: Expansion of multilineage progenitor cells. *Blood* **89(10):** 3624–3635.

10. Bradley, R. S. and A. M. C. Brown. 1995. A soluble form of Wnt-1 protein with mitogenic activity on mammary epithelial cells. *Mol. Cell. Biol.* **15:** 4616–4622.

11. Van Leeuwen, F., C. H. Samos, and R. Nusse. 1994. Biological activity of soluble *wingless* protein in cultured *Drosophila* imaginal disc cells. *Nature* **368:** 342–344.

12. Nusse, R. 1997. A versatile transcriptional effector of wingless signaling. *Cell* **89:** 321–323.

13. Kinzler, K. W. and B. Vogelstein. 1996. Lessons from hereditary colorectal cancer. Cell **87:** 159–170.

14. Korinek, V., N. Barker, P. J. Morin, D. vanWichen, R. deWeger, K. W. Kinzler, B. Vogelstein, and H. Clevers. 1997. Constitutive transcriptional activation by a β-catenin-Tcf complex in APC$^{-/-}$ colon carcinoma. *Science* **275:** 1784

15. van Genderen, C., R. M. Okamura, I. Farinas, R. G. Quo, T. G. Parslow, and R. Grosschedl. 1994. Development of several organs that require inductive epithelial-mesenchymal interactions is impaired in LEF-1-deficient mice. *Genes Dev.* **8:** 2691–2703.

16. Lee, F. S., T. F. Lane, A. Kuo, G. M. Shackleford, and P. Leder. 1995. Insertional mutagenesis identifies a member of the Wnt gene family as a candidate oncogene in the mammary epithelium of int–2/Fgf-3 transgenic mice. *Proc. Natl. Acad. Sci. USA* **92:** 2268–2272.

17. Roelink, H., E. Wagenaar, S. Lopes da Silva, and R. Nusse. 1990. *Wnt-3*, a gene activated by proviral insertion in mouse mammary tumors, is homologous to *int-1/Wnt-1* and is normally expressed in mouse embryos and adult brain. *Proc. Natl. Acad. Sci. USA* **87:** 4519–4523.

18. Dickson, C., R. Smith, S. Brookes, and G. Peters. 1984. Tumorigenesis by mouse mammary tumor virus: proviral activation of a cellular gene in the common integration region int–2. *Cell* **37:** 529–536.

19. Peters, G., S. Brookes, R. Smith, M. Placzek, and C. Dickson. 1989. The mouse homolog of the *hst/k-FGF* gene is adjacent to *int*-2 and is activated by proviral insertion in some virally induced mammary tumors. *Proc. Natl. Acad. Sci. USA* **86:** 5678–5682.

20. Robbins, J., B. J. Blondel, D. Gallahan, and R. Callahan. 1992. Mouse mammary tumor gene *int*-3: a member of the *notch* gene family transforms mammary epithelial cells. *J. Virol.* **66:** 2594–2599.

21. Asano, K., W. C. Merrick, and J. W. Hershey. 1997. The translation initiation factor eIF3-p48 sub-unit is encoded by int-6, a site of frequent integration by the mouse mammary tumor virus genome. *J. Biol. Chem.* **272(38):** 23,477–23,480.

22. Durgam, V. R. and R. R. Tekmal. 1994. The nature and expression of int–5, a novel mMTV integration locus gene in carcinogen-induced mammary tumors. *Ca. Lett.* **87(2):** 179–186.

23. Nusse, R., A. van Ooyen, D. Cox, Y. K. Fung, and H. E. Varmus. 1984. Mode of proviral activation of a putative mammary oncogene (int-1) on mouse chromosome 15. *Nature* **307:** 131–136.

24. Roelink, H., E. Wagenaar, and R. Nusse. 1992. Amplification and proviral activation of several *Wnt* genes during progession and clonal variation of mouse mammary tumors. *Oncogene* **7**: 487–492.

25. Tsukamoto, A. S., R. Grosschedl, R. C. Guzman, T. Parslow, and H. E. Varmus. 1988. Expression of the *int-1* gene in transgenic mice is associated with mammary gland hyperplasia and adenocarcinomas in male and female mice. *Cell* **55**: 619–625.

26. Lane, T. F. and P. Leder. 1997. Wnt-10b directs hypermorphic development and transformation in mammary glands of male and female mice. *Oncogene* **15**: 2133–2144.

27. Brown, A. M. C., R. A. Wildin, T. J. Prendergast, and H. E. Varmus. 1986. A retrovirus vector expressing the putative mammary oncogene int–1 causes partial transformation of a mammary epithelial cell line. *Cell* **46**: 1001–1009.

28. Ramakrishna, N. R. and A. M. C. Brown. 1993. Wingless, the Drosophila homolog of the mouse proto-oncogene Wnt-1, can cause transformation of mouse mammary epithelial cells. *Development* **119(Suppl.):** 95–103.

29. Rijsewijk, F., L. van Deemter, E. Wagenaar, A. Sonnenburg, and R. Nusse. 1987. Transfection of the int-1 mammary oncogene in cuboidal RAC mammary cell line results in morphological transformation and tumorigenicity. *EMBO J.* **6**: 127–131.

30. Bradbury, J. M., C. C. Niemeyer, T. C. Dale, and P. A. Edwards. 1994. Alterations of the growth characteristics of the fibroblast cell line C3H 10T1/2 by members of the Wnt gene family. *Oncogene* **9**: 2597–2603.

31. Young, C. S., M. Kitamura, S. Hardy, and J. Kitajewski. 1998. *Wnt-1* induces growth, cytosolic beta-catenin, and Tcf/Lef transcriptional activation in rat-1 fibroblasts. *Mol. Cell. Biol.* **18**: 2474–2485.

32. Jue, S. F., R. S. Bradley, J. A. Rudnicki, H. E. Varmus, and A. M. C. Brown. 1992. The mouse *Wnt-1* gene can act via a paracrine mechanism in transformation of mammary epithelial cells. *Mol. Cell. Biol.* **12**: 321–328.

33. Blasband, A., B. Schryver, and J. Papkoff. 1992. The biochemical properties and transforming potential of human *Wnt-2* are similar to *Wnt-1*. *Oncogene* **7**: 155–161.

34. Briskin, M. J., R.-Y. Hsu, T. Boggs, J. A. Schultz, W. Rishell, and R. A. Bosselman. 1991. Heritable retroviral transgenes are highly expressed in chickens. *Proc. Natl. Acad. Sci. USA* **88**: 1736–1740.

35. Wong, G. T., B. J. Gavin, and A. P. McMahon. 1994. Differential transformation of mammary epithelial cells by *Wnt* genes. *Mol. Cell. Biol.* **14**: 6278–6286.

36. Shimizu, H., M. A. Julius, Z. Zheng, M. Giarre, A. M. C. Brown, and J. Kitajewski. 1997. Mammary cell transformation by Wnt family proteins correlates with regulation of beta-catenin. *Cell Growth Diff.* **8**: 1349–1358.

37. Roelink, H. and R. Nusse. 1991. Expression of two members of the *Wnt* family during mouse development- restricted temporal and spatial patterns in the developing neural tube. *Genes Dev.* **5**: 381–388.

38. Humphreys, R. C. and J. M. Rosen. 1997. Stably transfected HC11 cells provide an in vitro and in vivo model system for studying Wnt gene function. *Cell Growth Diff.* **8**: 839–849.

39. Gavin, B. J. and A. P. McMahon. 1992. Differential regulation of the *Wnt* gene family during pregnancy and lactation suggests a role in postnatal development of the mammary gland. *Mol. Cell. Biol.* **12**: 2418–2423.

40. Weber-Hall, S. J., D. J. Phippard, C. C. Niemeyer, and T. C. Dale. 1994. Developmental and hormonal regulation of *Wnt* gene expression in the mouse mammary gland. *Differentiation* **57**: 205–214.

41. Bradbury, J. M., P. A. W. Edwards, C. C. Niemeyer, and T. C. Dale. 1995. Wnt–4 expression induces a pregnancy-like growth pattern in reconstructed mammary glands in virgin mice. *Dev. Biol.* **170**: 553–563.

42. Edwards, P. A. W., S. E. Hiby, J. Papkoff, and J. M. Bradbury. 1992. Hyperplasia of mouse mammary epithelium induced by expression of the *Wnt-1 (int-1)* oncogene in reconstituted mammary gland. *Oncogene* **7**: 2041–2051.

43. Bui, T. D., J. Rankin, K. Smith, E. L. Huguet, S. Ruben, T. Strachan, A. L. Harris, and S. Lindsay. 1997. A novel human Wnt gene, WNT10B, maps to 12q13 and is expressed in human breast carcinomas. *Oncogene* **14**: 1249–1253.

44. Huguet, E. L., J. A. McMahon, A. P. McMahon, R. Bicknell, and A. L. Harris. 1994. Differential expression of human *Wnt* genes 2, 3, 4, and 7B in human breast cell lines and normal and diseased breast tissue. *Cancer Res.* **54**: 2615–2621.

45. Iozzo, R. V., I. Eichstetter, and K. G. Danielson. 1995. Aberrant expression of the growth factor Wnt-5a in human malignancy. *Cell Regul.* **55**: 3495–3499.

46. Lejeune, S., E. L. Huguet, A. Hamby, R. Poulsom, and A. L. Harris. 1995. Wnt5a cloning, expression, and up-regulation in human primary breast cancers. *Clin. Cancer Res.* **1**: 215–222.

47. Meyers, S. L., M. T. O'Brien, T. Smith, and J. P. Dudley. 1990. Analysis of the *int-1, int-2*, c-*myc*, and *neu* oncogenes in human breast carcinomas. *Cancer Res.* **50**: 5911–5918.

48. Van de Vijver, M. J. and R. Nusse. 1991. The molecular biology of breast cancer. *Biochim. Biophys. Acta Rev. Cancer* **1072**: 33–50.

49. Dale, T. C., S. J. Weber-Hall, K. Smith, E. L. Huguet, H. Jayatliake, B. A. Gusterson, G. Shuttleworth, M. O'Hare, and A. L. Harris. 1996. Compartment switching of WNT-2 expression in human breast tumors. *Cell Regul.* **56**: 4320–4323.

50. Buhler, T. A., T. C. Dale, C. Kieback, R. C. Humphreys, and J. M. Rosen. 1993. Localization and quantification of Wnt-2 gene expression in mouse mammary development. *Dev. Biol.* **155**: 87–96.

51. Olson, D. J. and J. Papkoff. 1994. Regulated expression of Wnt family members during proliferation of C57MG mammary cells. *Cell Growth Diff.* **5**: 197–206.

52. He, X., J.-P. Saint-Jeannet, Y. Wang, J. Nathans, I. Dawid, and H. Varmus. 1997. A member of the frizzled protein family mediating axis induction by Wnt-5A. *Science* **275**: 1652–1654.

53. Moon, R. T., J. D. Brown, J. A. Yang-Snyder, and J. R. Miller. 1997. Structurally related receptors and antagonists compete for secreted Wnt ligands. *Cell* **88**: 725–728.

54. Rattner, A., J. C. Hsieh, P. M. Smallwood, D. J. Gilbert, N. G. Copeland, N. A. Jenkins, and J. Nathans. 1997. A family of secreted proteins contains homology to the cysteine-rich ligand-binding domain of frizzled receptors. *Proc. Natl. Acad. Sci. USA* **94(7)**: 2859–2863.

55. Kemler, R. 1993. From cadherins to catenins: cytoplasmic protein interactions and regulation of cell adhesion. *Trends Genet.* **9**: 317–321.

56. Berx, G., A. M. Cleton-Jansen, K. Strumane, W. J. deLeeuw, F. Nollett, F. vanRoy, and C. Cornelisse. 1996. E-cadherin is inactivated in a majority of invasive human lobular breast cancers by truncation mutations throughout its extracellular domain. *Oncogene* **13(9)**: 1919–1925.

57. Birchmeier, W. and J. Behrens. 1994. Cadherin expression in carcinomas: role in the formation of cell junctions and the prevention of invasiveness. *Biochim. Biophys. Acta.* **1198**: 11–26.

58. Birchmeier, W., J. Hulsken, and J. Behrens. 1995. Adherens junction proteins in tumour progression. *Cancer Surv.* **24**: 129–140.

59. Ochiai, A., S. Akimoto, Y. Shimoyama, A. Nagafuchi, S. Tsukita, and S. Hirohashi. 1994. Frequent loss of alpha catenin expression in scirrhous carcinomas with scattered growth. *Jpn J. Cancer Res.* **85**: 266–273.

60. Pierceall, W. E., A. S. Woodard, J. S. Morrow, D. Rimm, and E. R. Fearon. 1995. Frequent alterations in E-cadherin and alpha- and beta-catenin expression in human breast cancer cell lines. *Oncogene* **11(7)**: 1319–1326.

61. Sommers, C. L., E. P. Gelman, R. Kemler, P. Cowin, and S. W. Byers. 1994. Alterations in beta-catenin phosphorylation and plakoglobin expression in human breast cancer cells. *Cell Regul.* **54:** 3544–3552.

62. Zschiesche, W., I. Schonborn, J. Behrens, K. Herrenknecht, F. Hartveit, P. Lilleng, and W. Birchmeier. 1997. Expression of E-cadherin and catenins in invasive mammary carcinomas. *Anticancer Res.* **17(1B):** 561–567.

63. Dillon, D. A., T. D'Aquila, A. B. Reynolds, E. R. Fearon, and D. L. Rimm. 1998. The expression of p120ctn protein in breast cancer is independent of alpha- and beta-catenin and E-cadherin. *Am. J. Pathol.* **152:** 75–82.

64. Hashizume, R., H. Koizumi, A. Ihara, T. Ohta, and T. Uchikoshi. 1996. Expression of beta-catenin in normal breast tissue and breast carcinoma: a comparative study with epithelial cadherin and alpha-catenin. *Histopathology* **29(2):** 139–146.

65. Munemitsu, S., I. Albert, B. Souza, B. Rubinfeld, and P. Polakis. 1995. Regulation of intracellular beta-catenin levels by adenomatous polyposis coli (APC) tumor-suppressor protein. *Proc. Natl. Acad. Sci. USA* **92:** 3046–3050.

66. Inomata, M., A. Ochiai, S. Akimoto, S. Kiono, and S. Hiohashi. 1996. Alteration of beta-catenin expression in colonic epithelial cells of familial adenomatous polyposis patients. *Cancer Res.* **56:** 2213–2217.

67. Medeiros, A. C., M. A. Nagai, M. M. Neto, and R. R. Brentani. 1994. Loss of heterozygosity affecting the APC and MCC genetic loci in patients with primary breast carcinomas. *Ca. Epidemiol. Biomarkers Prev.* **3:** 331–333.

68. Thompson, A. M., R. G. Morris, M. Wallace, A. H. Wyllie, C. M. Steel, and D. C. Carter. 1993. Allele loss from 5q21 (APC/MCC) and 18q21 (DCC) and DCC mRNA expression in breast cancer. *Br. J. Cancer* **68:** 64–68.

69. Moser, A. R., E. M. Mattes, W. F. Dove, M. J. Lindstrom, J. D. Haag, and M. N. Gould. 1993. ApcMin, a mutation in the murine Apc gene, predisposes to mammary carcinoma and focal hyperplasias. *Proc. Natl. Acad. Sci. USA* **90:** 8977–8981.

70. Kashiwaba, M., G. Tamura, and M. Ishida. 1994. Aberrations of the APC gene in primary breast carcinoma. *J. Cancer Res. Clin. Oncol.* **120:** 727–731.

71. Candidus, S., P. Bischoff, K. F. Becker, and H. Hofler. 1996. No evidence for mutations in the alpha- and beta-catenin genes in human gastric and breast carcinomas. *Cancer Res.* **56(1):** 49–52.

72. Christiansen, J. H., S. J. Monkley, and B. J. Wainwright. 1996. Murine WNT11 is a secreted glycoprotein that morphologically transforms mammary epithelial cells. *Oncogene* **12:** 2705–2711.

73. Arheden, K., N. Mandahl, B. Strombeck, M. Isaksson, and F. Mitelman. 1988. Chromosomal localization of the human oncogene INT1 to 12q13 by in situ hybridization. *Cytogenet. Cell Genet.* **47:** 86–87.

74. Wainwright, B. J., P. J. Scambler, P. Stanier, E. K. Watson, G. Bell, C. Wicking, X. Estivill, M. Courtney, A. Boue, P. S. Pedersen, R. Williamson, and M. Farrall. 1988. Isolation of a human gene with protein sequence similarity to human and murine int-1 and the *Drosophila* segment polarity mutant *wingless. EMBO J.* **7:** 1743–1748.

75. Roelink, H., J. Wang, D. M. Black, E. Solomon, and R. Nusse. 1993. Molecular cloning and chromosomal localization to 17q21 of the human WNT-3 gene. *Genomics* **17:** 790–792.

76. Clark, C. C., I. Cohen, I. Eichstetter, L. A. Cannizzaro, J. D. McPherson, J. J. Wasmuth, and R. V. Iozzo. 1993. Molecular cloning of the human proto-oncogene Wnt-5A and mapping of the gene (WNT5A) to chromosome 3p14-p21. *Genomics* **18:** 249–260.

77. Ikegawa, S., Y. Kumano, K. Okui, T. Fujiwara, E. Takahashi, and Y. Nakamura. 1996. Isolation, chracterization and chromosomal assignment of the human WNT7A gene. *Cytogenet. Cell. Genet.* **74(1–2):** 149–152.

78. van Bokhoven, H., J. Kissing, M. Schepens, S. van Beersum, A. Simons, P. Riegman, J. A. McMahon, A. P. McMahon, and H. G. Brunner. 1997. Assignment of WNT7B to human chromosome band 22q13 by in situ hybrization. *Cytogenet. Cell Genet.* **77:** 288–289.
79. Hardiman, G., R. A. Kastelein, and J. F. Bazan. 1997. Isolation, characterization and chromosomal localization of human WNT10B. *Cytogen. Cell Genet.* **77:** 278–282.
80. Katoh, M., M. Hirai, T. Sugimura, and M. Terada. 1996. Cloning, expression, and chromosomal localization of Wnt-13, a novel member of the Wnt gene family. *Oncogene* **13:** 873–876.

I
Etiology
Breast Cancer Genes

9

Hereditary Breast Cancer Genes

Lynda B. Bennett, Joel D. Taurog, and Anne M. Bowcock

1. INTRODUCTION

Most breast cancers arise in women without a family history of the disease. However, in 5–10% of cases, or 25% of cases diagnosed before age 30 yr, an inherited predisposition is proposed. As long ago as 1866, Paul Broca documented aggregation of breast cancer in certain families. In 1978, Lynch et al. *(1)* described 86 families with a high incidence of breast cancer. Twelve families also had ovarian cancer, and there was evidence for a highly penetrant dominant gene predisposing to either type of cancer. Many of these families also had cancers at other sites and individuals with two or more primary cancers.

Large epidemiological studies (segregation analyses) in the 1980s indicated that the pattern of breast cancer occurrence in families is consistent with a dominant susceptibility gene or genes *(2,3)*. The frequency of this highly penetrant susceptibility allele was proposed to be 0.0006 to 0.0033, conferring a lifetime risk of breast cancer of 0.82–0.92. Such strong evidence for a predisposing breast cancer allele(s) was sufficient for a number of groups to embark on a positional cloning effort to isolate such a gene (reviewed by Bowcock, 1993) *(4)*.

2. ISOLATION OF BRCA1

2.1. Linkage to Chromosome 17q21

In 1990, Mary-Claire King and her co-workers made the seminal observation that susceptibility to early onset breast cancer was sometimes linked to a locus on human chromosome 17q12-21 *(5)*. Her group had been performing a genome-wide linkage scan with 23 extended Caucasian families with 146 cases of breast cancer and 329 unaffected relatives. These families had not been selected on the basis of age at onset, and evidence for linkage to a locus on chromosome 17 was seen in families where the average age at diagnosis was less than 46. When all families were considered, the combined maximum LOD (logarithm of the odds) score was 2.35 at $\theta = 0.20$ with D17S74 (by convention, evidence for linkage is only provided when LOD > 3.0). When only early onset cases were considered (diagnosis below 46 yr), the LOD score increased to 5.98 at $\theta = 0.001$. In an extension of this study, Narod et al. *(6)* confirmed this finding

From: Breast Cancer: Molecular Genetics, Pathogenesis, and Therapeutics
Edited by: A. M. Bowcock © Humana Press Inc., Totowa, NJ

in five families with both breast and ovarian cancer, also indicating that the altered gene at 17q21 conferred predisposition to ovarian cancer. This gene was subsequently named "BRCA1" (BReast CAncer 1). Linkage to BRCA1 was also demonstrated for seven of nine families with multiple cases of ovarian cancer, but without cases of breast cancer ("site-specific ovarian cancer") *(7)*.

To obtain estimates of risk of breast/ovarian cancer conferred by an altered BRCA1 allele, and to determine the proportion of breast/ovarian cancer families likely to harbor an altered BRCA1 gene, an international Breast Cancer Linkage Consortium was established. This was comprised of 214 families (157 with breast cancer, 57 with breast and ovarian cancer) ascertained by 13 groups in the U.S. and Europe. Linkage analysis indicated that approximately 45% of families with three or more cases of breast cancer were linked to BRCA1 *(8)* with an estimated 87% lifetime risk for women in these families of developing breast cancer. It was also suggested that 76% of breast cancer families with one case of ovarian cancer, or 92% of families with two or more cases of ovarian cancer, harbor a BRCA1 alteration *(9)*. With the isolation of the BRCA1 gene and the identification of multiple mutations, risk estimates could be more reliably determined. Initially they appeared to differ little from the original risk estimates, indicating that by the age of 70 BRCA1 mutation carriers from high-risk families have an overall breast cancer risk of approximately 85% and an ovarian cancer risk of around 60% *(10)*. However, determining reliable risks of breast/ovarian cancer in the general population would require over 100,000 individuals *(11)*. It is now thought that risks in the general population may be lower, possibly as a result of genetic background (i.e., protective genes in the general population or additional predisposing genes in the high-risk families such as HRAS1 rare alleles *[12]*) (*see* **Subheading 7.1.** for further discussion). Two independent reports also indicate that approximately 10% of women diagnosed with breast cancer under the age of 35 harbor a BRCA1 alteration *(13,14)*.

2.2. Identification of the BRCA1 Gene

A positional cloning strategy is the standard approach when there are no clues about the identity of the protein involved in a disease. Following localization with genetic linkage analysis, the disease locus was first refined with additional recombinants from BRCA1-linked families *(15–19)*. This ultimately refined the location of BRCA1 to ~600 kb. In order to identify genes from the region, large, overlapping, recombinant DNA molecules containing sequences from the BRCA1 region were isolated. These included yeast artificial chromosomes (YACs), P1 clones, and cosmids that were assembled into a physical map of the region. Expressed transcripts were isolated with a variety of techniques, and extended and characterized in 17q linked families. In October 1994, Miki et al. *(20)* described the successful isolation of BRCA1. Variations in this gene were described in 5/8 17q21 linked kindreds, segregating with the BRCA1-linked haplotype. These variants included an 11 base pair deletion in codon 24, one a nonsense mutation in exon 11, one a single base pair insertion in exon 20, and one missense mutation in exon 21. All of these variants were proposed to disrupt protein function and three resulted in premature chain termination. Mutations resulting in protein truncations have subsequently been shown to be the most common disease lesions for both BRCA1 and BRCA2 (*see* **Subheading 3.** and **6.2.**).

3. BRCA1 STRUCTURE

BRCA1 is a large gene spanning over 81 kb of genomic sequence *(21)*. BRCA1 intron lengths range from 403 bp to 9.2 kb and comprise 91% of the overall sequence. The coding sequence is unusually AT-rich and contains a remarkably high proportion of charged residues. The gene has a particularly high density of Alu repeats (41.5%) but a relatively low density (4.8%) of other repetitive sequences. Recent findings suggest that genomic deletions owing to inter-*Alu* recombination are common and they may account for BRCA1 mutations in 36–44% of Dutch families *(22,23)*.

BRCA1 consists of 24 exons, (22 coding) that encodes a protein of 1863 amino acids *(20)* and an mRNA of 7.8 kb. After the gene had initially been described, it was discovered that one of the cDNA clones used to reconstruct the open reading frame was aberrant and that exon 4 was in fact an Alu repeat not present in the normal transcript. Nonetheless, the exon numbering was retained so that all subsequent maps of the coding region of the gene skip from exon 3 to exon 5. Exon 11 is unusually large, extending for 3.4 kb. Alternative splicing of exon 1 (a noncoding exon) creates two different transcripts *(24)*, one of which is predominantly expressed in the mammary gland and the other in the placenta. Gudas et al. *(25)* proposed that alternate splicing of the large exon (exon 11) leads to transcripts of 8 and 4.6 kb. Multiple tissue-specific BRCA1 transcripts have been observed by Thakur et al. *(26)* who detected at least three BRCA1 protein isoforms, including those lacking exon 11. Full length BRCA1 localized to the nucleus, whereas BRCA1 lacking exon 11 was detected in the cytoplasm. It is possible that alternate splicing of BRCA1 may play a role in the regulation of its function by altering the subcellular localization of different isoforms in various tissues.

Comparison of the BRCA1 sequence to databases of already existing sequences revealed very little homology to any known genes. However, one feature that was noted from the outset was a RING finger domain near the N-terminus (residues 20–68; exons 2–5). This has the basis structure Cys3HisCys4 and binds two Zn^{2+} ions. The sequence in BRCA1 is Cys-X2-Cys-X11-Cys-X-His-X2-Cys-X2-Cys-X13-Cys-X2-Cys, where Xn represents n residues other than Cys or His *(20)*. RING domains have been proposed to serve as an interface for recognition of DNA or for protein–protein interactions *(27,28)*. Several lines of evidence suggest that this region of BRCA1 is critical for its function: (i) Several missense mutations in either of the cysteine residues at positions 61 and 64 within the RING domain are among the cancer-associated inherited BRCA1 mutations, despite the fact that most of the cancer-associated mutations result in truncation of the protein *(29)*. Stoppa-Lyonnet et al. *(30)* also recently reported two novel mutations in the RING domain, that change amino acids conserved in the human and mouse (Cys47Tyr and Lys56Arg). (ii) There is a high degree of homology in the mouse and rat counterparts, compared to most of the gene, which only shares 58% homology overall with the mouse homolog *(31,32)*; in fact the 49 amino acid N-terminal RING finger domain is completely conserved between human, mouse, and rat. (iii) Breast tumors from individuals with mutations that disrupt the RING-finger domain tend to be associated with a higher grade mitotic index than tumors from individuals with BRCA1 mutation in the middle of the gene *(33)*.

A novel protein termed BARD1 (BRCA1-associated RING domain), interacts in vitro and in vivo with the RING domain of BRCA1 *(27)*. BARD1 itself contains an N-terminal RING domain, and also shares a conserved C-terminal domain with BRCA1.

It also has a domain not shared with BRCA1 that contains three ankyrin repeats. The BARD1 gene encodes a protein of ~750 amino acids and maps to 2q33-34, a region not known to be a common site of alteration in cancer. BARD1 fails to interact with BRCA1 proteins that have point mutations at cysteine residues 61 or 64, strongly suggesting that these residues are critical for the interaction, and that the interaction is therefore critical in tumor suppression. The interaction with BARD1 requires the N-terminal 101 amino acids of BRCA1, a segment that includes, but is somewhat larger than, the RING domain itself. The biological function of BARD1 remains to be discovered, but it evidently involves binding to BRCA1 as a heterodimer or as two components of a larger complex, disruption of which predisposes to tumor formation.

The C-terminus of BRCA1 is similarly highly conserved in mouse. Mutations in this domain, now termed the BRCT domain (residues 1528-1863; *see* Chapter 10 by Chew et al.) are associated with an increased risk of familial breast cancer *(34,35)*, and removal of as little as the last 10 amino acids leads to early-onset breast cancer *(36,37)*. This region was proposed to act as a transcriptional activator *(38)* when fused to the GAL4 DNA binding domain. Transcriptional activation was abolished when four different mutations in this sequence were introduced: Ala1708Gln, Pro1749Arg, Met1775Arg, and Tyr1853ter. Recent studies indicate that the BRCT domains interact in vivo with CtIP, a protein originally isolated on the basis of its interaction with the CtBP transcriptional co-repressor *(129)*. This suggests that BRCA1 may regulate gene expression by modulating CtBP-mediated transcriptional repression. Most mutations affecting the BRCT domain are frameshift or nonsense mutations, including the prevalent 5382insC mutation *(39)*. Two missense mutations at highly conserved positions within the BRCT domain have also been observed in high-risk women from France *(30)*: Ala1708Glu, previously reported by Futreal et al. *(40)* and a novel mutation, Arg1751Gln. Both Ala1708 and Arg1751 are conserved in the mouse, reinforcing their potential importance. Another missense mutation, Met1775Arg, which is associated with development of breast cancer *(20,40)*, has been reported several times to date in the BIC database. This methionine residue is conserved in the murine *Brca1*. Pro1749Arg is another mutation altering a conserved amino acid within a region that is highly conserved in mouse, and may be responsible for ovarian cancer *(34)*. Other potentially important mutations leading to amino acid changes have been reported according to the latest data available from the BIC database *(39)* (*see* Fig. 1). Some changes have not been proven to be disease causing mutations, and these are referred to in the BIC as unclassified variants.

Jensen et al. *(41)* reported a granin consensus sequence at residues 1214-1223. Granins are secreted proteins, some of which are located in secretory granules, particularly associated with neuroendocrine tissue. These authors presented evidence that BRCA1 is a secreted protein, but this has not been found by others. These motifs are not well conserved in other species *(42)*, and the claim that they have any sequence specificity has been criticized *(43)*.

Putative nuclear localization signals (NLSs) were predicted at amino acids 499 to 508 (NKLKRKRRP) (NLS1) and 610 to 616 (NRLRRKS) (NLS2), which are similar to sequences found in steroid hormone receptor molecules such as estrogen and progesterone *(26,44)*. No missense mutations have been reported to date within these sequences. The human amino acid sequences at each putative nuclear localization signal are identical to the mouse protein for 7/9 and 7/7 residues, respectively. Thakur and co-workers

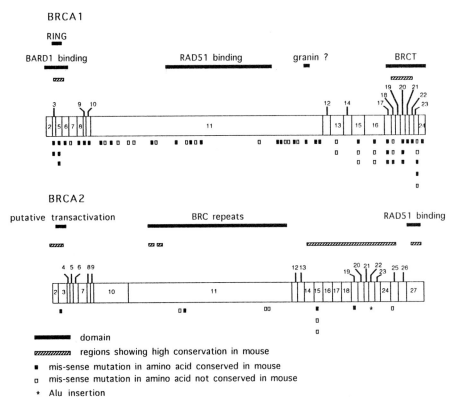

Fig. 1. Missense mutations in BRCA1 and BRCA2. The figure shows missense mutations reported in the BIC up to 6/98. Solid shaded bars indicate potentially functional domains in the two genes. Hatched bars indicate those regions shown to have high conservation between the human and mouse genes. Mutations that alter amino acids that are identical in mouse are shown as solid blocks, mutations that change nonconserved amino acids are shown as nonshaded blocks.

examined the functional significance of these two potential NLSs and found that deletion of NLS1 but not NLS2 disrupts nuclear localization *(26)*. Conservation between mouse and human indicates functional significance for these domains; however, this is not substantiated by the presence of any missense mutations within these regions.

Recent studies suggest that BRCA1 transactivates the expression of $p21^{WAF1/CIP1}$. Mutants of BRCA1, which lack a functional nuclear localization signal, C-terminal transactivation domain, or the *RAD51*-interacting domain are deficient in this activity. Activity was also deficient in the three tumor-associated transactivation-deficient mutants; Pro1749Arg, Tyr1753Arg, and Q1756insC *(45)*.

Brca1 and a DNA repair protein, *Rad51* colocalize in vivo and also co-immunoprecipitate in vitro *(46)* (*see also* Chapter 10 by Chew et al.). The region of BRCA1 shown to bind *Rad51* extends from amino acids 758-1064. Six missense mutations within this region have been reported (BIC 1997) (Fig. 1), three of which involve conserved amino acid residues.

4. ISOLATION OF BRCA2

Even before the BRCA1 gene was cloned, several lines of evidence pointed to at least one other dominant susceptibility gene. The main evidence was failure to show linkage to 17q21 for 45% of the high risk breast cancer families, particularly those without ovarian cancer. Another clue was the finding that of the several families with breast cancer in males as well as females, none showed linkage to BRCA1.

Linkage of HBC to a second locus, BRCA2, on chromosome 13q12-13 was reported in the fall of 1994, just a few weeks before the report identifying the gene for BRCA1 *(47)*. The work was the result of a large international collaboration, centered at the Institute of Cancer Research in the U.K., where a genome-wide linkage screen had been performed in 15 high-risk breast cancer families that failed to show linkage to BRCA1, and then in December 1995, Wooster and colleagues *(48)* reported the identification of BRCA2.

5. BRCA2 STRUCTURE

The open reading frame they described was 7.3 kb, but Northern analysis showed a transcript of 10–12 kb. The entire coding sequence and intron/exon structure was later elucidated by Tavtigian and co-workers *(49)*. The composite BRCA2 cDNA sequence consists of 11,385 bp, not including the polyadenylation signal or poly(A) tail. The gene is composed of 27 exons (26 coding exons) distributed over roughly 70 kb of genomic DNA, and like BRCA1 has an unusually high AT content. The predicted open reading frame begins at nucleotide 229 in exon 2 and encodes a protein of 3,418 amino acids. No similarity was detected with other proteins, there was no signal sequence at the N-terminus, and there were no obvious membrane-spanning regions. The only region where any previously described motif could be recognized lies in exon 11, which contains eight repeated domains, now termed BRC repeats *(50)*. Although the function of these BRC repeats has yet to be discerned, comparison of exon 11 sequences from six mammalian species showed a conserved 26 amino acid core within each of the eight BRC repeats found in all six species *(51)*, suggesting a conserved function for this region. There are four reported missense mutations within this region, but only one of these alters a conserved residue (Fig. 1).

Despite the lack of any sequence homology, remarkable similarities between BRCA2 and BRCA1 were immediately evident. The highest levels of BRCA2 expression were observed in breast, thymus, and testis, with slightly lower levels in lung, ovary, and spleen, a pattern very similar to that seen for BRCA1. Both genes are very large, with over 20 exons, both have a large exon 11, translational start sites in exon 2, and coding sequences that are AT-rich, both encode proteins that are highly charged with about one-fourth of the residues being acidic or basic, and both span >70 kb of genomic DNA.

Analysis of the BRCA2 gene in affected families by numerous groups showed that mutations in BRCA2, like those in BRCA1, are scattered throughout the coding region *(39,48,49,52–58)*.

Early estimates were that BRCA2 alterations exist in ~8% of families with three or more cases of breast cancer diagnosed in women < 50 years of age and in 18–25% of breast cancer families with least one case of male breast cancer *(55,56)*. More recently 73 women with breast cancer diagnosed at ≤32 yr of age were examined *(59)*. Only two BRCA2 mutations were found (3%), along with eight BRCA1 mutations (11%).

The mouse *Brca2* gene has been cloned and sequenced *(42,60)*. The gene is localized to mouse chromosome 5 in a region that is syntenic to human chromosome 13q12-13. Murine *Brca2* encodes a 3328 amino acid protein, 90 amino acids shorter than its human counterpart. Like *Brca1*, *Brca2* is relatively poorly conserved overall between human and mouse (59% identity; 72% similarity); however, there are several domains that show higher similarity *(60)*. A 100 amino acid region at the amino acid termini has 84% similarity between the mouse and human BRCA2. One missense mutation has been identified in this region (Tyr42Cys), which is at a conserved amino acid in the mouse gene, and may therefore be of functional importance. An 86% similarity exists between the two proteins from amino acids 2400 to 3075 near the carboxy terminus of the mouse gene. There are also three 50 amino acids regions that are highly conserved (90–96% similarity), two of which show 74% and 78% identity in mouse and human as well as in dog, African green monkey, and Chinese hamster which indicates that these domains may be functionally significant *(60)*. No missense mutations have been reported within these domains up to date.

BRCA2 protein has also been shown to associate with Rad51 *(61)*. In a yeast two-hybrid assay the C-terminal region (a.a. 3138–3232) of murine Brca2 interacts with Rad51. The interaction was confirmed in mammalian cells. This region shows 72% identity with human BRCA2, which suggests that it may be functionally significant.

When the BRCA2 sequence was initially reported, it was suggested that there was weak homology between residues 1094–1174 of BRCA2 and a region of BRCA1 *(48)*; however, judging by the poor conservation between the mouse and human homologs within this region, this may be coincidental rather than functionally significant.

6. MUTATIONAL ANALYSIS OF BRCA1 AND BRCA2

6.1. Techniques for Mutation Detection

The identification and sequencing of the BRCA genes has spurred many studies involving a search for BRCA2 mutations in familial and sporadic breast and ovarian cancers. So far, no functional assays are available, and therefore all mutation detection has to be carried out at the DNA level. This detection is not a trivial matter technically, since the genes are quite large and mutations are distributed throughout their length. The sizes of the genes generally precludes brute-force sequencing of the entire genomic sequence or even of all of the exons, as a screening procedure. Two major types of methods of detection have been used to screen for mutations. The first is the single strand conformation polymorphism (SSCP) assay *(62,63)*. Using this strategy, primer pairs can be used that will amplify short fragments of the gene in question, optimally ≤200 bp (*see*, for example, Friedman et al., 1994; Langston et al., 1996) *(13,36)*. The amplified product is denatured and then subjected to electrophoresis in a nondenaturing acrylamide gel. Secondary conformations of the DNA strands affect their migration in the gel, frequently permitting the identification of samples with slight alterations in DNA sequence on the basis of alteration in mobility. The aberrant band can then be isolated from the gel and sequenced to find the mutation. Overall, the sensitivity of this procedure is ~60%. Many investigators currently prefer heteroduplex methods that are predicted to have 95–99% sensitivity. Another major form of detection is the protein truncation test *(14,59,64)*. Since the majority of mutant BRCA1 and BRCA2 alleles encode truncated proteins, PCR products can be generated either from genomic DNA, as described above, or from cDNA fragments, and then studied in a transcription/translation system in which the protein products are generated and analyzed for size by gel electrophoresis.

The aforementioned methods for mutation detection are both time-consuming and expensive. Hacia and colleagues *(65)* described the use of a "DNA chip" to detect mutations in BRCA1. This could be a highly sensitive, high throughput assay for mutations. Similar approaches are being developed for the detection of mutations in the *CFTR* gene *(66)*, the HIV-1 reverse transcriptase and protease genes *(67,68)*, the β-globin gene *(69)*, and the mitochondrial genome *(70)*. Hacia and co-workers used was a two-color assay based on the hybridization of fluorescently labeled RNA targets to a high-density array of oligonucleotides on a solid surface. RNA from both the wild-type gene (fluorescein-labeled) and from a patient sample (biotinylated and subsequently stained with phycoerythrin–streptavidin conjugate) were competitively co-hybridized to a chip that had over 96,600 oligonucleotides designed to enable the detection of all possible single base substitutions or insertions, and 1–5 base deletions in exon 11. Relative ratios of fluorescent signals from wild-type and test samples were measured and analyzed. Either a gain or loss of signal indicates the presence of a mutation in the patient DNA. Mutations were successfully detected in 14 out of 15 patients known to harbor mutations in this exon. They reported no false positives.

As discussed below, in certain populations with a high frequency of a particular mutation, the situation can be simplified by screening for specific alterations. However, this can be problematic as illustrated in a study by Schubert et al. *(58)* where a set of 17 Ashkenazi Jewish women from families with ≥4 cases of breast or ovarian cancer were screened for alterations in BRCA1 or BRCA2 known to be common to this population. Mutations were only detected in half the women studied, leaving one with the question of whether these women had an alteration in an undiscovered BRCA gene, or whether they had a mutation in BRCA1/2 not yet described for this population.

6.2. Mutations in BRCA1 and BRCA2

Approximately 182 separate mutations have been reported in BRCA1 associated with breast or ovarian cancer *(39,71)*. BRCA2 mutations have been described by a number of groups *(35,48,49,56)*, but the most recent analysis of BRCA2 (D. Goldgar, personal communication) showed 111 distinct deleterious mutations, of which 84 (76%) have been reported in only one individual or family. In both genes, mutations are scattered throughout their length with the large exons containing a comparable share of the mutations. In an initial collaborative study *(29)* three primary mutations in BRCA1 were noted: A mutation in exon 2 within the ring finger domain (185delAG) that accounted for approximately 12% of BRCA1 mutations, a mutation in exon 20 (5382insC) that accounted for ~10% of mutations, and a mutation within exon 11 (4184del4) that was slightly less common. Table 1 summarizes the frequency of the different types of mutations found in BRCA1 and BRCA2. These include interstitial deletions or insertions of one or a few bases that generate frameshifts, base substitutions that generate a termination codon (nonsense mutations), mutations at splice junctions that result in a frameshift and premature termination or in deletion of an exon and missense mutations resulting in a single amino acid substitution. These proportions may be an underestimate if SSCP and PTT were used as neither of these methods are reliable for the detection of missense changes.

In the case of BRCA1 the most 5' mutation truncates all but the N-terminal 22 amino acids, whereas the most 3' mutation truncates only the C-terminal 10 amino acids. In

Table 1
Mutation Types in BRCA1 and BRCA2[a]

Gene	BRCA1	BRCA2
Mutation type		
Frameshifts	70%	68%
Nonsense mutations	20%	12%
Splice site	5%	7%
Missense	5%	13%

[a]Information on BRCA2 kindly provided by Dr. D. Goldgar (personal communication).

the case of BRCA2, no mutations have been reported in the two C-terminal exons (Fig. 1). A small number of families have been studied that show strong linkage of HB/OC (hereditary breast and/or ovarian cancer) to 17q21, but in which no abnormalities of the BRCA1 gene have been found. These appear to be predominantly genomic deletions *(36,72)*. Some of these alterations result in the absence of an mRNA transcript, with the site of the mutation being unknown. There is also an intriguing description of a woman from Scotland, U.K., who is homozygous for a BRCA1 mutation (2800delAA) and therefore homozygous for a truncated BRCA1 protein *(73)*.

Many polymorphisms have been described for both BRCA1 and BRCA2. In some cases it can be difficult to distinguish between a functional, normal polymorphism and a disease-associated missense mutation. In general, alterations resulting in premature termination of the polypeptide can be considered as mutations; however, this is not always the case and some protein truncation mutations can be shown to be polymorphisms. For example, a polymorphism at the 3' end of BRCA2 region has been described that deletes the terminal 93 amino acids with no apparent deleterious effects *(74)*. If the variant allele has a nonconservative substitution, particularly in a residue that is shared between the human and mouse genes, and if it cosegregates with cancer in families, then it seems reasonable to consider it at least provisionally as a disease-associated mutation *(30)*. This difficulty will presumably be obviated once functional assays for the wild-type proteins are established.

7. POPULATION GENETICS OF BRCA1 AND BRCA2 MUTATIONS

7.1. Distribution of BRCA1 and BRCA2 Inherited Mutations

To date, inherited mutations of BRCA1 and/or BRCA2 have been examined in HBC/HBOC families from the U.S., Austria, Belgium, Canada, Denmark, Finland, France, Germany, Holland, Israel, Italy, Japan, Norway, Russia, Sweden, and the U.K. In some of these studies, unselected patients with breast or ovarian cancer have also been examined. The results from these studies have been summarized in a recent review *(75)*, which examines the frequencies of particular mutations in high-risk families and populations of unselected patients. A number of interesting conclusions were drawn from these integrated data.

The proportion of high-risk HB/OC families with BRCA1 mutations varies widely, ranging from a high of 79% in Russia to ~10% in Japan and even less in Iceland. In European countries apart from Iceland, the proportion ranges from 14 to 29%. In the

U.S., Canada, and Israel, the proportions are 39, 40, and 47%, respectively. As discussed in more detail in **Subheading 7.3.**, there is a very high prevalence of mutant BRCA1 genes in Jewish populations, and the higher frequencies found in North American families may in part reflect inclusion of a number of Jewish families in these studies. Some of the variation may be due to ascertainment. For example, the Russian families all had at least two cases of ovarian cancer.

Couch et al. *(71)* examined 169 women with breast cancer and a familial risk factor (average of 4.0 breast, and 1.5 ovarian, cancer cases per family) for BRCA1 mutations; 15% reported Ashkenazi Jewish ancestry, and only the founder mutations 185delAG and 5382insC mutations were found in these families. The overall frequency of BRCA1 mutations was surprisingly low (16% overall vs 26% in the Jewish families), and did not correlate with either number of breast cancers per family or with number of cases of bilateral breast cancer. Higher frequencies of BRCA1 mutations in patients with familial breast cancer previously reported could be due to an ascertainment bias introduced by the selection of families with ovarian cancer cases as well as breast cancer. The authors predict that mutations in BRCA1 and BRCA2 may only account for 40–50% of hereditary breast cancer cases as opposed to previous estimates of 90%.

In almost all countries where mutations in both genes have been examined, the proportion of high-risk HB/OC families with BRCA1 mutations is higher than that for BRCA2, by a factor of ~1.5–2.0 The most dramatic exception is Iceland, where most families have been found to have a single BRCA2 mutation, and only one family has been reported with a BRCA1 mutation. In Israel, 24% of the HB/OC families were found to have a BRCA2 mutation. In U.S. and Canadian families, the percentages are 25 and 16, respectively.

Most studies where reduced penetrance has been observed for BRCA2 compared to BRCA1 have been with early onset cases. The lifetime risk is probably not different between BRCA1 and BRCA2, but the risk of developing breast cancer at an early age may be lower for BRCA2 carriers.

In at least 50–60% of high-risk families, no mutations in either BRCA1 or BRCA2 have been detected. This group includes some very striking families, including three Hungarian families with ≥6 cases of breast or ovarian cancer *(76)*; 4 of 25 Swedish families with breast cancer and ≥2 cases of ovarian cancer *(77)*; and 15 of 23 U.S. families with ≥3 cases of female breast cancer and ≥1 case at age <45 yr *(78)*. These observations support the possibility of at least one additional BRCA gene.

The nature of the mutations within different individual populations reveals some striking contrasts that reflect the widely differing histories of those populations. Perhaps the most dramatic example of a founder mutation that has become widespread within a population is the finding of a single mutation, BRCA2 999delTCAAA (999del5), in 16 of 21 high-risk families in Iceland *(49,57,79,80)*. Outside of Iceland, this mutation has only been found in two families in Finland *(81)*. Further studies of the BRCA2 999del5 mutation in Iceland are discussed in **Subheading 7.2.**

In Russia, 9 of 14 families with predominantly ovarian cancer shared the BRCA1 mutation, 5382insC, which is also widely distributed throughout Europe, whereas other mutant alleles, 4153delA (three families) and 2073delA (one family), have so far not been observed outside of Russia.

In a more extreme case of private alleles, most of the BRCA1 mutations found in Italian high-risk families have been uniquely found only in one family *(82–84)*. For example, in an analysis of 20 high-risk families from the Tuscany region, five separate mutations were found in seven families *(83)*. Three of the families shared one of the mutations, 1499insA. Although these families were thought to be unrelated, in two of them that could be tested, there was evidence for sharing of a common ancestral haplotype. Altogether, 19 of 25 Italian BRCA1 mutations are unique to individual families *(75)*.

The mutations can thus be classified as recurring or unique in distribution, although obviously mutations initially appearing as unique can subsequently be found to be recurring. Szabo and King *(75)* apply the term "ancient" to recurring mutations that are either national or international in distribution. Both types of recurrent mutations have been found in most European countries. For example, of eight recurrent BRCA1 and six recurrent BRCA2 mutations found in the U.K., six and three, respectively, have been found in other European countries, whereas the remainder have been found only within the U.K or in the U.K. and North America alone *(75)*. A study investigating 643 high-risk HBOC families from Holland and 23 from Belgium *(85)* identified BRCA1 mutations in approximately 10% of the families. Of 28 distinct mutations found, 17 have not been reported outside of the Low Countries. This included one, 2804delAA, which was found in 19 different families from six different centers in Holland, but has so far not been identified anywhere outside of Holland. Five other mutations have not been found in any other European country, and only two of these have been found outside of Holland, in each case in one family in the U.S. There was evidence for a common 17q21 haplotype for each of nine different recurring mutations, suggesting a common ancestor in each case. Different statistical methods were applied to the haplotype data to estimate the age of the 2804delAA mutation, with results ranging from 15 to 49 generations.

Of the recurrent mutations (27 BRCA1 and 14 BRCA2) described in Europe and Israel, approximately half (14 BRCA1 and 7 BRCA2) have been reported in the U.S. and/or Canada. In addition, 31 and 22 novel mutations in BRCA1 and BRCA2, respectively, have been reported in the U.S. and Canada.

As noted above, studies of familial aggregation of breast and ovarian cancer led to the prediction of a highly penetrant dominant allele predisposing to the HBOC syndrome, with a predicted population frequency of 0.0006 to 0.0033 and cumulative lifetime risk for breast cancer of ~80–90% within high-risk families *(2,3)*. The subsequent identification of BRCA1 and BRCA2, and the mutations in these genes associated with HBOC, strikingly confirmed most of these predictions. However, the frequency of these mutations in general populations has been more difficult to determine because of the great technical burden required to screen for large numbers of mutations in large numbers of individuals. An estimate based on assumptions from the family BRCA1 data placed the BRCA1 gene frequency at 0.0006 *(86)*.

7.2. An Icelandic Founder Mutation in BRCA2

Populations with a limited number of mutations are more amenable to population-based screening. As noted above, the BRCA2 999del5 mutation was found in a high proportion of familial breast cancer in Iceland. Iceland was settled in the 9th century by people from western Norway and from Ireland *(75,79)*. The population is thought to have remained at ~50,000–60,000 for several centuries until about 100 years ago, and the current population is comprised of ~265,000 members. The BRCA2 999del5 mutation appears to be a classic founder mutation, with a common haplotype harboring the mutant allele and at least six families traced back to a common ancestor in the 16th century (11–12 generations) *(57)*. To examine the frequency of this mutation in the general population and in patients with breast cancer Thorlacius *(57)* screened a random population of 520 Icelanders (~0.2% of the entire population), and tissue samples from 632 unselected women with breast cancer (23% of female breast cancer during the past 40 yr) and 30 men with breast cancer (100% of all cases during the past 40 yr) for the BRCA2 999del5 mutation. The mutant allele was found in three individuals of the sample population, i.e., 0.6%. This is 10-fold higher than the estimated frequency of all BRCA1 mutations *(86)*. The mutation was found in 16.6% of all women with breast cancer diagnosed at age ≤50 yr, and 7.7% of all women with breast cancer. This is similar to the 8.5% frequency of the mutation found in another sample of 459 Icelandic women with breast cancer *(80)*, although it is not clear how much overlap there was between the two populations. The median age of onset of breast cancer in the women with the mutation was 45 yr vs 60 yr for the women without the mutation. The oldest age of diagnosis for a mutation carrier was 77 yr. Of the cancer patients with the mutation, there were 61 whose family histories could be analyzed. Only nine had no first-, second-, or third-degree relatives with breast cancer. As will be seen, these data are largely consistent with those obtained from studies of BRCA1 and BRCA2 mutations in a population very different from Icelanders but also with a high population frequency of mutations, namely, Ashkenazi Jews.

7.3. BRCA1 and BRCA2 Founder Mutations in the Ashkenazi Jewish Population

7.3.1. The Origins of the Ashkenazi Jewish Population

The identification of two founder mutations, one in BRCA1 and the other in BRCA2, existing at frequencies of ~1% in the Ashkenazi Jewish population has been cause for concern and interest and is discussed in detail in **Subheadings 7.3.2.–7.3.5.** The term Ashkenazi is somewhat imprecise, but is generally used to refer to Jews originating, at least in recent centuries, from Europe, particularly Central and Eastern Europe. The name Ashkenaz is mentioned in *Genesis* as one of the descendants of Noah's son, Japheth (*Genesis 10:3*). Most classical commentators, including the Jerusalem Talmud, interpret this to be a reference to an Asiatic nation *(87)*. The name Ashkenaz is also mentioned in *Jeremiah 51:27*, as one of the kingdoms destined to conquer Babylon, again likely an Asiatic nation *(88)*. In later Jewish literature, Ashkenaz came to denote Germany. The first existing mention of the term in this context dates from the 9th century *(87)*. The term is definitely used with this meaning by the famous 11th century commentator, Rashi (Rabbi Shlomo ben Yitzhak, 1040–1105), who lived most of his life in northern France (*see* commentary to *Deut. 3:5*).

Jewish settlement in Western Europe dates back to antiquity, perhaps even before the return from the Babylonian exile ~350 BCE *(89)*. There were undoubtedly Jewish settlements throughout France and Germany during the era of Roman conquest of these areas. It is estimated that these settlements numbered approximately 1 million in population at the beginning of the 4th century CE, but their numbers diminished considerably following the rise of Christianity and fall of the Roman Empire, and it is estimated that at most a population of 10,000 survived as Jews by the end of the 8th century *(89,90)*. Modern recorded Jewish history in Western Europe dates from the time of Charlemagne (742–814). Under his reign, the Jewish population in France and Germany increased, with Jews immigrating to these communities from Italy, the Balkans, Babylonia (present day Iraq), and Asia Minor. This nuclear Ashkenazi population grew in succeeding centuries, but the founder population of "five to ten thousand souls who survived as Jews in Italy, Germany, and France by the end of the 8th century, were the true ancestors of the Ashkenazic Jews of the past 12 centuries...in the sense that all the Yiddish-speaking Jews of the year 1900, numbering more than 10 million, were the descendants of these five to ten thousand" *(89,90)*.

Between the 8th and 11th centuries, the Ashkenazi population in France and Germany grew and developed. However, beginning with the first crusade at the end of the 11th century, and continuing in subsequent centuries, frequent persecutions, expulsions, pogroms, and massacres at the hands of the larger population drove the surviving Ashkenazi population eastward. Throughout the 14th and 15th centuries, Jews from the west emigrated in increasing numbers to Poland, Lithuania, Bohemia, and neighboring areas of Central and Eastern Europe *(89,91)*. As previously noted, it is primarily these emigres who are thought to be the ancestors of the modern Ashkenazi population, members of which have been studied for BRCA mutations, as described in **Subheadings 7.3.2.–7.3.5.**

Much has been written regarding the Mendelian genetic disorders that have an increased prevalence in the Ashkenazi population, including Gaucher, Tay-Sachs, Niemann-Pick, and Canavan diseases, idiopathic torsion dystonia, cystic fibrosis, Bloom syndrome, mucolipidosis IV, familial dysautonomia, factor XI deficiency, pentosuria, and nonclassical 21-hydroxylase deficiency *(92,93)*. There is general agreement that founder effects probably account for much of the data, but the potential contributions of genetic drift and selective heterozygote advantage in some of these disorders has been controversial *(92,94–96)*.

7.3.2. The BRCA1 185delAG Mutation

Following the isolation of the BRCA1 gene, it was soon apparent that a number of families shared a single mutation, 185delAG. Further investigation revealed that these families were all of Ashkenazi Jewish origin *(29,97–101)*. Moreover, haplotype analysis indicated that the apparently unrelated families sharing this mutation also shared a common haplotype for the 17q21 chromosomal region carrying the mutation *(97,98,100)*. Struewing et al. *(98)* tested DNA samples from 858 unrelated Ashkenazi individuals from the U.S. and Israel who had previously sought genetic testing for Tay-Sachs disease and/or cystic fibrosis. A total of eight individuals with the 185delAG mutation were found, compared with none out of a mixed ethnic control group of 815 individuals. This result suggested a frequency of this single mutation of 0.9% in the Ashkenazi population, up to 15-fold higher than the predicted frequency of all BRCA1 mutations in the general population *(86)*.

The findings concerning 185delAG were rapidly confirmed and extended *(14,54, 102–104)*. The mutation is carried by 20% of Ashkenazi Jewish women diagnosed with breast cancer before age 42 yr, chosen without regard to family history; 35% of Ashkenazi

Jewish women with an affected first degree relative carry the mutation compared with 10% with no family history; and 30% of women with breast cancer diagnosed between 42 and 50 and with a family history of early onset breast or ovarian cancer carry the mutation. There is also a strong correlation of the mutation with familial ovarian cancer: 40% of women with ovarian cancer and a first-degree relative with breast or ovarian cancer have the 185delAG mutation, in contrast to 13% of women without an affected first degree relative. These studies contrast with a similar population-based study in a predominantly non-Jewish Caucasian group of women with breast cancer diagnosed before age 35 in which <10% of the women had a cancer-associated BRCA1 mutation *(13)*. The study of Modan et al. *(103)* is also significant in that one of the patients with the 185delAG mutation is from an Iraqi Jewish family, suggesting that the mutation may be prevalent in non-Ashkenazi Jews as well. The 185delAG mutation has also been seen on a haplotype distinct from the one found in the majority of Jewish families (including two families from Yorkshire, U.K., and four families of Moroccan origin), suggesting the likelihood of at least two independent origins for the mutation *(54,105,106)*.

A second BRCA1 mutation, 188del11 was reported by a single group, and was seen in 10 individuals, including 4 Jewish individuals with breast and/or ovarian cancer *(54)*. This mutation has not been found in any other study of Jewish or non-Jewish subjects.

7.3.3. The BRCA2 6174delT Mutation

Within months of the cloning of the BRCA2 gene, mutational analyses of additional HB/OC families were published. Tavtigian et al. *(49)* reported nine mutations in addition to the six described in the initial report by Wooster et al. *(48)*. Among these was a mutation in exon 11, 6174delT, identified in an individual of Ashkenazi Jewish descent. This prompted an analysis of Ashkenazi Jewish women with early onset breast cancer who had previously been examined for BRCA1 mutations. Investigators at Sloan Kettering in New York *(107)* selected Ashkenazi Jewish women who had had breast cancer before age 42, without regard to family history; 8% carried the BRCA2 6174delT mutation; and 38% of these had either a personal or family history of ovarian cancer.

7.3.4. Prevalence of Founder Mutations in the Ashkenazi Jewish Population

Oddoux et al. *(108)* and Roa et al. *(109)* found that 1–1.5% of Ashkenazi Jewish women harbored the BRCA2 6174delT mutation and did not find it among non-Jewish subjects. This frequency is comparable to that of the BRCA1 185delAG mutation, although as noted above, the studies of cancer patients and high risk families suggested a lower relative risk of breast or ovarian cancer associated with the BRCA2 mutation, compared with the BRCA1 mutation.

Roa et al. *(109)* also found the 5382insC mutation in 0.15% of the Ashkenazi Jewish women from the U.S., but did not find it in women from Israel.

When the three mutations, BRCA1 185delAG, 5382insC, and BRCA2 6174delT were considered in Jewish families from the U.S. and Canada with a minimum of two cases of breast cancer, and at least one diagnosed <50 yr *(110)*, 45.5% of families; were found to carry one of the three mutations; 41% carried the BRCA1 mutations, and only 4% carried the BRCA2 mutation, despite the higher frequency of this latter mutation in the Ashkenazi populations previously surveyed. This suggests a low penetrance for this allele. The prevalence of BRCA1 or BRCA2 mutations is substantially higher in families with both breast and ovarian cancer, and reaches an astounding 89% in families with two or more cases of ovarian cancer. Apart from this higher prevalence of ovarian cancer, there is little else that distinguishes the families with mutations from those in which no mutation was found. Rather strikingly, none of the four families in which there were cases of breast cancer at an extremely young age (<25 yr) showed mutations. These families also showed a high prevalence of other cancers

Abeliovich et al. *(111)* studied individual patients from Israel with breast or ovarian cancer and showed that approximately 50% of women with ovarian cancer and nearly all women with both breast and ovarian cancer harbor one of these changes. Nearly all carriers were found to have an affected first-degree relative. Both the 185delAG and 6174delT mutations had a similar prevalence among the carriers, but the 5382insC mutation was not found in any of the patients with ovarian cancer. Cancers at sites other than the breast or ovary were reported in many of the families.

7.3.5. Cancer Risk Conferred by BRCA Founder Mutations in the Ashkenazi Jewish Population

These studies examining both BRCA1 and BRCA2 confirmed that the recurrent BRCA mutations are very common in women in the Ashkenazi population with familial breast and ovarian cancer. However, the risk of breast or ovarian cancer in healthy carriers had not been determined. These findings emphasized the need for population-based studies to assess more accurately the true risk of carrying the BRCA1 and BRCA2 mutations and to provide further data to assess the feasibility of population screening and genetic counseling. In an effort to address this Struewing et al. *(112)* recruited over 5,000 Jewish men and women over age 20 in the Washington, DC area. Over half of these subjects were ≥50 yr old and 70% were women. A total of 120 participants were found to carry one of the three common mutations (2.26%). The overall frequencies of the BRCA1 185delAG and BRCA2 6174delT mutations, (0.8% and 1.2%) were similar to those previously reported, whereas the frequency of the BRCA1 5382insC mutation (0.4%) was substantially higher than previously found. A number of important conclusions could be drawn from this study, based on the personal and family histories of the participants: Mutations in both BRCA1 and BRCA2 were associated with a substantially increased risk of breast and ovarian cancer. The combined estimated risk of breast cancer by the age of 50 among carriers was 33%, compared with 4.5% for noncarriers; by age 70, these figures were 56% and 13%. For ovarian cancer, carriers showed a risk of 7% by age 50 and 16% by age 70, compared with risks of 0.4% and 1.2%, respectively, in noncarriers. A slightly lower estimated risk was observed among carriers of the BRCA2 6174delT mutation compared to BRCA1 185delAG carriers (26% vs 34% below age 50), however, the difference was small and the breast cancer risks associated with each of the three mutations were not significantly dissimilar. This observation was contrary to previous studies of small samples of Jewish women with early-onset breast cancer, which suggested that the risk of early-onset breast cancer was much lower for carriers of the 6174delT mutation compared to carriers of 185delAG *(14,102,108,109,113)*. Similarly, Struewing and colleagues saw no significant difference in risk estimates for ovarian cancer for the three mutations. Although subjects with a family history of breast or ovarian cancer were more likely to have a mutation, there were 31 carriers identified who did not report any breast or ovarian cancer in either first or second degree relatives. At least five of these carriers had three or more first degree female relatives over 40 *(112)*.

These data cannot be considered a completely unbiased sample of the Ashkenazi population, since over 5% of the participants were women who had survived breast or ovarian cancer, and 20% of the participants reported at least one first-degree relative with breast or ovarian cancer. This probable bias would tend to inflate the estimate of risk associated with the mutations. Nonetheless, these are the most comprehensive population data so far available. Considering the probable overestimate of true risk attributable to the nonrandom nature of the study population, the risk of cancer seems to be lower than lifetime risk of 85% attributed to BRCA1 carriers in high-risk families *(8)*. Various manipulations of the data to reduce the effects of biased sampling led to a predicted carrier-associated risk of breast cancer of 42–54% by age 70. Most likely, this difference from 85% is attributable to modifying genetic factors, but environmental or statistical factors may also explain part of the difference. Nonetheless, the sobering conclusion remains that at least 2.5% of Jewish women have up to a 60% lifetime risk of breast or ovarian cancer.

7.3.6. The BRCA1 185delAG Mutation in Non-Ashkenazi Jews

As noted in **Subheading 7.3.5.**, several studies have identified the BRCA1 185delAG mutation in women with breast or ovarian cancer living in Israel who are of Iraqi or Iranian Jewish descent *(103,111,113,114)*. There are as yet no published data on the prevalence of any of the mutations in non-Ashkenazi Jewish populations, but Modan et al., have unpublished data showing a 0.5% prevalence of the 185delAG mutation in Iraqi Jewish women in Israel (3 out of 600 in a population survey; with at least one 17q21 haplotype matching that of the Ashkenazi mutation) (B. Modan, personal communication). It is not currently clear if the 185delAG mutation antedates the dispersion of the Jewish people in Roman times or arose earlier, as proposed by Szabo and King *(75)*. At this point, one can only speculate on the basis of inadequate data. The Jewish communities of Iran and Iraq are among the oldest continuous Jewish communities, commencing with the Babylonian exile in the 5th century BCE and continuing up to our own time *(89)*. Following the destruction by the Romans of the Second Temple and subsequent Roman persecutions of the Jewish population in the Land of Israel in the 1st and 2nd centuries CE, the Jewish community in Babylonia (present day Iraq) became the dominant Jewish community in the world for the next eight centuries. The ascent of Islam after the 7th century coincided with somewhat of a decline in the fortunes of the Babylonian Jewish community, and over the next few centuries there was a substantial emigration from this community, primarily to North Africa and Spain. As noted in **Subheading 7.3.5.**, there was evidently also some immigration from Babylonia into the Ashkenazi population in the 8th and/or 9th century, and it is conceivable that the founder gene in the Ashkenazi population was actually introduced during this period of immigration. Alternatively, the mutation may have been transferred from West to East during the period when the Babylonian community was the center of the Jewish world *(111)*. However, as speculated by Szabo and King *(75)* and by Modan (personal communication), the mutation might have existed in the Jewish population in the time of the Second Temple or even before. Additional genetic epidemiologic studies are required to answer the question of the origin of this mutation.

8. MALE BREAST CANCER

As noted above, BRCA2 was originally mapped by studying families with cases of male breast cancer, since this entity did not seem to be a part of BRCA1-linked HBC. A number of cases of male breast cancer have indeed been found in families with BRCA2 mutations, as well as two cases in families with BRCA1 mutations *(48,49, 56,64,76,115–117)*. Since male breast cancer is rare (~1,000 new cases annually in the U.S.), it might be expected that a high percentage of apparently sporadic cases would have a genetic basis, and the role of germline mutations in the BRCA genes could be assessed by screening for mutations in patients unselected for family history. As described above, 40% of the 30 male breast cancer cases recorded in Iceland during the past 40 yr were associated with the BRCA2 999del5 mutation. However, in a study of a more diverse population, Friedman et al. *(118)* examined 54 male breast cancer cases from southern California. Sixteen had a first- or second-degree relative affected with breast and/or ovarian cancer. Two patients (4% of the total) carried a novel truncating mutation in the BRCA2 gene and only one of these had a family history of cancer. No BRCA1 mutations were found. These data suggest that most male breast cancer is not associated with germline mutations in BRCA1 or BRCA2, despite the clearly established increased susceptibility to male carriers of BRCA2 mutations, and in fact even with a family history, BRCA2 is only associated with male breast cancer in about 15% of families *(115)*. This low prevalence of BRCA mutations, even among the patients with a positive family history, would seem to provide additional evidence for the association of other genes with familial breast cancer.

9. OTHER CANCERS

A recurring theme as one reads descriptions of HC/OG families with or without known mutations, as well as the family histories of individuals found to have BRCA1 and BRCA2 mutations, is the high frequency of cancers at other sites. Cancers of the prostate and pancreas seem particularly frequent, but cancers of the adrenal cortex, brain, cervix, colon, endometrium, fallopian tube, gall bladder, lip, kidney, larynx, liver, lung, peritoneum, skin, stomach, testis, thyroid, and urethra, as well as leukemia, lymphoma, melanoma, mesothelioma, and myeloma have been reported in families with either BRCA1 or BRCA2 mutations *(49,56–58,78,79,111,119)*. Cancers of unknown primary site have also been noted. In the NIH study of a Jewish population in the Washington, DC area, a significantly elevated estimated risk of prostate cancer in BRCA1 carriers and their relatives was found, comparable to the risk for ovarian cancer. Family histories of some other cancers, including lung cancer, multiple myeloma, and Hodgkin's disease, were significantly elevated in carriers of mutations in BRCA1 or BRCA2, compared with noncarriers.

As noted above, somatic deletion of the chromosomal region carrying the BRCA2 gene in a pancreatic tumor aided in the original cloning of this gene, and BRCA2 mutations have recently been directly implicated in pancreatic cancer, an estimated 5% of which is thought to be associated with genetic predisposition *(120)*. Özçelik et al. *(121)* found two germline BRCA2 mutations in 41 unselected patients with pancreatic cancer. Of these, 13 were Jewish, and one of these carried the 6174delT mutation. Screening archival pancreatic cancers from 26 Jewish and 55 non-Jewish patients for this mutation identified three cases in the Jewish group, but none in the non-Jewish group. Thus, 4 of 39 (~10%) Jewish patients with pancreatic cancer unselected for family history had the BRCA2 6174delT mutation. These data specifically support the concept that BRCA2 predisposes to pancreatic cancer, as well as the more general concept that BRCA2 is a low penetrance cancer gene predisposing to a variety of cancers *(122)*.

A recent analysis by the Breast Cancer Linkage Consortium has identified an increased risk of other cancers, notably pancreas and prostate, in individuals with germline mutations of BRCA2, but with a lower penetrance than for breast or ovarian cancer (D. Goldgar, personal communication).

BRCA2 may function as a tumor suppressor gene in chronic B-cell lymphocytic leukemia (CLL). Garcia-Marco et al. *(123)* used fluorescence *in situ* hybridization to analyze deletions in chromosome 13 and found deletion of the 1-Mb 13q12.3 region that encompasses the BRCA2 gene in 28 of 35 cases of CLL (80%) and homozygous deletion of BRCA2 in 21 (60%).

10. GENOTYPE/PHENOTYPE CORRELATION

Attempts have been made to correlate the site of mutation with the phenotype of the associated tumors. Initial analysis of the mutations in BRCA1 led to the suggestion that the nearer the mutation to the 5' end of the gene, the more highly the gene is associated with ovarian cancer *(36)*, with a relatively sharp demarcation near the boundary of exons 12 and 13 *(34)*. It was also proposed that a higher incidence of breast cancers arose from mutations in the 3' portion of the gene. However, this has been disputed recently as other groups have failed to replicate these results *(13,29,105)*. A 3.3 kb region within exon 11 of BRCA2 between residues 3035-6629 was also identified as being associated with a higher incidence of ovarian cancers relative to breast cancers *(35)*; both truncating mutations and several missense mutations appear to be involved.

11. OTHER GENES

Germline mutations of several other genes have been shown to be associated with increased breast cancer susceptibility. These include the gene for the tumor suppressor p53 (Li-Fraumeni syndrome), the androgen receptor on chromosome Xq11.2-12, and a locus linked to HRAS1 on chromosome 11p15.5 *(124)*. Also, as noted above, the mutations in DNA mismatch repair genes that cause hereditary nonpolyposis colon cancer are also associated with an increased susceptibility to ovarian cancer *(125)*.

The gene responsible for Cowden disease (PTEN *[126,128]*; MMAC *[127]*) maps to 10q23.3 and is also altered in a variety of tumors *(126)* including sporadic breast, brain, and prostate cancers *(128)*. PTEN/MMAC is proposed to be a protein tyrosine phosphatase, and has a protein tyrosine phosphatase core motif and two potential tyrosine phosphatase acceptor sites. It also shows homology to the cytoskeletal proteins tensin and auxin *(126–128)*. Steck and colleagues *(127)* identified mutations in 2/14 (14%) of breast tumors. The first, a 25 base insertion in exon 3 causes premature truncation of the protein at codon 70; the second is a nine base deletion in exon 7, which changes LysPheMetTyr to Asn, and is within the first of the putative tyrosine phosphatase acceptor sites. Recent data suggest that germline mutations of PTEN/MMAC are found in 1/200 breast cancer families (B Weber, personal communication).

12. SUMMARY AND CONCLUSIONS

The identification of the BRCA1 and BRCA2 genes and the characterization of hundreds of mutations in these genes associated with breast and ovarian cancer constitute a triumph of modern clinical and molecular genetics.

The lifetime risks of developing breast cancer are approximately equal for BRCA1 and BRCA2 carriers; however, the age of onset in BRCA2 carriers is higher than that of BRCA1 carriers *(58)*. The frequency of BRCA1 mutations are 1.5–2-fold higher than BRCA2 mutations in all populations studied except for the Icelandic population.

BRCA1 and BRCA2 mutations together account for 6–10% of all breast cancer cases except in Israel, where this figure is somewhat higher at around 15%. The observation that neither BRCA1 nor BRCA2 mutations have been identified in around 50–60% of families with an increased risk of breast cancer is indicative of the possibility that there is another gene or genes responsible for familial breast cancer in these families. This and the extremely rare occurrence of somatic mutations in these genes in sporadic breast tumors is strong evidence that there are more genes involved in breast cancer development.

The majority of cancer-associated BRCA1 and BRCA2 mutations are small insertions or deletions that induce frameshifts and premature protein truncation. Mutations are located throughout both genes. The mutations range in prevalence from those that are widely dispersed throughout many populations, to those that are recurrent within individual populations, to those found only in single families or individuals. Most of the investigation of mutations has so far been carried out in Europe, North America, Israel, and Japan. Investigation of populations in other parts of the world are needed.

Women with mutations in either BRCA1 or BRCA2 are at significant lifetime risk for developing breast or ovarian cancer. The best estimates of this risk have come from studies of the Askhenazi Jewish population, which has an unusually high carrier frequency of ~2.5% for three recurrent mutations in BRCA1 and BRCA2. The lifetime risk of breast cancer in this population is probably at least 50%, and for ovarian cancer the risk probably approaches 20%. The three common mutations in BRCA1 and BRCA2 that have been identified in the Ashkenazi Jewish population do not account for all of the familial breast and/or ovarian cancer in this population, and therefore the absence of all three mutations does not necessarily reduce the breast/ovarian cancer risk to someone who has a family history breast or ovarian cancer.

A large majority of mutation carriers with breast and/or ovarian cancer have a history of a similarly affected first- or second-degree relative. This argues against screening of large populations without regard to family history.

Both BRCA1 and BRCA2 mutations are associated with other cancers, most notably of the pancreas and prostate, but probably others as well. The penetrance for any particular cancer appears to be lower than for breast or ovarian cancer. A formal assessment of the risk of other cancers to carriers of BRCA1 and BRCA2 mutations has not yet been done.

In many but not all studies comparing the two, the penetrance of BRCA1 mutations exceeds that of BRCA2 mutations, and in most populations, a greater proportion of hereditary breast and ovarian cancer is associated with BRCA1 mutations. Mutations in BRCA1 or BRCA2 appear to account for many but not all cases of hereditary breast cancer.

ACKNOWLEDGMENTS

L. B. B. is supported by a Susan G. Komen fellowship. Much thanks is owed to Drs. B. Weber and D. Haber for critical comments on this chapter.

REFERENCES

1. Lynch, H., R. Harris, H. Guirgis, K. Maloney, and L. Carmody. 1978. Familial association of breast/ovarian carcinoma. *Cancer* **41:** 1543–1549.

2. Claus, E. B., N. Risch, and W. D. Thompson. 1991. Genetic analysis of breast cancer in the Cancer and Steroid Hormone Study. *Am. J. Human Genet.* **48:** 232–242.

3. Newman, B., M. A. Austin, M. Lee, and M.-C. King. 1988. Inheritance of human breast cancer: evidence for autosomal dominant transmission in high-risk families. *Proc. Natl. Acad. Sci. USA* **85:** 3044–3048.

4. Bowcock, A. M. 1993. Molecular cloning of BRCA1: a gene for early onset familial breast and ovarian cancer. *Breast Cancer Research and Treatment.* **28:** 121–135.

5. Hall, J. M., M. K. Lee, B. Newman, J. E. Morrow, L. A. Anderson, B. Huey, and M.-C. King. 1990. Linkage of early-onset familial breast cancer to chromosome 17q21. *Science* **250:** 1684–1689.

6. Narod, S. A., J. Feunteun, H. T. Lynch, P. Watson, T. Conway, J. Lynch, and G. M. Lenoir. 1991. Familial breast-ovarian cancer locus on chromosome 17q12-q23. *Lancet* **338:** 82–83.

7. Steichen-Gersdorf, E., H. H. Gallion, D. Ford, C. Girodet, and D. F. Easton. 1994. Familial site-specific ovarian cancer is linked to BRCA1 on 17q12-21. *Am. J. Human Genet.* **55:** 870–875.

8. Easton, D. F., D. T. Bishop, D. Ford, and G. P. Crockford. 1993. Genetic linkage analysis in familial breast and ovarian cancer: results from 214 families. The Breast Cancer Linkage Consortium. *Am. J. Human Genet.* **52:** 678–701.

9. Narod, S. A., D. Ford, P. Devilee, R. B. Barkardottir, H. T. Lynch, and S. A. Smith. 1995. An evaluation of genetic heterogeneity in 145 breast-ovarian cancer families. *Am. J. Human Genet.* **56:** 254–264.

10. Easton, D. F., D. Ford, and D. T. Bishop. 1995. Breast and ovarian cancer incidence in BRCA1-mutation carriers. Breast Cancer Linkage Consortium. *Am. J. Human Genet.* **56:** 265–271.

11. Easton, D. 1997. Breast cancer genes—what are the real risks? *Nature Genet.* **16:** 210–211.

12. Phelan, C. M., T. R. Rebbeck, B. L. Weber, P. Devilee, M. H. Ruttledge, H. T. Lynch, et al. 1996. Ovarian cancer risk in BRCA1 carriers is modified by the HRAS1 variable number of tandem repeat (VNTR) locus. *Nature Genet.* **12:** 309–311.

13. Langston, A. A., K. E. Malone, J. D. Thompson, J. R. Daling, and E. A. Ostrander. 1996. BRCA1 mutations in a population-based sample of young women with breast cancer. *N. Engl. J. Med.* **334:** 137–142.

14. Fitzgerald, M. G., D. J. MacDonald, M. Krainer, I. Hoover, E. O'Neil, H. Unsal, et al. 1996. Germ-line BRCA1 mutations in Jewish and non-Jewish women with early-onset breast cancer. *N. Engl. J. Med.* **334:** 143–149.

15. Smith, S., D. Easton, D. Evans, and B. Ponder. 1992. Allele losses in the region 17q12-21 in familial breast and ovarian cancer involves the wild-type chromosome. *Nature Genet.* **2:** 128–131.

16. Kelsell, D. P., D. M. Black, D. T. Bishop, and N. K. Spurr. 1993. Genetic analysis of the BRCA1 region in a large breast/ovarian family: refinement of the minimal region containing BRCA1. *Human Mol. Genet.* **2:** 1823–1828.

17. Bowcock, A., L. Anderson, L. Friedman, D. Black, S. Osborne-Lawrence, S. Rowell, et al. 1993. THRA1 and D17S183 flank an interval of <4 cm for the breast-ovarian cancer gene (BRCA1) on chromosome 17q21. *Am. J. Human Genet.* **52:** 718–722.

18. O'Connell, P., H. Albertsen, N. Matsunami, T. Taylor, and J. E. Hundley. 1994. A radiation hybrid map of the BRCA1 region. *Am. J. Human Genet.* **54**: 526–534.

19. Albertsen, H., R. Plaetke, L. Ballard, E. Funimoto, and J. Connolly. 1994. Genetic mapping of the BRCA1 region on chromosome 17q21. *Am. J. Human Genet.* **54**: 516–525.

20. Miki, Y., J. Swensen, D. Shattuck-Eidens, P. A. Futreal, K. Harshman, S. Tavtigian, et al. 1994. A strong candidate for the breast and ovarian cancer susceptibility gene BRCA1. *Science* **266**: 66–71.

21. Smith, T. M., M. K. Lee, C. I. Szabo, N. Jerome, and M. McEuen. 1996. Complete genomic sequence and analysis of 117kb of human DNA containing the gene BRCA1. *Genome Res.* **6**: 1029–1049.

22. Gille, J., M. Strunk, R. van Schooten, R. Zweemer, R. Verheijen, F. Menko, and G. Pals. 1997. Outcome of BRCA1 and BRCA2 testing in 89 Dutch breast/ovarian cancer families. *Am. J. Human Genet.* **61**: A66.

23. Petrij-Bosch, A., T. Peelen, M. van Vliet, R. van Eijk, R. Olmer, M. Drusedau, F. B. L. Hogervorst, et al. 1997. BRCA1 genomic deletions are founder mutations in Dutch breast cancer patients. *Nature Genet.* **17**: 341–345.

24. Xu, C.-F., M. A. Brown, J. A. Chambers, B. Griffiths, H. Nicolai, and E. Solomon. 1995. Distinct transcription start sites generate two forms of BRCA1 mRNA. *Human Mol. Genet.* **4**: 2259–2264.

25. Gudas, J. M., T. Li, H. Nguyen, D. Jensen, F. J. Rauscher III, and K. H. Cowan. 1996. Cell cycle regulation of BRCA1 messenger RNA in human breast epithelial cells. *Cell Growth and Differentiation* **7**: 711–723.

26. Thakur, S., H. B. Zhang, Y. Peng, H. Le, B. Carroll, T. Ward, et al. 1997. Localization of BRCA1 and a splice variant identifies the nuclear localization signal. *Mol. Cell. Biology.* **17**: 444–452.

27. Wu, L. C., Z. W. Wang, J. T. Tsan, M. A. Spillman, A. Phung, X. L. Xu, et al. 1996. Identification of a RING protein that interacts in vivo with the BRCA1 gene product. *Nature Genet.* **14**: 430–440.

28. Saurin, A. J., K. L. B. Borden, M. N. Boddy, and P. S. Freemont. 1996. Does this have a familiar RING? *Trends Biochem. Sci.* **21**: 208–214.

29. Shattuck-Eidens, D., M. McClure, J. Simard, F. Labrie, S. Narod, F. Couch, et al. 1995. A collaborative survey of 80 mutations in the BRCA1 breast and ovarian cancer susceptibility gene: Implications for presymptomatic testing and screening. *JAMA* **273**: 535–541.

30. Stoppa-Lyonnet, D., P. Laurent-Puig, L. Essioux, S. Pages, G. Ithier, L. Ligot, et al. 1997. BRCA1 sequence variations in 160 individuals referred to a breast/ovarian family cancer clinic. *Am. J. Hum. Genet.* **60**: 1021–1030.

31. Lane, T. F., C. Deng, A. Elson, M. S. Lyu, C. A. Kozak, and P. Leder. 1995. Expression of Brca1 is associated with terminal differentiation of ectodermally and mesodermally derived tissues in mice. *Genes Dev.* **9**: 2712–2722.

32. Abel, K. J., J. Xu, G.-Y. Yin, R. H. Lyons, M. H. Meisler, and B. L. Weber. 1995. Mouse *Brca1*: localization, sequence analysis and identification of evolutionarily conserved domains. *Human Mol. Genet.* **4**: 2265–2273.

33. Sobol, H., D. Stoppa-Lyonnett, B. Bressasc-de-Paillerets, J.-P. Peyrat, F. Kerangueven, N. Janin, et al. 1996. Truncation at conserved terminal regions of BRCA1 protein is associated with highly proliferating hereditary breast cancers. *Cancer Res.* **56**: 3216–3219.

34. Gayther, S. A., W. Warren, S. Mazoyer, P. A. Russell, P. A. Harrington, M. Chiano, et al. 1995. Germline mutations of the BRCA1 gene in breast and ovarian cancer families provide evidence for a genotype-phenotype correlation. *Nature Genet.* **11**: 428–433.

35. Gayther, S. A., J. Mangion, P. Russell, S. Seal, R. Barfoot, B. A. J. Ponder, et al. 1997. Variation of risks of breast and ovarian cancer associated with different germline mutations of the BRCA2 gene. *Nature Genet.* **15**: 103–105.

36. Friedman, L. S., E. A. Ostermeyer, C. I. Szabo, P. Dowd, and E. D. Lynch. 1994. Confirmation of BRCA1 by analysis of germline mutations linked to breast and ovarian cancer in ten families. *Nature Genet.* **8:** 399–404.

37. Holt, J. T., M. E. Thompson, C. Szabo, C. Robinson Benion, C. L. Arteaga, M. C. King, and R. A. Jensen. 1996. Growth retardation and tumour inhibition by BRCA1. *Nature Genet.* **12:** 298–302.

38. Chapman, M. S. and I. M. Verma. 1996. Transcriptional activation by BRCA1. *Nature* **382:** 678–679.

39. BIC. 1997. http://www.nhgri.nih.gov/Intramural_research/Lab_transfer/Bic.

40. Futreal, P. A., Q. Liu, D. Shattuck Eidens, C. Cochran, K. Harshman, S. Tavtigian, et al. 1994. BRCA1 mutations in primary breast and ovarian carcinomas. *Science.* **266:** 120–122.

41. Jensen, R. A., M. E. Thompson, T. L. Jetton, C. I. Szabo, R. van der Meer, B. Helou, et al. 1996. BRCA1 is secreted and exhibits properties of a granin. *Nature Genet.* **12:** 303–308.

42. Connor, F., A. Smith, R. Wooster, M. Stratton, A. Dixon, E. Campbell, et al. 1997. Cloning, chromosomal mapping and expression pattern of the mouse BRCA2 gene. *Human Mol. Genet.* **6:** 291–300.

43. Koonin, E. V., S. F. Altschul, and P. Bork. 1996. BRCA1 protein products: functional motifs. *Nature Genet.* **13:** 266–267.

44. Chen, Y., C. F. Chen, D. J. Riley, D. C. Allred, P. L. Chen, D. Von Hoff, et al. 1995. Aberrant subcellular localization of BRCA1 in breast cancer. *Science* **270:** 789–791.

45. Somasundaram, K., H. Zhang, Y.-X. Zeng, Y. Houvras, Y. Peng, H. Zhang, et al. 1997. Arrest of the tumour-suppressor BRCA1 requires the CDK-inhibitor p21$^{WAF/CIP1}$. *Nature* **389:** 187–190.

46. Scully, R., J. Chen, A. Plug, Y. Xiao, D. Weaver, J. Feunteun, et al. 1997. Association of BRCA1 with Rad51 in mitotic and meiotic cells. *Cell* **88:** 265–275.

47. Wooster, R., S. L. Neuhausen, J. Mangion, Y. Quirk, D. Ford, N. Collins, et al. 1994. Localization of a breast cancer susceptibility gene, BRCA2 to chromosome 13q12-13. *Science* **265:** 2088–2090.

48. Wooster, R., G. Bignell, J. Lancaster, S. Swift, S. Seal, J. Mangion, et al. 1995. Identification of the breast cancer susceptibility gene BRCA2. *Nature* **378:** 789–792.

49. Tavtigian, S. V., J. Simard, J. Rommens, F. Couch, D. Shattuck Eidens, S. Neuhausen, et al. 1996. The complete BRCA2 gene and mutations in chromosome 13q-linked kindreds. *Nature Genet.* **12:** 333–337.

50. Bork, P., N. Blomberg, and M. Nilges. 1996. Internal repeats in the BRCA2 protein sequence. *Nature Genet.* **13:** 22–23.

51. Bignell, G., G. Micklem, M. R. Stratton, A. Ashworth, and R. Wooster. 1997. The BRC repeats are conserved in mammalian BRCA2 proteins. *Human Mol. Genet.* **6:** 53–58.

52. Lancaster, J., R. Wooster, J. Mangion, C. Phelan, C. Cochran, C. Gumbs, et al. 1996. BRCA2 mutations in primary breast and ovarian cancers. *Nature Genet.* **13:** 238–240.

53. Serova-Sinionikova, O. M., L. Boutrand, D. Stoppa-Lyonnet, B. Bressac-de-Paillerets, and V. Dubois. 1997. BRCA2 mutations in hereditary breast and ovarian cancer in France. *Am. J. Human Genet.* **60:** 1236–1239.

54. Berman, D. B., J. Costalas, D. C. Schultz, G. Grana, and M. Daly. 1996. A common mutation in BRCA2 that predisposes to a variety of cancers is found in both Jewish Ashkenazi and non-Jewish individuals. *Cancer Res.* **56:** 3409–3414.

55. Couch, F. J. and B. L. Weber. The Breast Cancer Information Core. 1996. Mutations and polymorphisms in the familial early-onset breast cancer (BRCA1) gene. *Human Mutation* **8:** 8–18.

56. Phelan, C., J. M. Lancaster, P. Tonin, C. Gumbs, C. Cochran, R. Carter, et al. 1996. Mutation analysis of the BRCA2 gene in 49 site-specific breast cancer families. *Nature Genet.* **13:** 120–122.

57. Thorlacius, S., G. Olafsdottir, L. Tryggvadottir, S. Neuhausen, J. G. Jonasson, S. V. Tavtigian, et al. 1996. A single BRCA2 mutation in male and female breast cancer families from Iceland with varied cancer phenotypes. *Nature Genet.* **13**: 117–119.

58. Schubert, E. L., M. K. Lee, H. C. Mefford, R. H. Argonza, J. E. Morrow, H. Judy, et al. 1997. BRCA2 in American families with four or more cases of breast or ovarian cancer: Recurrent and novel mutations, variable expression, penetrance and the possibility of families whose cancer is not attributable to BRCA1 or BRCA2. *Am. J. Human Genet.* **60**: 1031–1040.

59. Krainer, M., S. Silva-Arrieta, M. G. Fitzgerald, A. Shimada, C. Ishioka, R. Kanamaru, et al. 1997. Differential contributions of BRCA1 and BRCA2 to early-onset breast cancer. *N. Engl. J. Med.* **336**: 1416–1421.

60. Sharan, S. K. and A. Bradley. 1997. Murine BRCA2: Sequence, map position and expression pattern. *Genomics* **40**: 234–241.

61. Sharan, S. K., M. Morimatsu, U. Albrecht, D.-S. Lim, E. Regel, C. Dinh, et al. 1997. Embryonic lethality and radiation hypersensitivity mediated by Rad51 in mice lacking *Brca2*. *Nature* **386**: 804–810.

62. Orita, M., Y. Suzuki, T. Sekiya, and K. Hayashi. 1989. Rapid and sensitive detection of point mutations and DNA polymorphisms using the polymerase chain reaction. *Genomics* **5**: 874–879.

63. Orita, M., H. Wahana, H. Kanazawa, K. Hayashi, and T. Sekiya. 1989. Detection of polymorphisms of human DNA by gel electrophoresis as single-stranded conformation polymorphisms. *Proc. Natl. Acad. Sci. USA* **86**: 2766–2770.

64. Hogervorst, F. B. L., R. S. Cornelis, M. Bout, M. van Vliet, J. C. Oosterwiik, R. Olmer, et al. 1995. Rapid detection of BRCA1 mutations by the protein truncation test. *Nature Genet.* **10**: 208–212.

65. Hacia, J. G., L. C. Brody, M. S. Chee, S. P. A. Fodor, and F. S. Collins. 1996. Detection of heterozygous mutations in BRCA1 using high density oligonucleotide arrays and two-colour fluorescence analysis. *Nature Genet.* **14**: 441–447.

66. Cronin, M. T., R. V. Fucini, S. M. Kim, R. S. Masino, R. M. Wespi, and C. G. Miyada. 1996. Cystic fibrosis mutation detection by hybridization to light-generated DNA probe arrays. *Human Mutation* **7**: 244-255.

67. Lipshutz, R. J., D. Morris, M. Chee, E. Hubbell, M. J. Kozal, N. Shah, et al. 1995. Using oligonucleotide probe arrays to assess genetic diversity. *Biotechniques* **19**: 442–447.

68. Kozal, M. J., N. Shah, N. Shen, R. Yang, R. Fucini, T. Merigan, et al. 1996. Extensive polymorphisms observed in HIV-1 clade B protease gene using high density oligonucleotide arrays. *Nature Medicine* **2**: 753–759.

69. Yershov, G., V. Barsky, A. Belgovskiy, E. Kirillov, E. Kreindlin, I. Ivanov, et al. 1996. DNA analysis and diagnostics on oligonucleotide microchips. *Proc. Natl. Acad. Sci. USA* **93**: 4913–4918.

70. Chee, M., R. Yang, E. Hubbell, A. Berno, X. C. Huang, D. Stern, et al. 1996. Assessing genetic information with high density arrays. *Science* **274**: 610–614.

71. Couch, F. J., M. L. DeShano, A. Blackwood, K. Calzone, and J. Stopfer. 1997. BRCA1 mutations in women attending clinics that evaluate the risk of breast cancer. *N. Engl. J. Med.* **336**: 1409–1415.

72. Payne, S. and M.-C. King. 1997. Complex BRCA1 germline deletion and rearrangement of 1028 bp leads to deletion of exon 3 and disease predisposition: Splicing by exon definition in BRCA1. *Am. Soc. Human Genet.* **61**: A78.

73. Boyd, M., F. Harris, R. McFarlane, H. R. Davidson, and D. M. Black. 1995. A human BRCA1 gene knockout (letter). *Nature.* **375**: 541–542.

74. Mazoyer, S., A. M. Dunning, O. Serova, J. Dearden, N. Puget, C. S. Healey, et al. 1996. A polymorphic stop codon in BRCA2. *Nature Genet.* **14**: 253–254.

75. Szabo, C. I. and M.-C. King. 1997. Population genetics of BRCA1 and BRCA2. *Am. J. Human Genet.* **60**: 1013–1020.

76. Ramus, S. J., Z. Kote-Jarai, L. S. Friedman, M. van der Looij, and S. A. Gayther. 1997. Analysis of BRCA1 and BRCA2 mutations in Hungarian families with breast or breast-ovarian cancer. *Am. J. Human Genet.* **60:** 1242–1246.

77. Hakansson, S., O. Johannesson, U. Johansson, G. Sellberg, and N. Loman. 1997. Moderate frequency of BRCA1 and BRCA2 germ-line mutations in Scandinavian familial breast cancer. *Am. J. Human Genet.* **60:** 1068–1078.

78. Serova, O. M., S. Mazoyer, N. Puget, V. Dubois, and P. Tonin. 1997. Mutations in BRCA1 and BRCA2 in breast cancer families: are there more breast cancer-susceptibility genes? *Am. J. Human Genet.* **60:** 486–495.

79. Thorlacius, S., S. Sigurdsson, H. Bjarnadottir, G. Olafsdottir, J. G. Jonasson, L. Tryggvadottir, et al. 1997. Study of a single mutation with high carrier frequency in a small population. *Am. J. Human Genet.* **60:** 1079–1084.

80. Johannesdottir, G., G. Gudmundsson, and O. Johannsson. 1996. A high prevalence of the 999del5 mutation in Icelandic breast and ovarian cancer patients. *Cancer Res.* **56:** 3663–3665.

81. Vehmanen, P., L. S. Friedman, H. Eerola, L. Sarantaus, and S. Pyrhonen. 1997. A low proportion of BRCA2 mutations in Finnish breast cancer families. *Am. J. Human Genet.* **60:** 1050–1058.

82. Montagna, M., M. Santacatterina, B. Corneo, C. Menin, and O. Serova. 1996. Identification of seven new BRCA1 germline mutations in Italian breast and breast/ovarian cancer families. *Cancer Res.* **56:** 5466–5469.

83. Caligo, M. A., C. Ghimenti, G. Cipollini, S. Ricci, and I. Brunetti. 1996. BRCA1 germline mutational spectrum in Italian families from Tuscany: a high frequency of novel mutations. *Oncogene* **13:** 1483–1488.

84. De Benedetti, V. M., P. Radice, P. Mondini, G. Spatti, and A. Conti. 1996. Screening for mutations in exon 11 of the BRCA1 gene in 70 Italian breast and ovarian patients by protein truncation test. *Oncogene* **13:** 1353–1357.

85. Peelen, T., M. van Vliet, A. Petrij-Bosch, R. Mieremet, C. Szabo, A. van den Ouweland, et al. 1997. A high proportion of novel mutations in BRCA1 with strong founder effects among Dutch and Belgium hereditary breast and ovarian cancer families. *Am. J. Human Genet.* **60:** 1041–1049.

86. Ford, D., D. F. Easton, and J. Peto. 1995. Estimates of the gene frequency of BRCA1 and its contribution to breast and ovarian cancer incidence. *Am. J. Human Genet.* **57:** 1457–1462.

87. Zlotowitz, M. 1977. *Bereshis.* New York: Mesorah Publications, Inc.

88. Freedman, H. 1949. *Jeremiah.* London: Soncino Press.

89. Wein, B. 1993. *Herald of Destiny. The Story of the Jews in the Medieval Era 750-1058.* New York: Shaar Press.

90. Agus, I. A. 1969. *The Heroic Age of Franco-German Jewry.* Yeshiva University Press, New Jersey.

91. Greenbaum, M. 1995. *The Jews of Lithuania. A History of a Remarkable Community 1316–1945.* Jerusalem: Gefen Books

92. Motulsky, A. G. 1995. Jewish diseases and origins. *Nature Genet.* **9:** 99–101.

93. Bonne-Tamir, B. and A. Adam. 1992. *Genetic Diversity Among Jews.* New York: Oxford University Press.

94. Jorde, L. B. 1992. Genetic diseases in the Ashkenazi population: evolutionary considerations. In *Genetic Diversity Among Jews.* New York: Oxford University Press: pp. 305–318.

95. Risch, N., D. de Leon, L. Ozelius, P. Kramer, and L. Almasy. 1995. Genetic analysis of idiopathic torsion dystonia in Ashkenazi Jews and their recent descent from a small founder population. *Nature Genet.* **9:** 152–159.

96. Zoossmann-Diskin. 1995. ITD in Ashkenazi Jews—genetic drift or selection. *Nature Genet.* **11:** 13–14.

97. Friedman, L. S., E. A. Ostermeyer, C. I. Szabo, P. Dowd, L. Butler, T. Park, et al. 1995. Novel inherited mutations and variable expressivity of BRCA1 alleles, including the founder mutation 185 delAG in Ashkenazi Jewish families. *Am. J. Human Genet.* **57:** 399–404.

98. Struewing, J. P., D. Abeliovich, T. Peretz, N. Avishai, M. M. Kaback, F. S. Collins, and L. C. Brody. 1995. The carrier frequency of the BRCA1 185delAG mutation is approximately 1 percent in Ashkenazi Jewish individuals. *Nature Genet.* **11:** 198–200.

99. Takahashi, H., K. Behbakht, P. E. McGovern, H. C. Chiu, and F. J. Couch. 1995. Mutation analysis of the BRCA1 gene in ovarian cancers. *Cancer Res.* **55:** 2998–3002.

100. Simard, J., P. Tonin, F. Durocher, K. Morgan, J. Rommens, S. Gingras, C. Samson, et al. 1994. Common origins of BRCA1 mutations in Canadian breast and ovarian cancer families. *Nature Genet.* **8:** 392–398.

101. Tonin, P., O. Serova, G. Lenoir, H. Lynch, F. Durocher, J. Simard, et al. 1995. BRCA1 mutations in Ashkenazi Jewish women. *Am. J. Human Genet.* **57:** 189.

102. Offit, K., T. Gilewski, P. McGuire, A. Schluger, H. Hampel, K. Brown, et al. 1996. Germline BRCA1 185delAG mutations in Jewish women with breast cancer. *Lancet* **347:** 1643–1644.

103. Modan, B., E. Gak, R. B. Sade-Bruchim, G. Hirsh-Yechezkel, and L. Theodor. 1996. High frequency of BRCA1 185delAG mutation in ovarian cancer in Israel. National Israel Study of Ovarian Cancer. *JAMA* **276:** 1823–1825.

104. Muto, M. G., D. W. Cramer, J. Tangir, R. Berkowitz, and S. Mok. 1996. Frequency of the BRCA1 185delAG mutation among Jewish women with ovarian cancer and matched population controls. *Cancer Res.* **56:** 1250–1252.

105. Neuhausen, S. L., S. Mazoyer, L. Friedman, M. Stratton, K. Offit, A. Caligo, et al. 1996. Haplotype and phenotype analysis of six recurrent BRCA1 mutations in 61 families: results of an international study. *Am. J. Human Genet.* **58:** 271–280.

106. Barsade, R. B., A. Kruglikova, B. Modan, E. Gak, G. Hirshyechezkel, L. Theodor, et al. 1998. The 185delAG BRCA1 mutation originated before the dispersion of Jews in the Diaspora and is not limited to the Ashkenazim. *Human Mol. Genet.* **7:** 801–805.

107. Neuhausen, S., T. Gilewski, L. Norton, T. Tran, P. McGuire, J. Swensen, et al. 1996. Recurrent *BRCA2* 6147delT mutations in Ashkenazi women affected by breast cancer. *Nature Genet.* **13:** 126–128.

108. Oddoux, C., J. P. Struewing, C. M. Clayton, S. Neuhausen, L. C. Brody, M. Kaback, et al. 1996. The carrier frequency of the BRCA2 6174delT mutation among Ashkenazi Jewish individuals is approximately 1%. *Nature Genet.* **14:** 188–190.

109. Roa, B. B., A. A. Boyd, K. Volcik, and C. S. Richards. 1996. Ashkenazi Jewish population frequencies for common mutations in BRCA1 and BRCA2. *Nature Genet.* **14:** 185–187.

110. Tonin, P., B. Weber, K. Offit, F. Couch, T. Rebbeck, S. Neuhausen, and A. Godwin. 1996. Frequency of recurrent BRCA1 and BRCA2 mutations in Ashkenazi Jewish breast cancer families. *Nature Medicine* **2:** 1179–1183.

111. Abeliovich, D., L. Kaduri, I. Lerer, N. Weinberg, G. Amir, M. Sagi, and J. Zlotogora. 1997. The founder mutations 185delAG and 5382insC in BRCA1 and 6174delT in BRCA2 appear in 60% of ovarian cancer and 30% of early-onset breast cancer patients among Ashkenazi women. *Am. J. Human Genet.* **60:** 505–514.

112. Struewing, J. P., P. Hartge, S. Wacholder, S. M. Baker, and M. Berlin. 1997. The risk of cancer associated with specific mutations of BRCA1 and BRCA2 among Ashkenazi Jews. *N. Engl. J. Med.* **336:** 1401–1408.

113. Levy-Lahad, E., R. Catane, S. Eisenberg, B. Kaufman, G. Hornreich, E. Lishinsky, et al. 1997. Founder BRCA1 and BRCA2 mutations in Ashkenazi Jews in Israel: Frequency and differential penetrance in ovarian cancer and in breast-ovarian cancer families. *Am. J. Human Genet.* **60:** 1059–1067.

114. Sher, C., L. Sharabini-Gargir, and M. Shohat. 1996. Breast cancer and BRCA1 mutations. *N. Engl. J. Med.* **334:** 1199.

115. Couch, F. J., L. M. Farid, M. L. DeShano, S. V. Tavtigian, K. Calzone, L. Campeau, et al. 1996. BRCA2 germline mutations in male breast cancer cases and breast cancer families. *Nature Genet.* **13:** 123–125.

116. Struewing, J. P., L. C. Brody, M. R. Erdos, R. G. Kase, T. R. Giambarresi, S. A. Smith, et al. 1995. Detection of eight BRCA1 mutations in 10 breast/ovarian cancer families, including 1 family with male breast cancer. *Am. J. Human Genet.* **57:** 1–7.

117. Thorlacius, S., L. Tryggvadottir, G. H. Olafsdottir, J. G. Jonasson, and H. M. Ogmundsdottir. 1995. Linkage to BRCA2 region in hereditary male breast cancer. *Lancet* **346:** 544–545.

118. Friedman, L. S., S. A. Gayther, T. Kurosaki, D. Gordon, and B. Noble. 1997. Mutation analysis of BRCA1 and BRCA2 in a male breast cancer population. *Am. J. Human Genet.* **60:** 313–319.

119. Gudmundsson, J., G. Johannesdottir, A. Arason, J. Bergthorsson, and S. Ingvarsson. 1996. Frequent occurrence of BRCA2 linkage in Icelandic breast cancer families and segregation of a common BRCA2 haplotype. *Am. J. Human Genet.* **58:** 749–756.

120. Lynch, H. T., T. Smyrk, S. E. Kern, R. H. Hruban, and C. J. Lightdale. 1996. Familial pancreatic cancer: a review. *Semin Oncol.* **23:** 251–275.

121. Özçelik, H., B. Schmocker, N. Di Nicola, X.-H. Shi, and B. Langer. 1997. Germline BRCA2 6174delT mutations in Ashkenazi Jewish pancreatic cancer patients. *Nature Genet.* **16:** 17–18.

122. Boyd, J. 1996. BRCA2 as a low-penetrance cancer gene. *J. Natl. Cancer Inst.* **88:** 1408–1409.

123. Garcia-Marco, J. A., C. Caldas, C. M. Price, L. M. Wiedemann, and A. Ashworth. 1996. Frequent somatic deletion of the 13q12.3 locus encompassing BRCA2 in chronic lymphocytic leukemia. *Blood* **88:** 1568–1575.

124. Green, M. H. 1997. Genetics of breast cancer. *Mayo Clin Proc.* **72:** 54–65.

125. Boyd, J. and S. C. Rubin. 1997. Hereditary ovarian cancer: molecular genetics and clinical implications. *Gynecol. Oncol.* **64:** 196–206.

126. Li, J., C. Yen, D. Liaw, K. Podsypanina, S. Bose, S. I. Wang, et al. 1997. PTEN, a putative protein tyrosine phosphatase gene mutated in human brain, breast and prostate cancer. *Science.* **275:** 1943–1947.

127. Steck, P. A., M. A. Pershouse, S. A. Jasser, W. K. A. Yung, H. Lin, A. H. Ligon, et al. 1997. Identification of a candidate tumour suppressor gene, MMAC1, at chromosome 10q23.3 that is mutated in multiple advanced cancers. *Nature Genet.* **15:** 356–362.

128. Liaw, D., D. J. Marsh, J. Li, L. M. Dahia, S. I. Wang, Z. Zheng, et al. 1997. Germline mutations of the PTEN gene in Cowden disease, an inherited breast and thyroid cancer syndrome. *Nature Genet.* **16:** 64–67.

129. Yu, X., L. C. Wu, A. M. Bowcock, A. Aronheim, and R. Baer. 1998. The carboxy-terminal (BRCT) motifs of BRCA1 interact in vivo with CtIP, a protein implicated in the CtBP pathway of transcriptional repression. *J. Biol. Chem.* **273:** 35,388–35,392.

10

Biological Functions of the BRCA1 and BRCA2 Proteins

Helen K. Chew, Andrew A. Farmer, and Wen-Hwa Lee

1. INTRODUCTION

Breast cancer is the most commonly diagnosed nondermatologic cancer in women in the United States. It is second only to lung cancer as the most frequent cause of cancer-related deaths in American women. In 1996, the American Cancer Society projected over 184,000 newly diagnosed cases of breast cancer and over 44,000 deaths secondary to invasive breast cancer (1). The average American woman has a 1:8 lifetime risk of developing breast cancer. It is undoubtedly one of the most common malignancies in the Western world, yet there is currently no cure for metastatic breast cancer. For this reason, a tremendous effort has been focused on the prevention and early diagnosis of breast cancer.

In 1990, the first breast cancer susceptibility gene, BRCA1, was localized to chromosome 17q by linkage analysis of multiple families affected by early-onset breast and ovarian cancer (2). Four years after its localization, BRCA1 was identified by positional cloning (3). At about the same time that BRCA1 was cloned, a second breast-cancer susceptibility gene, BRCA2, was localized to chromosome 13q and cloned shortly thereafter (4,5).

Whereas mutations in BRCA1 are responsible for nearly all of the hereditary breast and ovarian cancer families, and up to 40–50% of families with hereditary breast cancer only (6), BRCA2 is strongly linked to hereditary breast cancer in both males and females (4,5). Together BRCA1 and BRCA2 account for the majority, although not all, of the hereditary breast cancer cases. (In this volume, Bennet et al. discuss hereditary breast cancer in Chapter 9.)

Although hereditary breast cancer families account for only 5–10% of all breast-cancer cases, there was hope that an understanding of BRCA1 and BRCA2 could be applied to benefit all breast cancer patients. This optimism led to speculation that improved screening of high-risk individuals through chromosomal analysis, and potential cures through gene therapy, were viable possibilities for the near future. However, this has not been the case. Despite an intense effort that has followed the discovery of these two genes, the roles of BRCA1 and BRCA2 in restraining the formation of breast cancer are not well understood. Moreover, their involvement in the majority of breast cancers, which are sporadic and not familial, has not been demonstrated.

From: Breast Cancer: Molecular Genetics, Pathogenesis, and Therapeutics
Edited by: A. M. Bowcock © Humana Press Inc., Totowa, NJ

Additionally, over 300 sequence variations have been reported in BRCA1; over 100 in BRCA2 (7). This has made quick and efficient mutational screening a challenge. As a result, there remains considerable controversy and speculation as to the function(s) and significance of these two genes.

This review will focus on what is currently known about the function of the BRCA1 and BRCA2 gene products. We will discuss the identification of the genes, the genetic data available, the characterization of the gene products, and their potential biological functions. Finally, we will comment on the current controversies and difficulties in our understanding of these two genes and their potential functions and suggest directions for future research.

2. BRCA1

2.1. Identification of the Gene

2.1.1. Gene Structure

In 1990, BRCA1 was localized to chromosome 17q21 by linkage analysis of families with early-onset breast and ovarian cancer (2). The cloning and sequencing of the gene was completed in 1994 (3). However, the structure of BRCA1 has provided only partial clues as to its function.

BRCA1 contains 24 exons that encode an 1863 amino-acid protein product (3). Exons 1 and 4 are noncoding. Exon 11 is unusually large, containing over half of the coding region of the gene. The BRCA1 sequence predicts an amino-terminal zinc RING finger domain of the C3HC4 structure. Although structurally different from the classic C2H2 zinc-fingers found in many transcription factors, similar zinc-fingers have been found in proteins that interact with DNA. However, it is not clear whether such RING domains are involved in direct DNA interactions or whether they permit such association indirectly through protein-protein interactions (8). In addition, an acidic carboxy-terminus suggests the presence of a transactivation domain. Because of these characteristics, the gene product is believed to be a transcription factor or cofactor that regulates the expression of specific target genes. The carboxy-terminal region encompassing the transactivation domain has also recently been described as containing a domain common to many proteins involved in DNA repair, including Rad 9, XRCC1, and three eukaryotic DNA-ligases (9–11). This domain, now termed the BRCT domain for BRCA1 C-Terminal domain, consists of a 95 amino acid sequence that can be repeated in tandem one or more times (9–11). It has been suggested that BRCT domains may be involved in protein:protein interactions, based on their structure and the observation that the minimal region of the p53 binding protein, p53BP1, required for binding to p53 contains a BRCT domain (9,12). The discovery of the BRCT domain in many proteins involved in DNA repair has fueled speculation that BRCA1 may have a role in the response to DNA damage.

2.1.2. Genetic Data

At press time, there have been over 300 reported sequence variations in BRCA1, with mutations scattered throughout this large gene (7). The majority of these mutations are either frameshift or nonsense mutations that result in a truncated protein product and provide few clues as to the function of the BRCA1 protein. However, a genotype-phenotype correlation has been proposed suggesting that mutations in the 3' end of the gene are less likely to be linked with ovarian carcinomas *(13,14)*. Of the few missense mutations, most are concentrated in the amino- or carboxy-termini, and disrupt either the RING domain or the putative transactivation domain *(7)*. The significance of some of mutations is unknown, implying a polymorphism that does not confer a malignant phenotype. However, other better characterized mutations, such as 185delAG in exon 2, found in the familial breast cancer of Ashkenazi Jews, are associated with a striking malignant phenotype. Two mutations, 185delAG and 5382insC, each account for nearly 10% of all known BRCA1 mutations *(7)*.

BRCA1 is linked to approximately 45% of breast-cancer-only families but to nearly all (79%) breast- and ovarian-cancer families *(6)*. The proportion of hereditary breast cancer has been estimated to be between 5–10% of all breast cancers. Of the large families studied in the Utah Population Database *(15)*, the percentage of breast cancers linked to family history approached 20%. However, in the Nurses' Health Study *(16)*, consisting of over 100,000 women followed for more than 20 yr, the percentage is much lower, closer to 6%. The actual number probably lies somewhere in the middle. In both of these large studies, hereditary breast cancer, linked to an autosomal dominant susceptibility gene, was not distinguished from simply having a family history of the disease without clear linkage to a susceptibility locus. A considerable problem in analyzing the genetics of breast cancer is that because the disease is fairly common within the general population, an inherited mutation may be difficult to distinguish from sporadic breast cancer in small- or even average-sized families.

The risk of a woman developing breast cancer, given a mutation in BRCA1, is difficult to quantify, because the frequency of mutations in the general population is unknown and penetrance of different mutations may vary. By studying high-risk families, Easton et al. *(17)* and Ford et al. *(18,19)* have estimated the cumulative risks of developing breast or ovarian cancer by age 70, given a mutation in the BRCA1 gene, to be 80% and 44%, respectively. More recently, Struewing et al. looked at a large population of Ashkenazi Jews, where the incidence of a BRCA1 or BRCA2 mutation is approximately 1% each *(20)*. Four specific mutations found in this ethnic group (185delAG, 5382insC, and 188del11 in BRCA1 and 6174delT in BRCA2) were screened in 5000 Ashkenazi Jews, and their risks assessed. In those with BRCA1 mutations, the risk of developing breast cancer or ovarian cancer by age 70 was 56% and 16%, respectively—much lower than first reported. The aforementioned risk assessment data are derived from women with the most highly penetrant genes. The risks for a woman without a family history, or specifically without a history of hereditary breast cancer (characterized by early onset, bilateral disease, and more than three first-degree relatives involved) are even lower. Currently, family history remains the single most important factor in determining risk.

Although hereditary breast cancers may only account for a small percentage of all breast cancers, inherited alterations may be involved in approximately 40% of breast cancers diagnosed before age 30 *(21)*. BRCA1 families have also been reported to have slightly increased incidences of colon and prostate cancer when compared to the general population. This implies that the function of BRCA1 may not be strictly limited to the breasts and ovaries. However, BRCA1's involvement in colon and prostate cancer has not been well-characterized.

2.1.3. BRCA1 as a Tumor Suppressor Gene

The pattern of inheritance of a tumor-suppressor gene is autosomal dominant. However, at the cellular level, the effects are recessive. In other words, both copies of an allele must be lost or mutated in order for a cell to lose the function of the tumor suppressor and ultimately progress to cancer. This is the so-called Knudson "two hit" hypothesis *(22,23)*. The likelihood that two separate genetic events will occur in one cell is very low. However, if one allele is inherited through the germline as a defective copy, only one additional "hit" is necessary in a somatic cell in order for the cell to lose that particular gene function *(22–24)*. Thus, germline mutations in tumor-suppressor genes effectively leave the individual genetically predisposed to developing cancer compared with the general population. This is apparent as dominantly inherited susceptibility. The second "hit" or loss of the wild-type allele is possible through a number of genetic events that may affect the somatic copy of the gene, including recombination, nondisjunction, or point mutation. These events may be influenced by factors such as hormonal status, environmental exposure, diet, and other risk factors. In addition, other genes linked to breast cancer, such as *p53 (25)* or RB *(24)* may also be involved and may alter a woman's risk compared with the risk of another woman with an identical BRCA1 mutation. The Ataxia Telangiectasia gene, ATM, has also been suggested to play a role in breast cancer *(26–28)*. However, some groups have not found a link *(29,30)*, and thus its role remains controversial. For a more detailed analysis of hereditary breast cancer, see the chapter by Bennet et al. in this volume. Analysis of tumors from patients with inherited BRCA1 mutations reveals loss of heterozygosity involving the wild-type allele *(31)*. This is consistent with Knudson's "two-hit" hypothesis, characteristic of the genetic behavior of classical cancer susceptibility genes.

The Knudson hypothesis argues that the same should be true for sporadic cancers, only that the rate of cancer formation will be lower because both "hits" must occur somatically. In this respect, however, BRCA1 does not behave as a classic tumor-suppressor gene. When Futreal et al. looked at sporadic breast and ovarian tumors with loss of heterozygosity in the BRCA1 region, expecting to find somatic mutations in these tumors, only 4 of the 44 tumor specimens studied had mutations and all four were in the germline *(15a)*. To date, only a few (10%) sporadic ovarian tumors and no sporadic breast cancer cells have been shown to carry mutations in BRCA1, despite a high frequency of loss of heterozygosity in the BRCA1 region in such tumors *(32)*. In contrast, classic tumor-suppressor genes, such as *p53* and the retinoblastoma gene *RB*, are mutated in both hereditary and sporadic cancer. It is possible that BRCA1 does not participate in the pathogenesis of nonfamilial breast cancer. This has been speculated *(33)* but is not particularly satisfying. The loss of genetic material in the region encompassing the wild-type allele in many tumors may be indicative of another tumor-suppressor gene in the region, distinct from BRCA1. Loss of heterozygosities studies indicting BRCA1 were actually done over a large region of chromosome 17q and thus may not be reflecting BRCA1 loss alone. Alternatively, the dosage of BRCA1 may affect breast-cancer development such that loss of one allele may be sufficient to promote cancer. It is reported that the level of BRCA1 mRNA is lower in many breast-cancer cells *(34)*. Finally, it is possible that potential mechanisms other than somatic mutation account for BRCA1's role in nonfamilial breast cancer. We will explore this possibility in depth later.

Table 1
Available BRCA1 Antibodies[a]

Antibody	Antigen	Serum source	Specificity (Band(s) on Western)	Reference
PAb 3' exon 11	A.A. 762–1315	Mouse	Single	Chen et al. *(31)*
MAb 17F8	A.A. 762–1315	Mouse	Single	This article (Table 2)
PAb A19	A.A. 1847–1863	Rabbit		
MAb MS	A.A. 1–304	Mouse	Multiple	Scully et al. *(40)*
MAb AP	A.A. 1313–1863	Mouse		
MAb SG	A.A. 1847–1863	Mouse		
pAb C-19	A.A. 1844–1863	Rabbit	Multiple	Jensen et al. *(58)*
B112	A.A. 2-355	Rabbit	Multiple	Wilson et al. *(76)*
C-20	A.A. 1843–1862	Rabbit	Multiple	Santa Cruz Biotechnology *(15a,19,27,83)*

[a]The BRCA1-region to which the antibodies were raised, the serum source, the number of protein bands detected by Western-blot analysis, and the references in which they are described are listed. Rabbit sera are all polyclonal. For the mouse antibodies, PAb, polyclonal serum, and MAb, monoclonal antibody.

2.2. Identification and Characterization of the BRCA1 Protein

2.2.1. Characterization of the BRCA1 Protein

Initial characterization of the BRCA1 protein product was possible with the availability of anti-BRCA1 antibodies. However, the antibodies available, both commercially and through independent laboratories, produced differing results that led to controversies concerning the size and the location of the BRCA1 protein. The specificity of the antibodies has been the most important factor in resolving these controversies. Table 1 summarizes the antibodies available and their specificity in detecting the BRCA1 protein by Western-blot analysis.

In 1995, Chen et al. first reported that BRCA1 was a 220-kilodalton protein using three distinct polyclonal antibodies (PAbs) raised against three different BRCA1 fragments *(35)*. This protein was localized to the nucleus of nonmalignant breast epithelial cells using the anti-BRCA1 antibody generated against the 3' end of exon 11 *(35)*. Nuclear staining of the protein was also seen in tumor cells that were not of breast or ovarian origin. In contrast, in many breast cancer and ovarian cancer cells, the same antiserum detected BRCA1 aberrantly located in the cytoplasm *(35)*.

Similarly, Scully et al. also characterized BRCA1 as a 220 kDa nuclear protein in nonmalignant breast cells using their own affinity-purified rabbit PAb and mouse monoclonal antibodies (MAbs) generated against a 20 amino acid carboxy-terminal peptide *(36)*. However, they found that BRCA1 was exclusively nuclear in both nonmalignant and malignant breast cells. Scully et al. attributed the cytoplasmic location of BRCA1 reported by Chen et al. *(35)* to staining and fixation artifacts.

The most surprising results were reported by Jensen et al. *(37)*. They found that BRCA1 was a 190 kDa protein secreted from vesicles. They used polyclonal antibodies raised against a C-terminal peptide containing 19 amino acids as well as the commercially available antibody from Santa Cruz Biotechnology Inc., C-20, generated against a carboxy-terminal 20 amino-acid peptide. These antibodies were similar to those generated by Scully et al. *(70)*, yet these two groups reported both a different molecular weight and a different subcellular location for the BRCA1 protein, leading to speculations as to the specificity of the antibodies used.

Other groups who used the C-20 antibody reported varying protein molecular weights and multiple bands on Western assays *(38–40)*, as well as molecular weights in agreement with Chen et al. and Scully et al. *(41)*. The utility of the C-20 antibody and similar sera raised against BRCA1 C-terminal peptides has been brought into question by Wilson et al. *(47)* who demonstrated that C-20 cross reacted with the 190 kDa epidermal growth-factor receptor (EGFR) in cell lines overexpressing the receptor. Because EGFR is commonly expressed in many mammary epithelial and breast-cancer cell lines and is a membrane-bound receptor, cross-reactivity of BRCA1 antibodies used by many investigators with this protein raises questions concerning the validity and reproducibility of their results.

Despite this controversy, most investigators have concurred that BRCA1 is a 220 kDa nuclear protein in normal human cells regardless of the antibodies used. However, the aberrant location of BRCA1 in the cytoplasm of advanced breast-cancer cells has remained controversial. To further address this issue, Chen et al. generated a Flag-tagged BRCA1 expression vector (pCEP4-Flag-BRCA1) *(43,44)*. The Flag-tag permitted detection of exogenous BRCA1 using the specific anti-Flag monoclonal antibody, M2 (Kodak). The M2 antibody detected a 220 kDa protein by Western-blot analysis in both nonmalignant breast epithelial cell lines and breast-cancer cell lines transfected with pCEP4-Flag-BRCA1. However, although immunostaining with M2 localized the tagged BRCA1 to the nuclei of normal cells, staining was seen in the cytoplasm of breast-cancer cells, in agreement with the initial findings of Chen et al. *(35)*. In addition, a Green Fluorescent Protein (GFP)-tagged BRCA1 fusion protein was created to allow direct viewing of the protein by fluorescence microscopy (Table 2). Again, the location of GFP-tagged BRCA1 in transfected cells was consistent with the initial observations of Chen et al. *(35)*. Significantly, detection of the GFP-BRCA1 fusion protein does not require fixation or staining, artifacts in which were suggested by Scully et al. *(36)* to explain the differences in location of BRCA1 in breast-cancer cells observed by Chen et al. *(35)*. More recently, a specific mouse MAb, 17F8, has been generated against the 3' region of exon 11 that recognizes a single 220 kDa protein in Western blots using cellular lysates of HBL100, an immortalized human breast epithelial cell line. Mislocation of BRCA1 in the cytoplasm of breast-cancer cells has also been observed with this antibody. Thus, four different methods for determining the molecular weight and subcellular location of BRCA1 consistently found that BRCA1 is normally a 220 kDa nuclear protein that is mislocated to the cytoplasm in many breast cancers (Table 2).

2.2.2. Biological Significance of BRCA1 Mislocation in Malignant Cells

Because BRCA1 is predominantly located in the nucleus of normal and nonbreast-cancer cells, its aberrant location in the cytoplasm of many breast cancer cells may be significant. If BRCA1 normally functions in the nucleus, retention of the protein in the

Table 2
Summary of the BRCA1 Localization Results Obtained
by Different Methods

Cell line	anti-BRCA1	flag-BRCA1	GFP-BRCA1	mAb 17f8
		Localization		
Non breast-cancer cell lines				
CV1	N[a]	N	N	N
DU145	N	N	N/D	N
T24	N	N	N	N
Saos-2	N	N/D[c]	N	N
5637	N	N/D	N/D	N
HBL100	N	N	N	N
Breast-cancer cell lines				
T47D	C[b]	C	C	C
MB468	C	C	C	C
MDA330	N, C[d]	C	N/D	N/D
MB231	C	C	C	C
ZR75	C	C	N/D	C
MCF7	N,C[d]	C	C	C
MB435S	C	N/D	C	C
MB415	C	N/D	C	C
SKBR-3	C	N/D	N/D	C
MB175-7	C	N/D	C	C
Hs578T	C	N/D	N/D	C
MB361	C	N/D	C	C
BT483	C	N/D	C	C
BT20	C	N/D	N/D	C

[a]N: nucleus C.
[b]Cytoplasm.
[c]N/D, not done.
[d]Small portion of cells shows nuclear localization.

cytoplasm may hamper the ability of the protein to execute its function. Thus, cytoplasmic retention of a nuclear protein may be an alternate method of protein inactivation, independent of direct mutation. In this regard, mislocation of wild-type, but not mutant, *p53* to the cytoplasm has also been observed in breast cancer *(45)*. Whether the cytoplasmic mislocation of BRCA1 significantly contributes to the progression of breast cancer remains unclear. It is possible that the aberrant cytoplasmic location of BRCA1 in advanced breast cancer cells may merely reflect the status of malignancy. In any event, determining the potential mechanism of protein mislocation will be of great interest to pursue.

Some clues are already forthcoming. Data from three groups has shown that amino-acid residues 503–508, which comprise an SV40 T-antigen-like nuclear localization sequence (NLS), are essential for the nuclear location of the BRCA1 gene product *(43,46,47)*. In addition, a yeast two-hybrid screen revealed that importin-α, a component of the NLS-receptor complex, interacts with the BRCA1 protein through this NLS

(43), and presumably this association is required for import of BRCA1 into the nucleus. Interestingly, a cytoplasmic protein with much stronger affinity for the NLS of BRCA1 than importin-α was found in the same two-hybrid screen *(48)*. It is possible that this cytoplasmic protein allows for regulation of BRCA1 transport into the nucleus, analogous to the function of IκB in sequestering NFκB *(49)*. Given the apparent high frequency of mislocation of BRCA1 in breast cancer cells, this finding is most exciting. Clearly, the nuclear transport of BRCA1 is under delicate regulation. Elucidation of the mechanism of regulation may shed light on how BRCA1 is normally transported into the nucleus and why it may be retained in the cytoplasm of many breast cancer cells.

2.2.3. Expression Pattern

The expression pattern of BRCA1 has also provided hints at possible function(s). At the cellular level, BRCA1 is phosphorylated *(50)* and its expression is cell cycle-dependent *(39,41,50)*, with the highest levels of both mRNA and protein expression occurring in late S through M phase. Phosphorylation of BRCA1 parallels its expression, suggesting that phosphorylation of BRCA1 may be important for its function *(50)*.

In the developing mouse, Brca1 is initially broadly expressed, later becoming more focused in different tissues in a pattern that follows their proliferation and differentiation. Thus, Brca1 appears to be expressed in cells undergoing rapid proliferation prior to differentiation *(51,52)*. Notably during puberty and pregnancy, there is considerable induction of Brca1 in mammary epithelium. Again these are periods of rapid proliferation and differentiation for this tissue. In ovariectomized animals, treatment with estradiol and progesterone restores the proliferation and the Brca1 expression. Similarly, human BRCA1 mRNA and protein expression are induced in cell culture when breast-cancer cells that are responsive to estradiol are treated with the hormone, and this response appears to be owing to the increase in cell proliferation *(39,53)*. Indeed, other mitogens such as insulin growth factor, epidermal growth factor, and retinoic acid, can also stimulate BRCA1 expression concordantly with their ability to induce S-phase entry *(53)*. Otherwise, this finding would be significant, because hormonal regulation of BRCA1 expression by estrogen would have been a convenient explanation as to why this gene, when mutated, should affect mainly reproductive organs such as the breast and ovary. Apparently, other pathways involved in tissue specificity exist and these will be important to explore.

2.3. Potential Biological Functions

The biological function of BRCA1 remains unclear. However, some clues have been provided by analysis of protein motifs, its expression pattern, and the properties of its interacting proteins. Important biological implications may also be inferred from gene-knockout models. Currently, there is no suitable biological system for addressing this question unequivocally. With this in mind, we will review the current information on the potential biological functions of BRCA1.

2.3.1. Transcriptional Activity

The carboxy-terminus of BRCA1 has been shown by three separate groups to be capable of activating transcription. Chapman and Verma *(54)* demonstrated transcriptional activation of a chloramphenicol acetyltransferase reporter gene in a kidney-derived cell line transfected with a construct expressing BRCA1 exons 16-24 (amino acids 1528-1863) fused to the GAL4-DNA-binding domain (DBD). Significantly, four separate mutants, corresponding to mutations of the carboxy-terminus seen in familial breast and ovarian cancers, failed to activate transcription. Montiero et al. *(55)* obtained similar results in both yeast and in mammalian cells, using nearly the same region of BRCA1 (amino acids 1560–1863) fused to the GAL4-DBD but with different reporter genes. Again familial mutations within this region abrogated transcriptional activity. Both groups also found that the distal C-terminus (amino acids 1760–1863) was capable of minimal transactivation activity, although Montiero et al. did not demonstrate this in mammalian cells. Finally, Chen et al. *(43)* fused different portions of the BRCA1 protein to the GAL4-DBD and tested for transactivation activity using a lacZ reporter in yeast. They found the highest level of activity to be between amino acids 1142–1643. The distal C-terminus also contained minimal transactivation activity. Combined, these three independent results suggest that there is definite transactivation activity in the carboxy-terminus of BRCA1. Slight differences between these groups in the precise location of the domain probably reflect the different cell systems and reporter genes used. However, this transactivation domain appears functionally significant, because familial point mutations in the region abolish transcriptional activity.

Although BRCA1 appears to have transcriptional activation potential, specific DNA-binding by BRCA1 has not been demonstrated. However, it has been proposed that the zinc RING domain at the amino-terminus may permit interaction with DNA either directly, or indirectly through protein-protein interaction *(8)*. Certainly this domain serves a critical function for BRCA1 because it is a site of frequent missense mutations in familial breast cancer, notably the Cys61Gly mutation. The current consensus is that BRCA1 may not recognize a specific DNA sequence. This being so, BRCA1 is most likely to act as either a coactivator or corepressor for sequence-specific DNA binding proteins, serving to link them to the transcriptional machinery *(8)*. In this model, the RING domain would serve as a protein-protein interaction domain to link BRCA1 to transcription factors bound to DNA. This hypothesis might be strengthened by the identification of proteins that interact with the RING finger. To date, only one such protein has been described. However, the function of this protein, designated BARD1 for BRCA1-associated RING-domain protein *(56)*, is unknown and its role in restraining tumor formation remains speculative.

2.3.2. Growth and Differentiation

BRCA1 appears to be important in cellular proliferation and/or differentiation. Consistent with a potential role in cell growth, BRCA1 has been shown to be phosphorylated and expressed in a cell-cycle-dependent manner *(39,41,50)*. In addition, the levels of BRCA1 mRNA appear to be reduced in both familial and sporadic breast cancer *(34)*. *Brca1*, the mouse homologue of BRCA1, is crucial for the growth and differentiation of the mouse embryo *(57–59)*. Three different groups have found that *Brca1* homozygous deletions (-/-) are lethal early in embryonic development. Both Liu et al. *(59)*, who generated a mutation in exon 11, and Hakem et al. *(58)*, who generated a deletion of exons 5 and 6 containing the zinc finger, produced embryos that failed to gastrulate and which differentiated poorly. These mice were resorbed by embryonic d 8.5 and 7.5 respectively. The third group also generated a mutation in exon 11 *(57)*, although this mutation was distinct from that of Liu et al. *(59)*. This mutation, although also lethal, generated embryos that survived until embryonic d 10–13. The mutant embryos were noted to have defects of neural development, including various degrees of anencephaly and spina bifida. These findings imply that the *Brca1* gene product likely plays a role in tissue growth and/or differentiation in mouse embryogenesis, consistent with the observed patterns of mRNA expression seen by *in situ* hybridization during development *(51,52)*. However, the molecular mechanisms driving this remain unknown. Terminal deoxynucleotide transferase-mediated dUTP-biotin nick end labeling (TUNEL) assays did not support increased apoptosis as the etiology of embryonic death. In addition, embryonic cells did incorporate BrdU (5-bromo-2'-deoxyuridine), implying that DNA synthesis is intact. However, mutant embryos were much smaller than their wild-type counterparts prior to their arrested development, implying that proliferation is defective. Interestingly, all these studies found mice carrying heterozygous deletions of *Brca1* (+/–) to be phenotypically normal with no evidence of increased predisposition to tumorigenesis through nearly two yr of observations *(60)*.

2.3.3. Repair Pathway

As previously discussed, the C-Terminus of BRCA1 contains a BRCT domain present in several proteins involved in DNA repair *(9–11)*. In addition, Scully et al. have described both colocalization and association of BRCA1 with Rad51, the human homolog of the bacterial RecA protein *(61)*. The role of human Rad51 is not clear, however, yeast Rad51 participates in the DNA double-strand-break repair pathway and in mitotic and meiotic recombination events *(62)*. Mutations of yeast *Rad51* result in chromosome loss *(62)*. In addition, mice deficient in *Rad51* cannot survive embryogenesis *(63)* implying that *Rad51* is also important for mouse embryonic development. A similar role in DNA repair and meiotic recombination has been proposed for human *Rad51*.

Using antibodies to BRCA1 and Rad51, Scully et al. stained MCF7 cells and found that both proteins exhibited an overlapping punctate-expression pattern in S-phase nuclei. However, this colocalization was transient and varied from cell to cell. In vitro binding of BRCA1 and Rad51 was suggested, but direct binding has not been confirmed. Finally, both BRCA1 and Rad51 colocalized on human synaptonemal complexes, suggesting a role for these two proteins in chromosomal recombination and maintenance of genome integrity *(61)*.

Although these findings are suggestive of an interaction between BRCA1 and human Rad51, several issues remain. First, reciprocal co-immunoprecipitation has to be demonstrated between BRCA1 and Rad51. Second, the specificity of the interaction needs to be confirmed by using mutants observed in familial breast cancer. Third, nonmalignant breast tissues need to be compared to provide functional evidence for these observations and to elucidate what the functional interaction of wild-type BRCA1 with Rad51 might be in normal breast tissue. The apparent colocalization of both proteins does not necessarily imply a biologically important interaction, and in fact, the interaction may be weak or not present at all. In a recent study by the same group, BRCA1 was copurified with RNA polymerase II holoenzyme, however, human Rad51 was not detected by copurification *(64)*. The lack of association of BRCA1 with human Rad51 in this latest study, and the absence of confirmation by other investigators are puzzling. Firm conclusions cannot be drawn.

2.4. Implications

Despite the wealth of genetic evidence linking BRCA1 to hereditary breast cancer, many difficulties remain in our understanding of the significance of a BRCA1 mutation.

First, BRCA1 appears to be a tumor-suppressor gene but does not completely behave like one, as previously discussed.

A second obstacle in understanding the genetics of BRCA1 is the observation that not all individuals with a family history of hereditary breast cancer have a mutation in the gene. This led to the speculation that another breast-cancer susceptibility gene must also be involved in familial breast cancer. This was confirmed by the localization and cloning of BRCA2, which appears to be linked with about the same percentage of hereditary breast cancers as BRCA1 *(4,5,65)*. However, these two genes together account for only 70–80% of all inherited breast cancers *(18)*. Speculation continues as to the future discovery of one or more additional breast cancer susceptibility genes.

Third, the absence of a family history does not preclude a mutation in BRCA1 in young women with breast cancer. Langston et al. *(66)* and Fitzgerald et al. *(67)* have each found that young women with breast cancer may harbor a BRCA1 mutation without necessarily having a family history of breast or ovarian cancer. Langston et al. looked at 80 women diagnosed with breast cancer before age 35. Approximately 10% had definite BRCA1 mutations in the germline and of these, one-third had no family history of either breast or ovarian cancer. Fitzgerald et al. looked similarly at 418 women with early-onset breast cancer (before age 40), not selected for family history. In the subgroup of women with unusually early-onset breast cancer at age 30 or younger, 15% harbored germline BRCA1 mutations. When a subgroup of 39 Jewish women were screened for the 185delAG mutation, it was found in 8 of them, or 21%, suggesting that BRCA1 mutations play a significant role in Jewish women with early-onset breast cancer. Seven of the 8 women in this subgroup, however, had at least one first- or second-degree relative with breast cancer. These two studies illustrate the complexity of the role of BRCA1 mutations in breast cancer with possible differences in penetrance, small families with limited histories, and mutations in noncoding regions accounting for the findings.

Although there remains much to learn and to clarify about the significance of a mutation in BRCA1, one cannot ignore that this gene is involved in hereditary breast cancer. The genetic data is by far the most compelling evidence that BRCA1 is an important gene in the pathogenesis of hereditary breast cancers.

3. BRCA2

Because its localization, identification, and cloning are more recent, there is less data available for BRCA2 concerning its possible function compared with its predecessor BRCA1. However, an emerging concept appears to be that BRCA2 shares similar expression patterns and potential function(s) with BRCA1. Although both play a substantial role in hereditary breast cancer in women, these genes diverge with respect to their roles in ovarian and male breast cancer. This may be explained by differing tissue specificity, hormonal influence, and penetrance among affected kindreds. This section will attempt to provide an outline of what is currently understood.

3.1. Identification of the Gene

3.1.1. Genetic Data

In 1994, BRCA2 was localized to chromosome 13q12–13 by linkage analysis of families with inherited breast cancer not attributed to mutations in BRCA1 *(4)*. A year later, the gene was successfully cloned *(5)*. By linkage studies, BRCA2 appeared to account for the same percentage of inherited female breast cancers as BRCA1 *(65)*. Together, these two breast cancer susceptibility genes were linked to the majority of familial breast cancer, approximately 70–80%. More recently, however, Krainer et al. *(68)* found a much lower incidence of BRCA2 mutations in a group of women with early-onset breast cancer. Of 73 females selected for a diagnosis of breast cancer before age 32, only 2 had a mutation in BRCA2 (2.7%) compared with 9 (12%) who had a mutation in BRCA1 *(67)*. In a separate study of 49 site-specific breast-cancer families, mutations in BRCA2 were found in only 8 families *(69)*, implying that the percentage of inherited breast cancers attributed to BRCA2 may be overestimated. This finding was supported by another group that examined 23 high-risk families and found that although a majority of hereditary breast cancers were owing to mutations in BRCA1 (61%), none were attributable to BRCA2, and 39% were not attributable to mutations in either gene *(70)*.

Interestingly, familial ovarian cancer is less commonly seen in BRCA2 kindreds, compared with BRCA1, although the risk of developing ovarian cancer with a mutated BRCA2 gene is still much higher than for the general population. Nearly all cases of inherited breast cancer and familial male breast cancer are owing to defects in BRCA2, although reports vary *(69,71)*. In addition, carcinomas of the pancreas, prostate, and colon occur at higher frequencies.

Mutations in BRCA2 confer an 85% lifetime risk of breast cancer and a 10% lifetime risk of ovarian cancer. The risk for male breast cancer, which is rare in the general population, is 6% *(71)*. Like the 185delAG mutation found in 1% of Ashkenazi Jews in BRCA1 kindreds, the 6174delT mutation in BRCA2 also affects up to 1.6% of Ashkenazi women. However, it appears that the penetrance of this mutation is much lower than the 185delAG mutation, as fewer women with this BRCA2 mutation develop breast cancer *(68)*.

3.1.2. Gene Structure

BRCA2 is nearly twice the size of BRCA1. It has 27 exons, 26 of which encode a large protein of 3418 amino acids. Like BRCA1, it has a large central exon 11. There have been over 100 distinct variants reported and like its predecessor, BRCA1, mutations span the sequence of this large gene *(7)*. The majority of these mutations lead to a truncated protein product (excluding the polymorphic stop codon at 3326), similar to BRCA1. Its sequence does not predict similarity to any known motif or cloned gene.

3.1.3. BRCA2 as a Tumor-Suppressor Gene

Mutations of BRCA2 are linked to a significant percentage of hereditary breast cancers, implying a loss of function that contributes to breast tumorigenesis in women, as well as men. The loss of heterozygosity at the wild-type locus seen in the tumors of patients with BRCA2-associated cancer also supports the role of this gene as a tumor suppressor *(72)*.

As was the case with BRCA1, however, mutations in BRCA2 occur infrequently in sporadic cases of breast cancer *(73)*. In 3 studies, the percentage of BRCA2 mutations in sporadic breast cancers was approximately 3% *(74–76)*. One study specifically looked at sporadic tumors with evidence of loss of heterozygosity in the region of BRCA2 *(74)*. However, only 2 out of 70 breast tumors had any alterations; one was a germline mutation, and the other was of unknown significance. Because BRCA2 lies on the same chromosome as the retinoblastoma susceptibility gene *RB*, mutations in *RB* were suggested to account for the loss of heterozygosity in these cases. However, this has not been borne out in studies of loss of heterozygosity on chromosome 13 in primary ovarian cancers *(77,78)*. Although loss of heterozygosity was seen in approximately 50% of ovarian tumors in both studies, RB protein expression was not diminished compared with normal tissue.

A possible explanation for these findings is that an undiscovered gene may regulate the expression of BRCA1 and BRCA2 in sporadic breast cancer and it is this gene that is mutated. As discussed in the case of BRCA1, a mechanism other than mutation may also explain BRCA2's role in sporadic tumors. Finally, the breast-cancer susceptibility genes may only be important in those genetically predisposed to the disease.

3.2. Expression Profile of BRCA2

Currently, there is no published data on the expression profile of the BRCA2 protein itself. However, the expression pattern of BRCA2 mRNA is similar to that of BRCA1, with highest levels in the testis, breast, thymus, and ovaries *(79)*. During mouse development, *Brca2* mRNA is first detected on embryonic d 7.5, a time of rapid proliferation *(80)*. At the cellular level, expression is regulated in a cell-cycle dependent manner and peak expression of BRCA2 mRNA is found in S phase *(81,82)*.

3.3. Potential Biological Functions

3.3.1. Transcriptional Activity

As with human BRCA1, BRCA2 shares only moderate homology with its mouse counterpart, Brca2, 58% overall. However, several areas are more highly conserved. One of these conserved regions is exon 3, which shares some similarity to the activation domain of the transcription factor c-Jun. Accordingly, this region appears to have transactivation activity when fused to the GAL4 DNA-binding domain in yeast and in two separate mammalian cell lines *(83)*. This is similar to the transactivation domain demonstrated in the carboxy-terminus of BRCA1 and has led to speculation that BRCA2 is also involved in regulating gene expression. Disruptions of both of these transcriptional activation domains by genetic mutations have been seen in familial breast cancers associated with BRCA1 and BRCA2.

3.3.2. Growth and Differentiation

Gene-knockout experiments involving *Brca2* have closely paralleled the findings of similar mouse models for *Brca1 (57–59)* and mouse *Rad51 (74)*. Three separate groups of investigators have demonstrated that homozygous *(Brca2–/–)* mutant mice cannot survive embryogenesis *(42,80,85)*. Sharan et al. *(80)* deleted exon 11 and noted that developmental arrest at embryonic d 6.5 coincides with the onset of detectable *Brca2* mRNA expression by *in situ* hybridization techniques. Prior to growth arrest, the embryos appear to be differentiating, and unlike *Brca1* homozygous knockouts, they do form mesoderm. This suggests that *Brca2* is important in mouse embryogenesis by influencing proliferation, more than differentiation. Suzuki et al. *(85)* deleted the 3' end of exon 10 and the 5' half of exon 11 and found arrest at embryonic d 9.5. Ludwig et al. *(42)* deleted a portion of exon 11, and embryos lived until d 8.5. Results from these three investigators imply that *Brca2*, like *Brca1*, plays an essential role in embryonic proliferation and differentiation. Similar to *Brca1*, *Brca2* heterozygotes (+/–) are phenotypically normal and fertile. Although they are predicted to be genetically predisposed to cancer, they show no evidence of increased tumor formation thus far.

3.3.3. Repair Pathway

Sharan and colleagues found that *Brca2* interacts with the mouse homologue of Rad51 in a yeast-two-hybrid assay and in mammalian cells *(80)*. Both gene products are expressed in embryonic tissue. Because of this association, homozygous-deficient embryos were examined for their sensitivity to gamma irradiation, which causes DNA double-strand breaks. *Brca2*-deficient homozygotes were more sensitive to radiation than their wild-type or heterozygous counterparts when inner-cell mass outgrowth and trophoblast cell numbers were measured.

3.4. Implications

The mapping and cloning of the second breast cancer susceptibility gene was accomplished quickly and gave rising hope that the function(s) of the these two gene products would soon become clear. However, BRCA2 presents similar dilemmas to BRCA1. Both are implicated as tumor-suppressor genes, but are not mutated in most sporadic tumors of the breast or ovaries. Although the genetic data substantiate the significant roles of BRCA1 and BRCA2, these two genes are not implicated in all hereditary breast cancers. Their possible shared functions and interactions will now be discussed.

4. INTERACTIONS BETWEEN BRCA1 AND BRCA2

Although they share little similarity to each other or to other known proteins, BRCA1 and BRCA2 have remarkably similar features. Both are highly linked to inherited breast cancer and to cancers involving the ovaries and male breasts, respectively. Both genes are large with a dominant central exon. BRCA1 and BRCA2 have been demonstrated to have transcriptional activity and the purported transactivation domains are conserved between mice and humans. Consistent with a role in growth and differentiation, both gene products are maximally expressed during cellular proliferation, and mouse embryos that lack *Brca1* or *Brca2* cannot complete embryogenesis.

Most recently, both proteins have been shown to associate with DNA-repair pathway proteins. The potential role(s) of BRCA1 and BRCA2 in DNA repair and meiotic recombination events may explain the apparent conflict between the knockout mice studies and the role of these genes in promoting human cancer. Whereas deletion of *Brca1* or *Brca2* in mice result in growth retardation and failed development of the embryo, loss of function of these genes in humans with hereditary breast cancer results in unrestricted growth and tumor formation. If mouse and human BRCA1 or BRCA2 participate in the DNA-repair pathway, then loss of *Brca1* or *Brca2* may be lethal to the developing mouse embryo at a time when growth and proliferation, as well as replication errors, are highest. In individuals with a germline alteration of BRCA1 or BRCA2, loss of the wild-type copy may predispose the individual to the accumulation of genetic insults. These may be further propagated with the mutation or loss of other genes. BRCA1-associated tumors have been found to have more histologically aggressive characteristics including higher S-phase fractions, higher mitotic index, and more aneuploidy *(75,84,86)*. If BRCA1 and BRCA2 are involved in genome stability through interactions with repair pathway proteins, such as Rad51, then mutations in these genes would be expected to have the more aggressive features discussed, particularly aneuploidy. This has been found to be the case *(87)*.

Taken together, these results suggest that BRCA1 and BRCA2 may have similar functions. Interestingly, *Brca2* homozygous deficient mice have normal levels of Brca1 and vice versa *(42)*. This implies that their functions are not redundant in mice, as normal levels of one protein do not rescue the mouse from embryonic lethality. In humans, one gene is more closely associated with ovarian carcinoma while the other is linked to male breast cancer. Why there is this divergence in the tumor spectrum associated with these two genes is not clear.

5. PERSPECTIVES

Whether mutations in either BRCA1 or BRCA2 are threshold events in breast cancer formation remain to be determined. In the case of BRCA1, where mechanisms other than mutation have been proposed to account for inactivation or reduced BRCA1 protein expression in sporadic tumors (i.e., decreased mRNA expression and cytoplasmic mislocation), loss of BRCA1 function in sporadic tumors is a late event, not present in all tumors. There is evidence that BRCA1 and BRCA2 may participate in repair pathways and in growth and differentiation. This role has been described by Kinzler and Vogelstein as that of a "caretaker" tumor-suppressor gene to distinguish it from a "gatekeeper" *(88)*. Caretakers maintain the integrity of the genome whereas gatekeepers, such as *RB*, regulate cellular proliferation and differentiation. In this model, the deletion of both copies of a gatekeeper gene are enough to induce tumorigenesis, as proliferation proceeds unregulated. Examples include the *RB*, *NF1*, and *APC* genes. In contrast, the deletion of both copies of a caretaker gene is not sufficient to initiate cancer. Rather, loss of caretaker gene function destabilizes the genome such that mutations in other genes occur more frequently. The subsequent loss of a gatekeeper gene then starts the malignant process.

Such a theory is intriguing and certainly other genes must play a role in restraining breast cancer formation in carriers of BRCA1 and BRCA2 mutations. However, the distinction of "gatekeepers" and "caretakers" is not clear-cut. For example, *p53* has been described as a "guardian of the genome" *(89)* that stops proliferation in response to DNA damage. Without *p53*, the genome is unstable in that mutations that occur are allowed to replicate *(89)*. Thus, *p53* appears to be part caretaker and part gatekeeper, and mutations in *p53* are common in sporadic cancers *(90)*. Genes such as *MSH2* and *ATM* are directly involved in DNA repair and their mutations also generate instabilities in the genome that promote cancer by increasing the event rate of mutation. They would then appear to fit the caretaker class more clearly. Both genes are highly conserved in evolution consistent with their role in the fundamental process of DNA repair. BRCA1 and BRCA2 are not so conserved, and their probable role as transcription factors suggest that they are not directly involved in DNA repair, but like *p53*, might be signaling the transcription of specific genes required for the response to damage. Notably, homozygous mutant *p53*, *Atm*, and *Msh2* mice are viable and have a higher frequency of tumor formation, whereas *Brca1* and *Brca2* mutant mice do not develop tumors as heterozygotes and are embryonic lethal as homozygotes. These differences may reflect differences in the precise molecular pathways in which these many genes reside or may be attributable to such genes having more than one function. BRCA1 and BRCA2 are large genes with a potential for multiple functional domains and for interactions with more than one gene. In addition, how these gene products are lost or altered to affect primarily reproductive organs is not known. All of the potential functions described may interplay with other environmental factors to produce breast cancer. Defining these functions and how they interact to prevent tumorigenesis remains a large but exciting task that promises to further our understanding of the of the mechanisms by which the disruption of normal cellular processes can lead to malignancy.

ACKNOWLEDGMENTS

The authors would like to thank the members of the Lee laboratory for sharing their unpublished data and for helpful discussions in preparing this review. We also wish to thank Dr. Gary Chamness for his helpful critique of the manuscript. This work was supported by grants from the National Institutes of Health (SPORE in Breast Cancer, Project 5, CA58183) and the Alice P. McDermott Endowment Fund.

REFERENCES

1. American Cancer Society. 1996. Cancer Facts and Figures, 1996. Publication no. 5008.96.
2. Hall, J. M., M. K. Lee, B. Newman, J. E. Morrow, L. A. Anderson, B. Huey, and M.-C. King. 1990. Linkage of early-onset familial breast cancer to chromosome 17q21. *Science* **250:** 1684–1689.
3. Miki, Y., J. Swensen, D. Shattuck-Eidens, P. A. Futreal, K. Harshman, S. Tavtigian, Q. Liu, C. Cochran, L. M. Bennett, W. Ding, R. Bell, J. Rosenthal, C. Hussey, T. Tran, M. McClure, C. Frye, T. Hattier, R. Phelps, A. Haugen-Strano, J. Katcher, K. Yakumo, Z. Gholalmi, D. Shaffer, S. Stone, S. Bayer, C. Wray, R. Bogden, P. Dayananth, J. Ward, P. Tonin, S. Narod, P. K. Bristow, F. J. Norris, L. Helvering, P. Morrison, P. Rosteck, M. Lai, J. C. Barrett, C. Lewis, S. Neuhausen, L. Cannon-Albright, D. Goldgar, R. Wiseman, A. Kamb, and M. H. Skolnick. 1994. A strong candidate for the breast and ovarian cancer susceptibility gene BRCA1. *Science* **266:** 66–71.
4. Wooster, R., S. L. Neuhausen, J. Mangion, Y. Quirk, D. Ford, N. Collins, K. Nguyen, S. Seal, T. Tran, D. Averill, P. Fields, G. Marshall, S. Narod, G. M. Lenoir, H. Lynch, J. Feunteun, P. Devilee, C. J. Cornelisse, F. H. Menko, P. A. Daly, W. Ormiston, R. McManus, C. Pye, C. M. Lewis, L. A. Cannon-Albright, J. Peto, B. A. J. Ponder, M. H. Skolnick, D. F. Easton, D. E. Goldgar, and M. R. Stratton. 1994. Localization of a breasst cancer susceptibility gene, BRCA2, to chromosome 13q12–13. *Science* **265:** 2088–2090.
5. Wooster, R., G. Bignell, J. Lancaster, S. Swift, S. Seal, J. Mangion, N. Collins, S. Gregory, C. Gumbs, G. Micklem, R. Barfoot, R. Hamoudi, S. Patel, C. Rice, P. Biggs, Y. Hashim,

A. Smith, F. Connor, A. Arason, J. Gudmundsson, D. Ficenec, D. Kelsell, D. Ford, P. Tonin, D. T. Bishop, N. K. Spurr, B. A. J. Ponder, R. Eeles, J. Peto, P. Devilee, C. Cornelisse, H. Lynch, S. Narod, G. Lenoir, V. Egilsson, R. B. Barkadottir, D. F. Easton, D. R. Bentley,. P. A. Futreal, A. Ashworth, and M. R. Stratton. 1995. Identification of the breast cancer susceptibility gene BRCA2. *Nature* (London) **378:** 789–792.

6. Easton, D. F., D. T. Bishop, D. Ford, G. P. Crockford, and the Breast Cancer Linkage Consortium. 1993. Genetic linkage analysis in familial breast and ovarian cancer: results from 214 families. Am. *J. Human Genet.* **52:** 678–701.

7. BCIC. Breast Cancer Information Core, Webmaster@nhgri.nih.gov.

8. Bienstock, R. J., T. Darden, R. Wiseman, L Pedersen, and J. C. Barrett. 1996. Molecular modeling of the amino-terminal zinc ring domain of BRCA1. *Cancer Res.* **56:** 2539–2545.

9. Koonin, E. V., S. F. Altschul, and P. Bork. 1996. Functional motifs. *Nature Genet.* **13:** 266–268.

10. Bork, P., K. Hofmann, P. Bucher, A. F. Neuwald, S. F. Altschul,. and E. V. Koonin. 1997. A superfamily of conserved domains in DNA damage-responsive cell cycle checkpoint proteins. FASEB J. **11:** 68–76.

11. Callebaut, I. and J.-P. Mornon. 1997. From BRCA1 to RAP1: a widespread BRCT module closely associated with DNA repair. *FEBS Lett.* **400:** 25–30.

12. Iwabuchi, K., P. L. Bartel, B. Li, R. Marraccino, and S. Fields. 1994. Two cellular proteins that bind to wild-type but not mutant p53. *Proc. Natl. Acad. Sci. USA.* **91:** 6098–6102.

13. Gayther, S. A., W. Warren, S. Mazoyer, P. A. Russell, P. A. Harrington, M. Chiano, S. Seal, R. Hamoudi, E. J. van Rensburg, A. M. Dunning, R. Love, G. Evans, D. Easton, D. Clayton, M. R. Stratton, and B. A. J. Ponder. 1995. Germline mutations of the BRCA1 gene in breast and ovarian cancer families provide evidence for a genotype-phenotype correlation. *Nature Genet.* **11:** 428–433.

14. Holt, J. T., M. E. Thompson, C. Szabo, C. Robinson-Benion, C. L. Arteaga, M.-C. King, and R. A. Jensen. 1996. Growth retardation and tumour inhibition by BRCA1. *Nature Genet.* **12:** 298–302.

15. Slattery, M. L. and R. A. Kerber. 1993. A comprehensive evaluation of family history and breast cancer risk. *JAMA* **270:** 1563–1568.

15a. Futreal, P. A., Q. Liu, D. Shattuck-Eidens, C. Cochran, K. Harshman, S. Tavtigian, L. M. Bennett, A. Haugen-Strano, J. Swensen, Y. Miki, K. Eddington, M. McClure, C. Frye, J. Weaver-Feldhaus, W. Ding, Z. Gholami, P. Soderkvist, L. Terry, S. Jhanwar, A. Berchuck, J. D. Iglehart, J. Marks, D. G. Ballinger, J. C. Barrett, M. H. Skolnick, A. Kamb, and R. Wiseman. 1994. BRCA1 mutations in primary breast and ovarian carcinomas. *Science* **266:** 120–122.

16. Colditz, G. A., W. C. Willett, D. J. Hunter, M. J. Stampfer, J. E. Manson, C. H. Hennekens, B. A. Rosner, and F. E Speizer. 1993. Family history, age, and risk of breast cancer. *JAMA* **270:** 338–343.

17. Easton, D. F., D. Ford, D. T. Bishop, and the Breast Cancer Linkage Consortium. 1995. Breast and ovarian cancer incidence in BRCA1-mutation carriers. Am. *J. Human Genet.* **56:** 265–271.

18. Ford, D. and D. F. Easton. 1995. The genetics of breast and ovarian cancer. *Br. J. Cancer* **72:** 805–812.

19. Ford, D., D. F. Easton, D. T. Bishop, S. A. Narod, D. E. Goldgar, and the Breast Cancer Linkage Consortium. 1994. Risks of cancer in BRCA1-mutation carriers. Lancet **343:** 692–695.

20. Struewing, J. P., P. Hartge, S. Wacholder, S. M. Baker, M. Berlin, M. McAdams, M. M. Timmerman, L. C. Brody, and M. A. Tucker. 1997. The risk of cancer associated with specific mutations of BRCA1 and BRCA2 among Ashkenazi Jews. *New Engl. J. Med.* **336:** 1401–1408.

21. Claus, E. B., N. Risch, and W. D. Thompson. 1991. Genetic analysis of breast cancer in the Cancer and Steroid Hormone Study. Am. *J. Human Genet.* **48:** 232–234.

22. Knudson, A. G. 1971. Mutation and cancer: statistical study of retinoblastoma. *Proc. Natl. Acad. Sci. USA* **68:** 820–823.

23. Knudson, A. G. 1993. Antioncogenes and human cancer. *Proc. Natl. Acad. Sci. USA* **90:** 10914–10921.

24. Riley, D. J., E. Y.-H. P. Lee, and W.-H. Lee. 1994. The retinoblastoma prtoein: more than a tumor suppressor. *Annu. Rev. Cell Biol.* **10:** 1–29.

25. Sidransky, D., T. Tokino, K. Helzlsouer, B. Zehnbauer, G. Rausch, B. Shelton, L. Prestigiacomo, B. Vogelstein, and N. Davidson. 1992. Inherited p53 gene mutations in breast cancer. *Cancer Res.* **52:** 2984–2986.

26. Swift, M., D. Morrell, R. B. Massey, and C. L. Chase. 1991. Incidence of cancer in 161 families affected by ataxia-telangiectasia. *New Engl. J. Med.* **325:** 1831–1836.

27. Swift, M., P. J. Reitnauer, D. Morrell, and C. L. Chase. 1987. Breast and other cancers in families with ataxia-telangiectasia. *New Engl. J. Med.* **316:** 1289–1294.

28. Athma, P., R. Rappaport, and M. Swift. 1996. Molecular genotyping shows that ataxia-telangiectasia heterozygotes are predisposed to breast cancer. *Cancer Genet. Cytogenet.* **92:** 130–134.

29. Wooster, R., D. Ford, J. Mangion, B. A. J. Ponder, J. Peto, D. F. Easton, and M. R. Stratton. 1993. Absence of linkage to the ataxia telangiectasia locus in familial breast cancer. *Human Genet.* **92:** 91–94.

30. Fitzgerald, M. G., J. M. Bean, S. R. Hegde, H. Unsal, D. J. MacDonald, D. P. Harkin, D. M. Finkelstein, K. J. Isselbacher, and D. A. Haber. 1997. Heterozygous ATM mutations do not contribute to early onset of breast cancer. *Nature Genet.* **15:** 307–310.

31. Chen, L. C., W. Kurisu, B. M. Ljung, E. S. Goldman, D. Moore II, and H. S. Smith. 1992. Heterogeneity for allelic loss in human breast cancer. J. Natl. Cancer Inst. **84:** 506–510.

32. Merajver, S. D., T. M. Pham, R. F. Caduff, M. Chen, E. L. Poy, K. A. Cooney, B. L. Weber, F. S. Collins, C. Johnston, and T. S. Frank. 1995. Somatic mutations in the BRCA1 gene in sporadic ovarian tumors. *Nature Genet.* **9:** 439–443.

33. Vogelstein, B. and K. W. Kinzler. 1994. Has the breast cancer gene been found? *Cell* **79:** 1–3.

34. Kainu, T., J. Kononen, O. Johansson, H. Olsson, A. Borg, and J. Isola. 1996. Detection of germline BRCA1 mutations in breast cancer patients by quantitative messenger RNA in situ hybridization. *Cancer Res.* **56:** 2912–2915.

35. Chen, Y., C.-F. Chen, D. J. Riley, D. C. Allred, P.-L. Chen, D. Von Hoff, C. K. Osborne, and W.-H. Lee. 1995. Aberrant subcellular localization of BRCA1 in breast cancer. *Science* **270:** 789–791.

36. Scully, R., S. Ganesan, M. Brown, J. A. De Caprio, S. A. Cannistra, J. Feunteun, S. Schnitt, and D. M. Livingston. 1996. Location of BRCA1 in human breast and ovarian cancer cells. *Science* **272:** 123–125.

37. Jensen, R. A., M. E. Thompson, T. L. Jetton, C. I Szabo, R. van der Meer, B. Helou, S. R. Tronick, D. L. Page, M.-C. King, and J. T. Holt. 1996. BRCA1 is secreted and exhibits properties of a granin. *Nature Genet.* **12:** 303–308.

38. Gudas, J. M., H. Nguyen, T. Li, and K. H. Cowan. 1995. Hormone-dependent regulation of BRCA1 in human breast cancer cells. *Cancer Res.* **55:** 4561–4565.

39. Gudas, J. M., T. Li, H. Nguyen, D. Jensen, F. J. Rauscher III, and K. H. Cowan. 1996. Cell cycle regulation of BRCA1 messenger RNA in human breast epithelial cells. *Cell Growth Differ.* **7:** 717–723.

40. Rao, V. N., N. Shao, M. Ahmad, and E. S. P. Reddy. 1996. Antisense RNA to the putative tumor suppressor gene BRCA1 transforms mouse fibroblasts. *Oncogene* **13:** 523–528.

41. Vaughn, J. P., P. L. Davis, M. D. Jarboe, G. Huper, A. C. Evans, R. W. Wiseman, A. Berchuck, J. D. Iglehart, P. A. Futreal, and J. R. Marks. 1996. BRCA1 expression is induced

before DNA synthesis in both normal and tumor-derived breast cells. *Cell Growth Differ.* **7:** 711–715.

42. Ludwig, T., D. L. Chapman, V. E. Papaioannou, and A. Efstratiadis. 1997. Targeted mutations of breast cancer susceptibility gene homologs in mice: lethal phenotypes of Brca1, Brca2, Brca1/Brca2, Brca1/p53, and Brca2/p53 nullizygous embryos. *Genes Dev.* **11:** 1226–1241.

43. Chen, C.-F., S. Li, Y. Chen, P.-L. Chen, Z. D. Sharp, and W.-H. Lee. 1996. The nuclear localization sequences of the BRCA1 protein interact with the importin-α subunit of the nuclear transport signal receptor. *J. Biol. Chem.* **271:** 32863–32868.

44. Chen, Y., P.-L. Chen, D. J. Riley, W.-H. Lee, D. C. Allred, and C. K. Osborne. 1996. Location of BRCA1 in human breast and ovarian cancer cells. *Science* **272:** 125–126.

45. Moll, U. M., G. Riou, and A. J. Levine. 1992. Two distinct mechanisms alter p53 in breast cancer: mutation and nuclear exclusion. *Proc. Natl. Acad. Sci. USA* **89:** 7262–7266.

46. Thakur, S., H. B. Zhang, Y. Peng, H. Le, B. Carroll, T. Ward, J. Yao, L. M. Farid, F. J. Couch, R. B. Wilson, and B. L. Weber. 1997. Localization of BRCA1 and splice variant identifies the nuclear localization signal. *Mol. Cell. Biol.* **17:** 444–452.

47. Wilson, C. A., M. N. Payton, G. S. Elliott,, F. W. Buaas, E. E. Cajulis, D. Grosshans, L. Ramos, D. M. Reese, D. J. Slamon, and F. J. Calzone. 1997. Differential subcellular localization, expression and biological toxicity of BRCA1 and the splice variant BRCA1-D11b. *Oncogene* **14:** 1–16.

48. Li, S., C.-Y. Ku, A. A. Farmer, Y. S. Cong, C.-F. Chen, and W.-H. Lee. 1998. Identification of a novel cytoplasmic protein that specifically binds to nuclear localization signal motifs. *J. Biol. Chem.* **273:** 6183–6189.

49. Ghosh, S. and D. Baltimore. 1990. Activation in vitro of NF-kappa B by phosphorylation of its inhibitor I-kappa B. *Nature* (London) **344:** 678–682.

50. Chen, Y., A. A. Farmer, C.-F. Chen, D. C. Jones, P.-L. Chen, and W.-H. Lee. 1996. BRCA1 is a 220-kDa nuclear phosphoprotein that is expressed and phosphorylated in a cell cycle-dependent manner. *Cancer Res.* **56:** 3168–3172.

51. Lane, T. F., C. Deng, A. Elson, M. S. Lyu, C. A. Kozak, and P. Leder. 1995. Expression of Brca1 is associated with terminal differentiation of ectodermally and mesodermally derived tissues in mice. *Genes Dev.* **9:** 2712–2722.

52. Marquis, S. T., J. V. Rajan, A. Wynshaw-Boris, J. Xu, G.-Y. Yin, K. J. Abel, B. L. Weber, and L. A. Chodosh. 1995. The developmental pattern of Brca1 expression implies a role in differentiation of the breast and other tissues. *Nature Genet.* **11:** 17–26.

53. Marks, J. R., G. Huper, J. P. Vaughn, P. L. Davis, J. Norris, D. P. McDonnell, R. W. Wiseman, P. A. Futreal, and J. D. Iglehart. 1997. BRCA1 expression is not directly responsive to estrogen. *Oncogene* **14:** 115–121.

54. Chapman, M. S. and I. M. Verma. 1996. Transcriptional activation by BRCA1. *Nature* (London) **382:** 678–679.

55. Monteiro, A. N. A., A. August, and H. Hanafusa. 1996. Evidence for a transcriptional activation function of BRCA1 C-terminal region. *Proc. Natl. Acad. Sci. USA* **93:** 13595–13599.

56. Wu, L. C., Z. W. Wang, J. T. Tsan, M. A. Spillman, A. Phung, X. L. Xu, M. W. Yang, L.-Y. Hwang, A. M. Bowcock, and R. Baer. 1996. Identification of a RING protein that can interact in vivo with the BRCA1 gene product. *Nature Genet.* **14:** 430–440.

57. Gowen, L. C., B. L. Johnson, A. M. Latour, K. K. Sulik, and B. H. Koller. 1996. Brca1 deficiency results in early embryonic lethality characterized by neuroepithelial abnormalities. *Nature Genet.* **12:** 191–194.

58. Hakem, R., J. L. de la Pompa, C. Sirard, R. Mo, M. Woo, A. Hakem, A. Wakeham, J. Potter, A. Reitmair, F. Billia, E. Firpo, C. C. Hui, J. Roberts, J. Rossant, and T. W. Mak. 1996. The tumor suppressor gene Brca1 is required for embryonic cellular proliferation in the mouse. *Cell* **85:** 1009–1023.

59. Liu, C.-Y., A. Flesken-Nikitin, S. Li, Y. Zeng, and W.-H. Lee. 1996. Inactivation of the mouse Brca1 gene leads to failure in the morphogenesis of the egg cylinder in early postimplantation development. *Genes Dev.* **10:** 1835–1843.

60. Liu, C.-Y. and W.-H. Lee. 1997. Unpublished results.

61. Scully, R., J. Chen, A. Plug, Y. Xiao, D. Weaver, J. Feuntuen, T. Ashlely, and D. M. Livingston. 1997. Association of BRCA1 with Rad51 in mitotic and meiotic cells. *Cell* **88:** 265–275.

62. Malkova, A.,E. L. Ivanov, and J. E. Haber. 1996. Double-strand break repair in the absence of RAD51 in yeast: a possible role for break-induced DNA replication. *Proc. Natl. Acad. Sci. USA.* **93:** 7131–7136.

63. Lim, D.-S. and P. Hasty. 1996. A mutation in mouse rad51 results in an early embryonic lethal that is suppressesd by a mutation in p53. *Mol. Cell. Biol.* **16:** 7133–7143.

64. Scully, R., S. F. Anderson, D. M. Chao, W. Wei, L. Ye, R. A. Young, D. M. Livingston, and J. D. Parvin. 1997. BRCA1 is a component of the RNA polymerase II holoenzyme. *Proc. Natl. Acad. Sci. USA* **94:** 5605–5610.

65. Tavtigian, S. V., J. Simard, J. Rommens, F. Couch, K. Shattuck-Eidens, S. Neuhausen, S. Merajver, S. Thorlacius, K. Offit, D. Stoppa-Lyonnet, C. Belanger, R. Bell, S. Berry, R. Bogden, Q. Chen, T. Davis, M. Dumont, C. Frye, T. Hattier, S. Jammulapati, T. Janecki, P. Jiang, R. Kehrer, J.-F. Leblanc, J. T. Mitchelll, J. McArthur-Morrison, K. Nguyen, Y. Peng, C. Samson, M. Schroeder, S. C. Snyder, L. Steele, M. Stringfellow, C. Stroup, B. Swedlund, J. Swensen, D. Teng, A. Thomas, T. Tran, T. Tran, M. Tranchant, J. Weaver-Feldhaus, A. K. C. Wong, H. Shĭzuya, J. E. Eyfjord, L. Cannon-Albright, F. Labrie, M. H. Skolnick, B. Weber, A. Kamb, and D. E. Goldgar. 1996. The complete BRCA2 gene and mutations in chromosome 13q-linked kindreds. *Nature Genet.* **12:** 333–337.

66. Langston, A. A., K. E. Malone, J. D. Thompson, J. R. Daling, and E. A. Ostrander. 1996. BRCA1 mutations in a population-based sample of young women with breast cancer. *New Engl. J. Med.* **334:** 137–142.

67. Fitzgerald, M. G., D. J. MacDonald, M. Krainer, I. Hoover, E. O'Neil, H. Unsal, S. Silva-Arrieto, D. M. Finkelstein, P. Beer-Romero, C. Englert, D. C. Sgroi, B. L. Smith, J. W. Younger, J. E. Garber, R. B. Duda, K. A. Mayzel, K. J. Isselbacher, S. H. Friend, and D. A. Haber. 1996. Germ-line BRCA1 mutations in Jewish and non-Jewish women with early-onset breast cancer. *New Engl. J. Med.* **334:** 143–149.

68. Krainer M., S. Silva-Arrieta, M. G. Fitzgerald, A. Shimada, C. Ishioka, R. Kanamaru, D. J. MacDonald, H. Unsal, D. M. Finkelstein, A. Bowcock, K. J. Isselbacher, and D. A. Haber. 1997. Differential contributions of BRCA1 and BRCA2 to early-onset breast cancer. *New Engl. J. Med.* **336:** 1461–1421.

69. Phelan, C. M., J. M. Lancaster, P. Tonin, C. Gumbs, C. Cochran, R. Carter, P. Ghadirian, C. Perret, R. Moslehi, F. Dion, M.-C. Faucher, K. Dole, S. Karimi, W. Foulkes, H. Lounis, E. Warner, P. Goss, D. Anderson, C. Larsson, S. A. Narod, and P. A. Futreal. 1996. Mutation analysis of the BRCA2 gene in 49 site-specific breast cancer families. *Nature Genet.* **13:** 120–122.

70. Rebbeck, T. R., F. J. Couch, J. Kant, K. Calzone, M. DeShano, Y. Peng, K. Chen, J. E. Garber, and B. L. Weber. 1996. Genetic heterogeneity in hereditary breast cancer: role of BRCA1 and BRCA2. *Am. J. Human Genet.* **59:** 547–553.

71. Couch, F. J., L. M. Farid, M. L. Deshano, S. V. Tavtigian, K. Calzone, L. Campeau, Y. Peng, B. Bogden, Q. Chen, S. Neuhausen, D. Shattuck-Eidens, A. K. Godwin, M. Daly, D. M. Radford, S. Sedlacek, J. Rommens, J. Simard, J. Garber, S. Merajver, and B. L. Weber. 1996. BRCA2 germline mutations in male breast cancer cases and breast cancer families. *Nature Genet.* **13:** 123–125.

72. Collins, N., R. McManus, R. Wooster, J. Mangion, S. Seal, S. R. Lakhani, W. Ormiston, P. A. Daly, D. Ford, D. F. Easton, and M. R. Stratton. 1995. Consistent loss of the wild type

allele in breast cancers from a family linked to the BRCA2 gene on chromosome 13q12–13. *Oncogene* **10:** 1673–1675.

73. Miki, Y., T. Katagiri, F. Kasumi, T. Yoshimoto, and Y. Nakamura. 1996. Mutation analysis in the BRCA2 gene in primary breast cancers. *Nature Genet.* **13:** 245–247.

74. Lancaster, J. M., R. Wooster, J. Mangion, C. M. Phelan, C. Cochran, C. Gumbs, S. Seal, R. Barfoot, N. Collins, G. Bignell, S. Patel, R. Hamoudi, C. Larsson, R. W. Wiseman, A. Berchuck, J. D. Iglehart, J. R. Marks, A. Ashworth, M. R. Stratton, and P. A. Futreal. 1996. BRCA2 mutations in primary breast and ovarian cancers. *Nature Genet.* **13:** 238–240.

75. Marcus, J. N., P. Watson, D. L. Page, S. A. Narod, G. M. Lenoir, P. Tonin, L. Linder-Stephenson, G. Salerno, T. A. Conway, and H. T. Lynch. 1996. Hereditary Breast Cancer. *Cancer* **77:** 697–709.

76. Teng, D. H.-F., R. Bogden, J. Mitchell, M. Baumgard, R. Bell, S. Berry, T. Davis, P. C. Ha, R. Kehrer, S. Jammulapati, Q. Chen, K. Offit, M. H. Skolnick, S. V. Tavtigian, S. Jhanwar, B. Swedlund, A. K. C. Wong, and A. Kamb. 1996. Low incidence of BRCA2 mutations in breast carcinoma and other cancers. *Nature Genet.* **13:** 241–244.

77. Dodson, M. K., W. A. Cliby, H.-J. Xu, K. A. DeLacey, S.-X. Hu, G. L. Keeney, J. Li, K. C. Podratz, R. B. Jenkins, and W. F. Benedict. 1994. Evidence of functional RB protein in epithelial ovarian carcinomas despite loss of heterozygosity at the RB locus. *Cancer Res.* **54:** 610–613.

78. Kim, T. K., W. F. Benedict, H.-J. Xu, S.-X. Hu, J. Gosewehr, M. Velicescu, E. Yin, J. Zheng, G. D'Ablaing, and L. Dubeau. 1994. Loss of heterozygosity on chromosome 13 is common only in the biologically more aggressive subtypes of ovarian epithelial tumors and is associated with normal retinoblastoma gene expression. *Cancer Res.* **54:** 605–609.

79. Rajan, J. V., M. Wang, S. T. Marquis, and L. A. Chodosh. 1996. Brca2 is coordinately regulated with Brca1 during proliferation and differentiation in mammary epithelial cells. *Proc. Natl. Acad. Sci. USA* **93:** 113078–13083.

80. Sharan, S. K., M. Morimatsu, U. Albrecht, D.-K. Lim, E. Regel, C. Dinh, A. Sands, G. Eichele, P. Hasty, and A. Bradley. 1997. Embryonic lethality and radiation hypersensitivity mediated by Rad51 in mice lacking Brca2. *Nature* (London) **386:** 804–810.

81. Sharan, S. K. and A. Bradley. 1996. Brca2 is coordinately regulated with Brca1 during proliferation and differentiation in mammary epithelial cells. *Proc. Natl. Acad. Sci. USA* **93:** 13078–13083.

82. Vaughn, J. P., F. D. Cirisano, G. Huper, A. Berchuck, P. A. Futreal, J. R. Marks, and J. D. Iglehart. Cell cycle control of BRCA2. 1996. *Cancer Res.* **56:** 4590–4594.

83. Milner, M., B. Ponder, L. Hughes-Davies, M. Seltmann, and T. Kouzarides. 1997. Transcriptional activation functions in BRCA2. *Nature* (London) **386:** 772–773.

84. Eisinger, F., D. Stoppa-Lyonnet, M. Longy, F. Kerangueven, T. Noguchi, C. Bailly, A. Vincent-Salomon, J. Jacquemier, D. Birnbaum, and H. Sobol. 1996. Germ line mutation at BRCA1 affects the histoprognostic grade in hereditary breast cancer. *Cancer Res.* **56:** 471–474.

85. Suzuki, A., J. L. de la Pompa, R. Hakem, A. Elia, R. Yoshida, R. Mo, H. Nishina, T. Chuang, A. Wakeham, A. Itie, W. Koo, P. Billia, A. Ho, M. Fukumoto, C. C. Hui, and T. W. Mak. 1997. Brca2 is required for embryonic cellular proliferation in the mouse. *Genes Dev.* **11:** 1242–1252.

86. Sobol, H., D. Stopppa-Lyonnet, B. Bressac-de-Paillerets, J.-P. Peyrat, F. Derangueven, N. Janin, T. Noguchi, F. Eisinger, J.-M. Guinebretiere, J. Jacquemier, and D. Birnbaum. 1996. Truncation at conserved terminal regions of BRCA1 protein is associated with highly proliferating hereditary breast cancers. *Cancer Res.* **56:** 3216–3219.

87. Beckman, M. W., F. Picard, H. X. An, C. R. C. vanRoeyen, S. I. Dominik, D. S. Mosny, H. G. Schnurch, H. G. Bender, and D. Niederacher. 1996. Clinical impact of detection of loss of heterozygosity of BRCA1 and BRCA2 markers in sporadic breast cancer. *Br. J. Cancer* **73:** 1220–1226.

88. Kinzler, K. W. and B. Vogelstein. 1997. Gatekeepers and caretakers. *Nature* (London) **386:** 761–763.

89. Lane, D. P. 1992. p53, guardian of the genome. *Nature* (London) 358: 15–16.

90. Hollstein, M., D. Sidransky, B. Vogelstein, and C. C. Harris. 1991. p53 mutations on human cancers. *Science.* **253:** 49–53.

11

Psychosocial Issues in BRCA1/2 Testing

Caryn Lerman and Beth N. Peshkin

1. INTRODUCTION

The availability of genetic testing for breast-cancer susceptibility provides an unprecedented opportunity for individuals to learn whether they carry cancer-predisposing mutations (*see* Chapters 8 and 9). Mutation carriers potentially can reduce their risk of cancer morbidity and mortality through increased surveillance and adoption of cancer-preventive practices. Noncarriers of mutations that are known to confer risk in their families may be relieved of persistent worry. However, it should be noted that testing is currently recommended only for high-risk families and is informative in only a subset of these. Nonetheless, participants in genetic testing research contribute to our evolving understanding of genetic and environmental factors that modify the penetrance of the major breast cancer genes and the efficacy of prevention options. Yet, genetic testing also has numerous psychological and social risks that must be considered so that the benefits of this new technology outweigh the risks of its application.

In this chapter, we address some of the emerging psychological and social issues posed by genetic testing for breast-cancer susceptibility. First, we present a brief overview of the genetic counseling process. Next, we present currently available data on patient decision-making about testing and the psychosocial and medical outcomes. We then discuss briefly the broader economic and social impact of genetic testing. Case illustrations are used to highlight pertinent clinical issues.

2. GENETIC-COUNSELING PROCESS

2.1. Overview of Process

Individuals interested in pursuing genetic testing are encouraged strongly to do so in the context of genetic counseling, both before and after testing *(1,2)*. The issues discussed during the genetic counseling session are an important part of the informed consent process and are outlined in Fig. 1. Although testing is commercially available and may be offered by community physicians, where available, a referral to a genetic counselor is appropriate given the time-intensive and complex nature of the counseling. In addition, genetic counseling and testing may be offered through research protocols or in conjunction with collaborative registries. Such programs are often designed

From: Breast Cancer: Molecular Genetics, Pathogenesis, and Therapeutics
Edited by: A. M. Bowcock © Humana Press Inc., Totowa, NJ

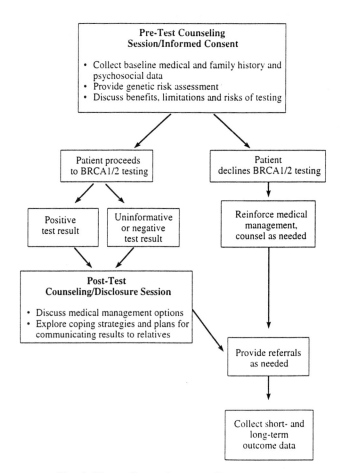

Fig. 1. Flow of genetic counseling process.

to collect detailed medical and family history information prospectively, as well as data on the long-term psychosocial and clinical outcomes *(3,4)*.

2.2. Intake

The genetic counseling process begins with an assessment of the patient's concerns, questions, and agenda. In order to provide an accurate risk assessment, a detailed family history in the form of a three-generation pedigree is obtained. Cancer histories are verified with medical-record documentation, when possible. A thorough medical history for the patient is also ascertained, which includes information about his or her current cancer screening and prevention practices.

The next section reviews the content of the genetic counseling session—components that are critical in order for patients to provide informed consent for testing. Patients should be able to consider and discuss questions such as: What are the pros and cons of testing? What is the likelihood that I have an alteration in a cancer-susceptibility gene? What medical options do I have if I test positive or negative? How will I and my family cope with this information?

2.3. Discussion of Testing Pros and Cons

It is crucial for patients to understand the complexities of genetic testing prior to providing a blood sample. Thus, as part of the informed consent process, a review of the potential benefits, limitations, and risks is essential, and it is often helpful for patients to explore their responses to different testing outcomes. Potential benefits of testing include gaining increased knowledge about cancer risks, which may help to tailor an appropriate screening and prevention regimen and to obtain information for relatives *(4)*. In addition, there may be psychological benefits owing to the reduction of uncertainty. Possible risks and limitations of testing include concerns about insurance and employment discrimination, negative emotional effects, and strained family relationships. A significant limitation of testing is that, regardless of the outcome, uncertainties remain about cancer risks and efficacy of preventive measures. A referral for additional counseling may be warranted for patients who may benefit from additional discussion of their personal responses to testing.

2.4. Genetic Risk Assessment

It is important for individuals considering testing to get a sense of the probability that they will test positive for a mutation in a cancer susceptibility gene such as BRCA1 or BRCA2. In general, the chance of obtaining an informative test result is maximized by first testing a woman with early-onset breast or ovarian cancer, and there are data available to guide the clinician as to the likelihood of obtaining a positive result in a particular individual or family *(5,6)*. If a mutation is identified, then autosomal dominant risks are applicable to first-degree relatives and may be extended throughout the pedigree, as appropriate. It is also important to emphasize that genetic risk can be transmitted through males. In families that are not suggestive of hereditary breast cancer, various empiric models may be used to assess breast-cancer risks *(7,8)*. The logistics of genetic testing with respect to blood drawing, turnaround time, type of testing available, and cost are explained to patients, as are the potential outcomes of testing, including the possibility that the test result may not be informative (e.g., a negative result after full BRCA1/2 testing in an affected individual may not rule out hereditary breast/ovarian cancer).

Because genetic testing results may be factored into an individual's medical management decisions, it is critical to review the cancer risks associated with altered breast-cancer genes and the uncertainties that exist with respect to these risks. No single number will be able to quantify precise cancer risks for an individual who tests positive, but taken in the context of a specific medical and family history, this information can be used qualitatively to target a screening and prevention program. Data on risks associated with specific BRCA1 or BRCA2 mutations are not yet available. Moreover, risk estimates have been derived largely from highly selected families in which multiple women have developed early onset breast and/or ovarian cancer *(9–11)*. Data from individuals with less striking family histories are beginning to emerge and suggest that on average, cancer risks are lower than those observed in the highest risk families *(12)*. Based on these studies, it is clear that women with a BRCA1 or BRCA2 mutation have a significantly elevated risk of breast cancer over the general population (i.e., 55–85% versus 12%, respectively), and to a lesser extent, also have an increased risk of ovarian cancer (i.e., 15–60% vs 1.5% in the general population). Increased risks for other cancers, such as those of the prostate, colon, pancreas, and breast cancer in men, have also been reported and research is underway to better characterize these risks.

2.5. Review of Medical Management Options

It is important to convey to patients that there are no proven methods of cancer screening and prevention in BRCA1/2 mutation carriers. However, prevention programs may be designed that are tailored to the risk level and resources of the individual, and should be considered in the context of his or her general health. These programs should also include standard age-appropriate guidelines as well as information about lifestyle modifications which, although not proven to reduce breast or ovarian cancer risks, may confer other health benefits. Men and women who test negative for a BRCA1/2 alteration identified in their family are often reassured that their cancer risks return to baseline. With respect to diseases like breast and colon cancer, these risks are not insubstantial.

In general, options for medical management may be divided into two categories. The first is early detection or surveillance, which generally involves more intensive screening and initiation of screening at an early age for breast and ovarian cancer. The following provisional guidelines in Table 1 were adapted from those proposed by the Cancer Genetics Studies Consortium *(13)*. These guidelines are based predominantly on expert opinion rather than epidemiologic outcome data. For example, between ages 25–35, it is recommended that women with a BRCA1/2 mutation obtain annual mammograms, coupled with clinician-performed breast exams every 6–12 mo. By contrast, women in the general population are advised to have mammograms every 1–2 yr between ages 40–50, and to obtain clinician breast exams every year. Women at high risk for ovarian cancer may wish to consider screening with pelvic exams, transvaginal ultrasounds, and CA-125 levels every 6–12 mo beginning at age 25–35. Owing in part to the significant limitations of this screening approach *(14)* and the relative rarity of ovarian cancer, ovarian screening is not offered to women at "average" risk (i.e., less than 2% in the general population). Where risks for colon and prostate cancer have been reported to be elevated, the absolute risks are not nearly as high as risks for breast and ovarian cancer, nor do the ages of onset appear to be significantly different from the general population *(10,12)*. Therefore, BRCA1/2 results usually do not affect screening guidelines for these cancers *(13)*.

The other category of cancer prevention is risk reduction. One method for potential risk reduction is the use of chemopreventive agents. Two drugs which may prove to be useful are Tamoxifen and the oral contraceptive pill *(13)*. Although both drugs may have possible adverse side effects, both also have appealing benefits aside from their potential to reduce cancer risks. A large randomized trial of Tamoxifen through the NSABPP-1 recently completed patient accrual. It remains to be seen whether this drug reduces breast-cancer risk in healthy women at increased risk for breast cancer, and if so, whether the magnitude of risk reduction is the same for women who are at high risk by virtue of their BRCA1/2 status. Although oral contraceptives appear to reduce ova-

Table 1
Medical Management Options for BRCA1/2 Mutation Carriers

Cancer Type	Provisional Guideline
Breast Cancer	Instruction and practice in monthly breast self-exam (BSE) by age 18–21
	Clinician performed exam every 6-12 mo and annual mammogram beginning between ages 25–35
	Consideration of chemoprevention trial
	Consideration of prophylactic mastectomy
Ovarian Cancer	CA-125 levels and transvaginal ultrasound with color Doppler every 6–12 mo beginning between ages 25-35
	Consideration of oral contraceptive use
	Consideration of prophylactic oophorectomy
Prostate Cancer	Rectal exam and PSA levels annually beginning at age 50
Colon Cancer	Fecal occult blood test annually and flexible sigmoidoscopy every 3–5 yr beginning at age 50
Other sites (e.g., cervix, skin, etc.)	Education about risk; standard age-appropriate guidelines

[a]Modified from ref. *13*.

rian cancer risk (15), it is unknown whether this is true also for women with BRCA1/2 mutations. It is likely that randomized trials of chemopreventive agents will become available to BRCA1/2 mutation carriers in the future.

The other method for potential risk reduction is surgery to remove the at-risk tissue or organ, such as prophylactic mastectomy or oophorectomy. Although these surgeries are thought to reduce the risk of developing breast and ovarian cancer *(16)*, they do not eliminate the risk *(13)*. The decision to undergo preventive surgery may also raise difficult questions regarding how a woman will obtain subsequent screening and how she will deal with the nebulous answers about the advisability of hormone-replacement therapy. Nevertheless, it is possible that women who opt for these procedures may obtain a decrease in anxiety, which enables them to enhance their quality of life. However, further research on the psychological benefits and costs of prophylactic surgery is needed.

2.6. Follow-up After Testing

Except in unusual circumstances, results of genetic testing are disclosed in person, at which time the clinician must balance the patient's desire for information as well as the importance of providing supportive counseling. Pertinent information about cancer risks, management options, and plans for communicating information are reviewed. When appropriate, referrals are made to specialists including oncologists and psychologists. For many patients, supplementing this session with written material and at least one follow-up phone call can serve to reinforce the information, answer questions, and provide further support as they begin to assimilate and accept the implications of their results.

3. EMPIRICAL RESEARCH ON GENETIC TESTING
FOR CANCER SUSCEPTIBILITY

3.1. Patient Decision-Making About Testing

As described above, to make informed decisions about genetic testing, patients must weigh the complex information about the benefits, limitations, and risks. According to models of consumer behavior, perceptions of the importance of the benefits (or pros) of testing would be expected to enhance intentions to be tested and actual test use, while concerns about the limitations and risks (or cons) should diminish intentions and hinder testing behavior. These models assume a "rational" process of decision-making in which an individual chooses the option which maximizes "expected utility"—or, in other words, the option for which he/she anticipates a higher likelihood of positive outcomes relative to negative outcomes.

The predictors of BRCA1 gene testing decisions were evaluated in a prospective cohort study of male and female members of hereditary breast-ovarian cancer (HBOC) families who were offered free BRCA1 testing *(4)*. Of 279 individuals, 43% decided to receive BRCA1 test results. It should be noted, however, that because testing was offered free of charge, rates of uptake of commercial testing (costing $200–$2400) may actually be lower. Reasons cited for wanting testing (pros) included: to learn about childrens' risks, to be reassured, and to make decisions about screening and surgery. Reasons for not wanting testing (cons) included: possible insurance discrimination, potential emotional effects on self and family, and concerns about test accuracy. Rates of BRCA1 test uptake were significantly greater among females, persons with higher levels of education, those with health insurance, and those who already had been affected with cancer. After controlling for these demographic and medical factors, test uptake was associated positively with knowledge of hereditary cancer and genetic testing and the perceived benefits of testing (pros). However, high levels of perceived limitations and risks (cons) did not deter testing. From a practical standpoint, this finding underscores the importance of emphasizing the limitations and risks of genetic testing to a greater degree in informed consent encounters.

The impact of alternate strategies to enhance informed decision-making for BRCA1 testing was examined in a recent randomized trial *(17)*. In this study, 400 women at low to moderate risk of breast or ovarian cancer were randomized to one of three pre-test education conditions: standard education only (educational approach) or education plus psychosocial counseling (counseling approach) or a wait-list control condition. The counseling approach provided standard education about BRCA1 testing and also asked participants to imagine how they would respond emotionally and behaviorally to positive and negative test results. Knowledge, perceived pros, perceived cons, and intentions were measured prior to education and at 1 mo. Because BRCA1 testing was not available for this population at the time of the study, provision of a blood sample for future testing served as a proxy measure of testing decisions. Compared to the wait-list control condition, both the educational and counseling approaches led to significant increases in knowledge. However, only the counseling approach led to increases in perceived limitations and risks of testing and decreases in perceived benefits. Because participants in the counseling approach had an opportunity to discuss the benefits and risks of testing more thoroughly and in a more personal way (i.e., by imagining their own reactions), they may have processed this information differently than those who received education only. However, contrary to expectations, neither the educational or counseling approach diminished intentions to have BRCA1 testing or to provide a blood sample. This finding suggests that other factors, such as patients' emotional states, may exert important influences on genetic testing decisions.

A recent study suggests that psychological distress may be an important determinant of patients' decisions to have genetic testing. In a study of women with a family history of breast-ovarian cancer, those who were more worried and distressed about their cancer risk were significantly more likely to participate in a breast-ovarian cancer risk counseling trial *(18)*. Similarly, among relatives of ovarian-cancer patients, cancer worries and mood disturbance were positively related to intentions to have BRCA1 testing *(19)*.

The association of psychological distress to actual use of BRCA1 testing was evaluated in the study of HBOC family members previously described *(20)*. Prior to the offer of testing, measures of cancer-specific and general distress were administered. Overall, levels of distress were not clinically significant in this population. After controlling for demographic factors and risk status, cancer-specific distress was found to be significantly and positively related to BRCA1/2 testing. Individuals with moderate to high levels of cancer-related distress were about three times more likely to receive BRCA1 testing than individuals with low distress levels. This suggests that the presence of even a moderate degree of distress can motivate BRCA1/2 test use. The implication of this finding is that patients who present for BRCA1/2 testing may represent a more psychologically vulnerable subgroup of the high-risk population.

3.2. Psychosocial Outcomes of Testing

Until recently, our knowledge of the psychosocial consequences of genetic testing for breast-ovarian cancer susceptibility was based entirely on anecdotal reports. These reports warned of negative emotional reactions in carriers and noncarriers of BRCA1 mutations *(2,21)*. However, in the past few years, several controlled investigations of the psychosocial impact of BRCA1 testing have been mounted, and interim data are available from a few of these studies.

The first of these studies focuses on the psychosocial effects of testing in a large HBOC kindred in Utah. The study protocol and measures were described *(22)*. Croyle and colleagues *(23)* recently reported preliminary findings from the first 60 women who received BRCA1 mutation test results. Study participants were interviewed by telephone before being scheduled for their initial meeting with a genetic counselor. Test results were provided at a second meeting with a genetic counselor and a psychosocial counselor (a psychiatrist, psychologist, or marriage and family therapist). One to two weeks later, participants were interviewed again to assess their reactions to learning their mutation status.

The report by Croyle et al. *(23)* focused on the impact of BRCA1 testing on generalized anxiety and on distress related specifically to genetic testing. There was no significant change from baseline to follow-up in the level of general anxiety reported by carriers. Among noncarriers, there was a small but significant decline in general distress. On the measure of specific distress, however, one group showed significantly

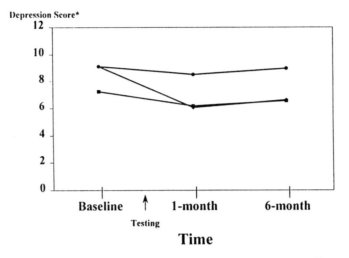

Fig. 2. Impact of BRCA1/2 testing on depressive symptoms in unaffected members of hereditary breast cancer families.

higher levels of disturbance when compared with the other participants. Even after controlling for baseline levels of general distress, women with no history of cancer or cancer-related prophylactic surgery reported higher levels of distress related to genetic testing. In contrast, mutation carriers who had already experienced cancer or prophylactic surgery showed no more distress than noncarriers.

Recently, we reported interim data from a prospective cohort study of members of several HBOC families in a registry maintained by Dr. Henry Lynch at Creighton University *(4)*. Changes in depressive symptoms and functional impairment from baseline to 1-mo post-testing were reported for 46 carriers of BRCA1 mutations, 50 noncarriers, and 44 decliners of BRCA1 testing. At baseline and 1-mo follow-up, all three groups scored in the normal ranges on these measures. Noncarriers of BRCA1 mutations exhibited significant decreases in depressive symptoms and role impairment and marginally significant decreases in sexual impairment, compared to carriers and decliners. Carriers and decliners of testing did not exhibit changes in any of these distress outcomes. Unpublished 6-mo follow-up data from this cohort suggest that this pattern of responses is maintained over time (*see* Fig. 2).

Although these two initial reports do not provide evidence for significant or pervasive adverse psychological effects of BRCA1 testing, caution is warranted in generalizing these findings to other populations and settings. Participants in these studies were members of high-risk families in hereditary cancer registries, many of whom were involved in prior cancer genetics studies. These families had been included in the registries because of their unusually high cancer rates. As a consequence of witnessing cancer in many close family members, emotional responses of study participants may have been blunted. In fact, levels of distress were lower in these HBOC families than in population-based samples of women with a family history of cancer and cancer patients *(20)*. In addition, most unaffected individuals in these high-risk families reported prior to testing that they expected to be mutation carriers. Thus, receiving a positive test result may have confirmed what they believed to be true all along. In some cases, worrying about the possibility of being a mutation carrier may be no less distressing than having that belief confirmed. Individuals who have less significant family histories, and who do not expect to receive positive results, may be more vulnerable to adverse psychological sequelae of BRCA1 testing. It should also be noted that all individuals in these studies were Caucasian (all of the Utah subjects were Mormon) and most had a high school education. In addition, all testing was provided as part of research protocols with extensive education and counseling. Such counseling may be responsible for the observed psychological benefits in the Lerman et al. study *(4)*.

3.3. Medical Outcomes of Testing

In order for BRCA1/2 testing to anticipated reductions in breast-ovarian cancer mortality, carriers must adopt recommendations for intensive and frequent surveillance *(13)*. To date, there are no published data on the impact of BRCA1/2 testing on adoption of recommended surveillance practices. However, our preliminary data from the cohort of HBOC family members suggest that screening adherence is suboptimal. Only 39% of eligible carriers had recommended mammograms during the 6 mo following testing and only 6% had transvaginal ultrasound or CA-125.

Rather than participate in frequent cancer surveillance, some female carriers of BRCA1/2 mutations are opting for prophylactic mastectomy and/or prophylactic oophorectomy. It is important to note that, although this procedure may reduce cancer risk, there may be a 5–10% or higher residual risk of cancer after these organs are removed *(24,25)*. In the cohort study previously described *(4)*, among unaffected female BRCA1 carriers, 18% intended to obtain prophylactic mastectomies and 33% intended to obtain prophylactic oophorectomies. Additional research is needed to document rates of surgery and to evaluate the psychosocial effects and efficacy of these medical procedures.

Preliminary data suggest that reproductive plans and choices may also be altered by genetic testing for breast-ovarian cancer susceptibility. In a survey of 56 women ages 40 and younger who had a family history of breast-ovarian cancer, 22% reported that they would be less likely to have children if they tested positive for a BRCA1 mutation and 17% reported being uncertain as to whether they would complete a pregnancy under these circumstances *(26)*. Moreover, 30% indicated that they would be interested in prenatal testing for BRCA1 and 30% would consider terminating a pregnancy if the fetus tested positive.

3.4. Economic Impact of Testing

In the current health care climate, the cost-effectiveness of genetic testing will be of paramount importance in the diffusion of this technology to clinical practice. To date, however, there has been limited attention to the cost-effectiveness of genetic testing for cancer susceptibility. In a recent analysis of the economic impact of genetic testing for hereditary nonpolyposis colon cancer, Brown and Kessler *(27)* estimated that the cost per year of life saved by testing is $55,000. This estimate is in the range of the cost per year of life saved for other cancer prevention practices such as mammography screening *(28)*. It should be noted, however, that any cost-effectiveness estimates for genetic testing for breast-cancer susceptibility or for other cancers would be highly speculative. Such estimates are affected strongly by the prevalence and penetrance of known mutations, as well as the efficacy of surveillance and prevention strategies in mutation carriers and their adoption of these practices. However, a reduction in health-care costs could be expected for individuals in high-risk families found to be noncarriers, because they would not longer require such intensive surveillance or surgical procedures. As yet, very little data on these parameters are available, making it difficult to calculate precise estimates.

3.5. Social Impact of Testing

One of the most significant social risks of genetic testing for breast-cancer susceptibility is the potential for discrimination by insurance companies on the basis of one's genetic status. As previously mentioned, fear of insurance discrimination is a potent barrier to participation in genetic testing and persons who lack health insurance are significantly less likely to be tested *(4)*. Although the experience with genetic testing for breast-cancer susceptibility is fairly recent, there are several documented cases of insurance discrimination on the basis of a variety of other genetic disorders *(29)*. In a recent survey of over 300 individuals from families with genetic disorders, 25% of respondents reported that they have been refused health insurance on the basis of their genetic risk, 22% had been refused life insurance, and 13% had been discriminated against in the employment setting *(30)*. A number of states in the U.S. have enacted legislation to address genetic discrimination *(31)* and recent federal legislation has enhanced the protection of genetic-testing participants. However, circumstances remain by which persons with increased genetic risk can be denied or refused insurance or be charged with excessively high premium rates.

4. CASE EXAMPLES TO ILLUSTRATE PSYCHOSOCIAL ISSUES

These vignettes are based on actual cases but have been modified to protect privacy.

Cases 1–3 are examples of informed consent/decision making issues about participation in testing.

4.1. Case #1

Annie is a 31-year-old married woman who was diagnosed with breast cancer at age 26. She underwent a unilateral mastectomy and chemotherapy and is now disease-free with a good long-term prognosis. Her paternal grandmother, who was diagnosed with ovarian cancer at age 60, is the only other case of cancer in the family. Her parents and her two older sisters are in good health (*see* pedigree in Fig. 3). The family is of Ashkenazi Jewish descent. Annie attended the genetic-counseling session with her husband, Jim. They were concerned mainly about cancer risks to future children based on Annie's medical and family history and were therefore very interested in pursuing genetic testing. Her oncologist had informed her that there was no medical contraindication for her to attempt pregnancy at this time. Jim's family history was noncontributory and he is not of Jewish descent.

During the genetic counseling session, they were informed that there have been three alterations in the BRCA1 and BRCA2 genes that occur with increased frequency in individuals of Jewish descent and that the chance of finding one of these alterations is

Case 1   Jewish

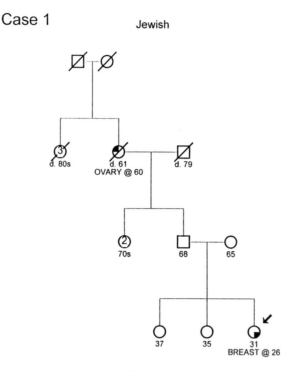

Fig. 3.

at least 20%, based primarily on Annie's young age at diagnosis. If an alteration was identified, then there would be a 50% chance of passing it down to future children. They were also counseled that a negative test result does not rule out the possibility of hereditary breast cancer, in which case future daughters would still face a somewhat increased risk of breast cancer based on empiric data. It was also explained that no one could guarantee the birth of a healthy child—that in fact, everyone has a few genes that do not work properly and it is not usually possible to know which genes are involved.

Much of the discussion focused on the couple's angst about the possibility of having a daughter who may be at risk for breast cancer. Jim also articulated his concern about Annie's prognosis. He wondered what would happen if she developed a recurrence and was not healthy enough to raise a child. He also was concerned about insurance issues. If Annie were to become ill again, he feared that losing or compromising their insurance because of a genetic test may deny them the resources they might need for state-of-the-art treatment such as bone-marrow transplant. Annie, however, was relatively unconcerned about developing cancer again. Nevertheless, these concerns about Annie provided the segue to discuss what genetic testing may be able to tell her, not about risk of metastatic disease as Jim had mentioned, but about her risk of developing breast cancer in her opposite breast and ovarian cancer, especially in the setting of a BRCA1 mutation. The conversation was then refocused to Annie, and secondarily to the issue of future children. Implications to her healthy parents and sisters were also considered. Annie was asked to imagine how she might cope with information that could affect her own health and the stability of relationships within her family. She imagined that her

Case 2

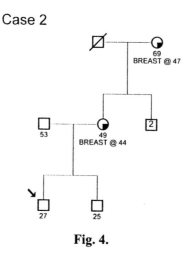

Fig. 4.

parent's feelings of guilt may be overwhelming, and as she considered her own future as a parent, she felt fearful and worried.

After several discussions with the genetic counselor over about a 12-mo period, Annie ultimately declined to get tested, and she is pregnant with her first child.

4.2. Case #2

Adam is a 27-year-old unmarried male whose mother and maternal grandmother recently learned that they have an alteration in the BRCA1 gene (*see* pedigree in Fig. 4). Adam's mother, a physician, reacted very positively upon learning her genetic testing results because she had always wanted to know why she and her mother developed early-onset breast cancer. She was very motivated to pursue early detection options for breast cancer (she had been treated with lumpectomy and radiation) and within 6 mo of learning her results, opted to have a prophylactic oophorectomy.

Adam presented for genetic counseling and testing, at his mother's strong urging, and said that he wanted to contribute a blood sample to "participate in research." He was somewhat indifferent about whether he wanted to receive results because he did not see that they would have any relevance to him. He did not perceive any "down sides" to testing and he specifically mentioned that he understood potential insurance risks but felt comfortable pursuing testing in a research setting where his results would be kept confidential.

Although it is recognized that many individuals choose to have genetic testing for a variety of reasons, including participating in research, he was not aware of at least two important issues that could impact him. One was that if he tested positive, current evidence suggests that his risk for prostate cancer and possibly colon cancer could be elevated. However, because these cancers do not appear to occur at early ages in male BRCA1 carriers, it is not clear that such information would affect his standard medical care in the future. In addition, if he were to test positive there would be a 50% chance that he could pass down the alteration to his children (boys and girls). He was also counseled about the fact that if he tested negative, his cancer risks

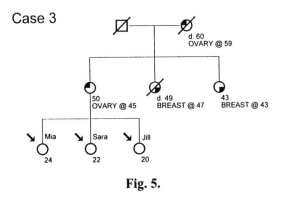

Fig. 5.

would be about the same as for other men in the general population and that he would know that the mutation could not be passed down to his children. He was also encouraged to consider the emotional implications should he test positive and to think through how his getting tested may affect decisions of his younger brother, how his mother may feel, and how he would communicate the information to a future spouse.

At the conclusion of the genetic counseling session, Adam decided to get tested, but articulated his main reason as concern for future children while also wanting to contribute to research. He was also very interested in obtaining his results. He later reported that while awaiting his results, he pursued discussions with his mother and brother about the potential impact on the family dynamics and was satisfied that these issues had been discussed openly and that he had a fuller appreciation for the potential impact of testing for himself and his family.

4.4. Case # 3

Three sisters, Jill, Sara, and Mia, ages 20, 22, and 24, attended a genetic counseling session together about 8 mo after learning that their mother had a BRCA1 alteration. Their mother, now age 50, is undergoing aggressive chemotherapy after a recent diagnosis of metastatic ovarian cancer. The family history is significant for two cases of early-onset breast cancer in their maternal aunts, and ovarian cancer in their maternal grandmother (*see* pedigree in Fig. 5). None of the sisters is married or has children. They are all in college or graduate school.

During the genetic counseling session, all the sisters verbalized their intentions to get tested and openly discussed their concerns about the implications of a positive result. For example, they were concerned about the lack of efficacy of cancer screening, particularly for ovarian cancer, and also for breast cancer in young women. They were not inclined to consider preventive surgery at this time. They wondered if a positive test result would affect decisions about oral contraceptive use, whether or when to have children, and how to raise the issue with future spouses. Although the sisters were participating in a free genetic counseling and testing research program with some measures in place to try to protect their privacy, they were also very worried about the potential effects of testing on their insurability. All of the sisters were covered at present under their parents' insurance and one sister had a part-time job with no benefits.

Another significant issue concerned the emotional implications of testing. The youngest sister, Jill, said that she hoped she would test positive because she felt that, as the youngest child, she had always gotten special attention, especially from her mother, and she felt best able to handle the information. Interestingly, the middle sister, Sara, remarked that she hoped they would all have the same result—that they should all learn that they have the alteration, or that they all do not have the alteration. She said that this way they could each understand what the others were experiencing— they would have a built-in support system, and no one would feel guilty or excluded. They commented that they have a very open relationship with their mother but were very concerned about her feeling guilty if any of them tested positive, and that she would become distracted from focusing on her own recovery. They were also aware of the large degree of reassurance they could obtain from negative test results. The oldest sister, Mia, was most certain about her decision to get tested. She had already been receiving more cancer screening than her younger sisters and also tried to reassure them that the potential benefits of testing outweighed the risks or limitations; even if the benefits were not immediate, she believed that the knowledge would be critical as they got older. She also comforted them by telling them that their mother has the emotional strength to support them in their decision about testing regardless of the outcome.

The genetic counseling session enabled the sisters to explore their feelings about testing outcomes and to consider the pros and cons of testing. Ultimately, they all suggested that the uncertainty associated with not knowing their genetic status would be more difficult than knowing one way or the other. Thus, Jill, Sara, and Mia all provided blood samples for testing, and were informed that the results would be available in about 1 mo, at which time they would be invited back for a disclosure visit.

When the results were available, Mia immediately scheduled her appointment. Before she learned of her results, Jill and Sara declined to schedule an appointment for follow-up. They cited concerns about insurance discrimination as their primary reason for declining at this time. They both said they wanted to wait to find out their results until they finished school and had jobs. Although they did not articulate concerns about feeling fearful or anxious about their results, it is quite likely that subsequent to these issues being raised and discussed openly during their initial session, they decided that this was perhaps information that they were not prepared to handle. Mia did test positive and expressed "relief" upon learning the result primarily owing to the reduction of uncertainty and interestingly, for solidifying a "bond" she had felt strongly to her mother—both emotionally and now genetically. She intended to share the information with her physicians in order to develop a plan for close surveillance and follow-up. In discussions with her over the next several weeks, Mia informed the genetic counselor that she communicated her test result to her sisters, and despite her own optimistic attitude, her sisters still chose not to receive their results.

Comment on cases 1–3: These cases illustrate that although it is important to address the issues presented by the patient, fully obtained informed consent means that the patient must be aware of the potential spectrum of issues that may arise, even if the information may be distressing. Helping patients to imagine how they would respond to this information, however, is a critical part of the genetic counseling process. Indi-

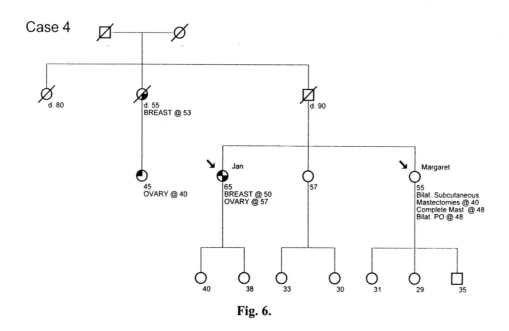

Fig. 6.

viduals considering testing do so for a variety of reasons, and their intentions and responses may change over time.

Cases 4 and 5 are examples of psychosocial and medical impact of genetic testing.

4.5. Case #4

Margaret is a 55-year-old woman who underwent bilateral prophylactic subcutane-ous mastectomies at age 40—within a year after her oldest sister, Jan, was diagnosed with invasive breast cancer. About 8 yr later, Jan developed ovarian cancer. In the setting of Jan's diagnosis and the strong family history of breast and ovarian cancer as represented on the pedigree (*see* Fig. 6), Margaret was counseled by her physician to have her ovaries removed as a preventive measure, especially because she had recently become menopausal. At age 48, she underwent an oophorectomy and also had addi-tional tissue removed from her breasts (in essence, she had "total mastectomies"). In 1996, Jan and Margaret participated in a genetic counseling session and were inter-ested in obtaining BRCA1/2 gene testing. Jan was interested primarily to gain informa-tion for her children and sister. Margaret wanted to get tested to learn about risks for her children, especially her daughters.

Because Jan had a history of two primary cancers, genetic testing for BRCA1 alter-ations was offered first to her. A common mutation in the gene was identified and then testing was extended to Margaret, who had a 50% chance of having inherited the muta-tion. In a second counseling session, Margaret was asked to explore how she would feel in the setting of learning that she tested positive and also to consider how she would feel if she tested negative. She said that she fully expected to learn that she has the mutation identified in her sister. She based this reasoning on a combination of factors in her medical history (she had a history of benign breast biopsies and always had difficult menses) as well as her perception that she looked like her older sister and that in general, "bad things seem to always happen" to her. Her decisions to undergo preventive surgery were based on these reasons as well as her anxiety about developing cancer. In the 7–15 yr since her surgeries, she remarked that she has enjoyed an exceptional and fulfilling quality of life. Her husband, family, friends, and coworkers have all provided support to her throughout this process. When asked to consider the implications of testing negative, she said that it would be the desirable, albeit unexpected, outcome because it would provide significant reassurance to her children and would eliminate the need to offer testing to them. The counseling session further reaffirmed that her decision to undergo surgery was an informed, reasonable choice, and for her was the best option. At the time, there was no way to help her to better quantify her risks for developing cancer other than that she could have a 50% chance of inheriting an altered gene that increased her cancer risk. She also realized that her satisfaction with this decision enabled her to be a productive, happy person in her personal and professional life.

During the next genetic counseling session, Margaret was informed that she did not carry the BRCA1 alteration identified in her family. She was delighted with this information because of the implications to her children. In several subsequent contacts with the genetic counselor, she has never expressed any regrets about her surgical decisions or choice to be tested.

4.6. Case #5

Two sisters, Rachel and Deborah, ages 40 and 45, tested positive for the BRCA2 alteration identified in their sister. As the pedigree illustrates (*see* Fig. 7), the family history of cancer other than their sister's diagnosis of breast cancer, is not very significant. Both Rachel and Deborah are accomplished, professional women. Rachel is married with three children; Deborah is single and has no children.

During the pre- and post-test counseling sessions, the sisters exhibited very different preferences for obtaining information. The elder sister wanted to get testing mostly owing to her curiosity, but was largely uninterested in hearing information about cancer risks associated with BRCA2 alterations and did not think that testing would affect her medical management or emotional well-being. She was already receiving breast exams every 3 mo along with annual mammograms. She also had regular gynecologic check-ups and because of the limited efficacy of ovarian cancer screening and the uncertainty about her ovarian-cancer risks, she did not think she would pursue ovarian screening or consider surgical options for risk reduction. Her sister, however, had a very different style of information seeking. She wanted to know many more details about the process of genetic testing, specific numerical risks associated with BRCA2 alterations and how they were derived, and data about screening and prevention options for breast and ovarian cancer. She was of the mind that, despite the uncertainties in cancer risks and efficacy of preventive measures, any heightened risk was too much to handle. She wanted to have prophylactic mastectomies and oophorectomy within the near future. She was also very concerned about her children, all of whom were too young to be tested. Whereas Rachel seemed very "panicked," Deborah seemed very complacent and did not appear to relate to Rachel's concerns.

During the counseling sessions, which both sisters attended together, their different perspectives were very evident. Deborah tried very hard to calm her sister whereas

Case 5

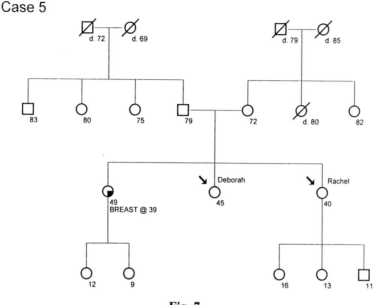

Fig. 7.

Rachel perceived Deborah as being apathetic and uninterested in the implications of their results. The ensuing discussion raised issues such as the idea that each person responds differently to this information, that there is no right or wrong way to feel, and that medical decision-making is a very personal matter. They were counseled to think carefully about the information, not to make any hurried decisions, and to realize that their decisions and feelings may vary over time. For example, one could opt for close screening now but consider surgical options in the future. One alternative that both sisters decided to investigate was a new chemopreventive agent for women at high risk for breast cancer. In so doing, Rachel was allowing herself to consider an option other than preventive surgery and Deborah was acknowledging that she was concerned about her cancer risks and would probably feel better if she knew she had carefully considered all alternatives for medical management.

In the 6 mo since their disclosure visit, both are still considering the chemoprevention trial, and Rachel is undecided about prophylactic surgery. She, however, continues to be very distressed and anxious, and was referred for follow-up psychological counseling.

Comment on cases 4–5: These cases illustrate that choices about medical management are highly individualized, as are the overall responses to learning genetic testing results. Psychological distress may make it difficult for patients to cope successfully with new information about their cancer risks, and may also hamper their ability to prioritize courses of action with respect to medical decisions, communication with family members, and dealing with their own emotions. The genetic counseling process can often help to prepare patients for these tasks by providing them with information and supportive counseling.

5. CONCLUSION

Discoveries of breast cancer susceptibility genes raise hopes concerning the public health benefit of genetic testing. However, before clinical counseling and testing programs are established on a widespread basis, effective and ethical means of communicating genetic risk information must be identified. Genetic counseling and testing protocols must be informed by empiric research that examines the psychosocial and clinical impact of testing programs on participants and their family members. In addition, further research is needed to elucidate individual differences in the psychosocial- and health-behavioral outcomes of genetic testing so that counseling strategies can be matched to individual patient needs. Consensus guidelines for surveillance and prevention should also be refined further as empiric data become available. At the same time, methods for enhancing patient adherence to recommended surveillance practices should be developed and validated. These issues will be best addressed if genetic testing for breast cancer susceptibility is conducted within the context of research that carefully assesses the immediate and long-term impact of participation in genetic counseling and testing programs.

ACKNOWLEDGMENTS

The authors would like to thank Henry Lynch, Steven Narod, and Stephen Lemon for their contributions to the work reported in this chapter, and Susan Marx for her assistance with manuscript preparation.

REFERENCES

1. American Society of Clinical Oncology. 1996. Statement of The American Society of Clinical Oncology: genetic testing for cancer susceptibility. *J. Clin. Oncol.* **14(5):** 1730–1736.
2. Biesecker, B. B., M. Boehnke, K. Calzone, D. S. Markel, J. E. Garber, F. S. Collins, and B. L. Weber. 1993. Genetic susceptibility for families with inherited susceptibility to breast and ovarian cancer. *JAMA* **269(15):** 1970–1974.
3. Jenks, S. 1996. NCI plans national cancer genetics network. *Natl. Cancer Inst.* **88:** 579–580.
4. Lerman, C., S. Narod, K. Schulman, C. Hughes, A. Gomez-Caminero, G. Bonney, K. Gold, B. Trock, D. Main, J. Lynch, C. Fulmore, C. Snyder, S. J. Lemon, T. Conway, P. Tonin, G. Lenoir, and H. Lynch. 1996. BRCA1 testing in families with hereditary breast-ovarian cancer: A prospective study of patient decision-making and outcomes. *JAMA* **275:** 1885–1892.
5. Berry, D. A., G. Parmigiani, J. Sanchez, J. Schildkraut, and E. Winer. 1997. Probability of carrying a mutation of breast-ovarian cancer gene BRCA1 based on family history. *J. Natl. Cancer Inst.* **89(3):** 227–238.
6. Couch, F. J., M. L. DeShano, M. A. Blackwood, K. Calzone, J. Stopfer, L. Campeau, A. Ganguly, T. Rebbeck, and B. L. Weber. 1997. BRCA1 mutations in women attending clinics that evaluate the risk of breast cancer. *N. Engl. J. Med.* **336(2):** 1409–1415.
7. Benichou, J., M. H. Gail, and J. J. Mulvihill. 1996. Graphs to estimate an individualized risk of breast cancer. *J. Clin. Oncol.* **14(1):** 103–110.
8. Claus, E. B., N. Risch, and W. D. Thompson. 1994. Autosomal dominant inheritance of early-onset breast cancer. *Cancer* **73(3):** 643–651.
9. Easton, D. F., D. Ford, D. T. Bishop, and the Breast Cancer Linkage Consortium. 1995. Breast and ovarian cancer incidence in BRCA1-mutation carriers. *Am. J. Human Genet.* **56:** 265–271.

10. Ford, D., D. F. Easton, D. T. Bishop, S. A. Narod, D. E. Goldgar, and the Breast Cancer Linkage Consortium. 1994. Risks of cancer in BRCA1-mutation carriers. *Lancet* **343:** 692–695.

11. Wooster, R., S. L. Neuhausen, J. Mangion, Y. Quirk, D. Ford, N. Collins, K. Nguyen, S. Seal, T. Tran, D. Averill, P. Fields, G. Marshall, S. Narod, G. M. Lenoir, H. Lynch, J. Feunteun, P. Devilee, C. J. Cornelisse, F. H. Menko, P. A. Daly, W. Ormiston, R. McManus, C. Pye, C. M. Lewis, L. A. Cannon-Albright, J. Peto, B. A. J. Ponder, M. H. Skolnick, D. F. Easton, D. E. Goldgar, and M. R. Stratton. 1994. Localization of a breast cancer susceptibility gene, BRCA2, to chromosome 13q12-13. *Science* **265:** 2088–2099.

12. Struewing, J. P., P. Hartge, S. Wacholder, S. M. Baker, S. M., Berlin, M. McAdams, M. M. Timmerman, L. C. Brody, and M. A. Tucker. 1997. The risk of cancer associated with specific mutations of BRCA1 and BRCA2 among Ashkenazi Jews. *N. Engl. J. Med.* **336(20):** 1401–1408.

13. Burke, W., M. Daly, J. Garber, J. Botkin, M. J. E. Kahn, P. Lynch, A. McTiernan, K. Offit, J. Perlman, G. Petersen, E. Thomson, C. Varricchio, and the Cancer Genetics Studies Consortium. 1997. Recommendations for follow-up care of individuals with an inherited predisposition to cancer. II. BRCA1 and BRCA2. *JAMA* **277(12):** 997–1003.

14. Carlson, K. J., S. J. Skates, and D. E. Singer. 1994. Screening for ovarian cancer. *Ann. Int. Med.* **121:** 124–132.

15. Hankinson, S. E., G. A. Colditz, D. J. Hunter, T. C. Spencer, B. Rosner, and M. J. Stampfer. 1992. A quantitative assessment of oral contraceptive use and risk of ovarian cancer. *Obstet. Gynecol.* **80:** 708–714.

16. Hartmann, L., R. Jenkins, D. Schaid, and P. Yang. 1997. Prophylactic mastectomy (PM): Preliminary retrospective cohort analysis. *Proc. Am. Assoc. Cancer Res.* **38:** 168.

17. Lerman, C., B. Biesecker, J. L. Benkendorf, J. Kerner, A. Gomez-Caminero, C. Hughes, and M. M. Reed. 1997. Controlled trial of pretest education approaches to enhance informed decision-making for BRCA1 gene testing. *J. Natl. Cancer Inst.* **89(2):** 148–157.

18. Lerman, C., B. K. Rimer, M. Daly, E. Lustbader, C. Sands, A. Balshem, A. Masny, and P. Engstrom. 1994. Recruiting high risk women into a breast cancer health promotion trial. *Cancer Epidemiol. Biomarkers Preven.* **3(3):** 271–276.

19. Lerman, C., M. Daly, A. Masny, and A. Balshem. 1994. Attitudes about genetic testing for breast-ovarian cancer susceptibility. *J. Clin. Oncol.* **12(4):** 843–850.

20. Lerman, C., M. D. Schwartz, T. H. Lin, C. Hughes, S. Narod, and H. T. Lynch. 1997. The influence of psychological distress on use of genetic testing for cancer risk. *J. Consult. Clin. Psychol.* **65(3):** 414–420.

21. Lynch, H. T., P. Watson, T. A. Conway, et al. 1993. DNA screening for breast/ovarian cancer susceptibility on linked markers: A family study. *Arch. Intern. Med.* **153:** 1979–1987.

22. Botkin, J. R., R. T. Croyle, K. R. Smith, B. J. Baty, C. Lerman, D. E. Goldgar, J. M. Ward, B. J. Flock, and N. E. Nash. 1996. A model protocol for evaluating the behavioral and psychological effects of BRCA1 testing. *J. Natl. Cancer Inst.* **88:** 872–882.

23. Croyle, R. T., K. R. Smith, J. R. Botkin, et al. 1997. Psychological responses to BRCA1 mutation testing: Preliminary findings. *Health Psychol.* **16:** 63–72.

24. Stefanek, M. E. 1995. Bilateral prophylactic mastectomy: Issues and concerns. *J. Natl. Cancer Inst. Monographs* **17:** 37–42.

25. Struewing, J. P., et al. 1995. Prophylactic oophorectomy in inherited breast/ovarian cancer families. *J. Natl. Cancer Inst.* **17:** 33–35.

26. Lerman, C., J. Audrain, and R. T. Croyle. 1994. DNA-testing for heritable breast cancer risks: Lessons from traditional genetic counseling. *Ann. Behav. Med.* **16(4):** 327–333.

27. Brown, M. L. and L. G. Kessler. 1995. The use of gene tests to detect hereditary predisposition to cancer: economic consideration. *J. Natl. Cancer Inst.* **87:** 1131–1135.

28. Brown, M. L. and L. Fintor. 1993. Cost-effectiveness of breast cancer screening: Preliminary results of a systematic review of the literature. *Breast Cancer Res. Treat.* **25:** 113–118.

29. Hudson, K. L., K. H. Rothenberg, L. B. Andrews, M. J. Ellis Kahn, and F. S. Collins. 1995. Genetic discrimination and health insurance: An urgent need for reform. *Science* **270:** 391–393.

30. Lapham, V., C. Kozma, and J. O. Weiss. 1996. Genetic discrimination: Perspectives of consumers. *Science* **274(5287):** 621–630.

31. Rothenberg, K. 1995. Genetic information and health insurance: state legislative approaches. *J. Law Med. Ethics* **23:** 312–319.

II
Biology of Tumor Progression
Breast Cancer Metastasis

12

Nm23, Breast Differentiation, and Cancer Metastasis

Patricia S. Steeg, Melanie T. Hartsough, and Susan E. Clare

1. TUMOR METASTASIS

The local control of breast cancer has been achieved for most patients by surgery and radiation therapy. Universally one of the greatest fears expressed by patients is "Has it spread?" The spreading of breast tumor cells from the primary tumor to colonize other sites of the body defines the metastatic process. Whether by direct organ compromise, or by side effects of their treatment, metastases remain significant contributors to patient morbidity and mortality. Our relative success at local control has been confounded by a general failure to progressively and substantially reduce breast cancer death rates *(1)*. Thus, a critical need exists to understand and develop effective treatments for those parameters contributing to breast cancer metastasis.

The metastatic process is complex, beginning with invasion at the primary site. The invasion process was initially described to include alterations in cell-cell and cell-extracellular matrix (ECM) attachments, proteolysis and motility *(2)*. A host of specific proteins have been identified for each of these component processes, including integrins, cell adhesion molecules, multiple classes of proteases, protease inhibitors, motility factors, and so on, that provide additional levels of complexity. While the presence of lymph node metastases is the best accepted predictor of high risk for poor prognosis, it is not known to what degree distant metastases actually result from lymphatic versus direct hematological dissemination. After arrival at a distant organ, colonization and angiogenesis are required for the development of a metastatic focus. Colonization remains understudied, but a body of literature suggests that tumor cell responses to growth factors may play a critical role. Angiogenesis is required for tumor cell growth beyond a size supported by diffusion of oxygen, and a host angiogenic stimulators and inhibitors have been identified (*see* refs. *3* and *4*).

Tumor metastasis is measured by in vivo assays using immunocompromised animals *(5)*. In experimental metastasis assays cells are injected into the tail vein and pulmonary metastases are quantitated several weeks postinjection. This assay is rapid and easily quantitated but only measures the last part of the metastatic process, as cells are placed directly into the circulation. Spontaneous metastasis assays involve the injection of tumor cells to form a primary tumor, which then seeds out distant metastases.

From: Breast Cancer: *Molecular Genetics, Pathogenesis, and Therapeutics*
Edited by: *A. M. Bowcock* © Humana Press Inc., Totowa, NJ

While recapitulating the metastatic cascade, this assay suffers from poor quantitation and requires relatively long times to complete. For breast cancer many of the cell lines used in research were derived from metastatic lesions but currently fail to exhibit metastatic behavior upon injection. Thus, long term culture has altered this important phenotype. The human MDA-MB-435 and MDA-MB-231 breast carcinoma cell lines have been extensively characterized for metastatic behavior *(6)*. For most individual parts of the metastatic process in vitro assays are available, including attachment, protease activity, motility, invasion, colonization, and angiogenesis.

One of the most promising avenues of breast cancer research is the development of biologically based therapies to thwart the progression of metastatic disease. Not all aspects of the metastatic process may be equally clinically applicable: It cannot be proven that, at the time of cancer diagnosis and therapy, a breast cancer patient has not already had metastatic cells invade from the primary tumor, intravasate and extravasate the circulatory system and lodge as an occult micrometastasis in distant organs. Thus, steps aimed at the colonization and angiogenesis involved in micrometastatic outgrowth may be most clinically applicable. Therapies targeting invasion (proteases, adherence, and so on) may be most applicable in targeting endothelial cell invasion in angiogenesis.

Of the many molecular events participatory in the tumor metastatic process, this chapter will focus on the *nm23* gene family. The metastasis suppressive capacity of *nm23* has provided a basic research framework on which to formulate translational developments.

2. THE NM23 GENE FAMILY

2.1. Trends in Expression

The first *nm23* gene was discovered on the basis of its reduced mRNA expression in highly metastatic murine K-1735 melanoma cell lines, as compared to lower metastatic potential variants of the same cell line series *(7)*. The *nm23* cDNA predicted a 17 kDa protein, and anti-peptide antibodies recognized two bands of 17 and 19 kDa on Western blots *(8)*. Nm23 protein levels were similarly reduced in the highly metastatic variants of the K-1735 murine melanoma cell line series *(8)*. Four human *nm23* genes have been reported, *nm23-H1*, *nm23-H2*, *nm23-DR*, and *nm23-H4 (8–11)*. Nm23-H1 is approx 90% identical to Nm23-H2, and >50% identical to the remaining members of the family. The most thoroughly studied in breast cancer is *nm23-H1*.

Homologs of *nm23* have been investigated in numerous other species, indicating its conservation through evolution. In various organisms the gene is known as *awd* (*Drosophila* abnormal wing discs) or nucleoside diphosphate kinase *(ndk/ndpk)*. Functions in differentiation, proliferation, signal transduction, DNA mutation, metabolism, and metastasis suppression have been investigated.

Reduced expression of *nm23* has been observed in highly metastatic tumor cells from other metastasis model systems. These include NMU induced rat mammary tumors *(7)*, mouse mammary tumor virus induced tumors *(12)*, ras or ras and adenovirus 2 E1a transfected rat embryo fibroblasts *(13,14)* and B16 murine melanomas *(15)*. In other systems no correlation was observed between *nm23* expression

Table 1
Correlation of Reduced Nm23 Expression with Indicators
of High Tumor Metastatic Potential in Breast Carcinoma Cohort Studies

Indicator of Metastatic Potential	N[a]	Additional Criteria[b]	P	Nm23 Expression Quantitator[c]
Survival				
Am. J. Pathol. 139:245, 1993	39	OS	0.05	Anti-P11
J. Natl. Cancer Inst. 83:281, 1991	71	OS	0.003	RNA
Int. J. Cancer 55:66, 1993	116	OS	0.014	MAb, Nm23-H1
J. Nat'l Cancer Inst. 86:1167, 1994	47	DFS	0.012	MAb, Nm23-H1
Br. J. Cancer 73:630, 1996	59	OS	0.001	MAb, Nm23-H1
J. Surg. Oncol. 65:22, 1997	100	DFS	0.0433	Anti-NDPKA
Nodal status				
Int. J. Oncol. 4:1353, 1994	124		0.04	MAb to Peptide
Cancer Lett. 101:137, 1996	33		0.00001	MAb, Nm23-H1
J. Natl. Cancer Inst. 85:727, 1993	127		0.0001	Anti-P11
Int. J. Cancer 74:102, 1997	128		0.007	RNA
Other histopathological indicators				
Jpn. J. Cancer Res. 84:871, 1993	77	ER	0.01	Anti-rat NDPK
Oncology Reports 3:183, 1996	76	Grade	0.02	Anti-NDPKA
No significant associations				
J. Pathol. 172:27, 1994	197			Anti-NDKA
Int. J. Cancer 50: 533, 1994	98			Anti-NDKA
Pathology 26:423, 1994	132			RNA
Cancer 79:1158, 1997	40			Anti-Nm23-H1

[a]Number of tumor specimens analyzed.
[b]OS, overall survival; DFS, disease-free survival; ER, estrogen receptor expression; Grade, Histologic grade.
[c]Anti-Nm23 antibodies, except where RNA is indicated.

and tumor metastatic potential, indicating that this gene is potentially relevant to only a subset of cancers.

Using human breast carcinoma cohorts, *nm23* expression, either at the RNA or protein levels, has been correlated with patient clinical course or tumor histopathologic data (Table 1). Six studies reported a significant correlation between reduced Nm23 expression and poor patient survival. Where tested, Nm23-H1 expression was a better predictor of poor patient survival than Nm23-H2 *(16)*. Another four studies reported low Nm23 expression to be significantly correlated with the presence of lymph node metastases, and an additional two reports found low expression correlated with other histopathologic indicators of high tumor metastatic potential. In contrast, four studies, two of which used the same antibody, failed to find any significant associations. Prognostic studies for many genes have yielded conflicting results and interpretation must take into account both biological and technical factors. For instance, given the existence of four Nm23 gene products, different antibodies may recognize various members of the gene family. Quantitation of low- vs high expression also varied among the studies reported. In some studies, the hypothesis predicted that a single area of low staining tumor cells could constitute a focus of highly metastatic tumor cells, of potential harm to the patient; in other studies, cutoffs or uniform low expression were used as criteria. Given these technical variables, the correlation of low Nm23 expression with parameters of aggressive behavior in 12/16 studies is indicative of a biologically relevant trend, subject to further testing in transfection experiments. In no case has Nm23 expression been shown to be an independent prognostic factor, and most analyses have not centered on the important node-negative breast tumors.

The relationship of Nm23 expression and proliferative activity of breast cells has been studied *(17)*. In certain cases Nm23-H1 expression was lower in tumor cells than in surrounding normal mammary epithelial cells, suggesting a role in proliferation in the tumorigenesis process. However, within tumor cell populations a different trend was noted, depending on their invasive and metastatic status. Thus, tumor cells which invaded the lymph nodes or were found in distant metastases exhibited a high proliferative rate and lower Nm23-H1 expression than those of the primary tumor. Similar trends for Nm23-H2 were not observed. The data suggest that *nm23* may be linked to proliferation under certain circumstances, not including invasive and metastatic behavior.

Simpson et al. analyzed Nm23 expression in ductal carcinoma in situ (DCIS) lesions, both pure DCIS and those with an accompanying invasive component *(18)*. For comedo DCIS, thought to be a relatively aggressive, possible precursor of invasive disease, pure lesions exhibited greater Nm23 expression than did lesions with an invasive component ($P = 0.04$). These data suggest that an initial decrease in Nm23 expression may occur early in tumor progression, with the invasion process.

2.2. Transfection Studies

Five transfection studies have confirmed that overexpression of *nm23* on a constitutive promoter can exert a metastasis suppressive effect in vivo *(19–23)*. Of these, two reports utilized breast carcinoma cells. Fukada et al. *(20)* transfected the rat α and β isoforms of *nm23* into highly metastatic MTLn3 rat mammary cells and examined spontaneous metastatic potential. Rats injected with the α isoform, the homolog of *nm23-H2*, exhibited an average 44% reduction in distant metastatic potential, while nodal metastases were equivalent to that of control transfectants. Primary tumor size remained unchanged between control and *nm23* transfectants.

Studies in human breast carcinoma cells used the human *nm23-H1* cDNA linked to a constitutive CMV promoter, transfected into the MDA-MB-435 breast carcinoma cell line. The *nm23-H1* transfectants exhibited a 50–90% reduction in spontaneous metastatic potential, to the lungs or lymph nodes, as compared to control transfectants *(22)*. No differences were observed in primary tumor size. Additionally, in vitro aspects of the metastatic cascade were examined. The *nm23-H1* transfectants exhibited less motility in Boyden chamber assays to a variety of stimulants including serum, IGF, PDGF, and autotaxin *(24,25)*. Colonization in soft agar was reduced in the *nm23-H1* transfectants. Moreover, in the presence of TGF-β, the colonization response of the metastatic control transfectants, but not the *nm23-H1* transfectants was stimulated *(22)*. These data confirm and extend work from several laboratories which showed that metastatically-competent cells can be stimulated in the colonization response by exogenous factors such as TGF-β and IL-6, originally termed the "clonal dominance" hypothesis *(26)*. These data may provide an important clue to the outgrowth of metastatic cells in a distant organ. Although endowed with oncogenes and inactivated suppressor genes, tumor cells must colonize in a distant organ independently of cell:cell and cell:ECM interactions, locally produced growth factors, and other regulatory interactions that were operative in the primary tissue. The ability to be stimulated in colonization by widely available paracrine signals such as TGF-β may represent a strategic advantage for metastatic cells.

Taken together, the transfection data in breast carcinoma cells indicate that overexpression of *nm23* can have a metastasis suppressive effect. In no case was metastatic potential abolished, indicating the participation of other regulatory events in this process. Data from in vitro assays suggest that *nm23* overexpression modifies or impairs the signal transduction response to a variety of signals, resulting in less aggressive behavior.

2.3. Role in Breast Differentiation

The role of *nm23-H1* in breast differentiation was investigated using a model system pioneered by Bissell et al. Previously a three dimensional culture system using reconstituted basement membrane was developed, in which normal human mammary epithelial cells exhibited several characteristics of the development and differentiation process, including formation of ascinar (duct-like) structures, production and basal deposition of basement membrane components and production and apical secretion of milk proteins *(27)*. Cell lines and cultures from human breast carcinomas failed to recapitulate this process. Using this culture system, *nm23-H1* transfectants of the MDA-MB-435 cell line formed duct-like structures with occasional central lumens, resembling breast ducts (Fig. 1) *(28)*. The basement membrane components type IV collagen and laminin were produced and deposited to the basal surface; sialomucin was produced but not apically secreted. After producing basement membrane, *nm23-H1* transfected colonies were growth inhibited, as measured by cells/colony or thymidine incorporation. These data provided strong evidence that *nm23-H1* overexpression can reverse the apparent de-differentiated state of a breast carcinoma cell line to establish aspects of normal development and differentiation. The basement membrane contains multiple proteins that signal through integrins, and binds growth factors, which could contribute to the altered signal responsiveness to the microenvironment evident in the differentiated *nm23-H1* transfectants. The data also serve to underscore the important role of the basement membrane in the maintenance of breast epithelial differentiation and growth.

The proposed role for *nm23* in differentiation originated from work in other species or cell types. Initially studied in *Drosophila* as *awd*, reduced expression or gene mutation resulted in normal development through metamorphosis, but lethal, aberrant differentiation of the brain, ovaries and imaginal discs post-metamorphosis *(29,30)*. More recently transfection of murine *nm23* into PC12 pheochromocytoma cells resulted in growth arrest and sympathetic neuron development in response to NGF *(31)*. Antisense oligonucleotides to *nm23* reversed the TGF-β dependent differentiation of HD3 colon carcinoma cells *(32)*.

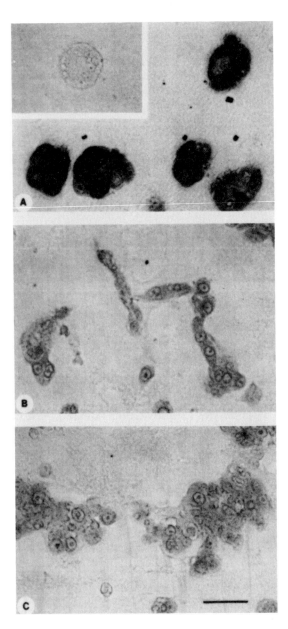

Fig. 1. Transfection of *nm23-H1* into human breast carcinoma cells promotes morphological differentiation in vitro. Twelve-day cultures of human MDA-MB-435 breast carcinoma cells within a basement membrane extract were stained for Nm23 expression (shown as dark or light intensities). **(A)** *nm23-H1* transfected H1-177 cells, exhibited spherical duct-like colonies with occasional central lumens. The inset shows Nm23 staining when the primary antibody was omitted as a control. **(B)** Control-transfected C-100 cells and **(C)** Parental MDA-MB-435 cells, failed to exhibit morphological evidence of differentiation *(28)*.

It can be hypothesized that the role of *nm23-H1* in differentiation may be central to its metastasis suppressive effect. During development, embryonic cells form differential adherences, move, invade, respond to growth factors and resemble metastatic cells, except that the process is both organized and terminable. Metastasis may therefore represent the aberrant reactivation of embryonic gene cascades.

2.4. Biochemical Functions of Nm23

The biochemical mechanism of action of Nm23 suppression of breast cancer metastasis is unknown to date. However, several exciting leads have developed which point to a potentially new role for this family of proteins. Summarized below are several interrelated biochemical functions known or proposed for Nm23, and site directed mutagenesis studies that attempt to link Nm23 structure and breast cancer metastasis suppressive activity.

2.4.1. Nucleoside Diphosphate Kinase (NDPK) Activity

All Nm23 isoforms and homologs of Nm23 exhibit a nonspecific nucleoside diphosphate kinase (NDPK) activity, in which Nm23 catalyzes a reversible phosphotransfer from a nucleoside triphosphate (NTP) to a nucleoside diphosphate (NDP), through a high energy Nm23-phosphohistidine intermediate *(33–38)*. The NDPKs are thought to be critical housekeeping enzymes that maintain the equilibrium of the cellular nucleotide pool *(38)*; however, other proteins also exhibit NDPK activity *(39)*. Nm23 may also provide a NTP regenerating system, supplying the necessary NTPs for G-protein regulation *(40)*. Similarly, NDPKs may aid the activation of a G protein-dependent, muscarinic potassium channel by supplying enough GTP in the immediate vicinity of the G-protein to ensure adequate receptor-mediated regulation of the channel *(41)*. Although the NDPK activity is the best characterized biochemical response of the Nm23 proteins, it is not sufficient to explain the effects of Nm23 on differentiation and metastasis *(42–44)*.

2.4.2. Histidine and Serine Protein Kinase

A second potential signaling option is the transfer of the phosphate from the phosphohistidine of the Nm23 intermediate to a serine or histidine residue on an acceptor protein. Engel and coworkers described the ability of purified Nm23 to transfer a phosphate from the phosphohistidine to serine/threonine residues of proteins in a colon carcinoma cell lysate containing urea *(45,46)*. Although none of the potential substrates of Nm23 have been isolated, the reaction reveals putative signaling pathways involving Nm23 kinase activity.

Second, incubation of PC12 cell lysate with bovine NDPK resulted in the histidine phosphorylation of a 120 kDa protein, identified as ATP-citrate lyase *(47)*. Histidine phosphorylation of Nm23-H2, Nm23-H1, and succinic thiokinase has been shown to occur in vitro by Nm23-H1 *(42)*. Histidine protein kinases represent a class of protein kinases relatively unstudied in mammalian cells, but which play a key role in signal transduction in prokaryotes *(see below)*.

2.4.3. Two-Component Signaling System

The two-component system is a class of histidine protein kinases and associated regulators which mediate bacterial responsiveness to external signals *(see ref. 48)*. The prototypical "two-component" phosphorelay system includes a sensor histidine kinase and a receiving protein. In response to a stimulus, such as a chemotactic signal, the sensor histidine kinase autophosphorylates on a histidine residue. The phosphate is then transferred from the phosphohistidine intermediate to an aspartate residue in the receiving protein, typically resulting in the stimulation or inhibition of transcriptional regulatory events. Thus far, the longest series of phosphotransfers consists of four phosphorylation events (His → Asp → His → Asp) on four separate proteins governing the initiation of sporulation in *Bacillus subtillus*.

Recent work indicates that eukaryotic organisms can also utilize histidine-mediated cascades. For example, in budding yeast *(Saccharomyces cerevisiae)* a variation of the prototypical "two component" system is important for osmosensing *(49,50)*. This particular system consists of three proteins each having a histidine kinase domain and receiving aspartate domain, resulting in the regulation of a HOG1 MAP kinase pathway.

Since Nm23 homologs are conserved from bacteria to mammals, it is possible that the Nm23 family governs analogous "two component" phosphorelay pathways. Lu et al. *(51)* have reported that Nm23 protein can participate in a Tar/EnvZ chimeric two component system in *Escherichia coli*. The first evidence suggesting Nm23 participation in a mammalian "two component " cascade was recently reported *(52)*. Nm23-H1 transferred a phosphate from its catalytic phosphohistidine to an aspartate or glutamate on a 43 kDa membrane bound protein from a brain extract. Many questions remain before this potentially exciting finding is understood, including the identity of physiological substrates and the mechanism of action, given a well defined but relatively small "active site" for Nm23 by x-ray crystallography. Thus, it is conceivable that a series of phosphorylation events exists that resembles those defined for two-component signal transduction systems in other organisms, and ultimately may have important implications physiologically.

2.4.4. Serine Autophosphorylation

Nm23 has been shown to autophosphorylate on serine residues in vitro and endogenously in human breast carcinoma and murine melanoma cells *(42,53–56)*. In vitro autophosphorylated Nm23 exhibited phosphoserine at amino acid 44 and on a peptide containing serines 120, 122, and 125; this phosphorylation may occur as an intramolecular transfer from an autophosphorylated histidine residue *(55)*. Moreover, Nm23 serine autophosphorylation can be inhibited in vitro by cAMP and cAMP analogs and in vivo by forskolin *(55,57)*.

2.4.5. Other Biochemical Activities

Nm23-H2 has been reported to bind and transactivate the CT/PuF element in the c-*myc* promoter *(58–60)*. There is no evidence that Nm23-H1 or other Nm23 family members bind or transactivate DNA. This activity remains debated, as Hildebrandt et al. *(61)* have reported that Nm23 can recognize a variety of single stranded polypyrimidine rich DNA and RNA sequences, and Michelotti et al. *(46)* have found no evidence for a direct role for Nm23-H2 or -H1 in CT/PuF binding or transactivation.

Binding of Nm23 to several proteins has been reported. A complex between heat shock complex 70 (hsc70) and a p16 cytosolic protein, related to Nm23-H1, was reported, which can influence the monomerization of the hsc70 complex *(63)*. Protein-protein interaction of Nm23 isoforms to nuclear orphan receptors has been reported utilizing a yeast two-hybrid screen *(64)*. Specific binding of a Nm23-H2 to RZRβ and Nm23-H1 to RORα occurred in vitro; endogenous complex formation of these proteins has, of, yet, to be described. Finally, complex formation of murine Nm23 and β-tubulin was reported in tumor cells in culture, regardless of metastatic potential, whereas this association was not observed in highly invasive primary tumor cells *(65)*.

2.4.6. Site Directed Mutagenesis Studies

In order to further identify which regions of Nm23-H1 are important for regulating breast cancer metastasis, site-directed mutants of Nm23-H1 were constructed and transfected into MDA-MB-435 breast carcinoma cells. The consequence of the overexpression of the wild type or mutant cDNAs on cell motility was determined in Boyden chamber assays *(25)*. The Nm23-H1 mutants utilized were: serine 44 (a potential phosphorylation site) to alanine (*nm23*[S44A]); proline 96 to serine (k-pn mutation in the *Drosophila nm23* homolog that participates in development defects) (*nm23*[P96S]); histidine 118 (required for NDPK and histidine kinase activity) to phenylalanine (*nm23*[H118F]); and serine 120 (a site of potential phosphorylation and of mutation in human neuroblastoma) to either glycine or alanine (*nm23*[S120G], *nm23*[S120A]).

While transfection of wild type *nm23-H1* and mutant *nm23*[S44A] suppressed MDA-MB-435 breast cancer cell motility, *nm23*[P96S], *nm23*[S120F], and *nm23*[S120G] abrogated this motility-suppressive effect. None of the transfectants regulated cellular proliferation.

Nm23-H1 wild type and mutant recombinant proteins were subsequently produced in bacteria, purified and assayed for the biochemical activities described herein *(66)*. Interestingly, those sites where biological suppression of breast cancer motility were observed, Proline 96 and Serine 120, were sites that disrupted a histidine dependent protein phosphotransferase pathway: Nm23[P96S] exhibited normal histidine and serine autophosphorylation and NDPK characteristics but was deficient in histidine protein kinase activity. Nm23[S120G] showed reduced autophosphorylation of histidine and downstream serine residues, as well as deficient histidine kinase activity; however, significant NDPK activity was retained. In contrast, Nm23-H1 wild type and Nm23[S44A] had normal activity in all assays. Taken together, these results indicate that a histidine-dependent protein phosphotransfer may represent an important signaling event in regulating the metastatic suppressive effects of Nm23-H1. This may include the histidine protein kinase activity of Nm23, in a histidine-to-histidine or two-component like transfer. Alternatively, it could result from a histidine dependent autophosphorylation, possibly to a downstream serine, which could influence kinase activity, binding to another protein, and so on. The identification of cellular Nm23 binding proteins and substrates is a current topic of intense research interest.

2.5. Translational Strategies Using Nm23

Significant improvement in breast cancer mortality rates will be realized when we can effect the two ends of the cancer spectrum, prevention of the disease and halting or eradicating metastatic disease, once breast cancer occurs. Toward the latter goal, we have asked how we can translate our observations and data concerning *nm23* into treatments.

2.5.1. Identification of Compounds Preferentially Inhibitory to Highly Metastatic Breast Carcinoma Cells Using COMPARE

The first strategy utilized the observation that low Nm23 expression was correlated with reduced patient disease free- or overall survival or other histopathologic indicators of high metastatic potential in cohorts of breast, ovarian, cervical, gastric, and hepatocellular carcinomas and in melanoma. Low expression of Nm23, therefore, can be considered to be a molecular marker of metastatic potential. Having this tool allowed us to ask the following question: Are there any existent compounds, either agents in clinical use, trial or development or compounds in a repository which have preferential inhibitory activity against low Nm23 expressing cell lines and therefore, by inference, are preferentially active against metastatic cells?

The NCI's Developmental Therapeutics Program (DTP) currently evaluates the in vitro efficacy of natural products and synthetic compounds on a panel of 60 human tumor cell lines. Analysis of the immense quantities of in vitro data generated is performed by a computer algorithm called COMPARE, which correlates the pattern of in vitro inhibitory activity of a seed compound on the 60 cell line panel to the corresponding inhibitory patterns of either 171 agents in clinical use, trial or development (Standard agents) or 30,000 compounds in a repository. This computer algorithm is able to correlate patterns of expression of a variable, such as the expression of Nm23, among the cell lines, with the sensitivities of the cell lines to the agents or compounds. Correlation is quantified by Pearson correlation coefficients which are generated by this program. Potential outcomes of this analysis are graphed on Fig. 2. Compounds which were inhibitory to only high Nm23 expressing cells lines (poorly metastatic) were defined as having a Pearson correlation coefficient of +1.0, compounds inhibitory only to low Nm23 expressing cell lines (highly metastatic) were designated with a correlation coefficient of –1.0, and compounds which exhibited no correlation with Nm23 expression had a correlation coefficient of 0 (Fig. 2).

Using the Nm23 expression levels of the breast carcinoma and melanoma subsets of the DTP cell line panel, the antiproliferative activity of 171 Standard agents on low- vs highly metastatic cell lines was estimated (22). None of the Standard agents exhibited a preferential inhibitory activity for low Nm23 expressing, highly aggressive cell lines with a Pearson correlation coefficient of ≤–0.64 (Fig. 2). Included in this list of Standard agents are those agents routinely administered for the adjuvant treatment of breast cancer. Pearson correlation coefficients for breast-active compounds ranged from +0.8 to –0.3, with Taxol being the most negative (Fig. 2). These results underscore the reality of the treatment of breast cancer: Although administration of these agents confers a disease-free and overall survival benefit *(1)*, survival curves never plateau and there is a significant rate of distant recurrence, i.e., metastasis, continuing for decades after initial treatment. These agents, although they unequivocally have an effect on rapidly proliferating cells, nevertheless, may have no effect on those processes related to metastatic competency which, therefore, may explain their limited efficacy.

A similar analysis of the 30,000 natural products and synthetic compounds in the DTP repository identified 40 compounds with a Pearson correlation coefficients of –0.70 to –0.9 *(66)*. Of these forty compounds, adequate supply of compound for additional studies existed for 34. Additional data was generated to determine whether these trends continued at multiple doses of the compounds, for longer culture periods, and with multiple human cell lines of known tumor metastatic potential. Four compounds emerged from these studies, and it is interesting to note that these compounds are structurally dissimilar from the standard chemotherapeutic agents and may represent heretofore unknown families of potentially therapeutic compounds.

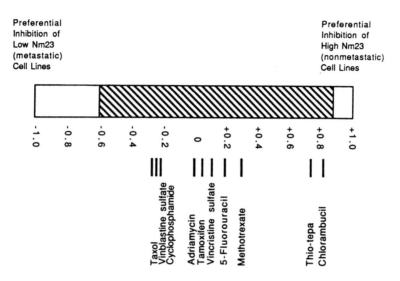

Fig. 2. COMPARE analysis of Nm23 expression of human breast carcinoma and melanoma cell lines vs in vitro antiproliferative response of 171 Standard agents *(66)*. The Nm23 expression levels of a panel of human breast carcinoma and melanoma cell lines was determined on western blots and quantitated by densitometry. The in vitro inhibitory effect of each chemotherapeutic agent on each cell line was determined using a Sulfohodamine B dye assay. The COMPARE program determined the correlation coefficient of the sensitivity of a cell line to each agent, versus its relative Nm23 expression level. Possible outcomes ranges from −1.0 to + 1.0. Shown in the cross hatched portion of the bar are the actual outcomes of the COMPARE analysis on the 171 Standard agents, all agents in clinical use, trial, or development. Noted below are the Pearson correlation coefficients of Standard agents used in the treatment of breast cancer.

None of the compounds elevated tumor cell Nm23 expression, suggesting that Nm23 was simply a marker of metastatic potential used in the study and not causally involved. Thus, COMPARE has identified four compounds which are both novel and preferentially inhibitory to human breast and melanoma cell lines which are distinguished by their metastatic competency.

In addition to studying the antiproliferative effects of these compounds, experiments were conducted to determine effects on activities particular to metastatic competency, such as motility. Boyden chamber assays demonstrated a significant inhibition of both random and stimulated motility with the addition to the chambers of NSC 680718, one of the four compounds identified. Initial in vivo testing of these compounds using the hollow fiber assay developed by DTP has shown inhibition of human tumor cell viability in subcutaneously implanted hollow fibers following the intraperitoneal injection of NSC 680718 (22). Inhibition was noted in five lines refractory to many conventional chemotherapeutic agents including two metastatically competent breast carcinoma cell lines, a colon carcinoma cell line, a melanoma cell line and a non-small cell lung carcinoma cell line. These promising results have led to approval for continued in vivo testing of efficacy and toxicity.

2.5.2. Increasing the Nm23 Expression of Metastatic Tumor Cells

Our second strategy has been to study the regulation of the expression of Nm23 with the eventual goal of finding a way of "turning on" the expression of Nm23 in low expressing cells and thereby abrogating or attenuating the metastatic potential of those metastatically competent cells. Coordinate examination of Nm23-H1 expression, allelic deletion status and patient clinical course data in a cohort study indicated that low Nm23-H1 protein expression was the best predictor of poor outcome *(67)*. Mutations in the *nm23-H1* coding region were not observed *(67)*. These data suggest that transcriptional control of *nm23-H1* may be an important regulatory event. Further study of the transcriptional regulation of Nm23-H1 was undertaken by cloning the *nm23-H1* promoter *(68)*. Progressive deletion mutations of this 2.1 kb fragment were constructed which and assayed for promoter activity using the CAT reporter gene *(69)*. Initial transfection experiments were performed with two human breast carcinoma cell lines: MCF-7, which exhibits relatively high Nm23-H1 expression and is virtually nonmetastatic upon injection into nude mice and MDA-MB-435, which exhibits lower Nm23-H1 expression and is metastatically competent in vivo. A second set of transfection experiments were subsequently carried out to investigate whether the trends of the MCF-7 and MDA-MB-435 set could be generalized, using the nonmetastatic ZR-75 and metastatic MDA-MB-231 breast carcinoma cell lines. Results of these two sets of transfection experiments demonstrated that the 2.1 kb fragment contains the sequences necessary to control differential *nm23-H1* expression between low- and high metastatic potential breast carcinoma cell lines *(69)*. Progressive deletion of restriction fragments has isolated a 443 base pair region which appears to be responsible for the differential transcription. Additionally, there appears to be a 544 bp region 5' to the 443 bp region which contains an inhibitory element. Further characterization of the 443 bp region responsible for differential transcriptional of *nm23-H1* has found no mutations, however changes in methylation patterns and differential patterns of transcription factor binding at the MAF site were observed which may be responsible for the differential transcription.

Our efforts currently are focused on finding a compound (natural or synthetic product) which will be able to "turn on" Nm23 expression by directly or indirectly interacting with the *nm23* promoter in vivo. We are fashioning a promoter construct, to be transfected into a low Nm23 expressing, metastatically competent human breast carcinoma cell line, which can be used for automated high-throughput drug screening efforts.

If successful, such a compound could potentially be used in an adjuvant setting to limit the colonization and metastatic outgrowth of occult micrometastases, potentially rendering these cells unable to form a life-threatening recurrence. In addition, we have reported that cells from three lineages, human breast carcinoma, human ovarian carcinoma and murine melanoma, are more sensitive to the in vitro growth inhibitory effect of cisplatin when *nm23* is overexpressed *(70)*. In vivo confirmation of this finding was provided in experimental metastasis assays using murine melanoma cells, where a single dose of cisplatin, after injection of implantation of melanoma cells, was more effective at reducing pulmonary metastasis formation on *nm23*-transfectants than controls. These conclusions are supported by the COMPARE analysis, in which 21/30

Standard agents with the highest Pearson correlation coefficients were alkylating agents *(66)*, which further suggests that *nm23* expression may have a similar relationship with additional alkylating agents. The mechanism remains unknown, but has been associated with the formation of increased numbers of interstrand DNA adducts by cisplatin in the *nm23* transfectants *(70)*. These data support that hypothesis that a Nm23 expressing elevating compound could also be used in combination with alkylating agents clinically.

3. CONCLUDING REMARKS

The development of relevant in vivo metastasis model systems, models for breast differentiation, and novel drug screening approaches as described herein can undoubtedly serve research on molecular markers other than *nm23*. It is hoped that this chapter will serve as a template for other molecular markers to progress from basic to pre-clinical research.

REFERENCES

1. EBCTCG. 1992. Systemic treatment of early breast cancer by hormonal, cytotoxic or immune therapy. *Lancet* **339:** 1–15, 71–85.
2. Liotta, L. A., P. S. Steeg, and W. G. Stetler-Stevenson. 1991. Cancer metastasis and angiogenesis: An imbalance of negative and positive regulation. *Cell* **64:** 327–336.
3. Folkman, J. 1997. Angiogenesis and angiogenesis inhibition: an overview. *EXS* **79:** 1–8.
4. Folkman, J. 1995. The influence of angiogenesis research on management of patients with breast cancer. *Br. Cancer Res. Treat.* **36:** 109–118.
5. Welch, D. 1997. Technical considerations for studying cancer metastasis in vivo. *Clin. Exp. Metast.* **15:** 272–306.
6. Price, J. E., A. Polyzos, R. D. Zhang, and L. M. Daniels. 1990. Tumorigenicity and metastasis of human breast carcinoma cell lines in nude mice. *Cancer Res.* **50:** 717–721.
7. Steeg, P. S., G. Bevilacqua, L. Kopper, U. P. Thorgeirsson, J. E. Talmadge, L. A. Liotta, and M. E. Sobel. 1988a. Evidence for a novel gene associated with low tumor metastatic potential. *J. Natl. Cancer Inst.* **80:** 200–204.
8. Rosengard, A. M., H. C. Krutzsch, A. Shearn, J. R. Biggs, E. Barker, I. M. K. Margulies, C. R. King, L. A. Liotta, and P. S. Steeg. 1989. Reduced Nm23/Awd protein in tumor metastasis and aberrant *Drosophila* development. *Nature* **342:** 177–180.
9. Milon, L., M.-F. Rosseau-Merck, A. Munier, M. Erent, I. Lascu, J. Capeau, and M.-L. Lacombe. 1997. nm23-H4, a new member of the family of human nm23/nucleoside diphosphate kinase gnes localised on chromosome 16p13. *Human Genet.* **99:** 550–557.
10. Stahl, J. A., A. Leone, A. M. Rosengard, L. Porter, C. R. King, and P. S. Steeg. 1991. Identification of a second human nm23 gene, nm23-H2. *Cancer Res.* **51:** 445–449.
11. Venturelli, D., R. Martinez, P. Melotti, I. Casella, C. Peschile, C. Cucco, G. Spampinato, Z. Darzynkiewicz, and B. Calabretta. 1995. Overexpression of DR-nm23, a protein encoded by a member of the nm23 gene family, inhibits granulocyte differentiation and induces apoptosis in 32Dc13 myeloid cells. *Proc. Natl. Acad. Sci. USA* **92:** 7435–7439.
12. Caligo, M. A., G. Cipollini, C. D. Valromita, M. Bistocchi, and G. Bevilacqua. 1992. Decreasing expression of nm23 gene in metastatic murine mammary tumors of viral etiology. *Anticancer Res.* **12:** 969–973.
13. Steeg, P. S., G. Bevilacqua, R. Pozzatti, L. A. Liotta, and M. E. Sobel. 1988b. Altered expression of nm23, a gene associated with low tumor metastatic potential, during adenovirus 2 E1a inhibition of experimental metastasis. *Cancer Res.* **48:** 6550–6554.

14. Su, Z.-Z., V. N. Austin, S. G. Zimmer, and P. B. Fisher. 1993. Defining the critical gene expression changes associated with expression and suppression of the tumorigenic and metastatic phenotype in Ha-ras-transformed cloned rat embryo fibroblast cells. *Oncogene* **8:** 1211–1219.

15. Lakshmi, M., C. Parker, and G. Sherbert. 1993. Metastasis associated mts1 and nm23 genes affect tubulin polymerisation in B16 melanomas: A possible mechanism of their regulation of metastatic behaviour of tumours. *Anticancer Res.* **13:** 299–304.

16. Tokunaga, Y., T. Urano, K. Furakawa, H. Kondo, T. Kanematsu, and H. Shiku. 1993. Reduced expression of Nm23-H1, but not of Nm23-H2, is concordant with the frequency of lymph-node metastasis of human breast cancer. *Int. J. Cancer* **55:** 66–71.

17. Caligo, M., G. Cipollini, A. Berti, P. Viacava, P. Collecchi, and G. Bevilacqua. 1997. NM23 gene-expression in human breast carcinomas—Loss of correlation with cell-proliferation in the advanced phase of tumor porgression. *Int. J. Cancer* **74:** 102–111.

18. Simpson, J. F., F. O'Malley, W. D. Dupont, and D. L. Page. 1994. Heterogeneous expression of nm23 gene product in noninvasive breast carcinoma. *Cancer* **73:** 2352–2358.

19. Baba, H., T. Urano, K. Okada, K. Furukawa, E. Nakayama, H. Tanaka, K. Iwasaki, and H. Shiku. 1995. Two isotypes of murine *nm23*/Nucleoside Diphosphate Kinse, *nm23-M1* and *nm23-M2*, are involved in metastatic suppression of a murine melanoma line. *Cancer Res.* **55:** 1977–1981.

20. Fukuda, M., A. Ishii, Y. Yasutomo, N. Shimada, N. Ishikawa, N. Hanai, N. Nagara, T. Irimura, G. Nicolson, and N. Kimura. 1996. Metastatic potential of rat mammary adenocarcinoma cells associated with decreased expression of nucleoside diphosphate kinase/nm23: Reduction by transfection of NDP Kinase a isoform, an nm23-H2 gene homolog. *Int. J. Cancer* **65:** 531–537.

21. Leone, A., U. Flatow, C. R. King, M. A. Sandeen, I. M. K. Margulies, L. A. Liotta, and P. S. Steeg. 1991. Reduced tumor incidence, metastatic potential, and cytokine responsiveness of nm23-transfected melanoma cells. *Cell* **65:** 25–35.

22. Leone, A., U. Flatow, K. VanHoutte, and P. S. Steeg. 1993. Transfection of human nm23-H1 into the human MDA-MB–435 breast carcinoma cell line: Effects on tumor metastatic potential, colonization, and enzymatic activity. *Oncogene* **8:** 2325–2333.

23. Parhar, R. S., Y. Shi, M. Zou, N. R. Farid, P. Ernst, and S. Al-Sedairy. 1995. Effects of cytokine mediated modulation of Nm23 expression on the invasion and metastatic behavior of B16F10 melanoma cells. *Int. J. Cancer* **60:** 204–210.

24. Kantor, J. D., B. McCormick, P. S. Steeg, and B. R. Zetter. 1993. Inhibition of cell motility after nm23 transfection of human and murine tumor cells. *Cancer Res.* **53:** 1971–1973.

25. MacDonald, N., J. Freije, M. Stracke, R. Manrow, and P. Steeg. 1996. Site directed mutagenesis of nm23-H1: Mutation of proline 96 or serine 120 abrogates its motility inhibitory activity upon transfection into human breast carcinoma cells. *J. Biol. Chem.* **271:** 25,107–25,116.

26. Kerbel, R. S. 1990. Growth dominance of the metastatic cancer cell: cellular and molecular aspects. *Adv. Cancer Res.* **55:** 87–132.

27. Petersen, O. W., L. Rønnov-Jessen, A. R. Howlett, and M. J. Bissel. 1992. Interaction with basement membrane serves to rapidly distinguish growth and differentiation patterns of normal and malignant human breast epithelial cells. *Proc. Natl. Acad. Sci. USA* **89:** 9064–9068.

28. Howlett, A. R., O. W. Petersen, P. S. Steeg, and M. J. Bissell. 1994. A novel function for Nm23: Overexpression in human breast carcinoma cells leads to the formation of basement membrane and growth arrest. *J. Natl. Cancer Inst.* **86:** 1838–1844.

29. Dearolf, C., E. Hersperger, and A. Shearn. 1988a. Developmental consequences of awdb3, a cell autonomous lethal mutation of *Drosophila* induced by hybrid dysgenesis. *Dev. Biol.* **129:** 159–168.

30. Dearolf, C., N. Tripoulas, J. Biggs, and A. Shearn. 1988b. Molecular consequences of awdb3, A cell autonomous lethal mutation of Drosophila induced by hybrid dysgenesis. *Dev. Biol.* **129**: 169–178.

31. Gervasi, F., I. D'Agnano, S. Vossio, G. Zupi, A. Sacchi, and D. Lombardi. 1996. nm23 influences proliferation and differentiation of PC12 cells in response to nerve growth factor. *Cell Growth Diff.* **7**: 1689–1695.

32. Hsu, S., F. Huang, L. Wang, S. Banerjee, S. Winawer, and E. Friedman. 1994. The role of nm23 in transforming growth factor β1-mediated adherence and growth arrest. *Cell Growth Diff.* **5**: 909–917.

33. Biggs, J., E. Hersperger, P. S. Steeg, L. A. Liotta, and A. Shearn. 1990. A *Drosophila* gene that is homologous to a mammalian gene associated with tumor metastasis codes for a nucleoside diphosphate kinase. *Cell* **63**: 933–940.

34. Wallet, V., R. Mutzel, H. Troll, O. Barzu, B. Wurster, M. Veron, and M. L. Lacombe. 1990. Dictyostelium nucleoside diphosphate kinase highly homologous to Nm23 and Awd proteins involved in mammalian tumor metastasis and drosophila development. *J. Natl. Cancer Inst.* **82**: 1199–1202.

35. Berg, P. and W. K. Joklik. 1953. Transphosphorylation between nucleoside polyphosphates. *Nature* **172**: 1008–1009.

36. Edlund, B., L. Rask, P. Olsson, O. Wålinder, Ö. Zetterqvist, and L. Engström. 1969. Preparation of crystalline nucleoside diphosphate kinase from baker's yeast and identification of 1-[32P]phosphohistidine as the main phosphorylated product of an alkaline hydrolysate of enzyme incubated with adenosine [32P] triphosphate. *Eur. J. Biochem.* **9**: 451–455.

37. Krebs, H. A. and R. Hems. 1953. Some Reactions of Adenosine and Inosine Phosphates in Animal Tissues. *Biochimica et Biophysica Acta* **12**: 172–180.

38. Parks, R. E. and R. P. Agarwal. 1973. *Nucleoside diphosphokinases*, vol. 8. Academic Press, New York.

39. Lu, Q., and M. Inouye. 1996. Adenylate kinase complements nucleoside diphosphate kinase deficiency in nucleotide metabolism. *Proc. Natl. Acad. Sci. USA* **93**: 5720–5725.

40. Randazzo, P. A., J. K. Northup, and R. A. Kahn. 1992. Regulatory GTP binding proteins (ARF, Gt and RAS) are not activated directly by nucleoside diphosphate kinase. *J. Biol. Chem.* **267**: 18182–18189.

41. Heidbuchel, H., G. Callewaert, J. Vereecke, and E. Carmeliet. 1993. Acetylcholine-mediated K+ channel activity in guinea-pig atrial cells is supported by nucleoside diphosphate kinase. *Pflugers Arch.* **422**: 316–324.

42. Freije, J. M. P., P. Blay, N. J. MacDonald, R. E. Manrow, and P. S. Steeg. 1997. Site-directed mutation of Nm23-H1. Mutations lacking motility suppressive capacity upon transfection are deficient in histidine-dependent protein phosphotransferase pathways in vitro. *J. Biol. Chem.* **272**: 5525–5532.

43. Golden, A., M. Benedict, A. Shearn, N. Kimura, A. Leone, L. A. Liotta, and P. S. Steeg. 1993. Nucleoside diphosphate kinase, nm23 and tumor metastasis: possible biochemical mechanisms. Kluwer Academic Publishers, Boston.

44. Xu, J., L. Liu, F. Deng, L. Timmons, E. Hersperger, P. Steeg, M. Veron, and A. Shearn. 1996. Rescue of the awd mutant phenotype by expression of human Nm23/NDP kinase in Drosophila. *Develp. Biol.* **177**: 544–557.

45. Engel, M., M. Veron, B. Theisinger, M.-L. Lacombe, T. Seib, S. Dooley, and C. Welter. 1995. A novel serine/threonine-specific protein phosphoransferase activity of Nm23/nucleoside-diphosphate kinase. *Eur. J. Biochem.* **234**: 200–207.

46. Hossler, F. E. and R. Rendi. 1971. Molecular species of a soluble nucleoside diphosphokinase related to the Na+. K+-ATPase. *Biochem. Biophys. Res. Comm.* **43**: 530–536.

47. Wagner, P. and N.-D. Vu. 1995. Phosphorylation of ATP-Citrate Lyase by Nucleoside diphosphate kinase. *J. Biol. Chem.* **270**: 21758–21764.

48. Appleby, J. L., J. S. Parkinson, and R. B. Bourret. 1996. Signal transduction via the multi-step phosphrelay: not necessarily a road less traveled. *Cell* **86:** 845–848.

49. Maeda, T., S. Wurgler-Murphy, and H. Saito. 1994. A two-component system that regulates an osmosensing MAP kinase cascade in yeast. *Nature* **369:** 242–245.

50. Posas, F., S. M. Wurgler-Murphy, T. Maeda, E. A. Witten, T. C. Thai, and H. Saito. 1996. Yeast HOG1 MAP kinase cascade is regulated by a multistep phosphorelay mechanism in the SLN1-YPD1-SSK1 "two component" osmosensor. *Cell* **86:** 865–875.

51. Lu, Q., H. Park, L. Egger, and M. Inouye. 1996. Nucleoside-diphosphate kinase-mediated signal transduction via histidyl-aspartyl phosphorelay systems in Escherichia coli. *J. Biol. Chem.* **271:** 32,886–32,893.

52. Vu, N.-D., P. D. Wagner, and P. S. Steeg. 1997. Two-component kinase like activity of Nm23 correlates with its motility suppressing activity. *Proc. Natl. Acad. Sci. USA* **94:** 9000–9005.

53. Biondi, R., M. Engel, M. Sauane, C. Welter, O. Issinger, L. d. Asua, and S. Passeron. 1996. Inhibition of nucleoside diphosphate kinase by in vitro phosphorylation by protein kinase CK2. Differential phosphorylation of NDP kinases in He La cells in culture. *FEBS Lett.* **399:** 183–187.

54. Hemmerich, S. and I. Pecht. 1992. Oligomeric structures and autophosphorylation of nucleoside diphosphate kinase from rat mucosal mast cells. *Biochemistry* **31:** 4580–4587.

55. MacDonald, N. J., A. DeLaRosa, M. A. Benedict, J. M. P. Freije, H. Krutsch, and P. S. Steeg. 1993. A novel phosphorylation of Nm23, and not its nucleoside diphosphate kinase activity, correlates with suppression of tumor metastasis. *J. Biol. Chem.* **269:** 25,780–25,789.

56. Muñoz-Dorado, J., N. Almaula, S. Inouye, and M. Inouye. 1993. Autophosphorylation of nucleoside diphosphate kinase from *Myxococcus xanthus. J. Bacteriol.* **175:** 1176–1181.

57. Anciaux, K., K. V. Dommelen, R. Willems, D. Roymans, and H. Slegers. 1997. Inhibition of nucleosides diphosphate kinase (NDPK/nm23) by cAMP analogues. *FEBS Lett.* **400:** 75–79.

58. Berberich, S. and E. Postel. 1995. PuF/NM23-H2/NDPK-B transactivates a human c-myc promoter-CAT gene via a functional nuclease hypersensitive element. : 2343–2347.

59. Postel, E. H., S. J. Berberich, S. J. Flint, and C. A. Ferrone. 1993. Human c-myc transcription factor PuF identified as Nm23-H2 nucleoside diphosphate kinase, a candidate suppressor of tumor metastasis. *Science* **261:** 478–480.

60. Postel, E. H., V. H. Weiss, J. Beneken, and A. Kirtanes. 1996. Mutational analysis of Nm23-H2/NDP kinase identifies the structural domains critical to recognition of c-myc regulatory element. *Proc. Natl Acad. Sci. USA* **93:** 6892–6897.

61. Hildebrandt, M., M. Lacombe, S. Mesnildrey, and M. Veron. 1995. A human NDP-Kinase-B specifically binds single-stranded poly-pyrimidine sequences. *Nucleic Acids Res.* **23:** 3858–3864.

62. Michelotti, E., S. Sanford, J. Freije, N. MacDonald, P. Steeg, and D. Levens. 1997. Nm23/PuF does not directly stimulate transcription through the CT element in vivo. *J. Biol. Chem.* **272:** 22526–22530.

63. Leung, S.-M. and L. E. Hightower. 1997. A 16-kDa protein functions as a new regulatory protein for Hsc70 molecular chaperone and is identified as a member of the Nm23/nucleoside diphosphate kinase family. *J. Biol. Chem.* **272:** 2607–2614.

64. Paravicini, G., M. Steinmayr, E. André, and M. Becker-André. 1996. The metastasis suppressor candidate nucleoside diphosphate kinase Nm23 specifically interacts with members of the ROR/RZR nuclear orphan receptor subfamily. *Biochem. Biophys. Res. Comm.* **227:** 82–87.

65. Lombardi, D., A. Sacchi, G. D'Agostino, and G. Tibursi. 1995. The association of the Nm23-M1 protein and beta-tubulin correlates with cell differentiation. *Exp. Cell Res.* **217:** 267–271.

66. Freije, J. M. P., J. A. Lawrence, M. G. Hollingshead, A. D. L. Rosa, V. Narayanan, M. Grever, E. A. Sausville, K. Paull, and P. S. Steeg. 1997. Identification of compounds with preferential in vitro inhibitory activity against low Nm23 expressing human breast carcinoma and melanoma cell lines. *Nature Med.* **3:** 395–401.

67. Cropp, C., R. Lidereau, A. Leone, D. Liscia, A. Cappa, G. Campbell, E. Barker, V. L. Doussal, P. Steeg, and R. Callahan. 1994. NME1 protein expression and loss of heterozygosity mutations in primary human breast tumors. *J. Natl. Cancer Inst.* **86:** 1167–1169.

68. DeLaRosa, A., B. Mikhak, and P. Steeg. 1996. Identification and characterization of the promoter for the human metastasis suppressor gene nm23-H1. *Archives Med. Res.* **27:** 395–401.

69. Clare, S., A. DeLaRosa, R. Kurek, N. MacDonald, R. Lidereau, M. Hartsough, and P. Steeg. Submitted for publication. The nm23-H1 promoter in breast cancer metastasis: Identification and characterization of regions mediating high versus low gene expression levels. *J. Biol. Chem.*

70. Ferguson, A., U. Flatow, N. MacDonald, F. Larminant, V. Bohr, and P. Steeg. 1996. Increased sensitivity to cisplatin by nm23-transfected tumor cell lines. *Cancer Res.* **56:** 2931–2935.

13

Role of Integrins in the Development and Malignancy of the Breast

Edward C. Rosfjord and Robert B. Dickson

1. INTRODUCTION

In the developing breast, there are structural and functional changes that are unlike those seen in any other adult tissue. These changes, range from the branching morphogenesis of the developing gland, through proliferation in pregnancy, to milk production in its fully differentiated state, and conclude with postlactational involution (apoptosis). Each of these processes require a delicate interplay between the ductal epithelial cells, the myoepithelial cells, and the surrounding basement membrane and stroma. Integrins appear to play a major role in this intricate control. During the onset and progression of breast cancer, this delicate interplay is disrupted. Ductal hyperplasia may be characterized by curious perturbations in cellular adhesion and migration, extending columns of epithelial cells into the lumen. Throughout hyperplasia, the epithelial cells appear to respond to their extracellular environment and remain organized with respect to each other and to the basement membrane. In contrast, in ductal or lobular carcinoma, cells no longer respond appropriately to their extracellular environment and grow in random orientation with no appropriate axis or orientation (1). During breast cancer progression, certain populations of cells gain the ability to migrate along extracellular matrix and basement membrane and invade through these connective tissues (2,30).

The alterations in epithelial architecture associated with tumorigenesis are accompanied by changes in expression of integrins. In general, integrins are expressed at points of cell-cell and cell-matrix attachment in normal and hyperplastic breast tissue. In carcinoma, however, there is a dramatic decrease in expression of most integrin subunits. An added complexity is that in invasive carcinomas, subpopulations of cells exhibit polarized expression of integrins on their subcellular processes involved in migration and invasion. This variability of expression and localization causes difficulty when using integrins as a marker for breast cancer. In ductal carcinoma *in situ*, high expression of β_1 integrins may indicate a well-differentiated tumor and correlate with other markers of differentiation such as estrogen-receptor progesterone-receptor (ER/PR) expression. In an invasive carcinoma, high expression of integrins may correlate with a metastatic phenotype and may even suggest possible sites of metastasis (Table 1). Therefore, for integrin expression to provide any diagnostic information, it must be used in conjunction with histology and pathology data.

From: Breast Cancer: Molecular Genetics, Pathogenesis, and Therapeutics
Edited by: A. M. Bowcock © Humana Press Inc., Totowa, NJ

Table 1
Integrin Expression in the Normal and Neoplastic Breast

Integrin[a]	Ligand[a]	Cellular expression in the normal mammary gland	Knock out mammary[b]	Expression in breast-cancer progression[c]						References
				Normal	FA	DCIS	IDC	ILC	MET	
$\alpha_1\beta_1$	Col, Lam	Myoepithelia, vascular endothelia, stroma	Normal	++	++	+	+	++		(3,14,17,18,22,44,45)
$\alpha_2\beta_1$	Col, Lam	Basal epithelia, luminal epithelia	No KO	+++	+++	+	+/-	+/-	+/-	(15,16,18–22,36,39,41,47–51,58–60)
$\alpha_3\beta_1$	Col, Ent, Fn, Lam	Myoepithelia, smooth muscle	Normal	++	++	+	+	+		(15,17–19,22,27,36,40–42,44,48, 80,81,84,93,97,99,100,101,120)
$\alpha_4\beta_1$	Fn, VCAM-1, MAdCAM-1	Lymphocytes Fibroblasts	Lethal[d]	+	+	+				(3,18,44,74–76,78)
$\alpha_5\beta_1$	Fn	Epithelial, smooth muscle, vascular endothelium	Lethal[d]	+	+++	++	+	+	+	(3,16,20,22,73,76,77)
$\alpha_6\beta_1$	Lam	Basal epithelia	?[e]	+++	++	+	+++	+++	+++	(15,16,18–22,36,39,41,47–51,58–60)
$\alpha_6\beta_4$	Lam	Basal epithelia myoepithelia[f]	?[e]	+++	++	+	+/-	+/-	g	(15,22,23,27,85,90–93,98)
$\alpha_v\beta_3$	Vn, Fb, Fn, Lam,Ost, vWFV	Basal epithelia, Vascular endothelium	No KO[h]	+	+	+	++	++	+++	(19,20,22,59,102–109,112–117,119)

[a]Ligands: Col, Collagen; Ent, Entactin; Fb, Fibrinogen; Fn, Fibronectin; Lam, Laminin; Ost, Osteopontin; Vn, Vitronectin; vWF, von Willebrand factor.

[b]Mammary-gland development in gene-knockout mice: Normal, no apparent malformations and normal function in mouse ($\alpha_1\beta_1$) or mammary-gland transplant ($\alpha_3\beta_1$); No KO, a gene knockout mouse has not been created for this integrin.

[c]Breast cancer progression abbreviations: DCIS, ductal carcinoma *in situ*; FA, fibroadenoma; IDC, invasive ductal carcinoma; ILC, invasive lobular carcinoma; MET, metastases; +++ high level of expression, ++ moderate level, + low but detectable, +/– weak or absent.

[d]Integrin $\alpha_4\beta_1$ and $\alpha_5\beta_1$ knockout mice are embryonic lethals (76–78).

[e]Both α_6 and β_4 knockout mice have been created but their impact on mammary development has not been determined.

[f]Expression of $\alpha_6\beta_4$ likely associated with hemidesmosomes.

[g]Hemidesmosomes present in myoepithelial carcinoma suggesting expression of $\alpha_6\beta_4$.

[h]Although a mouse knockout has not been created, humans that have a mutation in β_3 integrin are viable and there is no mention of malformed mammary-gland development.

Integrins are membrane proteoglycan receptors that mediate interactions between the cell and the extracellular matrix (ECM). Proper function of the integrin receptor requires the formation of a heterodimer between an α and β integrin subunit. At present, there are 15 different α subunits and 8 different β subunits that combine to form 21 different $\alpha\beta$ heterodimers with different substrate specificities *(2–4)*. Integrin molecules participate in receptor signal transduction (outside-in) via the Ras, $pp125^{FAK}$, and protein kinase C (PKC) pathways *(3,5)*. In addition, integrins also display inside-out signal transduction whereby the distribution and affinity of the integrins for ligand is adjusted by cytoplasmic proteins such as actin and talin *(3,6,7)*. Integrins have been shown to function in cellular invasion, metastasis, migration, adhesion, neovascularization, and apoptosis *(8–13)*.

2. EXPRESSION OF INTEGRINS IN BREAST DEVELOPMENT AND BREAST CANCER

2.1. Expression of β_1 Integrin

2.1.1. Expression of β_1 Integrin in Mammary-Gland Development

β_1 integrin is the most promiscuous integrin, forming heterodimers with 10 different α subunits *(3)*. In general, expression of β_1 integrin in the breast is stable. Integrin β_1 is expressed in the newborn rat mammary gland by the basal epithelial cells and at points of cell-cell contact between luminal epithelial cells *(14)*. Expression of β_1 integrin on the basal myoepithelial cells increases by 1.5 wk after birth and expression remains high throughout prepubertal development, puberty, pregnancy, and lactation. Anbazagan et al. described β_1 integrin expression in the newborn human breast *(15)*. There is strong expression of β_1 integrin in the basal cells and in cell-cell contacts between luminal epithelial cells of ducts. Expression in terminal end buds appears to be limited to myoepithelial cells with very weak staining of the ductal epithelial cells *(15)*.

In the adult breast, high levels of β_1 integrin mRNA are observed in both myoepithelial cells and luminal epithelial cells *(16)*. Expression of β_1 integrin protein is highest in myoepithelial cells with distinct expression on myoepithelial processes *(17–20)*. Ductal and luminal epithelial cells express β_1 integrin protein weakly, with stronger expression toward the basal surface of these cells *(18–21)*. Strong expression is also observed in the surrounding fibroblasts and myofibroblasts, smooth muscle, neural bodies, and in capillary endothelium *(17,22,23)*. The extensive expression of β_1 integrins and the numerous α subunits with which it forms heterodimers, suggest that β_1 integrin is essential to the proper growth and function of the mammary gland.

Recently, two separate investigators have created gene knock out mice to specifically examine the role of β_1 integrin in development *(24,25)*. Unfortunately, removal of this gene results in embryonic lethality shortly after implantation. Therefore, the function of β_1 integrin in the mammary gland has been examined in vitro by growing normal mammary epithelial cell lines on purified ECM. Normal breast epithelial cells form complex three dimensional structures, such as ridges, balls, and acini, when grown on or in purified reconstituted ECM *(26–28)*. The formation of the acinar structures is part of a process of differentiation that ultimately results in the production of milk proteins such as β-casein. These acinar structures express β_1 integrins along their "basal" surface (outside) and at sites of cell-cell contact between the cells. Neutralizing antibodies to β_1 integrins dramatically inhibit the formation of these structures and block production of β-casein *(28)*. Growth of normal mammary epithelial cells in culture appears to require their attachment to extracellular matrix *(29–31)*. Consistent with this concept, neutralizing antibodies to β_1 integrins inhibited thymidine incorporation by mammary epithelial cells and induced apoptosis of mammary epithelial cells *(32–34)*. In summary, the β_1 integrin appears to be essential for the growth and differentiation of normal mammary epithelial cells.

2.1.2. Expression of β_1 Integrin in Breast Cancer

Since β_1 integrin plays such a central role in the growth and differentiation of breast epithelial cells, its expression might be expected to decrease during breast cancer. Expression of β_1 integrin mRNA decreases in breast cancer, with the highest expression observed in fibroadenoma and other well-differentiated tumors. Expression decreases in poorly differentiated, invasive cancer and metastases *(16)*. Expression of β_1 integrin protein also decreases in breast cancer but not to the same extent as its mRNA *(16)*. Expression remains high in the myoepithelial cells of nonmalignant conditions such as fibrocystic disease, fibroadenomas, and cystosarcoma phylloides *(17,18,20,35,36)*. Expression continues to remain high in the normal myoepithelial component of intraductal carcinomas with reduced expression in luminal epithelial cells where expression is either lost or is primarily cytoplasmic *(17,25,36)*. One exception to this is in cribriform ductal carcinoma, where the cell-cell contacts that form bridges across the lumen stain strongly for β_1 integrin *(23)*, suggesting that β_1 integrins are participating in cell-cell contacts.

In invasive ductal carcinomas, there is focal expression of β_1 integrin at sites of cell-cell and cell-matrix contact *(17)*. Expression of β_1 integrin was weak or cytoplasmic in Grades I and II invasive ductal carcinomas with little to no expression of this integrin in Grade III invasive ductal carcinomas 11/15 ($p < 0.002$) *(19,36,37)*. Reduction in expression of β_1 integrin correlated with a transition to a malignant phenotype in ductal carcinoma ($p < 0.01$) and reduced expression of β_1 integrin correlated with the presence of axillary nodal metastases ($p < 0.001$) (22). Limited study of both local and distant breast-cancer metastases suggests that both express β_1 integrin at low to moderate levels *(16,20,22)*. Noninvolved breast tissue in breast-cancer patients continues to strongly express β_1 integrin *(36)*. Invasive lobular carcinomas retain expression of β_1 integrin with focal, polarized staining of pseudopodia *(17,39)*.

All breast-cancer cell lines studied to date appear to express low to moderate levels of functional β_1 integrin on their surfaces *(33,38–40)*. In these cells, β_1 integrin mediates adhesion to laminin, type I collagen, type IV collagen, and fibronectin. When breast-cancer cell lines are grown in reconstituted ECM, they do not form round acinar structures; instead, they form disorganized collections of cells with random membrane staining of β_1 integrin *(33)*. Unlike the case for normal breast epithelial cells, neutralizing antibodies to β_1 integrin do not effect the growth or apoptosis of breast-cancer cells *(33)* suggesting that in breast-cancer cell lines there is a disregulation or failure of signaling from β_1 integrin.

Recent analysis of a spontaneous human breast-tumor cell line suggests that signalling disregulation occurs in stages. Weaver et al. describe a breast tumor cell line, T4-2, that has undergone apparent disregulation of β_1 integrins and forms disorganized collections of cells in reconstituted ECM *(34)*. Neutralizing antibodies to β_1 integrin do not induce apoptosis, but they do revert the disorganized cells into round acinar structures. These structures have decreased growth rates and contain fewer cells than untreated or control treated cells. Neutralizing antibodies to β_1 integrin also inhibit the formation of tumors when these cells are injected into nude mice. This phenotype is completely reversible and removal of neutralizing antibodies to β_1 integrin results in reversion to a disorganized growth pattern. These studies suggest that the regulation of growth and apoptosis by β_1 integrin may utilize independent pathways. For some breast cancers, an initial disregulation may occur where cells fail to apoptose. Additional disregulation of this integrin may render breast-cancer cells independent of structural regulation by ECM *(33)*.

There is some direct evidence that β_1 integrins may actually participate in the migration and invasion of breast-cancer cells. Neutralizing antibodies to β_1 integrins can inhibit migration and invasion of invasive breast-cancer cells through laminin *(40)*, fibronectin, and type IV collagen *(38,41,42)*. In a detailed study, neutralizing antibodies to β_1 integrins inhibited the number and size of pulmonary metastases in a mouse breast-cancer model *(43)*. The inhibitory antibodies blocked formation of both macrometastases and micrometastases from a parental SP1 cell line, but not from the cell line SP1-3M that had been selected and propagated based on its metastatic properties. Lastly, this study determined that neutralizing antibodies to β_1 integrin did not greatly alter the growth of the primary tumor or the tumor take of either cell line. These studies suggest that β_1 integrin may play an important role in the invasion or metastasis of breast cancer, however, analysis of SP1-3M cells suggests that more advanced cancers may utilize alternative adhesion pathways to form pulmonary metastases.

2.2. Expression of $\alpha_1\beta_1$ Integrin

2.2.1. Expression of $\alpha_1\beta_1$ Integrin in Mammary-Gland Development

Integrin α_1 is a receptor for collagen and laminin *(3)*. In the developing rat mammary gland, integrin α_1 is expressed on the basal surface of myoepithelial cells by 1.5 wk after birth *(14)*. It continues to be expressed at moderate levels through puberty, postpuberty, and pregnancy. Expression of integrin α_1 is present on the basal surface of myoepithelial cells of lactating breast alveoli. This integrin is also expressed in the stroma, smooth muscle, and by vascular endothelium in the adult human breast *(17,22,44)*. With all of this stable expression of α_1 integrin during breast development, there is no evidence that α_1 integrin participates in breast development or breast cancer. Gene-knock-out studies have been performed on the α_1 integrin and there is no obvious mammary phenotype. Mice homozygous for the α_1 knockout bear viable young and have raised as many as six litters. The mammary glands of these mice appear normal histologically and they function properly. There is no change in the ability of these mice to feed and litter survival is normal *(45,46)*. Together, the fact that α_1 expression does not fluctuate during breast development and remodeling, and that mice homozygous for a loss of α_1 do not appear to have altered gland structure or function suggest that α_1 integrin does not participate in the development or function of the breast.

2.2.2. Expression of $\alpha_1\beta_1$ Integrin in Breast Cancer

Integrin α_1 is primarily expressed by myoepithelial cells, and these cells, in general, do not contribute to ductal carcinoma. Expression of integrin α_1 appears to be restricted to the myoepithelial cells in fibroadenoma, benign tumors and ductal carcinoma *(17,18,44)*. Expression of α_1 integrin changes in invasive carcinoma. There is peripheral expression of α_1 integrin on some luminal epithelial cells in invasive ductal carcinoma, suggesting that α_1 integrin may participate in the migration of these cells *(15,44)*. Curiously, in invasive breast cancer there is increased expression of α_1 integrin by the surrounding normal stroma that is manifesting a desmoplastic response to the invading tumor *(44)*. In contrast to ductal carcinoma, invasive lobular carcinoma is characterized by strong expression of α_1 integrin in pseudopodia *(17)*, again suggesting that α_1 integrin may participate in the migration of breast-cancer cells. In summary, α_1 integrin appears to be restricted to the myoepithelia in normal and benign breast tissue. In some invasive ductal and lobular carcinomas, there appears to be fine, polar expression of α_1 integrin that may correspond to migratory projections.

2.3. Expression of $\alpha_2\beta_1$ Integrin

2.3.1. Expression of $\alpha_2\beta_1$ Integrin in Mammary Gland Development

In vitro analysis has demonstrated that $\alpha_2\beta_1$ functions as a cellular receptor for collagen I, collagen IV, and laminin *(41,47–51)*. All three molecules are major components of the breast epithelial basement membrane *(26,49,52,53)*. Several lines of evidence suggest that integrin $\alpha_2\beta_1$ is essential to the normal growth, differentiation, and development of the mammary gland. Integrin $\alpha_2\beta_1$ is expressed in the basolateral and basal epithelia of many tissues, including breast, colon, prostate, sweat glands, and keratinizing skin epithelium *(21)*. Recently, immunohistochemistry and *in situ* hybridization have determined that expression of α_2 mirrors the expression of collagen I, collagen IV, and laminin during infant breast development and pregnancy *(15,49)*. A detailed immunohistochemical examination of integrin expression in the infant breast determined that α_2 expression is lowest in rudimentary ductal systems with little or no branching. As duct branching increases to form a mammary tree with terminal lobules, there is increased expression of α_2 in both luminal and basal epithelial cells. Maximal expression of β_1 was observed in apocrine epithelial cells *(15)*. Together, these observations suggest that coordinated expression of α_2 integrin and ECM proteins are necessary for proper mammary-gland development and lactation.

In the normal adult breast, expression of $\alpha_2\beta_1$ is highest in the ducts at the basal-cell layer, where the ductal epithelia contacts the basement membrane, and in intercellular junctions *(16,20,37)*. This suggests that α_2 integrin may participate in cell-cell adhesion and there is some evidence that α_2 may interact with α_3 or other cell-adhesion molecules in intercellular adhesion *(54)*. However, recent evidence suggests that this may not be a general phenomenon and overexpression of integrins may actually inhibit intercellular adhesion *(55)*. $\alpha_2\beta_1$ has been shown to be the principle β_1 integrin expressed on MTSV1-7 immortalized mammary epithelial cells *(26,56)*. These cells form three-dimensional structures in collagen gels and ridges and balls around collagen fibers. Neutralizing antibodies to integrin α_2 inhibit the formation of these structures, but neutralizing antibodies to α_3 integrin and nonneutralizing antibodies to α_2 do not *(26,56)*.

Recently, the role of $\alpha_2\beta_1$ in breast epithelial differentiation has been examined in vitro by using antisense oligonucleotides directed against integrin α_2 in the human breast-cancer cell line T47D *(57)*. T47D cells express high levels of integrin α_2 and form duct-like structures when grown in a reconstituted ECM. Antisense inhibition of α_2 resulted in an inability of these cells to form these duct-like structures, in increased cellular motility in vitro, and in decreased cellular adhesion to collagen and laminin *(57)*.

2.3.2. Expression of $\alpha_2\beta_1$ Integrin in Breast Cancer

Several studies have examined the expression of integrin $\alpha_2\beta_1$ in breast cancer *(16,18–20,22,36,37,58)*. All studies to date have identified strong expression of α_2 in the normal adult breast. Expression is limited to basolateral epithelial or to myoepithelial cells within the ducts *(16,19,20,37)*. Expression remains high in fibroadenoma and well-differentiated intraductal carcinomas. Expression decreases in Grade I invasive ductal carcinomas and in invasive lobular carcinomas. Expression is greatly reduced in Grades II and III invasive ductal carcinomas, in mucinous carcinomas, and in metastasis. Immunohistochemical analysis of bone metastasis identified weak or no expression of $\alpha_2\beta_1$ integrin *(59)*. In contrast, noninvolved breast tissue retained high expression of α_2 *(36)*. Several studies have identified a correlation between loss of α_2 and the transition to a more invasive or metastatic phenotype. Integrin α_2 expression correlated with estrogen-receptor expression ($p = 0.0327$ *[18]*), loss of integrin α_2 correlated with transition to malignant breast cancer ($p < 0.01$ *[22]*); and loss of α_2 expression was prognostic for higher histopathologic grading ($p = 0.0134$ *[18]* $p = 0.048$ *[21]*) or for axillary nodal metastasis ($p < 0.001$ *[22]*). Gui et al. 1995 extended these findings and demonstrated that neutralizing antibodies to α_2 and β_1 integrin are able to inhibit laminin adhesion by breast-cancer cells obtained from women with negative lymph nodes ($p < 0.001$) Laminin adhesion by breast-cancer cells obtained from women with positive lymph nodes was not significantly influenced by neutralizing antibodies to α_2 or β_1 integrin *(41)*. Similar correlations have been observed in vitro. Noninvasive, well-differentiated breast-cancer cell lines, like T47D, express high levels of integrin $\alpha_2\beta_1$ and adhere well to collagen and laminin *(39)*. In contrast, less-differentiated invasive breast-cancer cell lines, such as MDA-MB-435 and MDA-MB-231, express little or no $\alpha_2\beta_1$ and do not adhere well to collagen *(38,39,40)*.

There is some evidence that expression of $\alpha_2\beta_1$ can directly influence the migratory and invasive characteristics of breast-cancer cells *(60)*. Expression of α_2 integrin in Mm5MT cells, a mouse mammary tumor cell line that lacks α_2 integrin, decreased their motility and invasion in an in vitro transwell invasion assay. Cells expressing α_2 integrin were no longer capable of anchorage independent growth and formed smaller tumors in vivo *(60)*. In summary, $\alpha_2\beta_1$ integrin appears to be a marker for breast epithelial-cell differentiation and may function as a tumor suppressor gene by suppressing the growth, migration, and invasion of breast-cancer cells. This is the only known integrin that fluctuates in response to changing amounts of ECM during mammary-gland development and lactation *(49)*. Furthermore, loss of α_2 integrin during breast cancer progression appears to be permanent, and α_2-expressing populations are not frequently observed among invasive cells or metastases.

2.4. Expression of $\alpha_3\beta_1$ Integrin

2.4.1. Expression of $\alpha_3\beta_1$ Integrin
in Mammary-Gland Development and Breast Cancer

Integrin $\alpha_3\beta_1$ is a heterogeneous receptor for laminin-5, collagen, fibronectin, and entactin *(51,62–67)*. Genetic knockout studies have determined that this integrin plays a crucial role in the development of epidermal basement membrane *(68)* and in the organization of basement membrane in tissues with extensive branching morphogenesis, such as kidney and lung *(69)*.

To examine the role of α_3 integrin in the development of the mammary gland, mammary fat pads from α_3 knockout mice were transplanted to recipient female mice *(70)*. These studies determined that mammary glands that lack α_3 integrin develop the same as control mammary glands through pregnancy. There is normal casein expression in the α_3-deficient glands, suggesting that these glands can fully differentiate. Immunohistochemical analysis of the expression of the other major laminin receptor, α_6 integrin, suggests that it is not effected by loss of α_3. Similarly, expression and distribution of laminin-5 was not effected by the loss of α_3 integrin *(70)*. Together, these results suggest that other integrins, possibly α_6, may serve compensatory roles to α_3 in the proper development of the mammary gland.

Numerous investigators have identified strong expression of α_3 integrin along the basement membrane, on myoepithelial cells, and on smooth muscle of normal breast tissue and fibroadenomas *(18,20,22,37,44,70)*. Weak staining was also observed on luminal epithelial cells. There was little to no expression of α_3 integrin in invasive ductal carcinomas and invasive lobular carcinomas. Loss of integrin α_3 expression correlated with malignant progression of breast cancer ($p < 0.001$) and the presence of axillary nodal metastases ($p < 0.001$) *(22)*. Two studies further evaluated the expression of α_3 integrin in invasive breast cancer *(18,44)*. In both studies, expression of α_3 integrin was retained on ductal epithelial cells in invasive ductal carcinoma. Even still, expression of α_3 positively correlated with the presence of estrogen receptors ($p = 0.0399$) *(18)*, suggesting that α_3 integrin correlates with a more differentiated breast cancer phenotype.

2.4.2. Role of $\alpha_3\beta_1$ Integrin in Breast Cancer Metastasis

Integrin α_3 may play some role in the migration of metastatic breast-cancer cells. Tawil et al. examined the ability of metastatic breast-cancer cells to adhere to cryostat sections of lymph-nodes *(71)*. They determined that this adhesion was primarily mediated by fibronectin. Neutralizing antibodies to α_3 integrin inhibited the attachment of the breast-cancer cells to the lymph-node material. Immunohistochemical analysis identified both integrin α_3 and β_1 at sites of focal adhesion between breast-cancer cells and fibronectin. Lastly, Coopman et al. determined that in the invasive breast-cancer cell line MDA-MB-231, integrin $\alpha_3\beta_1$ participates in the phagocytosis of gelatin and reconstituted ECM *(52,72)*. In summary, expression of $\alpha_3\beta_1$ decreases during breast-cancer progression, however, expression of $\alpha_3\beta_1$ integrin in invasive breast-cancer cells may provide the capacity to invade through connective tissue and migrate within the lymphatics.

2.5. Expression of $\alpha_4\beta_1$ and $\alpha_5\beta_1$ Integrin

2.5.1. Expression of $\alpha_4\beta_1$ and $\alpha_5\beta_1$ Integrin in Mammary Gland Development and Breast Cancer

Integrin $\alpha_5\beta_1$ is a fibronectin receptor and binds to the Arg-Gly-Asp containing region of fibronectin *(3,73)*. Integrin α_4 recognizes an alternatively spliced form of fibronectin as well as vascular cell adhesion molecule (VCAM-1) and mucosal addressin cell adhesion molecule (MAdCAM-1) *(3,74,75)*. Integrin α_4 is primarily expressed by lymphocytes and fibroblasts within and around normal breast tissue. There is no information on developmental expression of either α_4 or α_5 integrin in the breast and both the α_4 and α_5 knockout mice are embryonic lethals *(76–78)*. In breast cancer, integrin α_4 is not expressed on epithelial cells; instead it appears to be restricted to infiltrating lymphocytes *(18,44)*. Integrin α_5 is expressed weakly on epithelial cells, myoepithelial cells, smooth muscle, and vascular endothelium *(20,22)*. Immunohistochemical and *in situ* evaluation of integrin α_5 in breast cancer determined that α_5 expression appears to roughly correlate with the differentiation of the tumor *(16,20)*. Integrin α_5 is expressed at high levels in fibroadenoma and in well differentiated ductal carcinomas; and expression diminishes, but remains detectable in poorly differentiated breast cancers and in metastatic breast cancers. Expression of integrin α_5 appears to correlate with expression of estrogen-receptor expression *(16,18,20)*. Reduction of expression of α_5 appears to correlate with the transition of breast cancer to a malignant phenotype ($p < 0.001$), but it does not appear to correlate with the presence of axillary nodal metastases *(22)*.

There is some evidence that expression of α_5 integrin may influence metastatic spreading. Murthy et al. examined two metastatic mouse mammary-carcinoma cell lines, TA3Ha and TA3AD *(79)*. TA3Ha cells express much higher levels of α_5 than TA3AD. TA3Ha cells preferentially metastasize to sites of surgical injury in the spleen ($p < 0.00001$) or liver ($p < 0.00001$). Metastasis to sites of wound healing was inhibited in a dose-dependent manner by preincubating TA3Ha cells with fibronectin or with synthetic fibronectin peptides ($p < 0.005$). Together, these studies suggest that $\alpha_4\beta_1$ and $\alpha_5\beta_1$ do not participate strongly in the early events of breast cancer but expression of $\alpha_5\beta_1$ may foster a transition to an invasive or metastatic phenotype.

2.6. Expression of $\alpha_6\beta_1$ and $\alpha_6\beta_4$ Integrin

2.6.1. Expression of $\alpha_6\beta_1$ and $\alpha_6\beta_4$ Integrin in Mammary-Gland Development

Integrin α_6 is primarily a laminin receptor *(48,80,81)*. It is also the only integrin that forms a heterodimer with integrin β_4 and preferentially associates with β_4 integrin *(82)*. In the absence of integrin β_4, integrin α_6 does associate with the β_1 integrin *(40,83,84)*. In the newborn and infant human breast, α_6 integrin is primarily expressed on basal cells along the basement membrane, with lighter expression on luminal epithelial cells *(15)*. Similarly, integrin β_4 is exclusively expressed by basal cells at the basement membrane in both the infant and the adult breast *(15,23,27,120)*. The lactating mammary gland retains strong expression of α_6 and β_4 at the basement membrane *(85)*. It is probable that much of the expression of α_6 and β_4 observed in the developing and lactating breast are contained within hemidesmosomes. Hemidesmosomes are a complex multiprotein structure that attach basal epithelial and myoepithelial cells to the underlying basement membrane *(86,87)*. Integrin $\alpha_6\beta_4$ is the primary integrin component of hemidesmosomes *(88,89)*. Genetic knock out studies have established that mice lacking either α_6 or β_4 integrin are unable to form hemidesmosomes *(90–92)*. Immunohistochemical and Western-blot analyses of β_4 knockout mice have determined that in β_4 –/– mice there is a dramatic downregulation of α_6 integrin protein to barely detectable levels. Expression of integrin β_1 and the other major laminin receptor, integrin α_3, were not affected *(90,92)*. Similarly, immunohistochemical analysis determined that there was reduced expression of β_4 integrin in α_6 –/– mice *(91)*. These results suggest that the primary function of α_6 and β_4 integrin in developing epithelial cells is in the formation of hemidesmosomes. All of the knockout mice die soon after birth of skin defects; this has made examination of mammary glands difficult. Therefore, it is uncertain what role $\alpha_6\beta_4$ plays in breast development. Bergstraesser et al. examined hemidesmosome expression in normal adult mammary cells by electron microscopy *(93)*. These studies determined that both luminal and myoepithelial mammary epithelial cells express hemidesmosomes at their basal plasma membrane where they contact the basement membrane.

Howlett et al. and Weaver et al. examined the expression of $\alpha_6\beta_1$ and $\alpha_6\beta_4$ in normal breast epithelium grown in vitro in reconstituted ECM *(33,34)*. These cells form organized round acini with a defined lumen. Integrin α_6, β_1 and β_4 were expressed on the basal (outside) surface of these acini. Treatment of these acini with neutralizing antibodies to either α_6, β_1, or β_4 resulted in their disruption and the formation of disorganized cellular masses. These observations suggest that α_6 and β_4 integrins help to maintain the basal-luminal orientation of breast epithelial cells and that disruption of this orientation may lead to disorganized growth.

2.6.2. Expression of $\alpha_6\beta_1$ and $\alpha_6\beta_4$ Integrin in Breast Cancer

Numerous studies have identified strong expression of integrin $\alpha_6\beta_1$ in normal breast myoepithelial and luminal epithelial cells at the basement membrane *(17–19,22,36,44, 85,94)*. These cell types also strongly express laminin, the ligand for α_6 integrin *(94–96)*. d'Ardenne et al. determined that expression of $\alpha_6\beta_1$ correlated with the expression of laminin ($p < 0.001$) and was inversely related to tumor grading ($p < 0.01$) *(44)*. Natali et al. determined that the cellular distribution of α_6 models the state of the basement membrane *(94)*. Normally $\alpha_6\beta_1$ integrin is expressed along the basolateral side along the basement membrane. When the laminin rich basement membrane is disrupted in cancer, expression of $\alpha_6\beta_1$ decreases, and the remaining expression is no longer polarized. In general, most studies have observed a loss of α_6 staining during breast cancer progression *(36)* and recent studies suggest that laminin adhesion decreases dramatically in breast-cancer cells *(41,42)*. Indeed, Sager et al. used differential display and identified α_6 integrin as a candidate tumor suppressor gene in mammary epithelial cells *(97)*. In a study of 73 patient samples, Gui et al. determined that a loss of $\alpha_6\beta_1$ correlated with malignant tumors ($p < 0.01$) and with axillary nodal metastases ($p < 0.001$). The same study determined that a loss of β_4 integrin correlated with malignant tumors ($p < 0.05$) *(22)*. One possible exception is in myoepithelial carcinoma of the breast. This is a very malignant cancer of the myoepithelial cells with a poor prognosis. Electron-microscopic examination of a myoepithelial tumor determined that they continue to express hemidesmosomes, arguing that $\alpha_6\beta_4$ is expressed in these tumors *(98)*.

2.6.3. Expression of $\alpha_6\beta_1$ Integrin in Invasive Breast Cancer

Invasive ductal and lobular carcinoma appears to have very different expression of α_6 integrin. Pignatelli et al. observed strong polarized expression of α_6 integrin in 27% (5/18) of invasive lobular carcinomas *(19)*. Expression is weak to nonexistent in Grades I and II ductal carcinomas, however, approximately 36% of Grade III invasive ductal carcinomas express strong or polarized expression of α_6 integrin. Koukoulis et al. identified strong staining of $\alpha_6\beta_1$ in pseudopodia of infiltrating lobular carcinomas *(17)*. Similarly, Pignatelli et al. observed expression of α_6 integrin in 78% of invasive lobular carcinomas *(19)*. Most of these invasive lobular carcinomas expressed low levels of β_4 integrin. Friedrichs et al. performed a prognostic study with 119 frozen tumor biopsies of invasive ductal carcinomas with survival data *(99,100)*. In this study, integrin α_6 was expressed both at the luminal and basal surfaces of epithelial cells. In invasive carcinomas, low expression of α_6 integrin (less than 5% positive staining cells) was a strong predictor of patient survival ($p < 0.0192$). Furthermore, this study observed high α_6 integrin expression in 30 of 34 distant metastases. Together, these studies suggest that there appears to be a gradual decrease in expression of integrin α_6 in ductal breast cancer. However, once the tumor has become invasive, higher expression of α_6 becomes a strong predictor of metastatic progression and death.

One complication in the study of integrin α_6 in breast cancer is that there are two known splice variants. Patriarca et al. examined the expression of each variant in the normal breast and breast cancer by immunohistochemistry *(101)*. The normal breast appears to express only integrin α_{6A}. However, there appears to be a transition to expression of integrin α_{6B} in advanced invasive ductal carcinoma. This was also examined in Friedrichs et al.; they observed a slightly higher ratio (albeit insignificant) of α_{6A} to α_{6B} in surviving patients, as opposed to deceased patients *(99)*.

Shaw et al. expanded on the observations in Friedrichs et al. *(40)*. They inhibited $\alpha_6\beta_1$ function in the invasive and metastatic breast-cancer cell line MDA-MB-435 (a β_4 integrin-negative line) by a dominant-negative approach. They transfected these cells with a construct that encodes a mutant β_4 integrin, lacking its large (100 kDa) cytoplasmic tail. MDA-MB-435 cells transfected with this mutant β_4 integrin exhibited decreased adhesion to laminin, decreased migration on laminin, and decreased invasion through reconstituted ECM in a transwell invasion assay (40). This is consistent with studies by Murthy et al., which described expression of α_6 integrin on metastatic mouse mammary carcinoma cells *(79)*. Incubation of these cells with laminin prior to their injection into mice inhibited the formation of metastases ($p < 0.005$). Together, these studies suggest that α_6 integrin may contribute to a invasive metastatic phenotype and that β_4 integrin may play an important role in regulating this phenotype.

2.7. Expression of $\alpha_V\beta_3$ Integrin

2.7.1. Expression of $\alpha_V\beta_3$ Integrin in Mammary-Gland Development

Integrin $\alpha_V\beta_3$ is primarily a vitronectin receptor *(102,103)* but it can also serve as a receptor for laminin *(104)*, fibronectin *(105)*, fibrinogen, von Willebrand factor *(103)*, thrombospondin *(106,107)*, osteopontin *(108,109)*, and PECAM-1 *(110,111)*. Pechox et al. examined the expression of integrin α_V in the human embryonic breast *(112)*. Integrin α_V was not expressed in budding or sprouting ductal epithelial cells through the 20th week of gestation. Expression of integrin α_V was first observed in the malpighian epithelium and in preadipocytes at 28 wk of gestation. This is consistent with studies in the developing mouse *(113)* where integrin $\alpha_V\beta_3$ is not expressed until mid- to late-gestation. Immunohistochemical examination of breast biopsies identified very weak expression of integrin $\alpha_V\beta_3$ in the normal adult breast. Expression of this integrin was primarily basolateral, along the basal surface at the basement membrane and at sites of cell-cell contact *(20)*. Integrin α_V is primarily expressed in the myoepithelium and in vascular endothelial cells, where it can heterodimerize with β_3 and β_5 integrins *(114)*. It is also expressed on luminal epithelial cells and stromal cells where it is likely to form heterodimers with β_1 integrin *(22)*. It is unlikely that integrin β_3 is required for mammary gland development. Loss of function mutations in β_3 integrin can give rise to the bleeding disorder Glanzmann's thrombasthenia. This disease effects both men and women. Numerous women with Glanzmann's thrombasthenia have been observed through puberty and childbirth and mammary gland abnormalities have not been noted in this population *(115,116)*.

2.7.2. Expression of $\alpha_V\beta_3$ Integrin in Breast Cancer

Similar to the expression patterns of α_1 and α_6, Zutter et al. described a mild decrease in α_V expression in ductal carcinomas. Expression of α_V integrin decreases during the progression to malignant breast cancer ($p < 0.01$) *(20,22)*, and loss of α_V correlated with the presence of axillary nodal metastases ($p < 0.001$) *(22)*. Its expression appears to increase dramatically within invasive breast cancers. Koukoulis et al. and Pignatelli et al. describe high expression of α_V integrin in 65% invasive ductal and 85% of lobular breast carcinomas *(17,19)*. Pignatelli further determined that the $\alpha_V\beta_3$ heterodimer was expressed in 10% invasive ductal carcinomas and in approximately 50% of invasive lobular carcinomas *(19)*. Serre et al. examined the expression of integrin α_V in breast cancer by electron microscopy. In both ductal carcinoma and invasive lobular carcinoma, there is narrow expression of integrin α_V within the endoplasmic reticulum and on the plasma membrane at the basement membrane *(117)*.

2.7.3. Role of $\alpha_V\beta_3$ Integrin in Neovascularization and Metastasis of Breast Cancer

The high expression of $\alpha_V\beta_3$ integrin in breast tumors may contribute to two different components of breast cancer progression: angiogenesis and metastasis. Integrin $\alpha_V\beta_3$ is expressed by microvascular endothelial cells *(101)* and this expression increases 4-fold during angiogenesis in vitro (in a chick chorioallantoic membrane assay) and in wound tissue compared to normal tissue *(8,9,13)*. Neutralizing antibodies to $\alpha_V\beta_3$ can block growth factor-induced angiogenesis in vitro. In a severe combined immunodeficient (SCID)-mouse breast-tumor-xenograft model, neutralizing antibodies to $\alpha_V\beta_3$ decreased the number of infiltrating blood vessels within the tumor approximately 3–4 fold and decreased the tumor mass and volume by approximately 4-fold *(10)*. Together, these studies argue that expression of $\alpha_V\beta_3$ by the breast cancer stroma may participate in the neovascularization of the tumor, promoting growth and metastatic spread.

Perhaps the most important characteristic of $\alpha_V\beta_3$ expression is its correlation with bone metastases. As previously mentioned, $\alpha_V\beta_3$ is a receptor for osteopontin and is expressed by osteoclasts, presumably because it is a osteopontin receptor *(118)*. Immunohistochemical examination of 22 breast-cancer metastases that localized to the bone found strong expression of $\alpha_V\beta_3$ protein in all samples. In contrast, these same samples did not express $\alpha_2\beta_1$ integrin. *In situ* analysis confirmed that these metastases expressed β_3 integrin mRNA *(59)*. These results are in agreement with the results of Kitazawa and Maeda who used *in situ* hybridization to identify β_3 integrin mRNA in breast cancer and breast-cancer metastases *(119)*. This study identified heterogeneous or low expression of β_3 mRNA in the primary tumor and lymph-node metastases, but high expression of β_3 mRNA in skeletal metastases. These studies suggest two possible roles for the β_3 integrin: either breast-cancer cells that express β_3 integrin are more invasive and metastatic or breast-cancer cells that express β_3 simply get caught in the bone. In summary, upregulation of integrin $\alpha_V\beta_3$ in the stroma may promote the vascularization of breast tumors. These vascularized tumors may then migrate out of the tumor and extravasate in the bone where they form metastases.

3. CONCLUSION

In the normal tissue, integrins are primarily expressed along the basal laminal surface closest to the basement membrane. Integrin α_6 and β_4 are primarily contained in hemidesmosomes forming strong focal attachment to the basement membrane. Some integrins, β_1, α_2, α_3, and α_6 appear to also be expressed at cell-cell contacts. There is great fluctuation in expression of α_2 during breast development, pregnancy and lactation, suggesting that this integrin participates in the functional differentiation and development of the breast. Further analysis of the contribution of various integrins to breast-cancer development must await additional analysis of knockout mice using inducible promoters or surgical transfer of mammary glands lacking these genes from neonatal integrin knockout mice to viable hosts.

In general, during tumor progression there is a decrease in the expression of most integrin subunits. This may correlate with the histologic transformation, where cells no longer adopt a polarized organized orientation from the basement membrane to the lumen and adopt a more disorganized random orientation. For α_2 integrin, this downregulation appears permanent and may provide a growth advantage or allow for invasion or metastasis. Similarly, expression of β_4 integrin decreases and probably allows for a dissolution of hemidesmosomes and detachment from the basement membrane. Integrins that bind laminin (α_3 and α_6) appear to decrease during early cancer, but they may be then expressed by more invasive cells, enabling them to invade through the laminin-rich basement membrane. Lastly, the α_V integrins may promote neovascularization of the tumor and actively direct metastasis to the bone. The use of integrins as a marker for breast-cancer progression requires a detailed examination of the cellular localization of the integrin as well as the level of expression. For example, high α_6 expression may indicate a tissue that is well-differentiated and expressing hemidesmosomes, or it may indicate a cell type that is rampantly disorganized, has lost basal-luminal orientation, and is displaying an invasive/metastatic phenotype. Analysis of a panel of integrins α_1, α_2, α_6, and α_V together with histopathology may provide a very accurate depiction of the ability of a breast cancer to progress and metastasize.

ACKNOWLEDGMENTS

Edward C. Rosfjord was supported by a Susan G. Komen Breast Cancer Foundation Postdoctoral Fellowship, Grant # 9703. Edward C. Rosfjord and Robert B. Dickson were supported by a SPORE in Breast Cancer (NIH #1P50CA5185).

REFERENCES

1. Rosen, P. P. and H. A. Oberman. 1993. *Atlas of Tumor Pathology (Third Series, Fascicle 7) Tumors of the mammary gland.* Armed Forces Institute of Pathology, Washington DC.
2. Dedhar, S. 1990. Integrins and tumor invasion. *BioEssays* **12**: 583–590.
3. Hynes, R. O. 1992. Integrins: versatility, modulation, and signaling in cell adhesion. *Cell* **69**: 11–25.
4. Luscinskas, F. W. and J. Lawler. 1994. Integrins as dynamic regulators of vascular function. *FASEB J.* **8**: 929–938.
5. Schlaepfer, D. D., S. K. Hanks, T. Hunter, and P. van der Geer. 1994. Integrin-mediated signal transduction linked to ras pathway by GRB2 binding to focal adhesion kinase. *Nature* **372**: 786–791.
6. Lewis, J. M. and M. A. Schwartz. 1995. Mapping in vivo associations of cytoplasmic proteins with integrin β_1 cytoplasmic domain mutants. *Mol. Biol. Cell* **6**: 151–159.
7. Miyamoto, S., S. K. Akiyama, and K. M. Yamada. 1995. Synergistic roles for receptor occupancy and aggregation in integrin transmembrane function. *Science* **267**: 883–885.
8. Brooks, P. C., R. A. F. Clark, D. A. and Cheresh. 1994. Requirement of vascular integrin $\alpha_v\beta_3$ for angiogenesis. *Science* **264**: 569–571.
9. Brooks, P. C., A. M. Montgomery, M. Rosenfeld, R. A. Reisfeld, T. Hu, G. Klier, and D. A. Cheresh. 1994. Integrin $\alpha_v\beta_3$ agonists promote tumor regression by inducing apoptosis of angiogenic blood vessels. *Cell* **79**: 1157–1164.
10. Brooks, P. C., S. Stromblad, R. Klemke, D. Visscher, F. H. Sarkar, and D. A. Cheresh. 1995. Antiintegrin $\alpha_v\beta_3$ blocks human breast cancer growth and angiogenesis in human skin. *J. Clin. Invest.* **96**: 1815–1822.
11. Montgomery, A. M., R. A. Reisfeld, and D. A. Cheresh. 1994. Integrin $av\beta_3$ rescues melanoma cells from apoptosis in three-dimensional dermal collagen. *Proc. Natl. Acad. Sci. USA* **91**: 8856–8860.
12. Rouslahti, E. and J. C. Reed. 1994. Anchorage dependence, integrins and apoptosis. *Cell* **77**: 477–478.
13. Varner, J. A., P. C. Brooks, and D. A. Cheresh. 1995. Review: The integrin $\alpha_v\beta_3$: angiogenesis and apoptosis. *Cell Adh. Comm.* **3**: 367–374.
14. Deugnier, M. A., E. P. Moiseyeva, J. P. Thiery, and M. Glukhova. 1995. Myoepithelial cell differentiation in the developing mammary gland: progressive acquisition of smooth muscle phenotype. *Dev. Dyn.* **204**: 107–117.
15. Anbazhagan, R., J. Bartek, G. Stamp, M. Pignatelli, and B. Gusterson. 1995. Expression of integrin subunits in the human infant breast correlates with morphogenesis and differentiation. *J. Pathol.* **176**: 227–232.
16. Zutter, M. M., H. R. Krigman, and S. A. Santoro. 1993. Altered integrin expression in adenocarcinoma of the breast. Analysis by *in situ* hybridization. *Am. J. Pathol.* **142**: 1439–1448.
17. Koukoulis, G. K., I. Virtanen, M. Korhonen, L. Laitinen, V. Quaranta, and V. E. Gould. 1991. Immunohistochemical localization of integrins in the normal, hyperplastic, and neoplastic breast. *Am. J. Pathol.* **139**: 787–799.
18. Mechtersheimer, G., M. Munk, T. Barth, K. Koretz, and P. Moller. 1993. Expression of beta 1 integrins in non-neoplastic mammary epithelium, fibroadenoma and carcinoma of the breast. *Virchows Arch. A Pathol. Anat. Histopathol.* **422**: 203–210.
19. Pignatelli, M., M. R. Cardillo, A. Hanby, and G. W. Stamp. 1992. Integrins and their accessory adhesion molecules in mammary carcinomas: loss of polarization in poorly differentiated tumors. *Human Pathol.* **23**: 1159–1166.
20. Zutter, M. M., G. Mazoujian, and S. A. Santoro. 1990. Decreased expression of integrin adhesive protein receptors in adenocarcinoma of the breast. *Am. J. Pathol.* **137**: 863–870.

21. Zutter, M. M. and S. A. Santoro. 1990. Widespread histologic distribution of the $\alpha_2\beta_1$ integrin cell- surface collagen receptor. *Am J. Pathol.* **137:** 113–120.

22. Gui G. P., C. A. Wells, P. D. Browne, P. Yeomans, S. Jordan, J. R. Puddefoot, G. P. Vinson, and R. Carpenter. 1995. Integrin expression in primary breast cancer and its relation to axillary nodal status. *Surgery* **117:** 102-108.

23. Hanby, A. M., C. E. Gillett, M. Pignatelli, and G. W. Stamp. 1993. β_1 and β_4 integrin expression in methacarn and formalin-fixed material from in situ ductal carcinoma of the breast. *J. Pathol.* **171:** 257–262.

24. Fassler, R. and M. Meyer. 1995. Consequences of lack of beta 1 integrin gene expression in mice. *Genes Dev.* **9:** 1896–1908

25. Stephens, L. E., A. E. Sutherland, I. V. Klimanskaya, A. Andrieux, J. Meneses, R. A. Pedersen, and C. H. Damsky. 1995. Deletion of β_1 integrins in mice results in inner cell mass failure and peri-implantation lethality. *Genes Dev.* **9:** 1883–1895.

26. Berdichevsky, F., C. Gilbert, M. Shearer, and J. Taylor-Papadimitriou. 1992. Collagen-induced rapid morphogenesis of human mammary epithelial cells: the role of the $\alpha_2\beta_1$ integrin. *J. Cell Sci.* **102:** 437–446.

27. Berdichevsky, F., D. Alford, B. D'Souza, and J. Taylor-Papadimitriou. 1994. Branching morphogenesis of human mammary epithelial cells in collagen gels. *J. Cell Sci.* **107:** 3557–3568.

28. Streuli, C. H., N. Bailey, and M. J. Bissel. 1991. Control of mammary epithelial differentiation: basement membrane induces tissue-specific gene expression in the absence of cell-cell interaction and morphological polarity. *J. Cell Biol.* **115:** 1383–1395.

29. Boudreau, N., C. J. Sympson, Z. Werb, and M. J. Bissell. 1995. Suppression of ICE and apoptosis in mammary epithelial cells by extracellular matrix. *Science* **267:** 891–893

30. Liotta, L. A., P. S. Steeg, and W. G. Stetler-Stevenson. 1991. Cancer metastasis and angiogenesis: an imbalance of positive and negative regulation. *Cell* **64:** 327–336.

31. Pullan, S., J. Wilson, A. Metcalfe, G. M. Edwards, G. M., N. Goberdhan, J. Tilly, J. A. Hickman, C. Dive, and C. Streuli. 1996. Requirement of basement membrane for the suppression of programmed cell death in mammary epithelium. *J. Cell Sci.* **109:** 631–642.

32. Boudreau, N., Z. Werb, and M. J. Bissell. 1996. Suppression of apoptosis by basement membrane requires three-dimensional tissue organization and withdrawal from the cell cycle. *Proc. Natl. Acad. Sci. USA* **93:** 3509–3513.

33. Howlett A. R., N. Bailey, C. Damsky, O. W. Petersen, and M. J. Bissell. 1995. Cellular growth and survival are mediated by beta 1 integrins in normal human breast epithelium but not in breast carcinoma. *J. Cell Sci.* **108:** 1945–1957.

34. Weaver, V. M., O. W. Petersen, F. Wang, C. A. Larabell, P. Briand, C. Damsky, and M. J. Bissell. 1997. Reversion of the malignant phenotype of human breast cells in three-dimensional culture and in vivo by integrin blocking antibodies. *J. Cell Biol.* **137:** 231–245.

35. Gould, V. E., G. K. Koukoulis, and I. Virtanen. 1990. Extracellular matrix proteins and their receptors in the normal hyperplastic and neoplastic breast. *Cell Diff. Dev.* **32:** 409–416.

36. Jones, J. L., D. R. Critchley, and R. A. Walker. 1992. Alteration of stromal protein and integrin expression in breast—a marker of premalignant change? *J. Pathol.* **167:** 399–406.

37. Pignatelli, M., A. M. Hanby, G. W. H. and Stamp. 1991. Low expression of β_1, α_2 and α_3 subunits of VLA integrins in malignant mammary tumors. *J. Pathol.* **165:** 25–32.

38. Gui, G. P. H., J. R. Puddefoot, G. P. Vinson, C. A. Wells, and R. Carpenter. 1995. In vitro regulation of human breast cancer cell adhesion and invasion via integrin receptors to the extracellular matrix. *Br. J. Surgery* **82:** 1192–1196.

39. Maemura, M., S. K. Akiyama, V. L. Woods, and R. B. Dickson. 1995. Expression and ligand binding of $\alpha_2\beta_1$ integrin on breast carcinoma cells. *Clin. Exp. Metast.* **13:** 223–235.

40. Shaw, L. M., C. Chao, U. M. Wewer, and A. M. Mercurio. 1996. Function of the integrin $\alpha_6\beta_1$ in metastatic breast carcinoma cells assessed by expression of a dominant-negative receptor. *Cancer Res.* **56:** 959–963.

41. Gui, G. P. H., J. R. Puddefoot, G. P. Vinson, C. A. Wells, and R. Carpenter, R. 1995. Modulation of very late activation-2 laminin receptor function in breast cancer metastasis. *Surgery* **118:** 245–250.

42. Gui, G. P. H., Puddefoot, J. R., Vinson, G. P., Wells, C. A., and Carpenter, R. 1997. Altered cell-matrix contact: a prerequisite for breast cancer metastasis? *Br. J. Cancer* **75:** 623–633.

43. Elliot, B. E., P. Ekblom, H. Pross, A. Niemann, and K. Rubin. 1994. Anti-β_1 integrin IgG inhibits pulmonary macrometastasis and the size of micrometastases from a murine mammary carcinoma. *Cell Adh. Comm.* **1:** 319–332

44. d'Ardenne, A. J., P. I. Richman, M. A. Horton, A. E. Mcaulay, and S. Jordan. 1991. Co-ordinate expression of the alpha–6 integrin laminin receptor subunit and laminin in breast cancer. *J. Pathol.* **165:** 213–220.

45. Gardner, H., J. Kreidberg, V. Koteliansky, and R. Jaenisch. 1996. Deletion of integrin α1 by homologous recombination permits normal murine development but gives rise to a specific deficit in cell adhesion. *Dev. Biol.* **175:** 301–313.

46. Gardner, H., personal communication.

47. Hemler, M. E. 1988. Adhesive protein receptors on hemopoietic cells. *Immunol. Today* **9:** 109–113.

48. Lotz, M. M., C. A. Korzelius, and A. M. Murcurio. 1991. Human colon carcinoma cells use multiple receptors to adhere to laminin: involvement of $\alpha_6\beta_4$ and $\alpha_2\beta_1$ integrins. *Cell Regul.* **1:** 249–257.

49. Keely, P. J., J. E. Wu, and S. A. Santoro. 1995. The spatial and temporal expression of the $\alpha_2\beta_1$ integrin and its ligands, collagen I, collagen IV, and laminin, suggest important roles in mouse mammary morphogenesis. *Differentiation* **59:** 1–13

50. Takada, Y. and M. E. Hemler. 1989. The primary structure of the VLA–2/collagen receptor α_2 subunit (platelet GPIa): homology to other integrins and the presence of a possible collagen-binding domain. *J. Cell Biol.* **109:** 397–406.

51. Wayner E. A. and W. G. Carter. 1987. Identification of multiple cell adhesion receptors for type IV collagen and fibronectin in human fibrosarcoma cells possessing unique a and common b subunits. *J. Cell Biol.* **105:** 1873–1884

52. Kleinman, H. K., M. L. McGarvey, J. R. Gassell, V. L. Star, F. B. Cannon, G. W. Laurie, and G. R. Martin. 1986. Basement membrane complexes with biological activity. *Biochemistry* **25:** 312–318.

53. Kleinman, H. K., B. S. Weeks, H. W. Schnaper, M. C. Kibbey, K. Yamamura, and D. S. Grant. 1993. The laminins: a family of basement membrane glycoproteins important in cell differentiation and tumor metastases. *Vitam. Horm.* **47:** 161–186.

54. Symington B. E., Y. Takada, and W. G. Carter. 1993. Interaction of integrins $\alpha_3\beta_1$ and $\alpha_2\beta_1$: potential role in keratinocyte intercellular adhesion. *J. Cell Biol.* **120:** 523–535.

55. Weitzman J. B., A. Chen, and M. E. Hemler. 1995. Investigation of the role of beta 1 integrins in cell-cell adhesion. *J. Cell Sci.* **108:** 3635–3644

56. D'Souza, B., F. Berdichevsky, N. Kyprianou, and J. Taylor-Papadimitriou. 1992. Collagen-induced morphogenesis and expression of the α_2-integrin subunit is inhibited in c-erbB2-transfected human mammary epithelial cells. *Oncogene* **8:** 1797–1806.

57. Keely, P. J., A. M. Fong, M. M. Zutter, and S. A. Santoro. 1995. Alteration of collagen-dependent adhesion, motility, and morphogenesis by the expression of antisense α_2 integrin mRNA in mammary cells. *J. Cell Sci.* **108:** 595–607

58. Maemura, M. and R. B. Dickson. 1994. Are cellular adhesion molecules involved in the metastasis of breast cancer? *Breast Cancer Res. Treat.* **32:** 239–260.

59. Liapis, H., A. Flath, and S. Kitazawa. 1996. Integrin $\alpha V\beta_3$ expression by bone-residing breast cancer metastases. *Diagn. Mol. Pathol.* **5:** 127–135.

60. Zutter, M. M., S. A. Santoro, W. D. Staatz, and Y. L. Tsung. 1995. Re-expression of the $\alpha_2\beta_1$ integrin abrogates the malignant phenotype of breast carcinoma cells. *Proc. Natl. Acad. Sci.* **92:** 7411–7415.

61. Carter, W. G., M. C. Ryan, and P. J. Gahr. 1991. Epiligrin, a new cell adhesion ligand for integrin $\alpha_3\beta_1$ in epithelial basement membranes. *Cell* **65:** 599–610.

62. Dedhar, S., K. Jewell, M. Roijani, and V. Gray. 1992. The receptor for the basement membrane glycoprotein entactin is the integrin alpha 3/beta 1. *J. Biol. Chem.* **267:** 18,908–18,914.

63. Delwel, G. O., A. de Melker, F. Hogervorst, L. H. Jaspars, D. L. Fles, I. Kuikman, A. Lindblom, M. Paulsson, R. Timpl, and A. Sonnenberg. 1994. Distinct and overlapping ligand specificities of the alpha 3A beta 1 and alpha 6A beta 1 integrins: recognition of laminin isoforms. *Mol. Biol. Cell* **5:** 203–215.

64. Elices, M. J., L. A. Urry, and M. E. Hemler. 1991. Receptor function for the integrin VLA-3: fibronectin, collagen, and laminin binding are differentially influenced by Arg-Gly-Asp peptide and by divalent cations. *J. Cell Biol.* **112:** 169–181.

65. Gehlsen, K. R., P. Sriramarao, L. T. Furcht, and A. P. Skubitz. 1992. A synthetic peptide derived from the carboxy terminus of the laminin A chain represents a binding site for the alpha 3 beta 1 integrin. *J. Cell Biol.* **117:** 449–459.

66. Hemler, M. E., M. J. Elices, B. M. C. Chan, B. Zetter, N. Matsuura, and Y. Takada. 1990. Multiple ligand binding functions for VLA-2 ($\alpha_2\beta_1$) and VLA-3 ($\alpha_3\beta_1$) in the integrin family. *Cell Diff. Dev.* **32:** 229–238.

67. Weitzman, J. B., R. Pasqualini, Y. Takada, and M. E. Hemler. 1993. The function and distinctive regulation of the integrin VLA-3 in cell adhesion, spreading, and homotypic cell aggregation. *J. Cell Biol.* **268:** 8651–8657.

68. DiPersio, C. M., K. M. Hodivala-Dilke, R. Jaenisch, J. A. Kreidberg, and R. O. Hynes. 1997. $\alpha_3\beta_1$ integrin is required for normal development of the epidermal basement membrane. *J. Cell Biol.* **137:** 729–742.

69. Kreidberg, J. A., M. J. Donovan, S. L. Goldstein, H. Rennke, K. Shepard, R. C. Jones, and R. Jaenisch. 1996. Alpha 3 beta 1 integrin has a crucial role in kidney and lung organogenesis. *Development* **122:** 3537–3547.

70. Alexander, C. M., S. Goldstein, C. Daniel, and J. Kreidberg. Children's Hospital, Boston MA. In preparation.

71. Tawil, N. J., V. Gowri, M. Djoneidi, J. Nip, S. Carbonetto, and P. Brodt. 1996. Integrin $\alpha_3\beta_1$ can promote adhesion and spreading of metastatic breast carcinoma cells on the lymph node stroma. *Int. J. Cancer* **66:** 703–710.

72. Coopman, P. J., D. M. Thomas, K. R. Gehlsen, and S. C. Mueller. 1996. Integrin $\alpha_3\beta_1$ participates in the phagocytosis of extracellular matrix molecules by human breast cancer cells. *Mol. Biol. Cell* **7:** 1789–1804.

73. Pytela, R., M. D. Piershbacher, and E. Ruoslahti. 1985. Identification and isolation of a 140 kd cell surface glycoprotein with properties expected of a fibronectin receptor. *Cell* **40:** 191–198.

74. Guan, J.-L., and R. O. Hynes. 1990. Lymphoid cells recognize an alternatively spliced segment of fibronectin via the integrin receptor $\alpha_4\beta_1$. *Cell* **60:** 51–63.

75. Mould, A. P., L. A. Wheldon, A. Komoriya, E. A. Wayer, K. M. Yamada, and M. J. Humphries. 1990. Affinity chromatographic isolation of the melanoma adhesion receptor for the IIICS region of fibronectin and its identification as the integrin $\alpha_4\beta_1$. *J. Biol. Chem.* **265:** 4020–4024.

76. Hynes, R. O. 1996. Targeted mutations in cell adhesion genes: What have we learned from them? *Dev. Biol.* **180:** 402–412.

77. Yang, J. T., H. Rayburn, and R. O. Hynes. 1993. Embryonic mesodermal defects in α_5 integrin-deficient mice. *Development* **119:** 1093–1105.

78. Yang, J. T., H. Rayburn, and R. O. Hynes. 1995. Cell adhesion events mediated by α_4 integrins are essential in placental and cardiac development *Development* **121:** 549–560.

79. Murthy, M. S., S. E. Reid, Jr., X. F. Yang, and E. P. Scanlon. 1996. The potential role of integrin receptor subunits in the formation of local recurrence and distant metastasis by mouse breast cancer cells. *J. Surg. Oncol.* **63:** 77–86.

80. Sonnenberg, A., P. W. Modderman, and F. Hogervorst. 1988. Laminin receptor on platelets is the integrin VLA-6. *Nature* **336:** 487–489.

81. Sonnenberg, A., C. J. T. Linders, P. W. Modderman, C. H. Damsky, M. Aumailley, and R. Timpl. 1990. Integrin recognition of different cell-binding fragments of laminin (P1, E3, E8) and evidence that $\alpha_6\beta_1$ but not $\alpha_6\beta_4$ functions as a major receptor for fragment E8. *J. Cell Biol.* **110:** 2145–2155.

82. Hemler, M. E., C. Crouse, and A. Sonnenberg, A. 1989. Association of the VLA-α_6 subunit with a novel protein. *J. Biol. Chem.* **264:** 6529–6535.

83. Hall, D. E., L. F. Reichardt, E. Crowley, B. Holley, H. Moezzi, A. Sonnenberg, and C. H. Damsky. 1990. The alpha 1/beta 1 and alpha 6/beta 1 integrin heterodimers mediate cell attachment to distinct sites on laminin. *J. Cell Biol.* **110:** 2175–2184.

84. Ruiz, P., D. Dunon, A. Sonnenberg, and B. A. Imhof. 1993. Suppression of mouse melanoma metastasis by EA-1, a monoclonal antibody specific for α_6 integrins. *Cell Adh. Comm.* **1:** 67–81.

85. Sonnenberg, A. and C. J. T. Linders. 1990. The $\alpha_6\beta_1$ (VLA-6) and $\alpha_6\beta_4$ protein complexes: tissue distribution and biochemical properties. *J. Cell Sci.* **96:** 207–217.

86. Green, K. J. and J. C. R. Jones. 1996. Desmosomes and hemidesmosomes: structure and function of molecular components. *FASEB* **10:** 871–880.

87. Jones, J. C. R., J. Asmuth, S. E. Baker, M. Langhofer, S. I. Roth, and S. B. Hopkinson, S. B. 1994. Hemidesmosomes: extracellular matrix/intermediate filament connectors. *Exp. Cell. Res.* **213:** 1–11.

88. Sonnenberg, A., J. Calafat, H. Janssen, H. Daams, J. D. Aplin, M. H. Liesbeth, M. H. van der Raaij-Helmer, R. Falcioni, S. J. Kennel, J. D. Aplin, J. Baker, M. Loizdou, and D. Garrod. 1991. Integrin α_6/β_4 complex is located in hemidesmosomes, suggesting a major role in epidermal cell-basement membrane adhesion. *J. Cell Biol.* **113:** 907–917.

89. Stepp, M. A., M. S. Spurr, A. Tisdale, J. Elwell, and I. K. Gipson. 1990. $\alpha_6\beta_4$ integrin heterodimer is a component of hemidesmosomes. *Proc. Natl. Acad. Sci. USA* **87:** 8970–8974.

90. Dowling, J., Q. C. Yu, and E. Fuchs. 1996. β_4 integrin is required for hemidesmosome formation, cell adhesion and cell survival. *J. Cell Biol.* **134:** 559–572.

91. Georges-Labouesse, E., N. Messaddeq, G. Yehia, L. Cadalbert, A. Dierich, and M. Le Meur. 1996. Absence of integrin α_6 leads to epidermolysis bullosa and neonatal death in mice. *Nature Gen.* **13:** 370–373.

92. van der Neut, R., P. Krimpenfort, J. Calafat, C. M. Niessen, and A. Sonnenberg. 1996. Epithelial detachment due to absence of hemidesmosomes in integrin β_4 deficient mice. *Nature Gen.* **13:** 366–369.

93. Bergstraesser, L. M., G. Srinivasan, J. C. R. Jones, S. Stahl, and S. A. Weitzman. 1995. Expression of hemidesmosomes and component proteins is lost by invasive breast cancer cells. *Am. J. Pathol.* **147:** 1823–1839.

94. Natali, P. G., M. R. Nicotra, C. Botti, M. Mottolese, A. Bigotti, and O. Segatto. 1992. Changes in expression of $\alpha_6\beta_4$ integrin heterodimer in primary and metastatic breast cancer. *Br. J. Cancer* **66:** 318–322.

95. Charpin, C., J. C. Lissitzky, J. Jacqumier, M. N. Lavaut, F. Kopp, N. Pourreau-Schneider, P. M. Martin, and Toga, M. 1986. Immunohistochemical detection of laminin in 98 human breast carcinomas: a light and electron microscopic study. *Human Pathol.* **17:** 355–365.

96. d'Ardenne, A. J. and N. J. Barnard. 1989. Paucity of fibronectin in invasive lobular carcinoma of the breast. *J. Pathol.* **157:** 219–224.

97. Sager, R., A. Anisowicz, M. Neveu, P. Liang, and G. Sotiropoulou. 1993. Identification by differential display of alpha 6 integrin as a candidate tumor suppressor gene. *FASEB* **7:** 964–970.

98. Lakhani, S. R., M. J. O'Hare, P. Monaghan, J. Winehouse, J.-C. Gazet, and J. P. Sloane. 1995. Malignant myoepithelioma (myoepithelial carcinoma) of the breast: a detailed cytokeratin study. *J. Clin. Pathol.* **48:** 164–167.

99. Friedrichs, K., P. Ruiz, F. Franke, I. Gille, H. J. Terpe, and B. A. Imhof. 1995. High expression level of α_6 integrin in human breast carcinoma is correlated with reduced survival. *Cancer Res.* **55:** 901–906.

100. Imhof, B. A., L. Piali, R. H. Gisler, and D. Dunon. 1996. Involvement of alpha 6 and alpha v integrins in metastasis. *Curr. Top. Microbiol. Immunol.* **213:** 195–203

101. Patriarca, C., D. Ivanyi, D. Fles, A. de Melker, G. van Doornewaard, L. Oomen, R. M. Alfano, G. Coggi, and A. Sonnenberg. 1995. Distribution of extracellular and cytoplasmic domains of the α_3 and α_6 integrin subunits in solid tumors. *Int. J. Cancer* **63:** 182–189.

102. Cheresh, D. A. 1987. Human endothelial cells synthesize and express an Arg-Gly-Asp-directed adhesion receptor involved in attachment to fibrinogen and von Willebrand factor. *Proc. Natl. Acad. Sci. USA* **84:** 6471-6475.

103. Cheresh, D. A. and R. C. Spiro. 1987. Biosynthetic and functional properties of an Arg-Gly-Asp-directed receptor involved in human melanoma cell attachment to vitronectin, fibrinogen, and von Willebrand factor. *J. Biol. Chem.* **262:** 17,703–17,711.

104. Kramer, R. H., Y. F. Cheng, and R. Clyman. 1990. Human microvascular endothelial cells use β_1 and β_3 integrin receptor complexes to attach to laminin. *J. Cell Biol.* **111:** 1233–1243.

105. Charo, I. F., L. Nannizzi, J. W. Smith, and D. A. Cheresh. 1990. The vitronectin receptor alpha v beta 3 binds fibronectin and acts in concert with alpha 5 beta 1 in promoting cellular attachment and spreading on fibronectin. *J. Cell Biol.* **111:** 2795–2800.

106. Lawler, J., R. Weinstein, and R. O. Hynes, R. O. 1988. Cell attachment to thrombospondin: the role of ARG-GLY-ASP, calcium, and integrin receptors. *J. Cell Biol.* **107:** 2351–2361.

107. Lawler, J. and R. O. Hynes. 1989. An integrin receptor on normal and thrombasthenic platelets that binds thrombospondin. *Blood* **74:** 2022–2027.

108. Miyauchi, A., J. Alvarez, E. M. Greenfield, A. Teti, M. Grano, S. Colucci, A. Zambonin-Zallone, F. P. Ross, S. L. Teitelbaum, and D. Cheresh. 1993. Binding of osteopontin to the osteoclast integrin alpha v beta 3. *Osteoporos Int.* **3:** 132–135.

109. Ross, F. P., J. Chappel, J. E. Alvarez, D. Sander, W. T. Butler, M. C. Farach-Carson, K. A. Mintz, P. G. Robey, S. L. Teitelbaum, and D. A. Cheresh. 1993. Interactions between the bone matrix proteins osteopontin and bone sialoprotein and the osteoclast integrin alpha v beta. *J. Biol. Chem.* **268:** 9901–9907.

110. Buckley, C. D., R. Doyonnas, J. P. Newton, S. D. Blystone, E. J. Brown, S. M. Watt, and D. L. Simmons. 1996. Identification of alpha v beta 3 as a heterotypic ligand for CD31/PECAM-1. *J. Cell Sci.* **109:** 437–445.

111. Piali, L., P. Hammel, C. Uherek, F. Bachmann, R. H. Gisler, D. Dunon, and B. A. Imhof. 1995. CD31/PECAM-1 is a ligand for $\alpha_v\beta_3$ integrin involved in adhesion of leukocytes to endothelium. *J. Cell Biol.* **130:** 451–460.

112. Pechoux, C., P. Clezardin, R. Dante, C. M. Serre, M. Clerget, N. Bertin, J. Lawler, P. D. Delmas, J. Vauzelle, and L. Frappart. 1994. Localization of thrombospondin, CD36 and CD51 during prenatal development of the human mammary gland. *Differentiation* **57:** 133–141.

113. Yamada, S., K. E. Brown, and K. M. Yamada. 1995. Differential mRNA regulation of integrin subunits α_V, β_1, β_3, and β_5 during mouse embryonic organogenesis. *Cell Adh. Comm.* **3:** 311–325.

114. Clezardin, P., L. Frappart, M. Clerget, C. Pechoux, and P. D. Delmas. 1993. Expression of thrombospondin (TSP1) and its receptors (CD36 and CD51) in normal, hyperplastic, and neoplastic human breast. *Cancer Res.* **53:** 1421–1430.

115. Coller, B. S., U. Seligsohn, H. Peretz, and P. J. Newman. 1994. Glanzmann thrombasthenia: new insights from an historical perspective. *Semin. Hematol.* **31:** 301–311

116. George, J. N., J. P. Caen, and A. T. Nurden. 1990. Glanzmann's thrombasthenia: the spectrum of clinical disease. *Blood* **75:** 1383–1395

117. Serre, C. M., P. Clezardin, L. Frappart, G. Boivin, and P. D. Delmas. 1995. Distribution of thrombospondin and integrin av in DCIS, invasive ductal and lobular human breast carcinomas. Analysis by electron microscopy. *Virchows Arch.* **427:** 365–372.

118. Nesbitt, S., A. Nesbit, M. Helfrich, and M. Horton. 1993. Biochemical characterization of human osteoclast integrins. Osteoclasts express avβ_3, $\alpha_2\beta_1$ and $\alpha_v\beta_1$. *J. Biol. Chem.* **268:** 16,737–16,745.

119. Kitazawa, S. and S. Maeda. 1995. Development of skeletal metastases. *Clin. Orthaped. Related Res.* **312:** 45–50.

120. Terpe, H. J., H. Stark, P. Ruiz, and B. A. Imhof. 1994. Alpha 6 integrin distribution in human embryonic and adult tissues. *Histochemistry* **101:** 41–49.

14

Matrix Metalloproteinases
in the Pathogenesis of Breast Cancer

John R. MacDougall and Lynn M. Matrisian

1. INTRODUCTION

This chapter will focus on a class of molecules, the matrix metalloproteinases (MMPs), and their role in the biological behavior of breast cancers. Following a brief overview of the characteristics of MMPs, the chapter will summarize the literature on MMPs as malignancy-associated molecules, and their role in the progression of cancers in general. The focus will then switch to the association between MMPs and breast cancer based on information regarding both spatial (i.e., *in situ* localization of MMPs in tumors) and temporal (i.e., MMP expression as a function of tumor stage and grade) patterns of MMP expression in breast cancers. The regulation of MMPs will be discussed in an attempt to understand how molecular lesions associated with the genesis and progression of breast cancer can modulate the expression and activity of MMPs. The MMPs as functional mediators of malignant behavior will next be addressed, with particular emphasis on direct lines of evidence, such as gene transfection and transgenic and knock-out approaches, to understand MMP function. This section will also draw from data analyzing the role of MMPs in the normal functioning mammary gland. Finally, the use of MMP inhibitors, both as further evidence of a functional role for MMPs in the pathogenesis of breast cancer and as potential therapeutic modalities, will be mentioned, although a more complete discussion of the application of MMP inhibitors to the clinical treatment of breast cancer is found in Chapter 20.

2. MMPS AS MALIGNANCY-ASSOCIATED MOLECULES

2.1. The MMP Family of Molecules

The MMP family of enzymes at present is composed of at least 16 members. The members of this family of enzymes share several defining characteristics, including reliance on a metal ion (Zn^{2+}) for catalytic activity, activity at a physiological pH, and characteristic functional domains. These common domains include a propeptide, characterized by the amino acid sequence PRCGVPDV, which is responsible for latency, and the common sequence in the catalytic domain HEXGHXXGXXHS, in which the histidine residues are responsible for co-ordination of the Zn^{2+}. Other regions not

From: Breast Cancer: *Molecular Genetics, Pathogenesis, and Therapeutics*
Edited by: A. M. Bowcock © Humana Press Inc., Totowa, NJ

common to all MMPs are the hemopexin-like and hinge region domains found in all family members except matrilysin, the fibronectin-like domain found in the gelatinases, and a transmembrane domain found in the membrane-type MMPs. In addition to the PRCGVPDV activation domain, it has recently been found that some MMPs have a furin cleavage site, which, in some cases, can also function as an activation signal. For a more complete review of MMP structure, *see* ref. *1*.

As their name suggests, the MMPs degrade molecules of the basement membrane (BM) and extracellular matrix (ECM). In fact, taken as a whole, the family of MMPs is able to degrade virtually every component of the ECM. In addition, it is evident that these enzymes can act on a wide variety of substrates outside of the ECM, including growth factors and their receptors (*2,3*, for example). The activity of MMPs for various substrates has traditionally been the basis for the subclassification of various family members. The collagenases, composed of interstitial collagenase (MMP-1), neutrophil collagenase (MMP-8), and collagenase-3 (MMP-13) degrade fibrillar type I, II, and III collagens. The gelatinases, including gelatinase A (MMP-2) and gelatinase B (MMP-9), degrade denatured collagen (i.e., gelatin), as well as type IV collagen, hence their historical name, type IV collagenases. The stromelysins, made up of stromelysin-1 (MMP-3), stromelysin-2 (MMP-10), and matrilysin (MMP-7), have the widest range of substrate specificities, including proteoglycans, laminin, fibronectin, and a variety of collagens. Other members of the MMP family for which substrate specificity has been examined include metalloelastase (MMP-12), a macrophage enzyme that degrades elastin, myelin, and other matrix proteins, and is also responsible for the generation of the angiogenesis inhibitor angiostatin *(4–6)*; stromelysin-3 (MMP-11), which has relatively weak catalytic activity against matrix substrates *(7)*; and the membrane-type MT1-MMP, which activates gelatinase A, as well as having activity against ECM substrates *(8–10)*. New members of the MMP family have recently been added. MMP-18, cloned from Xenopus, has activity against fibrillar collagen *(11)*; MMP-19 has been cloned from several sources, including a mammary-gland cDNA library *(12,13)*; and enamelysin (MMP-20) is a porcine enzyme whose expression is restricted to the enamel organ *(14)*. With considerable overlap in activity against various substrates, it has become more attractive to classify members of this family based on common protein domain structures (as discussed above, and in ref. *15*). The characteristics of the MMP family members are summarized in Fig. 1., along with domain assignments.

The MMP family is also associated with a family of endogenous inhibitors, the tissue inhibitors of metalloproteinases, or TIMPs. Composed of four members, TIMPs 1–4, these relatively low mol wt (approx 20–30 kDa) inhibitors are expressed by a wide variety of tissues and cell types. In general, all of the TIMPs are able to inhibit the active site of all of the MMPs, although there is evidence to suggest that there may be slight differences among various TIMP/MMP combinations *(16)*. It has also been observed that TIMP-1 and TIMP-2 are found associated with latent gelatinase B and A, respectively. The exact function of this association remains poorly understood, although it has been speculated that, at least in the case of gelatinase A and TIMP-2, this association may facilitate molecular activation through a complex that includes MT1-MMP *(17)*.

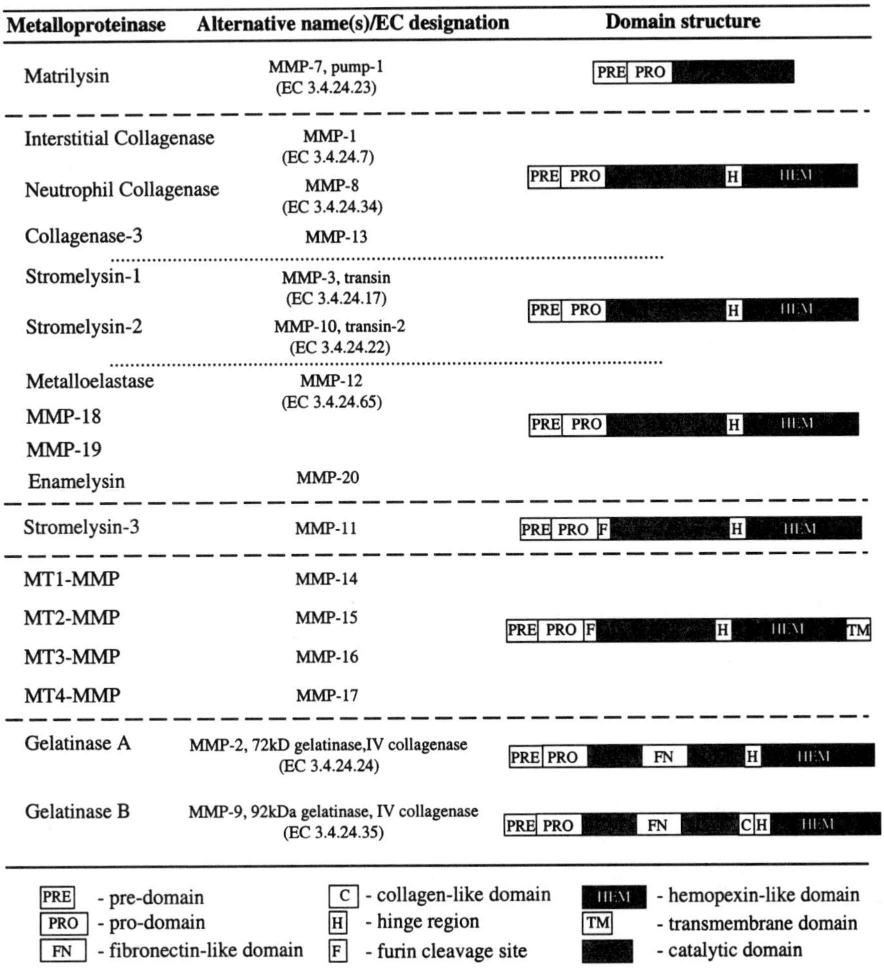

Metalloproteinase	Alternative name(s)/EC designation	Domain structure
Matrilysin	MMP-7, pump-1 (EC 3.4.24.23)	
Interstitial Collagenase	MMP-1 (EC 3.4.24.7)	
Neutrophil Collagenase	MMP-8 (EC 3.4.24.34)	
Collagenase-3	MMP-13	
Stromelysin-1	MMP-3, transin (EC 3.4.24.17)	
Stromelysin-2	MMP-10, transin-2 (EC 3.4.24.22)	
Metalloelastase	MMP-12 (EC 3.4.24.65)	
MMP-18		
MMP-19		
Enamelysin	MMP-20	
Stromelysin-3	MMP-11	
MT1-MMP	MMP-14	
MT2-MMP	MMP-15	
MT3-MMP	MMP-16	
MT4-MMP	MMP-17	
Gelatinase A	MMP-2, 72kD gelatinase, IV collagenase (EC 3.4.24.24)	
Gelatinase B	MMP-9, 92kDa gelatinase, IV collagenase (EC 3.4.24.35)	

PRE - pre-domain C - collagen-like domain HEM - hemopexin-like domain
PRO - pro-domain H - hinge region TM - transmembrane domain
FN - fibronectin-like domain F - furin cleavage site - catalytic domain

Fig. 1. The members of the MMP family can be grouped according to domain structure. The accepted name of each MMP is given, as well as other common names. The MMP number and EC classification assigned by the enzyme commission are also given. The protein domain structure is outlined for each MMP, including the common domains, as well as domains unique to individual MMPs. MMPs -4, -5, and -6 are not shown. Initially, a collagen telopeptidase activity was assigned to MMP-4. However, this enzyme remains to be purified and unambiguously identified as a new MMP. MMP-5 and MMP-6, although initially thought novel family members at the time of discovery, were found to be MMP-2 and MMP-3, respectively.

2.2. MMPs as Malignancy-Associated Molecules

The defining characteristics of MMPs make this family of enzymes likely candidates to be involved in tumor progression, since they are extracellular enzymes capable of matrix degradation, and are optimally active at neutral pH. It is thought that this capacity to degrade ECM allows for cellular movement and invasion in the process of metastasis *(18),* as well as access to growth factors liberated from degraded ECM *(19).* This potential role for MMPs was first described by Liotta et al. *(20),* when it was discovered that highly metastatic variants of the B16 melanoma cell line displayed an enhanced ability to degrade type IV or BM collagen. Historically, this was an important observation, because, as it was thought, metastatic cancer cells must cross two or three BMs containing type IV collagen. Since then, countless studies have addressed the expression and function of virtually all of the MMP family members in a variety of tumor systems (reviewed in ref. *21*).

Conclusions drawn from the literature over the past decade indicate the following general patterns for MMP involvement in tumor progression:

1. MMPs are often associated with advanced, malignant cancers, and not early, benign ones, although some interesting exceptions to this rule exist. The number of different MMPs and their relative levels also tend to increase with more aggressive stages of tumor progression. MMPs can be expressed by the malignant cells themselves, or, quite commonly, as a stromal response to the presence of the tumor.
2. MMP gene expression is controlled both positively and negatively by a number of factors also known to be involved in malignant disease progression, including growth factors, cytokines, tumor promoters and oncogenes. In addition to transcriptional regulation, both posttranscriptional and posttranslational mechanisms of MMP regulation are recognized, including the requirement for activation and subsequent susceptibility to inhibition by TIMPs.
3. Inhibition of MMP activity or expression in tumor cells leads to diminished malignancy, and MMP overexpression leads to the acquisition of a more malignant phenotype. In addition to genetic approaches to regulating MMP levels or activity, more recent studies with synthetic MMP inhibitors have not only provided proof-of-principle data for the role of MMPs in tumor aggressiveness, but also provided a vehicle for the application of this knowledge to the treatment of human disease.

Recently, understanding of the role of MMPs in neoplastic progression has taken a turn. Evidence, direct and indirect, from a variety of systems suggests that MMP expression and/or activity may also be associated with the primary growth of tumors and the competence for clonogenic growth of metastases, and not simply the requirement for an invasive phenotype to complete the metastatic journey. Evidence for this is suggested from the work of Chambers et al., who used intravital microscopy *(22)*. In addition, experiments addressing the role of the MMP matrilysin in tumor progression have suggested that it may in fact be involved in the development of early-stage tumors (i.e., adenomas) *(23)*, thus emphasizing the potential importance of these molecules in not only the end stage of cancer, but also the early pathogenesis of this disease. This subject has recently been reviewed by Chambers and Matrisian *(24)*.

3. MMPS IN BREAST CANCER

3.1. Spatial and Temporal Expression of MMPs in Breast Cancer

MMP expression in breast cancer in general follows the same trends seen in other cancers. A number of MMPs have been shown to be expressed by breast cancer cells, but not expressed by their normal counterparts. These include the gelatinases A and B, membrane-type metalloproteinases, stromelysin-3, and matrilysin, and, to a lesser degree, interstitial collagenase and collagenase-3. The tissue pattern of MMP expression demonstrates an interesting, predominantly stromal pattern of expression, at least at the mRNA level, which has important implications for the eventual understanding of the role of MMPs in the biological behavior of breast cancer. The only MMP not showing a primarily stromal pattern of expression is matrilysin *(25)*, which implies special consideration, and possibly unique functions, for this MMP. There are also a number of intriguing interactions between MMP subfamilies, which add to the complexity of the biology of MMPs. The MMPs of particular relevance to breast cancer are discussed individually below.

3.1.1. Stromelysin-3

The MMP stromelysin-3 was initially cloned as a gene differentially expressed in malignant, compared to fibroadenomatous, breast tissue *(26)*. When the tissue distribution of this gene was examined, it was found to be expressed exclusively in the stroma of breast cancers, an observation which has been confirmed by several groups *(27–29)*. This observation heralded a shift in the paradigm for MMPs in tumor progression. Until that time, MMPs had primarily been assumed to be tumor-cell associated, although some evidence for host–tumor interactions had been described (ref. *30* and references therein). A wide range of tumor cell lines expressed MMP activity, and, intuitively, if a tumor cell invaded a distant organ site, it was felt that it would have to supply its own machinery to do so. The counterintuitive spatial pattern of stromal expression has been repeated for other MMPs, in addition to stromelysin-3, and is now a common theme, although the consequences of such a pattern of expression to the progression of breast cancers remains to be clearly understood.

Stromelysin-3 expression correlates well with the progression of breast cancers to aggressive disease. Hahnel et al. *(28)* found that, although only 10% of ductal carcinoma *in situ* (DCIS) samples showed expression of stromelysin-3 mRNA by Northern blot analysis, approx 65% of primary and metastatic breast carcinomas showed such expression. Heppner et al. *(29)* noted a similar expression pattern in DCIS vs invasive cancers, and observed that, in contrast to other stromal MMPs, the pattern of hybridization for stromelysin-3 mRNA was only evident in the stromal cells directly adjacent to the tumor, rather than a diffuse staining throughout the entire tumor stroma. Wolf et al. *(31)* reported that *in situ* carcinomas of the comedo type, which show an increased tendency to progress toward invasiveness, stained positive for stromelysin-3 more frequently than lobular *in situ* carcinomas, which show a decreased tendency toward progression. The role of stromelysin-3 in the progression of breast cancers has been strengthened by several reports of its power as a prognostic marker in patient samples. Engel et al. *(32)* found, by *in situ* hybridization combined with quantitative techniques, that overexpression of stromelysin-3 was correlated with poor outcome and a shorter time to disease progression. In addition, they found that the correlation of outcome and stromelysin-3 overexpression was not correlated with other prognostic factors, including estrogen receptor status, tumor size, or microvessel counts, suggesting that stromelysin-3 expression in breast cancers could act as an independent prognostic marker.

3.1.2. Gelatinases

The gelatinase subfamily of MMPs has received considerable attention as the enzymes responsible for the type IV collagenolytic activity associated with metastatic cells. Gelatinase A levels, as measured by a variety of techniques, including gelatin zymography, ELISA, RT-PCR, immunolocalization, and *in situ* hybridization, has been demonstrated to be elevated in breast cancer and breast cancer-derived cell lines (*see* ref. *33* for review).

The stage-specific expression of gelatinase A protein in breast cancer has been described by Monteagudo et al. *(34)*, using immunolocalization techniques. Although normal tissues showed immunoreactivity restricted to myoepithelial cells of lobules and ducts, increasing progession from benign through *in situ*, invasive, and to metastatic carcinomas showed an increasing degree of tumor-cell-associated staining. Although the frequency of positive tumors did not change with increasing stage, the frequency of positive cells within a lesion did (*in situ* 10%, invasive carcinoma 80%, metastases 100%). This pattern is reminiscent of the clonal dominance model of tumor progression, in which, as a tumor cell population progresses toward metastatic competence, the tumor becomes increasingly populated by metastatically competent cells. Further studies have confirmed the tumor-cell-specific localization of gelatinase A immunostaining. For example, Hoyhtya et al. *(35)* found that gelatinase A staining was predominantly cytoplasmically located in tumor cells, and, in one-third of tumor samples, the localization could be found associated with the tumor cell membrane.

The mRNA *in situ* hybridization pattern of gelatinase A, in contrast to the immunolocalization pattern, has consistently been found to be associated with cells of the stroma *(29,36–40)*. Soini et al. *(38)* describe moderate-to-strong hybridization seen in both fibroblasts and endothelial cells of tumors, but not the tumor cells themselves. Heppner et al. *(29)* report that 100% of cases examined showed stromal gelatinase A mRNA hybridization, which, in contrast to stromelysin-3, displayed a wide, diffuse pattern within the stroma of the tumor.

The immunolocalization and mRNA *in situ* analyses of gelatinase A expression suggest that, although the mRNA for gelatinase A is associated with the stromal elements within a tumor, the protein associates with the tumor cells. This generalization suggested that tumor cells might express a gelatinase receptor, in order to have localized the protein of a stromally synthesized MMP. In vitro studies confirmed this speculation, with the demonstration of a high-affinity binding site for gelatinase A on the surface of breast cancer cells *(41)*.

Gelatinase B has also been studied in breast cancer, although not to the same extent as gelatinase A. It has been localized, like gelatinase A, to the stromal elements of the tumor, including fibroblastic cells, as well as infiltrating inflammatory cells *(42)*, which are a common site of localization for gelatinase B. In addition, Heppner et al. *(29)* reported strong gelatinase B mRNA hybridization associated with the vasculature of breast cancers. In one study, however, gelatinase B mRNA could be localized to the cells of the tumor parenchyma *(38)*. Overall expression of gelatinase B has been correlated with grade of disease; that is, aggressive disease tended to be consistently positive for gelatinase B mRNA and protein *(27)*. The plasma levels of gelatinase B also correlated with the presence of breast cancer, compared to healthy individuals or individuals hospitalized for noncancer-related illness *(43)*.

3.1.3. Membrane-Type Metalloproteinases

The recently described membrane-type subfamily of MMPs is characterized by their localization to the plasma membrane via a transmembrane spanning domain. The substrate specificity of this subfamily of enzymes includes gelatins, but, most important, it seems clear that a major function for the MT-MMPs is to activate other MMPs, including gelatinase A. This interaction will be discussed in Subheading 3.2.2. This has important implications for breast cancer, because, as will be discussed, one major switch in breast cancer progression is the ability of metastatic breast cancer cells to activate gelatinase A, but nonmetastatic breast cancers are unable to do so *(44)*.

The expression of MT-MMP mRNAs in breast cancers is also associated with stromal elements within the tumors *(29,45,46)*. The diffuse pattern of hybridization for MT1-MMP mRNA within the tumor stroma is similar, but not identical, to the pattern observed for gelatinase A *(29,45)*. Polette et al. *(46)* described the induction of MT1-MMP in fibroblasts when they were co-cultured with breast cancer cell lines. The tissue distribution of MT2- and MT3-MMPs indicates that these molecules do not play a significant role in breast cancers *(47)*. MT4-MMP was recently cloned from a cDNA library derived from a breast carcinoma *(48)*. This family member shows expression in a number of tumor cell lines, although the tissue distribution remains to be determined *(49)*. It has recently been demonstrated that the immunohistological localization of MT1-MMP is associated with cells of the tumor parenchyma *(47)*.

3.1.4. Matrilysin

Matrilysin represents an unusual member of the MMP family, because it is the only MMP that seems to be expressed by the cells of the tumor parenchyma, rather than those of the stroma *(29,31)*. In addition, matrilysin transcripts are detected in fibroadenomas, in ductal carcinoma *in situ* specimens, and in apparently normal glandular epithelial cells adjacent to malignant tissue *(26,29,31)*. The tissue distribution and the expression of matrilysin in early lesions represents a clear divergence from the expression of the other MMPs relevant in breast cancer. These differences prompt speculation about the potential role matrilysin might have in very early stages of breast pathogenesis, as opposed to participation in late-stage tumor invasion and metastasis.

3.1.5. Other MMPs

Heppner et al. *(29)* summarized the expression of nine MMPs in a small set of breast cancers, and found that, in general, most of the MMP expression represents a host response to the tumor. Intersitial collagenase and collagenase-3 were both found in a minority of the samples (4 of 13 each). However, although interstitial collagenase was found to be associated with stromal elements, the expression of collagenase-3 was found to be associated with isolated tumor cells. The expression of interstitial collagenase in a minority of cases (9 of 34) has been confirmed by Okada et al. *(45)*. Metalloelastase was also found to be expressed in a subset of cases (5 of 13), and was localized to macrophages and necrotic areas *(29)*.

3.2. Regulation of MMPs in Breast Cancer Cells

Under normal conditions, MMPs are a tightly regulated class of molecules that are rarely detected in adult tissues. Exceptions to this are situations in which adult tissues are undergoing dramatic morphological and functional changes, such as in the cycling and postpartum uterus, during wound healing, and postlactational mammary gland involution *(50,51)*. In addition, since MMPs are produced as zymogens, regulation of their activation and control of their ultimate activity by endogenous MMP inhibitors must be considered in understanding MMP regulation. The following will focus on an understanding of MMP regulation as it pertains to breast cancer.

3.2.1. Regulation of MMP Expression

The control of MMP gene expression has been studied *in vitro* in some detail. Most of the MMP gene 5' promoter sequences contain AP-1 and *ets* binding sites (reviewed in ref. *52*). The presence of such promoter elements make the MMP genes responsive to oncogenic stimuli, such as *ras*, or growth factor signaling, such as EGF, via the upregulation of members of the *fos*, *jun*, and *ets* families of transcription factors. Since the presence of such oncogenic signals is a hallmark of cancer progression, it is not a surprise that MMPs can be described as malignancy-associated genes.

An example of the role of oncogenes in the regulation of MMP expression has been demonstrated by Giunciuglio et al. *(53)*, using MCF-10A cells, a cell line derived from normal mammary epithelium, which were then infected with retroviruses harboring the Ha-*ras* oncogene and/or the *erb*B-2 oncogene. In this study, the doubly transformed cells showed a higher invasive index in the Boyden chamber assay, compared to either of the single transfectants. This increase in invasive index corresponded to an increase in gelatinase A expression, as well as to a decrease in TIMP-2 expression, supporting the hypothesis that it is the balance between MMP and inhibitor expression that determines the phenotype of cancer cells. This work is reminiscent of several studies with breast cancer patients that indicate that the overexpression of gelatinase A *(42,54)*, and, more specifically, a shift in the ratio of gelatinase A: TIMP-2 in their tumors, is associated with a poor outcome *(55)*.

Growth factors appear to influence the expression of MMPs in breast cancer cells. Welch et al. *(56)* found that TGF-β could stimulate the metastatic potential, and both gelatinase A and B expression and activation, in metastatic mammary carcinoma cells. Himmelstein and Muschel *(57)* found that co-culture of human breast cancer cells with rat embryo fibroblasts, or exposure of breast cancer cells to fibroblast-derived conditioned media, led to the induction of gelatinase B expression by the cancer cells. Korczak et al. *(58)* found that metastatic sublines of a murine mammary carcinoma cell line expressed approx 15-fold more stromelysin-1 and threefold less TIMP-1 than the nonmetastatic parental cells. The mechanism regulating stromelysin-1 expression in the metastatic variants was autocrine in nature, since conditioned medium from the metastatic cells, when applied to the nonmetastatic parental cells, was able to induce stromelysin-1 gene expression *(59)*. The authors of this chapter have found a role for growth factor receptors in the regulation of MMP expression in MDA-MB-468 breast cancer cells. These cells, which overexpress the EGF-receptor (EGF-R), also constitutively express matrilysin. Sublines selected for diminished levels of EGF-R expression, through the use of antisense RNA or ligand/toxin fusion protein-mediated selection *(60)*, show a concomitant loss of matrilysin expression, suggesting an intimate dependence of matrilysin expression on EGF-R expression and/or activity (manuscript in preparation).

Studies have also addressed the paracrine influence of breast cancer cells on the stromal expression of MMPs. Ito et al. *(61)* co-cultured the human breast cancer cell lines MCF-7 and BT-20 with dermal fibroblasts, and found that the former cell line was able to induce interstitial collagenase, gelatinase A, stromelysin-1, and TIMP-1 in the fibroblasts, and the latter cell line was able to induce gelatinase A and TIMP-1. Normal mammary epithelial cells in co-culture with fibroblasts were found to induce

TIMP-1 only in the fibroblasts, suggesting that specific signals are sent from the tumor to the stromal cells, as first suggested by Biswas et al. (*30* and refs. therein), and supported by *in situ* localization data (*see* ref. *29*, for example). Further analysis in this system demonstrated that both membrane associated and soluble factors produced by the MCF-7 cells were responsible for the observed response in the fibroblasts (*61*). Similar results have been observed with induction of MT1-MMP in stromal fibroblasts. Polette et al. (*46*) found that MT1-MMP expression could be induced in fibroblasts by conditioned medium derived from MDA-231 cells, but not from MCF-7 cells. This induction was also associated with a concomitant activation of gelatinase A, as will be discussed below.

3.2.2. Regulation of MMP Activity

The MMPs are generally secreted in a zymogen form, and become activated following a conformational change that disrupts the interaction of the unpaired cysteine residue in the pro domain with the catalytic zinc (*62*). Activation of the cysteine switch in vivo is believed to occur primarily by a proteolytic cascade involving serine proteases in particular, although other mechanisms have also been suggested. MMP family members can activate other MMP family members by cleavage of the pro domain, so that a cascade of events can result in enzymatic activities capable of digestion of all components of an ECM. Stromelysin-3 is distinct from the other secreted MMPs, in that it contains a conserved furin recognition sequence, and can be secreted in an activated form following intracellular cleavage by this processing enzyme (*63*). Since this discovery, the MT-MMPs have also been shown to contain this domain, and MT1-MMP can be processed by furin (*48,64*). This observation has interesting implications for the biological consequences of the expression of these specific MMPs in tumors. For example, intracellular activation suggests the potential for a wide range of new substrates available for catalysis. Secretion of active stromelysin-3 suggests the possibility that this enzyme might be responsible for initiating a cascade of events that results in the activation of all available MMPs. This distinct activity may shed light on the observation that stromelysin-3 is an independent prognostic marker (*32*), and therefore presumably an important effector of the malignant phenotype of breast cancers.

Gelatinase A activation also occurs through a mechanism distinct from that of other MMPs. For gelatinase A, activation seems to require the assembly of an activation complex localized at the cell surface that is anchored by a furin-activated (i.e., intracellularly activated) MT-MMP molecule (*8,65*). The latent complex of gelatinase A and TIMP-2, an interaction mediated through the C-terminus of gelatinase A and the N-terminus of TIMP-2 (*66,67*), is thought to be localized to the cell surface by the ability of the C-terminus of TIMP-2 to bind the membrane-localized MT1-MMP (*68*). It is speculated that the association of these three molecules then leads to an additional MT-MMP molecule, subsequently activating the anchored gelatinase A. The assembly of this complex involving TIMP-2 may explain why this molecule, although a metalloproteinase inhibitor, has been observed to be a poor prognostic factor in breast cancers in one study (*39*).

In breast cancer, the activation of gelatinase A has been a focus of much attention. This was first described by Azzam et al. (*44*), who reported that activation of gelatinase A, and not simply its expression, was correlated with disease aggressiveness in a large number of breast cancer cell lines, as indicated by markers such as cellular estrogen receptor negativity and vimentin positivity. Gelatinase A activation is mediated by cellular membranes *(44,54,69)*, and the observation that the activator could be associated with the membrane fraction of cells assisted in identifying MT1-MMP as being involved in gelatinase A activation *(8)*. The activation of gelatinase A by breast cancer cell lines could also be correlated with an epithelial-to-mesenchymal transition; i.e., the cells that showed the ability to activate gelatinase A also displayed characteristics of mesenchymal rather than epithelial cells, including the loss of cytokeratin, estrogen receptor, and E-cadherin expression, and the appearance of vimentin immunoreactivity. These markers are poor prognostic factors in breast cancers. It is intriguing that the constitutive expression of MT1-MMP was also strictly correlated with those cells that had undergone the epithelial-to-mesenchymal transition *(70)*. These data suggest that gelatinase A activation may be a consequence of the expression of a package of genes involved in the epithelial-to-mesenchymal phenotypic transition. These genes might be co-ordinately regulated, possibly by one or only a few molecular master switches, whose oncogenic activation or inactivation might be a crucial step to the determination of malignancy in breast cancers. The regulation of MT-MMP and gelatinase A activation is far from being understood, and remains a very complex and controversial area. For example, the significance of secreted forms of MT1-MMP, the role of MT4-MMP *(48)*, and the interaction with collagen I, which has been reported to influence the activation of gelatinase A *(71)*, are all areas yet to be fully explored and understood.

4. MMPS AS MEDIATORS OF MALIGNANT BEHAVIOR IN BREAST CANCER

4.1. MMPs in Cell Culture Models of Breast Cancer

MMPs have been associated with tumor invasion and metastasis, since the observation that metastatic B16 melanoma cells demonstrate an enhanced type IV collagenase activity, compared to nonmetastatic B16 melanoma cells *(20)*. Similar observations were made by Nakajima et al., who found that type IV collagen and lung subendothelial matrix degradation, and serum and plasma levels of gelatinase B, correlated with the metastatic potential of a series of rat mammary adenocarcinoma cells *(72,73)*. Stromelysin-1 has also been demonstrated to influence the invasive phenotype of breast cancer cells. Cells derived from mammary tumors arising in WAP stromelysin-1 transgenic mice display an enhanced invasive ability in vitro *(74)*. This invasive phenotype could be inhibited through the use of an MMP-specific inhibitor GM6001, but not inhibitors of other protease classes, and antisense oligodeoxynucleotides against stromelysin-1, but not collagenase-3 or stromelysin-3, were found to mimic the effect of the MMP inhibitor.

The overexpression of TIMPs in cultured cells also provides evidence for a role for MMPs in mammary tumor progression. A study by Wang et al. *(75)* describes transfection of the recently identified TIMP-4 into human MDA-MB-435 breast carcinoma cells. Overexpression of TIMP-4 reduced in vitro invasiveness, using the Boyden chamber assay, and in vivo metastasis to lymph nodes and lungs in nude mice. Overexpression of TIMP-4 also negatively influenced the growth of MDA-MB-435 cells, as well as angiogenesis, when assayed by histological microvessel counts.

There is growing evidence for a role for MMPs in early stages of tumor formation. The overexpression of stromelysin-3 by gene transfection in human MCF-7 breast cancer cells resulted in an enhancement in tumor growth, and, more specifically, tumor take, in immunodeficient mice *(76)*. In addition, stromelysin-3 expression was reduced by antisense RNA technology in NIH3T3 cells that endogenously expressed stromelysin-3, reducing the tumorigeniticy of these cells. In both cases, the effect was an alteration in the tumor take, and not in the growth rate of the tumor cells.

4.2. MMPs in In Vivo Models of Breast Cancer

An early clue that MMPs were a functional component of the mammary gland was the observation that type IV collagenase activity was upregulated in the involuting mammary gland, and possibly was responsible for the removal of BM in this process *(77)*. With the mouse as the model, a great deal has been learned about the role of MMPs in mammary gland biology. In addition, advances have been made in the area of in vivo models of breast cancer, with the development of tissue-specific promoters that target the expression of oncogenes to the mammary gland.

4.2.1. MMPs in Mammary Gland Biology

The pioneering work by Bissell et al. *(78)* has demonstrated that the ECM contains cues important for the differentiated function of mammary epithelial cells. Given the importance of the ECM to mammary gland function, it follows that remodeling of the ECM carries with it equal importance. Talhouk et al. *(79)* have described the role of MMPs in the function of the normal mammary gland, and how the expression of MMPs alters the cellular interaction with the BM, which consequently has effects on cellular function. Mammary epithelial cells produce a wide range of enzymatic activities, including both gelatinolytic and caseinolytic metalloproteinases. The activity of these enzymes is lowest during lactation and highest during glandular involution when matrix is degraded and differentiated function ceases, and the gelatinolytic activity was secreted toward the basal lamina in reconstituted glands in vitro. The expression of MMPs and their inhibitors was inversely related, and tightly associated with the differentiated state of the gland, as measured by β-casein expression. In particular, when the level of TIMP-1 in the mammary gland was elevated through the use of slow release pellets, the high-level casein expression was prolonged, and alveolar regression was delayed, supporting the contention that MMPs and their inhibitors were responsible for controlling involution and differentiated function in the mammary gland *(80)*.

MMPs were also considered likely effectors of the development and branching morphogenesis of the mammary gland. Witty et al. *(81)* found that stromelysin-1, stromelysin-3, and gelatinase A all were expressed in the developing gland, and stromelysin-1 in particular was associated with stromal fibroblasts in the elongating ducts. It is unlikely, however, that this enzyme is determining the sites of branch points as a result of its matrix-degrading activity, because stromelysin-1 expression was distributed in cleft structures, and not in end buds, and appeared to be associated with a reparative process, rather than active clearing of pathways for ductal advancement. These same enzymes are expressed in the mammary gland during early pregnancy, and are localized by *in situ* hybridization to the stromal components surrounding the developing alveoli of the pregnant mammary gland *(81,82)*.

4.2.2. MMP Transgenic Mice

The generation of transgenic mice expressing MMPs, under the control of mammary-specific promoters, has been useful in the evaluation of the roles of MMPs in mammary gland function. Both the mouse mammary tumor virus long-terminal repeat (MMTV-LTR) and the whey acidic protein (WAP) promoters have been used to target expression of an activated form of stromelysin-1 to the mammary gland, and MMTV-matrilysin mice have also been generated and characterized. The differences in the regulation of these promoters, with the MMTV-promoter being regulated by hormones that appear at the time of puberty, and the WAP promoter responsive to lactational hormones, has resulted in some differences in the phenotypic presentation of these mice with respect to normal mammary gland form, function, and tumorigenesis.

4.2.2.1. MAMMARY GLAND DIFFERENTIATION AND DEVELOPMENT

The MMTV-stromelysin-1 transgenic mice generated by Witty et al. *(81)* expressed a phenotype referred to as "inappropriate alveolar development". At 13 wk, the glands of virgin female transgenic mice were composed of approximately twice the number of cells, compared to their nontransgenic controls, and had the morphological features of a 10-d pregnant animal. This increase in the number of cells was also associated with an increase in the frequency of cells undergoing DNA synthesis, as measured by Bromo-deoxyuridine incorporation, suggesting that expression of stromelysin-1 and the alterations in morphogenesis seen in these transgenic mice might be related to increases in cellular proliferation. Expression of β-casein mRNA was also noted in the glands of virgin transgenic mice overexpressing stromelysin-1, indicating that expression of this gene also had an influence on cellular differentiation. Degradation of matrix components was evident by the replacement of obvious basal lamina structures with an amorphous material, as visualized by electron microscopy.

Using the WAP promoter to direct stromelysin-1 gene expression to the mammary gland, Sympson et al. *(82)* observed a strikingly similar phenotype to that of Witty et al. *(81)*. Specifically, there was an enhancement of lateral branching, in addition to alveolar abnormalities. Expression of β-casein was also observed in virgin glands of transgenic mice, emphasizing the important relationship between ECM, protease action, and cellular differentiation. During lactation, transgene expression was high, and was accompanied by alterations in BM integrity, as well as modifications in the morphology of alveoli, characterized by a reduction in size. In both pregnant and lactating glands, the expression of milk proteins was reduced, supporting the contention that cellular interaction with the ECM and BM influence the differentiated function of mammary epithelial cells. The use of the WAP-stromelysin-1 transgenic mice has further demonstrated that the reduction in gland size and cell number during lactation is through an apoptotic mechanism involving the loss of cell/ECM contact mediated through β_1 integrins *(83)*. This was further supported through the use of TIMP-1 transgenic mice, in that the introduction of the TIMP-1 transgene into WAP-stromelysin-1 mice rescued the mammary epithelial cells from apoptosis *(84)*. Effects of stromelysin-1 expression on mammary epithelial cell apoptosis were also observed in the MMTV-stromelysin-1 mice *(85)*.

It is difficult to reconcile the observations that stromelysin-1 expression results in an increase in mammary epithelial cell proliferation, differentiation, and death, since these appear to be opposing activities. Perhaps the most palatable view of this complexity lies in the realization that the BM and ECM contains information vital to the identity and activity of the cell. Signals to grow, die, or differentiate come from the external environment, and the cell is influenced by the interface with this environment through its association with structural proteins. Thus, hormonal instructions can be perceived in a different context if normal cell–cell and cell–matrix interactions are disrupted. Further analysis of the action of MMPs in the developing mammary gland provide exceptional opportunities to understand the contributions of matrix and matrix degradation to the control of basic cellular processes such as proliferation, differentiation, and apoptosis.

4.2.2.2. TUMORIGENESIS

Using the MMTV-stromelysin-1 mice, Witty et al. *(85)* examined chemically induced mammary tumor formation in these animals. It was discovered that these animals showed a decreased tendency to form DMBA-induced mammary tumors. Approximately 65% of wild-type animals developed tumors, but stromelysin-1 transgenic animals developed tumors in 35% of mice. This reduction in tumor incidence was paralleled by a delay in the time to tumor onset. However, there seemed to be no significant effect of stromelysin-1 expression on tumor formation in mice that contained both the stromelysin-1 transgene and the MMTV-driven TGF-α transgene. These results suggested that the growth effect of TGF-α eliminated the inhibitory effect of stromelysin-1 on DMBA-induced mammary tumorigenesis. An evaluation of transgenic mammary glands at the time of DMBA administration revealed a 1.6-fold increase in the proliferative index of stromelysin-1-expressing mammary glands, compared to wild-type controls, and a 4-fold increase in the apoptotic index, as determined by using terminal deoxytransferase labeling techniques. These results suggested that the ectopic expression of stromelysin-1 increased the turnover rate of the mammary epithelial cells targeted by the chemical carcinogen, resulting in an elimination of a higher percentage of mutated cells through an apoptotic mechanism. The negating effect of the TGF-α transgene is apparently caused by a normalization of the ratio of proliferation:apoptosis in the bigenic mice. The results obtained by these studies are therefore likely to be influenced by the tumor induction protocol used, and appears to reflect an effect of stromelysin-1 on target cell populations, rather than an effect on cells that have already initiated tumorigenic events.

Positive effects of stromelysin-1 on mammary tumor formation have been revealed in preliminary reports that the WAP-stromelysin-1 transgenic mice develop spontaneous mammary adenocarcinomas *(86–88)*. These mammary tumors, which have been observed in four independent lines of transgenic mice, all display reactive stromas and phenotypic abnormalities ranging from severe hyperplasia to adenocarcinomas. Tumor formation has been observed in virgin animals as young as 4 mo, suggesting that extensive hormonal fluctuations are not required for tumorigenesis.

Matrilysin has recently been targeted to the mammary gland in vivo, under the control of the MMTV-LTR. Although no obvious morphological consequences of matrilysin expression were observed in the development of the mammary gland, there was an enhancement of tumor formation when these animals were crossed with MMTV-*neu* animals. This enhancement displayed itself as a decreased time to tumor formation, and as a reduced frequency of disease-free animals over time, but involved no obvious differences in growth or apoptosis rates. In addition, older MMTV-matrilysin animals were observed to spontaneously develop hyperplastic alveolar nodules (HANs), but older wild-type animals did not *(89)*. It has also been recently demonstrated that extinction of matrilysin expression, through the use of knock-out technology, leads to an approx 50% decrease in the formation of intestinal adenomas in *min* mice *(23)*. This observation suggests that matrilysin expression is important to the formation and growth of early intestinal lesions. Experiments involving matrilysin overexpression in the mammary glands of mice leads to a similar conclusion.

5. MMPS AS THERAPEUTIC TARGETS FOR BREAST CANCER

The evidence presented so far suggests that MMPs are candidate players in the pathogenesis of breast cancer, not only at the level of invasion and metastasis, but also at earlier stages of tumor progression. This makes MMPs attractive targets for breast cancer therapies. As was discussed in Subheading 4.1., TIMPs are able to retard the invasive and growth potential of mammary tumors in vivo *(75)*. Sledge et al. *(90)*, using the synthetic MMP inhibitor BB-94, have also demonstrated that MMP inhibition can influence the growth and metastasis of breast tumors, and, in this case, the regrowth of breast tumors after surgical resection. Inhibition of mammary tumor metastasis has also been observed utilizing the same MMP inhibitor, and the effect appeared to be at the level of metastasis outgrowth *(91)*. In an experimental model of breast cancer bone metastasis, TIMP-2 alone, or in combination with an inhibitor of bone resorption, resulted in a decrease of radiologically detectable bone lesions *(92)*. In studies involving other tumor systems, there also seems to be a connection between MMP inhibition and tumor growth *(22–24)*, which may be through the inhibition of tumor angiogenesis *(93)*. If so, this would be particularly exciting in light of the results from Weidner et al. *(94)*, in which tumor angiogenesis was strongly predictive for recurrence in women presenting with node-negative breast cancer. As clinical trials with synthetic MMP inhibitors continue, there is optimism that the low toxicities and biological effects of these compounds will prove attractive for the treatment, and perhaps even the prevention, of breast malignancies. Additional discussions of this topic can be found in Chapter 20.

6. SUMMARY AND KEY UNANSWERED QUESTIONS

This chapter has made an attempt to describe the role of MMPs as mediators of the malignant phenotype, with specific emphasis on breast cancer. Breast cancers express a variety of MMPs, and, in several cases, expression correlates with stage and grade of disease. Preclinical studies support a causal role for MMPs in several stages of tumor progression. There are, however, a number of areas in which questions remain unanswered.

One area requiring further investigation is the tissue localization pattern of MMP expression. MMP mRNA tends to be expressed in cells within the stroma of cancers, but in only a few instances has tumor-cell-associated expression been demonstrated. It is possible that these results are influenced by limitations in the specificity and/or sensitivity of the techniques currently employed. In addition, the information ultimately required is the localization of active forms of MMP family members, a task that requires the generation of reagents not currently available. These studies, and careful genetic manipulation of stromal and tumor MMPs in animal-model systems, are required to understand the contribution of host and tumor MMPs to various stages of mammary tumor progression.

Another key area of investigation is the mechanism by which MMP expression alters the phenotype of cancer cells. It has been widely thought that MMP expression by tumor cells would enhance the invasive and metastatic capacity of cancer cells, by virtue of its ability to degrade BM and ECM components. However, recent experimental evidence suggests that MMPs may also act to modulate the growth of primary tumors and metastatic foci. The mechanism underlying this phenomenon is poorly understood, although several hypotheses are conceivable. For instance, potential substrates for MMPs could affect the activity of growth factors and cytokines, which in turn enhance tumorigenicity. These potentially novel functions for MMPs could enhance understanding of the malignant behavior of cancers, and provide new therapeutic approaches to the prevention and treatment of breast cancer.

ACKNOWLEDGMENTS

L. M. M.'s laboratory is supported by funds from the National Institutes of Health (R01-CA 60867 and R01-CA 46843) and the D.O.D. (DAMD17-94-J-4226). J. R. M. is supported by a fellowship from the Susan G. Komen Breast Cancer Foundation.

REFERENCES

1. Birkedal-Hansen, H. 1995. Proteolytic remodeling of extracellular matrix. *Curr. Opin. Cell Biol.* **7**: 728–735.
2. Levi, E., R. Fridman, H. Miao, Y. Ma, A. Yayon, I. Vlodavsky, H. Q. Miao, Y. S. Ma. 1996. Matrix metalloproteinase 2 releases active soluble ectodomain of fibroblast growth factor receptor 1. *Proc. Natl. Acad. Sci. USA* **93**: 7069–7074.
3. Gearing, A. J. H., P. Beckett, M. Christodoulou, M. Churchill, J. M. Clements, M. Crimmin, A. H. Davidson, A. H. Drummond, W. A. Galloway, R. Gilbert, et al. 1995. Matrix metalloproteinases and processing of pro-TNF-Alpha. *J. Leukocyte Biol.* **57**: 774–777.
4. Belaaouaj, A., J. M. Shipley, D. K. Kobayashi, D. B. Zimonjic, N. Popescu, G. A. Silverman, S. D. Shapiro. 1995. Human macrophage metalloelastase. Genomic organization, chromosomal location, gene linkage, and tissue-specific expression. *J. Biol. Chem.* **270**: 14,568–14,575.
5. Dong, Z., R. Kumar, X. Yang, I. J. Fidler. 1997. Macrophage-derived metalloelastase is responsible for the generation of angiostatin in Lewis lung carcinoma. *Cell* **88**: 801–810.
6. Chandler, S., J. Cossins, J. Lury, G. Wells. 1996. Macrophage metalloelastase degrades matrix and myelin proteins and processes a tumor necrosis factor-alpha fusion protein. *Biochem. Biophys. Res. Commun.* **228**: 421–429.
7. Murphy, G., J.-P. Segain, M. O'Shea, M. Cockett, C. Ioannou, O. Lefebvre, P. Chambon, P. Basset. 1993. The 28-kDa N-terminal domain of mouse stromelysin-3 has the general properties of a weak metalloproteinase. *J. Biol. Chem.* **268**: 15,435–15,441.
8. Sato, H., T. Takino, Y. Okada, J. Cao, A. Shinagawa, E. Yamamoto, M. Seiki. 1994. A matrix metalloproteinase expressed on the surface of invasive tumour cells. *Nature* **370**: 61–64.
9. Imai, K., E. Ohuchi, T. Aoki, H. Nomura, Y. Fujii, H. Sato, M. Seiki, Y. Okada. 1996. Membrane-type matrix metalloproteinase 1 is a gelatinolytic enzyme and is secreted in a complex with tissue inhibitor of metalloproteinase 2. *Cancer Res.* **56**: 2707–2710.

10. Ohuchi, E., K. Imai, Y. Fujii, H. Sato, M. Seiki, Y. Okada. 1997. Membrane type I matrix metalloproteinase digests interstitial collagens and other extracellular matrix macromolecules. *J. Biol. Chem.* **272**: 2446–2451.

11. Stowlow, M. A., D. D. Bauzon, J. Li, T. Sedgwick, V. C. Liang, Q. A. Sang, Y. B. Shi. 1996. Identification and characterization of a novel collagenase in Xenopus laevis: possible roles during frog development. *Mol. Biol. Cell* **7**: 1471–1483.

12. Pendas, A. M., V. Knauper, X. S. Puente, E. Llano, M. G. Mattei, S. Apte, G. Murphy, C. Lopez-Otin. 1997. Identification and characterization of a novel human matrix metalloproteinase with unique structural characteristics, chromosomal location and tissue distribution. *J. Biol. Chem.* **272**: 4281–4286.

13. Cossins, J., T. J. Dudgeon, G. Catlin, A. J. H. Gearing, J. M. Clements. 1996. Indentification of MMP-18, a putative novel human matrix metalloproteinase. *Biochem. Biophys. Res. Commun.* **228**: 494–498.

14. Bartlett, J. D., J. P. Simmer, J. Xue, H. C. Margolis, E. C. Moreno. 1996. Molecular cloning and mRNA tissue distribution of a novel matrix metalloproteinase isolated from porcine enamel organ. *Gene* **183**: 123–128.

15. Powell, W. C., L. M. Matrisian. 1996. Complex roles of matrix metalloproteinases in tumor progression, in *Attempts to Understand Metastasis Formation I: Metastasis-Related Molecules* (Gunthert, U. and W. Birchmeier, eds.), Springer-Verlag, Berlin, pp. 1–21.

16. Denhardt, D. T., B. Feng, D. R. Edwards, E. T. Cocuzzi, U. M. Malyankar. 1993. Tissue inhibitor of metalloproteinases (TIMP, aka EPA): Structure, control of expression and biological functions. *Pharmacol. Ther.* **59**: 329–341.

17. Yu, M., H. Sato, M. Seiki, E. W. Thompson. 1995. Complex regulation of membrane-type matrix metalloproteinase expression and matrix metalloproteinase-2 activation by concanavalin A in MDA-MB-231 human breast cancer cells. *Cancer Res.* **55**: 3272–3277.

18. MacDougall, J. R., L. M. Matrisian. 1995. Contributions of tumor and stromal matrix metalloproteinases to tumor progression, invasion and metastasis. *Cancer Metastasis Rev.* **14**: 351–362.

19. Vlodavsky, I., G. Korner, R. Ishai-Michaeli, P. Bashkin, R. Bar-Shavit, Z. Fuks. 1990. Extracellular matrix-resident growth factors and enzymes: possible involvement in tumor metastasis and angiogenesis. *Cancer Metastasis Rev.* **9**: 203–226.

20. Liotta, L. A., K. Tryggvason, S. Garbisa, I. Hart, C. M. Foltz, S. Shafie. 1980. Metastatic potential correlates with enzymatic degradation of basement membrane collagen. *Nature* **284**: 67–68.

21. Stetler-Stevenson, W. G., R. Hewitt, M. Corcoran. 1996. Matrix metalloproteinases and tumor invasion: from correlation and causality to the clinic. *Semin. Cancer Biol.* **7**: 147–154.

22. Koop, S., R. Khokha, E. E. Schmidt, I. C. MacDonald, V. L. Morris, A. F. Chambers, A. C. Groom. 1994. Overexpression of metalloproteinase inhibitor in B16F10 cells does not affect extravasation but reduces tumor growth. *Cancer Res.* **54**: 4791–4797.

23. Wilson, C. L., K. J. Heppner, P. A. Labosky, B. L. M. Hogan, L. M. Matrisian. 1997. Intestinal tumorigenesis is suppressed in mice lacking the metalloproteinase matrilysin. *Proc. Natl. Acad. Sci. USA* **94**: 1402–1407.

24. Chambers, A. F., L. M. Matrisian. 1997. Changing views of the role of matrix metalloproteinases in metastasis. *J. Natl. Cancer Inst.* **89**: 1260–1270.

25. Wilson, C. L., L. M. Matrisian. 1996. Matrilysin: An epithelial matrix metalloproteinase with potentially novel functions. *Int. J. Biochem. Cell. Biol.* **28**: 123–136.

26. Basset, P., J. P. Bellocq, C. Wolf, I. Stoll, P. Hutin, J. M. Limacher, O. L. Podhajcer, M. P. Chenard, M. C. Rio, P. Chambon. 1990. A novel metalloproteinase gene specifically expressed in stromal cells of breast carcinomas. *Nature* **348**: 699–704.

27. Kossakowska, A. E., S. A. Huchcroft, S. J. Urbanski, D. R. Edwards. 1996. Comparative analysis of the expression patterns of metalloproteinases and their inhibitors in breast neo-

plasia, sporadic colorectal neoplasia, pulmonary carcinomas and malignant non-Hodgkin's lymphomas in humans. *Br. J. Cancer* **73:** 1401–1408.

28. Hahnel, E., J. M. Harvey, R. Joyce, P. D. Robbins, G. F. Sterrett, R. Hahnel. 1993. Stromelysin-3 expression in breast cancer biopsies: Clinico-pathological correlations. *Int. J. Cancer* **55:** 771–774.

29. Heppner, K. J., L. M. Matrisian, R. A. Jensen, W. H. Rodgers. 1996. Expression of most matrix metalloproteinase family members in breast cancer represents a tumor-induced host response. *Am. J. Pathol.* **149:** 273–282.

30. Kataoka, H., R. DeCastro, S. Zucker, C. Biswas. 1993. Tumor cell-derived collagenase-stimulatory factor increases expression of interstitial collagenase, stromelysin, and 72-kDa gelatinase. *Cancer Res.* **53:** 3154–3158.

31. Wolf, C., N. Rouyer, Y. Lutz, C. Adida, M. Loriot, J.-P. Bellocq, P. Chambon, P. Basset. 1993. Stromelysin 3 belongs to a subgroup of proteinases expressed in breast carcinoma fibroblastic cells and possibly implicated in tumor progression. *Proc. Natl. Acad. Sci. USA* **90:** 1843–1847.

32. Engel, G., K. Heselmeyer, G. Auer, M. Bäckdahl, E. Eriksson, S. Linder. 1994. Correlation between stromelysin-3 mRNA level and outcome of human breast cancer. *Int. J. Cancer* **58:** 830–835.

33. Tryggvason, K., M. Höyhtyä, C. Pyke. 1993. Type IV collagenases in invasive tumors. *Breast Cancer Res. Treatment* **24:** 209–218.

34. Monteagudo, C., M. J. Merino, J. San-Juan, L. A. Liotta, W. G. Stetler-Stevenson. 1990. Immunohistochemical distribution of type IV collagenase in normal, benign, and malignant breast tissue. *Am. J. Pathol.* **136:** 585–592.

35. Höyhtyä, M., R. Fridman, D. Komarek, K. Porter-Jordan, W. G. Stetler-Stevenson, L. A. Liotta, C.-M. Liang. 1994. Immunohistochemical localization of matrix metalloproteinase 2 and its specific inhibitor TIMP-2 in neoplastic tissues with monoclonal antibodies. *Int. J. Cancer* **56:** 500–505.

36. Daidone, M. G., R. Silvestrini, A. D'Errico, G. Di Fronzo, E. Benini, A. M. Mancini, S. Garbisa, L. A. Liotta, W. F. Grigioni. 1991. Laminin receptors, collagenase IV and prognosis in node-negative breast cancers. *Int. J. Cancer* **48:** 529–532.

37. Poulsom, R., A. M. Hanby, M. Pignatelli, R. E. Jeffery, J. M. Longcroft, L. Rogers, G. W. H. Stamp. 1993. Expression of gelatinase A and TIMP-2 mRNAs in desmoplastic fibroblasts in both mammary carcinomas and basal cell carcinomas of the skin. *J. Clin. Pathol.* **46:** 429–436.

38. Soini, Y., T. Hurskainen, M. Höyhtyä, A. Oikarinen, H. Autio-Harmainen. 1994. 72 KD and 92 KD type IV collagenase, type IV collagen, and laminin mRNAs in breast cancer: a study by in situ hybridization. *J. Histochem. Cytochem.* **42:** 945–951.

39. Visscher, D. W., M. Höyhtyä, S. K. Ottosen, C.-M. Liang, F. H. Sarkar, J. D. Crissman, R. Fridman. 1994. Enhanced expression of tissue inhibitor of metalloproteinase-2 (TIMP-2) in the stroma of breast carcinomas correlates with tumor recurrence. *Int. J. Cancer* **59:** 339–344.

40. Iwata, H., S. Kobayashi, H. Iwase, A. Masaoka, N. Fujimoto, Y. Okada. 1996. Production of matrix metalloproteinases and tissue inhibitors of metalloproteinases in human breast carcinomas. *Jpn. J. Cancer Res.* **87:** 602–611.

41. Emonard, H. P., A. G. Remacle, A. C. No'l, J.-A. Grimaud, W. G. Stetler-Stevenson, J.-M. Foidart. 1992. Tumor cell surface-associated binding site for the M_r 72,000 type IV collagenase. *Cancer Res.* **52:** 5845–5848.

42. Davies, B., D. W. Miles, L. C. Happerfield, M. S. Naylor, L. G. Bobrow, R. D. Rubens, F. R. Balkwill. 1993. Activity of type IV collagenases in benign and malignant breast disease. *Br. J. Cancer* **67:** 1126–1131.

43. Zucker, S., R. M. Lysik, M. H. Zarrabi, U. Moll. 1993. M_r 92,000 type IV collagenase is increased in plasma of patients with colon cancer and breast cancer. *Cancer Res.* **53:** 140–146.

44. Azzam, H. S., G. A. Arand, M. E. Lippman, E. W. Thompson. 1993. Association of MMP-2 activation potential with metastatic progression in human breast cancer cell lines independent of MMP-2 production. *J. Natl. Cancer Inst.* **85:** 1758–1764.

45. Okada, A., J. Bellocq, M. Chenard, M. Rio, P. Chambon, P. Basset. 1995. Membrane-type matrix metalloproteinase (MT-MMP) gene is expressed in stromal cells of human colon, breast and head and neck carcinomas. *Proc. Natl. Acad. Sci. USA* **92:** 2730–2734.

46. Polette, M., C. Gilles, V. Marchand, M. Seiki, J. M. Tournier, P. Birembaut. 1997. Induction of membrane-type matrix metalloproteinase 1 (MT1-MMP) expression in human fibroblasts by breast adenocarcinoma cells. *Clin. Exp. Metastasis* **15:** 157–163.

47. Ueno, H., H. Nakamura, M. Inoue, K. Imai, M. Noguchi, H. Sato, M. Seiki, Y. Okada. 1997. Expression and tissue localization of membrane-types 1,2, and 3 matrix metalloproteinases in human invasive breast carcinomas. *Cancer Res.* **57:** 2055–2060.

48. Puente, X. S., A. M. Pendas, E. Llano, G. Velasco, C. Lopez-Otin. 1996. Molcular cloning of a novel membrane-type matrix metalloproteinase from a human breast carcinoma. *Cancer Res.* **56:** 944–949.

49. Gilles, C., M. Polette, M. Seiki, P. Birembaut, E. W. Thompson. 1997. Implication of collagen type 1-induced membrane-type 1 matrix metalloproteinase expression and matrix metalloproteinase-2 activation in the metastatic progression of breast carcinoma. *Lab. Invest.* **76:** 651–660.

50. Hulboy, D. L., L. A. Rudolph, L. M. Matrisian. 1996. Matrix metalloprotienases as mediators of reproductive function. *Mol. Hum. Reprod.* **3:** 27–45.

51. Sinclair, R. D., T. J. Ryan. 1997. Proteolytic enzymes in wound healing: the role of enzymatic debridement. *Australasian J. Dermatol.* **35:** 35–41.

52. Crawford, H. C., L. M. Matrisian. 1996. Mechanisms controlling the transcription of matrix metalloproteinase genes in normal and neoplastic cells. *Enzyme Protein* **49:** 20–37.

53. Giunciuglio, D., M. Culty, G. Fassina, L. Masiello, A. Melchiori, G. Paglialunga, G. Arand, F. Ciardiello, F. Basolo, E. W. Thompson, et al. 1995. Invasive phenotype of MCF10A cells overexpressing c-Ha-ras and c-erbB-2 oncogenes. *Int. J. Cancer* **63:** 815–822.

54. Brown, P. D., R. E. Bloxidge, E. Anderson, A. Howell. 1993. Expression of activated gelatinase in human invasive breast carcinoma. *Clin. Exp. Metastasis* **11:** 183–189.

55. Onisto, M., M. P. Riccio, P. Scannapieco, C. Caenazzo, L. Griggio, M. Spina, W. G. Stetler-Stevenson, S. Garbisa. 1995. Gelatinase A/TIMP-2 imbalance in lymph-node-positive breast carcinomas, as measured by RT-PCR. *Int. J. Cancer* **63:** 621–626.

56. Welch, D. R., Á. Fabra, M. Nakajima. 1990. Transforming growth factor § stimulates mammary adenocarcinoma cell invasion and metastatic potential. *Proc. Natl. Acad. Sci. USA* **87:** 7678–7682.

57. Himelstein, B. P., R. J. Muschel. 1996. Induction of matrix metalloproteinase 9 expression in breast carcinoma cells by a soluble factor from fibroblasts. *Clin. Exp. Metastasis* **14:** 197–208.

58. Korczak, B., R. S. Kerbel, J. W. Dennis. 1991. Constitutive expression and secretion of proteases in non-metastatic SP1 mammary carcinoma cells and its metastatic sublines. *Int. J. Cancer* **48:** 557–561.

59. Korczak, B., R. S. Kerbel, J. W. Dennis. 1991. Autocrine and paracrine regulation of tissue inhibitor of metalloproteinases, transin, and urokinase gene expression in metastatic and nonmetastatic mammary carcinoma cells. *Cell Growth Differ.* **2:** 335–341.

60. Dixit, M., J. L. Yang, M. C. Poirier, J. O. Price, P. A. Andrews, C. L. Arteaga. 1997. Abrogation of cisplatin-induced programmed cell death in human breast cancer cells by epidermial growth factor antisense RNA. *J. Natl. Cancer Inst.* **89:** 365–373.

61. Ito, A., S. Nakajima, Y. Sasaguri, H. Nagase, Y. Mori. 1995. Co-culture of human breast adenocarcinoma MCF-7 cells and human dermal fibroblasts enhances the production of matrix metalloproteinases 1, 2 and 3 in fibroblasts. *Br. J. Cancer* **71:** 1039–1045.

62. Van Wart, H. E., H. Birkedal-Hansen. 1990. The cysteine switch: A principle of regulation of metalloproteinase activity with potential applicability to the entire matrix metalloproteinase gene family. *Proc. Natl. Acad. Sci. USA* **87:** 5578–5582.

63. Pei, D., S. J. Weiss. 1995. Furin-dependent intracellular activation of the human stromelysin-3 zymogen. *Nature* **375:** 244–247.

64. Sato, H., T. Kinoshita, T. Takino, K. Nakayama, M. Seiki. 1996. Activation of a recombinant membrane type 1-matrix metalloproteinase (MT1-MMP) by furin and its interaction with tissue inhibitor of metalloproteinases (TIMP)-2. *FEBS Lett.* **393:** 101–104.

65. Kolkenbrock, H., A. Heckerkia, D. Orgel, N. Ulbrich, H. Will. 1997. Activation of progelatinase A and progelatinase A TIMP-2 complex by membrane type 2 matrix metalloproteinase. *Biol. Chem.* **378:** 71–76.

66. Kolkenbrock, H., D. Orgel, A. Hecker-Kia, W. Noack, N. Ulbrich. 1991. The complex between a tissue inhibitor of metalloproteinases (TIMP-2) and 72-kDa progelatinase is a metalloproteinase inhibitor. *Eur. J. Biochem.* **198:** 775–781.

67. Goldberg, G., B. Marmer, G. Gregory, A. Eisen, S. Wilhelm, C. He. 1989. Human 72-kilodalton type IV collagenase forms a complex with a tissue inhibitor of metalloproteinases designated TIMP-2. *Proc. Natl. Acad. Sci. USA* **86:** 8207–8211.

68. Strongin, A. Y., I. E. Collier, G. Bannikov, B. L. Marmer, G. A. Grant, G. I. Goldberg. 1995. Mechanism of cell surface activation of 72-kDa type IV collagenase. Isolation of the activated form of the membrane metalloprotease. *J. Biol. Chem.* **270:** 5331–5338.

69. Brown, P. D., R. E. Bloxidge, N. S. A. Stuart, K. C. Gatter, J. Carmichael. 1993. Association between expression of activated 72-kilodalton gelatinase and tumor spread in non-small-cell lung carcinoma. *J. Natl. Cancer Inst.* **85:** 574–578.

70. Pulyaeva, H., J. Bueno, M. Polette, P. Birembaut, H. Sato, M. Seiki, E. W. Thompson. 1997. MT1-MMP correlates with MMP-2 activation potential seen after epithelial to mesenchymal transition in human breast carcinoma cells. *Clin. Exp. Metastasis* **15:** 111–120.

71. Thompson, E. W., M. Yu, J. Bueno, L. Jin, S. N. Maiti, F. L. Palao-Marco, H. Pulyaeva, J. W. Tamborlane, R. Tirgari, I. Wapnir, et al. 1994. Collagen induced MMP-2 activation in human breast cancer. *Breast Cancer Res. Treatment* **31:** 357–370.

72. Nakajima, M., D. R. Welch, P. N. Belloni, G. L. Nicolson. 1987. Degredation of basement membrane type IV collagen and lug subendothelial matrix by rat mammary adenocarcinoma cell clones of differing metastatic potentials. *Cancer Res.* **47:** 4869–4876.

73. Nakajima, M., D. R. Welch, D. M. Wynn, T. Tsuruo, G. L. Nicolson. 1993. Serum and plasma M_r 92,000 progelatinase levels correlate with spontaneous metastasis of rat 13762NF mammary adenocarcinoma. *Cancer Res.* **53:** 5802–5807.

74. Lochter, A., A. Srebrow, C. J. Sympson, N. Terracio, Z. Werb, M. J. Bissell. 1997. Misregulation of stromelysin-1 expression in mouse mammary tumor cells accompanies acquisition of stromelysin-1-dependent invasive properties. *J. Biol. Chem.* **272:** 5007–5015.

75. Wang, M., Y. E. Liu, J. Greene, S. Sheng, A. Fuchs, E. M. Rosen, Y. E. Shi. 1997. Inhibition of tumor growth and metastasis of human breast cancer cells transfected with tissue inhibitor of metalloproteinase 4. *Oncogene* **14:** 2767–2774.

76. Noel, A. C., O. Lefebvre, E. Maquoi, L. Van Hoorde, M. P. Chenard, M. Mareel, J. M. Foidart, P. Basset, M. C. Rio, L. Vanhoorde. 1996. Stromelysin-3 expression promotes tumor take in nude mice. *J. Clin. Invest.* **97:** 1924–1930.

77. Martinez-Hernandez, A., L. M. Fink, G. B. Pierce. 1976. Removal of basement membrane in the involuting breast. *Lab. Invest.* **31:** 455–462.

78. Lin, C. Q., M. J. Bissell. 1993. Multi-faceted regulation of cell differentiation by extracellular matrix. *FASEB J.* **7:** 737–743.

79. Talhouk, R. S., J. R. Chin, E. N. Unemori, Z. Werb, M. J. Bissell. 1991. Proteinases of the mammary gland: developmental regulation in vivo and vectorial secretion in culture. *Development* **112:** 439–449.

80. Talhouk, R. S., M. J. Bissell, Z. Werb. 1992. Coordinated expression of extracellular matrix-degrading proteinases and their inhibitors regulates mammary epithelial function during involution. *J. Cell Biol.* **118:** 1271–1282.

81. Witty, J. P., J. Wright, L. M. Matrisian. 1995. Matrix metalloproteinases are expressed during ductal and alveolar mammary morphogenesis, and misregulation of stromelysin-1 in transgenic mice induces unscheduled alveolar development. *Mol. Biol. Cell* **6:** 1287–1303.

82. Sympson, C. J., R. S. Talhouk, C. M. Alexander, J. R. Chin, S. M. Clift, M. J. Bissell, Z. Werb. 1994. Targeted expression of stromelysin-1 in mammary gland provides evidence for a role of proteinases in branching morphogenesis and the requirement for an intact basement membrane for tissue-specific gene expression. *J. Cell Biol.* **125:** 681–693.

83. Boudreau, N., C. J. Sympson, Z. Werb, M. J. Bissell. 1995. Suppression of ICE and apoptosis in mammary epithelial cells by extracellular matrix. *Science* **267:** 891–893.

84. Alexander, C. M., E. W. Howard, M. J. Bissell, Z. Werb. 1996. Rescue of mammary epithelial cell apoptosis and entactin degradation by a tissue inhibitor of metalloproteinase-1 transgene. *J. Cell Biol.* **135:** 1669–1667.

85. Witty, J. P., T. Lempka, R. J. Coffey, Jr., L. M. Matrisian. 1995. Decreased tumor formation in 7,12-dimethylbenzanthracene-treated stromelysin-1 transgenic mice is associated with alterations in mammary epithelial cell apoptosis. *Cancer Res.* **55:** 1401–1406.

86. Sympson, C. J., M. J. Bissell, Z. Werb. 1995. Mammary gland tumor formation in transgenic mice overexpressing stromelysin-1. *Semin. Cancer Biol.* **6:** 159–163.

87. Sympson, C. J., R. S. Talhouk, M. J. Bissell, Z. Werb. 1994. The role of metalloproteinases and their inhibitors in regulating mammary epithelial morphology and function in vivo. *Perspect. Drug Discovery Design* **2:** 401–411.

88. Sternlicht, M. D., J. Xie, C. Sympson, M. Bissell, Z. Werb. 1997. Mice that express an autoactivating stromelysin-1 transgene develop progressive mammary gland lesions. *Proc. Am. Assoc. Cancer Res.* **38:** 257.

89. Rudolph-Owen, L. A., R. Clian, W. J. Muller, L. M. Matrisian. 1997. The matrix metalloproteinase matrilysin accelerates mammary tumorigenesis in MMTV-*neu* transgenic animals, submitted.

90. Sledge, G. W., Jr., M. Qulali, R. Goulet, E. A. Bone, R. Fife. 1995. Effect of matrix metalloproteinase inhibitor batimastat on breast cancer regrowth and metastasis in athymic mice. *J. Natl. Cancer Inst.* **87:** 1546–1550.

91. Eccles, S. A., G. M. Box, W. J. Court, E. A. Bone, W. Thomas, P. D. Brown. 1996. Control of lymphatic and hematogenous metastasis of a rat mammary carcinoma by the matrix metalloproteinase inhibitor batimastat (BB-94). *Cancer Res.* **56:** 2815–2822.

92. Yoneda, T., A. Sasaki, C. Dunstan, P. J. Williams, F. Bauss, Y. A. DeClerck, G. R. Mundy. 1997. Inhibition of osteolytic bone metastasis of breast cancer by combined treatment with the bisphosphonate ibandronate and tissue inhibitor of the matrix metalloproteinase-2. *J. Clin. Invest.* **99:** 2509–2517.

93. Brown, P. D., R. Giavazzi. 1995. Matrix metalloproteinase inhibition: a review of antitumour activity. *Ann. Oncol.* **6:** 967–974.

94. Weidner, N., J. Folkman, F. Pozza, P. Bevilacqua, E. N. Allred, D. H. Moore, S. Meli, G. Gasparini. 1992. Tumor angiogenesis: a new significant and independent prognostic indicator in early-stage breast carcinoma. *J. Natl. Cancer Inst.* **84:** 1875–1887.

15

The Urokinase Plasminogen Activation System in Breast Cancer

Anders N. Pedersen, Claus Holst-Hansen, Thomas L. Frandsen, Boye Schnack Nielsen, Ross W. Stephens, and Nils Brünner

1. INTRODUCTION

Cancer invasion is a complex process in which degradation of the extracellular matrix plays a crucial role. This degradation is accomplished by the concerted action of several proteolytic enzyme systems, including generation of plasmin by the urokinase pathway of plasminogen activation, matrix metalloproteases and other extracellular proteases. Increased expression and secretion of urokinase plasminogen activator (uPA) strongly correlates with the malignant phenotype of many types of cells, and the central role of uPA in tumor invasion is now well established (1–3).

Immunohistochemical and *in situ* hybridization data suggest a complex interaction between the proteases, their receptors, and inhibitors, as it has been shown that some of the components are expressed by the epithelial carcinoma cells while others are expressed by the cells constituting the tumor stroma, e.g., fibroblasts, macrophages, and endothelial cells.

It has also been shown that cancer tissue contains higher concentrations of proteases than the non-malignant tissue in which the tumor arises, and that the level of the proteases in the cancerous tissue is related to patient outcome, i.e., high protease content is related to poor prognosis. With these findings in mind it is tempting to hypothesize a functional role for proteolytic enzymes in facilitating cancer invasion and metastasis. In support of this hypothesis is the emerging amount of experimental and clinical data demonstrating the inhibition of invasion and metastatic tumor spread as a result of interfering with the proteolytic enzyme systems.

In this chapter, we will first give a short introduction to the urokinase plasminogen activation system and then review the literature with regard to the biological role of this proteolytic system in breast cancer.

2. BIOCHEMISTRY OF THE UROKINASE PLASMINOGEN ACTIVATION SYSTEM

uPA is a 52 kDa serine protease (1,4) that is secreted as an inactive single chain proenzyme (pro-uPA) (5,6). This immature form has only 1/250 the activity of the

From: Breast Cancer: *Molecular Genetics, Pathogenesis, and Therapeutics*
Edited by: A. M. Bowcock © Humana Press Inc., Totowa, NJ

mature enzyme *(7)*. Pro-uPA can be activated to uPA by plasmin, cathepsin B and kallikrein *(1,8)*, which all cleave the single chain pro-uPA within an intrachain loop held closed by a disulfide bridge. Thus the active enzyme consists of two chains (A+B) held together by this disulfide bridge. Active uPA has high specificity for the Arg560-Val561 bond in plasminogen, and cleavage between these residues gives rise to active plasmin. Plasminogen *(1,4)* is present at high concentration (1.5–2.0 μM) in plasma and interstitial fluids, and represents a plentiful potential source of plasmin activity. Unlike uPA, plasmin is a relatively nonspecific protease, cleaving many glycoproteins and proteoglycans of the extracellular matrix, as well as fibrin *(66)*. In addition, it is important to note that plasmin can activate some of the metalloproteases which also degrade tissue matrix *(10,11)*, and plasmin is known to activate growth factors, i.e., TGF-β *(21)*, which may further modulate stromal interactions in the expression of enzymes and tumor neo-angiogenesis.

Pro-uPA and uPA bind to a specific cell-surface receptor (uPAR) *(12,13)*. This receptor consists of a glycolipid-anchored three-domain 60 kDa glycoprotein whose N-terminal domain 1 contains the high affinity binding site for a growth factor domain within the A-chain of uPA. Since uPAR also has another important interaction with vitronectin *(14)*, these two interactions explain the observed localization of pro-uPA and thus potential uPA activity at the focal contacts and junctions formed between cells and with the extracellular matrix *(15)*. Indeed uPA binding to uPAR promotes binding of uPAR to the matrix protein vitronectin *(14)*, and thus adhesion of cells to a vitronectin substratum. A soluble form of uPAR has also been detected in body fluids of cancer patients *(16,17)*, and it seems plausible that this form has been released from the surface of cells. Cleavage of the glycolipid anchor by a phospholipase *(12)*, or proteolytic cleavage between domains 1 and 2 *(13)* are two known ways in which release of soluble receptor forms may occur. Indeed, the proteolytic activity of uPA can cleave its own receptor both in vitro and in vivo *(18,19)*.

Low affinity, high capacity binding of plasminogen to cell-surface proteins through the lysine binding sites of plasminogen kringles *(20)* enhances considerably the rate of plasminogen activation by uPA *(8,22)*. This is probably owing to the proximity of bound plasminogen to the laterally mobile uPAR *(23)* on the cell-surface. Furthermore, plasmin formed on the cell surface is able to catalyse the activation of uPAR-bound pro-uPA *(8)*, while remaining protected from plasma proteinase inhibitors, especially α-2-antiplasmin. Cell-surface bound plasmin can then mediate the nonspecific matrix proteolysis which facilitates migration of tumor cells through restraining tissue structures and activates or releases growth factors in the matrix.

Plasminogen activation by uPA is regulated by two important inhibitors, PAI-1 and PAI-2 *(4,15)*. PAI-1, a 52 kDa single chain protein, is secreted in an active but conformationally unstable form, whose inhibitory activity is stabilized and prolonged by binding to vitronectin *(24,25)*. PAI-1 is the most abundant fast-acting inhibitor of uPA in tumor tissues, and it is also able to inactivate uPA which is bound to uPAR. Formation of PAI-1 or PAI-2 complexes with uPA on the cell-surface leads to internalization of the uPAR/uPA/PAI complex *(26)* and probably drives uPAR cycling through the endosomal compartment back to the cell surface *(27)*. uPA activity may also be lost from the cell-surface by plasmin cleavage at Lys135-Lys136 in the A-chain of uPA, leaving only the so-called amino terminal fragment (ATF) bound on the cell. The general plasma proteinase inhibitor, α2-macroglobulin, inactivates soluble uPA relatively slowly, but uPA bound to uPAR is apparently protected by a steric effect *(28)*, thus allowing plasminogen activation to occur on the surface of cells even in the presence of serum *(8)*.

The interaction between PAI-1 and the cell-surface uPA system is now also appreciated as a modulator of cell adhesion and migration *(29)*. The basis of this effect is competition by active PAI-1 for uPAR binding sites on matrix vitronectin. Thus a high local concentration of PAI-1 can overcome uPAR-mediated adhesion and promote cell detachment, increased motility and migration. This may be most important for transformed epithelial cells which have reduced adhesion interactions with other matrix proteins, i.e., fibronectin *(30)*.

3. CELLULAR LOCALIZATION OF COMPONENTS OF THE UROKINASE PLASMINOGEN ACTIVATION SYSTEM IN BREAST CANCER

Histochemical studies have contributed substantially to a better understanding of the biological mechanisms of the plasminogen activation system during cancer invasion. A number of groups have reported on the cellular localization of the components of the uPA system in breast cancer; it is clear from these studies that while the epithelial cells may contribute with some of the essential components of this system, uPA, uPAR, and PAI-1 are predominantly expressed by stromal cells which are recruited or induced by the tumor cells to actively participate in tissue destruction and remodeling.

3.1. uPA

In situ hybridization studies have shown that uPA mRNA is expressed by fibroblast-like cells surrounding nests of cancer cells *(31,32)*. In a study by Wolf et al. *(32)* uPA mRNA was found in this cell type in all of 11 cases investigated, and in a study by Nielsen et al. *(31)* uPA mRNA was detected in stromal cells in 26 of 28 cases of invasive ductal carcinoma and in four of six cases of invasive lobular carcinoma. Only one of the 28 cases of invasive ductal carcinoma exhibited uPA-positive cancer cells. Comparison of *in situ* hybridization for uPA with the localization of macrophages, endothelial cells, and myofibroblasts, suggested that the myofibroblast was the main contributor of uPA expression *(31)*.

The suggested localization of uPA mRNA in breast cancer is in agreement with recent immunohistochemical studies performed by Nielsen et al. *(33)*. Six monoclonal antibodies with different uPA-epitopes and three preparations of polyclonal antibodies from three different rabbits showed an identical staining pattern, although no immunoreactivity was seen with three different irrelevant monoclonal control antibodies and a preparation of anti-uPA polyclonal antibodies depleted of uPA immunoreactivity. The study comprised 25 cases of invasive ductal carcinoma, and uPA immunoreactivity was identified in stromal cells in all of the 25 samples. The strongest immunoreactivity was observed in fibroblast-like cells surrounding nests of cancer cells (Fig. 1A), as it has been reported for uPA mRNA. Only three of the cases had positive staining for uPA in cancer cells, and in these three cases only a minority of the cancer cells were uPA-positive.

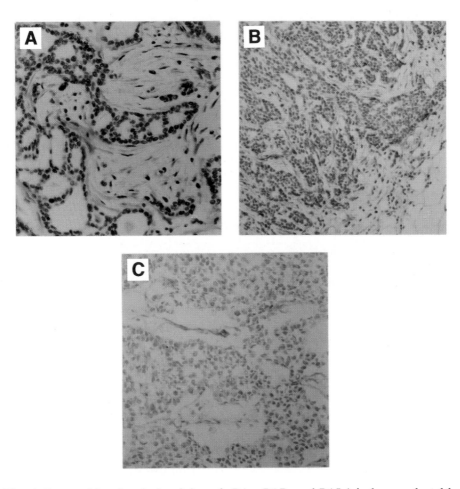

Fig. 1. Immunohistochemical staining of uPA, uPAR, and PAI-1 in human ductal breast cancer. Paraffin sections **(A)** and **(B)** and cryostat sections **(C)** were incubated with polyclonal antibodies to uPA (A), polyclonal antibodies to uPAR (B), and a monoclonal antibody (#380) to PAI-1 (C). uPA immunoreactivity is seen in cells (myofibroblasts) surrounding nests of cancer cells (A: red-brown color), uPAR immunoreactivity in scattered macrophage-like cells in the stroma - here, at the tumor periphery (B: red-brown color), and PAI-1 immunoreactivity in vascular structures (C: red-brown color).

These findings clearly indicate that the main producer of uPA in breast cancer tissue is the myofibroblast. Originally, the myofibroblast was identified in healing wounds as a fibroblastic cell with features of smooth muscle cell differentiation *(34)*. In ductal mammary carcinomas and intraductal papillomas, these cells may constitute up to 80% of the stromal cells, but it is less abundant in other benign breast lesions, and is absent from normal breast tissue *(35)*.

The observation of a general absence of uPA immunoreactivity in cancer cells in breast tumors, however, is in contrast to a number of other reports, where uPA immunoreactivity was mainly seen in the cancer cells *(36–43)*. For example, while stromal uPA immunoreactivity was reported by Carriero et al. *(36)*, who observed staining confined to the stroma using one monoclonal antibody only, the use of five other monoclonal anti-uPA antibodies showed uPA immunoreactivity confined to the tumor cells, and in a recent report by Christensen et al. *(44)*, normal and malignant epithelial cells as well as stromal cells, including fibroblasts, macrophages, endothelial cells and mast cells were found to be positive for uPA immunoreactivity. The reason for the discrepancies is intriguing. It is likely that different fixation and/or detection procedures influence the immunohistochemical staining pattern, but a thorough study is clearly needed to resolve these conflicting results.

3.2. uPAR

In a report by Pyke et al. *(45)* uPAR immunoreactivity was assessed by two different monoclonal antibodies. uPAR was detected in 51 of 60 cases of invasive ductal carcinoma. In 49 of the cases macrophage-like cells closely surrounding malignant epithelium were identified as uPAR-positive (Fig. 1B). In only eight of 51 cases carcinoma cells were positive for uPAR and in 2 of 34 cases vessels were identified as positive. Similar results were reported by Bianchi et al. *(46)* and Luther et al. *(47)*. Using another monoclonal antibody and rabbit polyclonal antibodies, Bianchi et al. *(46)* detected uPAR in 49 cases of invasive ductal carcinoma. uPAR immunoreactivity was seen in macrophage-like cells (48/49), cancer cells (21/49) and endothelial cells (8/49). In the recent study by Luther et al. *(47)* antibodies directed specifically against domains 1, 2, and 3 were used in immunohistochemistry. Two out of five antibodies specific for domain 2 showed strong immunoreactivity, two of three domain 1 specific antibodies weak immunoreactivity, while three of three antibodies specific for domain 3 showed no immunoreactivity. Although it is difficult to make firm conclusions from this latter study in regard to accessibility of the specific epitopes, it is tempting to speculate whether such domain specific antibodies could be used in immunohistochemistry to identify epitopes that are only accessible in processed forms of uPAR, or only accessible due to interactions between uPAR and other molecules such as uPA and vitronectin. A number of other reports *(36,37,40,41,44)* also describe the immunohistochemical localization of uPAR in breast cancer, while there is a lack of studies using *in situ* hybridization.

3.3. PAI-1

Bianchi et al. *(48)* detected PAI-1 immunoreactivity in 15 of 20 cases of invasive breast carcinoma, using monoclonal antibodies. PAI-1 immunoreactivity was seen in all 15 cases in stromal cells which were described as endothelial cells (5/15) and macrophages (13/15). Extensive tumor cell staining was seen in 2 cases, while a few cancer cells exhibited PAI-1 immunoreactivity in eight cases. In a study by Reilly et al. *(49)* of 43 cases of invasive breast carcinoma, PAI-1 immunostaining was seen in cancer cells and vascular cells. Results obtained in our laboratory by immunohistochemistry and in situ hybridization *(50)* have shown PAI-1 mRNA and immunoreactivity mainly in the stromal component, especially vascular cells (Fig. 1C), while PAI-1 positive cancer cells were a rare observation. Other groups have also reported on PAI-1 immunohistochemistry in breast cancer *(37,39,41,43,44)*.

3.4. PAI-2

Few studies have investigated the cellular localization of PAI-2 in breast cancer tissue. In immunohistochemical studies by Costantini et al. *(38)* and Damjanovich et al. *(39)* PAI-2 was barely detectable. Thorough histochemical studies are still awaited to clarify the relation between PAI-2 as a marker of good prognosis and the cellular expression pattern in human breast cancer tissue.

In conclusion, studies on the cellular localization of the uPA system in breast cancer suggest that tumor-infiltrating stromal cells together with the epithelial cancer cells form a cell population which is collectively responsible for the extracellular proteolytic activity. Although uPA is produced predominantly by myofibroblasts, the uPA mediated matrix degradation may take place on the cell surface of macrophages and cancer cells. Cancer invasion should therefore be considered as a multicellular process rather than as an attribute of individual tumor cells.

4. PROGNOSTIC IMPLICATIONS
OF THE UROKINASE PLASMINOGEN ACTIVATION SYSTEM
IN BREAST CANCER

The identification of patients at high risk of relapse is currently one of the most important issues in breast cancer research. However, the selection of high-risk patients continues to be difficult owing to the unpredictable course of this disease. Axillary lymph node status is currently recognized as the best clinical discriminant between good and poor prognosis, yet almost 30% of node-negative patients and 65% of node-positive patients will experience a relapse. Additional prognostic markers are therefore urgently needed *(51)*.

Since metastatic disease is the main cause of cancer patient morbidity and mortality, the measurement of molecules functionally involved in the regulation of tumor invasion and metastasis is attractive as a means to predict prognosis.

Quantitation of uPA can principally be performed in two ways: by measurement of its enzymatic activity or by immunological assay. For prognostic studies the measurement of uPA-activity has been of limited use *(52,53)*, while determination of immunoreactive uPA by ELISA has proven to be the superior method for these types of analyses *(54–56)*. At least six different ELISAs for uPA determination are available *(57)*. These assays employ different standards as well as different antibody combinations, with different affinities for the various forms of uPA. In order to harmonize studies on uPA tumor content, a European study group under BIOMED-1 has recently established a uPA standard and quality assured reference material *(57)*.

PAI-1 can be determined either by assay of its inhibitory activity or by immunoassays. So far only one prognostic study has been conducted using determination of patient plasma PAI-1 activity *(58)*. Five different PAI-1 ELISAs are available *(55,59–62)*. These assays display the same multiplicity of variations as described for the uPA ELISAs. Therefore the European study group is also in the process of establishing an international PAI-1 standard as well as reference material *(62)*. In contrast to the existing studies described below, future studies on uPA and PAI-1 should be standardized with these reference materials, as we have earlier suggested *(50)*, allowing direct comparison of absolute antigen levels between different studies to be performed.

PAI-2 determination has been performed in breast cancer tissue by the use of two different ELISAs *(63,76)*, and uPAR determination in prognostic studies has so far been performed by two ELISA formats *(65,66)*. Recently, a modification of one of the existing uPAR ELISAs was applied to plasma from stage IV breast cancer patients *(17)*.

In the published studies, different buffers have been used for the extraction of uPA, uPAR, PAI-1, and PAI-2 from tumor tissue. The buffers can be grouped as follows: neutral buffers without detergent (steroid hormone receptor buffer) *(55,59,63,65,67–70)*, neutral buffers with detergent *(61,67,69)*, and detergent buffers with a low pH *(66,70)*. The type of extraction buffer used is probably less important for PAI-1 than for uPA. Jänicke et al. *(69)* found that addition of detergent to the extraction buffer resulted in a twofold increase in extractable uPA, while the PAI-1 concentration remained almost the same. Similarly, Rønne et al. *(66)* found that the uPA concentration in extracts made with a detergent buffer with a low pH was about eightfold higher than with a neutral buffer without detergent, while the PAI-1 concentration remained unchanged. However, in both studies a good correlation between uPA immunoreactivity in detergent and nondetergent extracts was observed. With respect to prognostic impact, uPAR extraction in a nondetergent buffer appears to be more favorable *(67)*.

When assessing the prognostic impact of uPA, uPAR, PAI-1, and PAI-2, one of two approaches to divide patients into prognostic groups is generally chosen: division of the tumor levels either by the median value, or by an optimized cut-off value. It cannot readily be determined which method to favor in each case. However, it should be emphasized that when using the optimized cut-off point to dichotomize patients into those with good and poor prognosis, the clinical relevance of the chosen cut point can be validated only in an independent, comparable group of patients.

In the following sections several prognostic studies are described. Each study has used its own definition of cut point, prognostic endpoint, as well as which patient stages to include. Therefore the conclusions of the individual studies cannot be directly compared.

4.1. uPA

uPA levels have been reported to be increased in primary breast cancer tissue as compared to normal breast tissue *(71)*. Also, direct associations between primary tumor uPA content and tumor size, uPA content and number of tumor positive axillary lymph nodes *(52)* as well as uPA content and tumor microvessel density *(72)* have been demonstrated, suggesting that the quantitation of uPA may yield valuable prognostic information. The first preliminary study to demonstrate uPA as a prognostic marker in breast cancer was performed by Duffy et al. *(52)*, who reported that when using an optimized cut point, high primary tumor uPA-activity was significantly associated with shorter disease-free interval in a group of 52 node-negative and node-positive patients. They confirmed their findings in another retrospective study of 166 patients *(54)*, where immunoreactive uPA was found to be an independent marker of recurrence-free and overall survival. Other groups have also demonstrated the prognostic impact of uPA, as determined by various ELISAs *(55,56,61,63,68,73)* including a luminometric immunoassay *(64)*. In a larger study of 671 node-negative and -positive patients by Foekens et al. *(73)* the prognostic value of uPA was also found to apply to the clinically important node-negative subgroup of patients, a finding which has been confirmed by others *(61,74,75)*. It has also been shown that high uPA content is an indicator of poor response to first line endocrine therapy in recurrent breast cancer *(76)*.

4.2. uPAR

uPAR is present in breast cancer tissue but undetectable in normal breast tissue *(77)*, and uPAR also appears to be a prognostic marker. Grøndahl-Hansen et al. *(67)* were the first to report on the prognostic value of ELISA-determined uPAR in detergent and nondetergent extracts prepared from the same 505 primary breast tumors. Univariate analysis showed that uPAR levels above the median value in the set of nondetergent extracts were significantly associated with a shorter overall survival. In a clinically relevant subgroup of 201 node-positive postmenopausal patients, uPAR in nondetergent extracts had a particularly strong prognostic impact, and in this group uPAR appeared to be an independent and the single most important biochemical marker of both relapse-free and overall survival. By the use of a different ELISA, Duggan et al. *(65)* confirmed the prognostic impact of uPAR in nondetergent extracts of 141 primary tumors. It is intriguing that the uPAR determination in nondetergent extracts provides a stronger prognostic parameter than measurement of uPAR in detergent extracts. The uPAR in nondetergent extracts probably represents a soluble form released from the cell surface *(16,66)*, a fraction that is particularly interesting from a functional point of view, since active uPA and plasmin can cleave uPAR within the three domains, and phospholipases C and D can release uPAR by cleaving the glycolipid anchor.

4.3. PAI-1

PAI-1 content was found to be 74-fold increased in breast cancer tissue as compared to normal breast tissue *(71)*. Similar findings were reported by Reilly et al. *(49)* and by Sumiyoshi et al. *(78)*, who also found that the levels of PAI-1 were directly proportional to the number of tumor positive axillary lymph nodes. Jänicke et al. *(71)* were the first to describe the prognostic significance of PAI-1 in breast cancer. Including tumor extracts from 113 node-negative and -positive patients, high PAI-1 level as determined by ELISA was shown to be an independent and significant predictor of poor prognosis, and even better than uPA. Later retrospective studies *(55,59,63)* confirmed this prognostic impact of PAI-1. The paradox that high—and not low—tumor content of PAI-1 (a strong, fast-acting inhibitor of uPA) is associated with poor prognosis is possibly explained by the finding of PAI-1 predominantly in the extracellular matrix of the tumor stroma and in many cases in areas surrounding the tumor vessels, where high PAI-1 levels are proposed to protect the tumor from auto-degradation by uPA-catalyzed plasmin formation *(79,80)*. Of particular interest is that PAI-1 appears as an independent prognostic variable, implying that determination of tumor PAI-1 contributes significantly to the prognostic information obtained by other markers. For example, in a subgroup of patients with steroid hormone receptor positive tumors, who have a better prognosis than patients with receptor negative tumors, PAI-1 tumor measurements enabled further prognostic stratification *(55,59)*. A later study by Foekens et al. *(76)* showed further that in a group of 235 tamoxifen-naive patients with recurrent breast cancer, PAI-1 predicted poor response to tamoxifen as first line endocrine therapy.

In the study by Foekens et al. *(59)* PAI-1 was found to be the strongest biochemical prognostic marker when compared to uPA, cathepsin D, pS2, estrogen and progesterone receptors. A recent study by Grøndahl-Hansen et al. *(68)*, including 295 low-risk patients, showed PAI-1 to be the single most important prognostic factor as compared

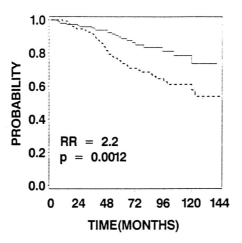

Fig. 2. Impact of PAI-1 level in cytosolic tumor extracts on overall survival in 295 low-risk breast cancer patients. Patients were divided into two groups with PAI-1 levels below (——) and above (----) the median value. The P value was calculated by the log-rank test, and the relative risk (RR) was calculated by the Cox regression model.

to uPA, uPAR, and other established prognostic variables. In this latter study, with a median follow-up of 7.4 yr, low-risk patients with high tumor PAI-1 content experienced a relative risk of death 2.2 times that of patients with low tumor PAI-1 (Fig. 2), indicating the clinical value of PAI-1 determination as one of the important factors in the complex system that predicts patient outcome.

4.4. PAI-2

High PAI-2 tumor levels seem, at least in some patient groups, to be related to good prognosis. High tumor PAI-2 levels were found to be inversely correlated to axillary lymph node involvement *(78)*, and in a study of 314 patients Bouchet et al. *(63)* found that high levels of immunoreactive tumor PAI-2 correlated with longer metastasis-free survival in both node-negative and -positive groups of patients. Foekens et al. *(76)* used a different PAI-2 ELISA and did not find any significant association between PAI-2 and prognosis in the overall patient group. However, in patients with high tumor uPA content, high PAI-2 level correlated significantly with a better prognosis.

uPA, uPAR, and PAI-1 tumor levels correlate to each other, but have also been reported to be mutually independent prognostic markers. For example, Jänicke et al. *(61)* found that by combining uPA and PAI-1 levels, node-negative patients with high tumor content of both molecules experienced a 45% risk of relapse after three years in contrast to only a 7% risk for patients with low tumor levels of both molecules. Recently, a prospective study was initiated *(81)* where node-negative patients are postoperatively randomized to adjuvant therapy or observation on the basis of their tumor content of uPA and PAI-1.

uPA, uPAR, and PAI-1 have also been shown to be prognostic markers in other types of cancer, including lung cancer *(82–84)*, colon cancer *(60,85)*, gastric cancer *(86–88)*, ovarian cancer *(89)*, cervical cancer *(90)*, renal cancer *(91)*, bladder cancer *(92)*, and brain tumors *(93)*.

Future studies will focus on the determination of the various components of the urokinase plasminogen activation system in blood. The development of sensitive assays for markers in blood will replace the requirement for a tissue sample with an easily and readily accessible sampling of peripheral blood, thus allowing screening of total populations and high-risk groups, and also the monitoring of relapse and prediction of treatment response. We have recently found that stage IV breast cancer patients have significantly elevated plasma levels of uPAR as compared to healthy controls *(17)*, indicating that a soluble form of uPAR is released from the cancer tissue into the blood stream. The prognostic significance of uPAR in blood from breast cancer patients remains, however, to be established. von Tempelhoff et al. *(58)* have reported that plasma PAI-1 activity was elevated in a group of 183 patients compared to healthy controls, and that high PAI-1 activity was significantly associated with poor prognosis.

Additionally, future studies will focus on modifications of ELISAs to achieve more selective measurements. The existing ELISAs have been developed in such a way as to measure all forms of the given molecule, including pro-forms and other inactive forms. However, the amount of the active forms of a molecule may more closely reflect the ongoing level of proteolytic activity in a tumor and thereby be particularly related to prognosis. There are at present no assays available that selectively measure active uPA or active PAI-1. However, since the complex between uPA and PAI-1 can only be formed from the active forms of both molecules, quantitation of this complex may represent a method for the indirect measurement of the level of active components. Therefore, we have recently developed a uPA:PAI-1 complex ELISA *(70)*, and are currently evaluating the prognostic significance of this complex within breast cancer extracts. Similarly, since plasminogen activation is strongly enhanced by uPA:uPAR complex formation, the tumor level of uPA:uPAR complex may better reflect the ongoing proteolytic activity. In order to evaluate the prognostic value of this complex in tumor extracts an ELISA for the quantitation of uPA:uPAR complex has also recently been developed *(94)*.

5. THERAPEUTIC INTERVENTIONS

The establishment of a basic role for proteolytic enzymes in facilitating cancer invasion and metastasis through breakdown of basement membranes and extracellular matrix has resulted in the search for and development of protease inhibitors or receptor antagonists as a means of blocking this proteolytic activity. We will in the following review the in vitro and in vivo data on intervention with the uPA-system.

5.1. Plasmin

Plasmin has received much attention in the past years in relation to tumor invasion and metastasis. There is an extensive literature on inhibition of plasmin activity in both in vitro and in vivo model invasion systems. It is evident that direct blocking of plasmin activity in vitro leads to inhibition of degradation of extracellular matrix as shown in amniotic membrane assays *(95)*, fibrin gel assays *(96)*, and in Matrigel invasion assays *(96–101)*. In vivo inhibition of plasmin leads to impaired primary tumor growth and decreased local invasion *(102–104)*. Moreover, it was shown that treatment with a plasmin inhibitor (urinary trypsin inhibitor) significantly reduced formation of lung metastases in a spontaneous metastasis model *(99)*.

5.2. uPA

Already in 1983 it was shown that inhibition of uPA activity in a model of human tumor cells growing on the chorioallantoic membrane of chicken embryos, lead to impaired ability of the tumor cells to metastasize *(105)*. Several studies have repeated this effect on tumor cell invasion and metastasis, both *in vitro* and *in vivo,* either through antibody inhibition of the catalytic activity of uPA or by antisense expression *(95,106–109)*. Recently, it was shown that when cellular blue nevi were chemically induced on the skin of mice genetically deficient in uPA, they had a significantly reduced ability to progress to malignant melanomas as compared to nevi on wild-type mice *(140)*, suggesting a causative role for uPA in transformation to malignancy.

5.3. uPAR

uPAR has the ability to localize and enhance proteolytic activity on the surface of cells *(110)*, and it also plays an important role in tumor cell adhesion and migration *(29)*. Therefore, a new intervention strategy based on the use of uPAR antagonists seems attractive, and interference with uPA:uPAR binding is likely to cause less toxic side-effects than direct inhibition of the catalytic activity of uPA or plasmin. In fact, in vitro studies have shown that inhibition of uPA binding to uPAR on the surface of cultured cells leads to diminished plasmin formation *(109,111)* and inhibition of tumor cell invasion in vitro. uPA:uPAR interaction can be blocked by using monoclonal anti-uPAR antibodies *(97,109,112,113)*, monoclonal anti-uPA antibodies *(14)*, noncatalytic fragments of uPA (i.e., ATF) *(97,100,115–117)*, a soluble form of uPAR as a scavenger for uPA *(118)*, and by inhibiting uPAR gene expression using antisense oligonucleotides *(119,120)*. For example, antisense inhibition of uPAR in a squamous cell carcinoma resulted in inhibition of local invasion and an increase in tumor latency *(121)*. Antagonists of uPA:uPAR binding have also been studied in animal tumor models, and these antagonists have shown both anti-invasive and anti-metastatic effects *(97,115,121)*. Significant reduction of spontaneous metastases in two tumor models could be demonstrated using treatment with a noncatalytic fragment of uPA *(115)* and by inoculation of cancer cells expressing a mutated inactive form of uPA *(97)*. Recently, another study showed that treatment with a uPAR antagonist inhibited angiogenesis and tumor growth in a syngeneic tumor model *(122)*.

5.4. PAI-1

Although prognostic studies in breast cancer consistently show that high tumor PAI-1 levels are associated with shorter survival, the exact role of PAI-1 in cancer as well as the rationale for the inhibition of the uPA:PAI-1 interaction are still controversial.

Although one study has shown that PAI-1 inhibits in vitro invasion in a Matrigel assay *(123)*, others have reported that co-expression of uPA, uPAR, and PAI-1 is needed for optimum invasiveness through the Matrigel *(124)*. In the latter work, it was shown that inhibition of PAI-1 activity by an antibody could significantly reduce the in vitro invasive capacity of lung cancer cells. Results from in vivo models have not clarified whether or not PAI-1 promotes or inhibits invasion and metastasis. Eitzman and coworkers *(125)* found no significant difference between mice overexpressing PAI-1 and mice genetically deficient in PAI-1 with respect to growth and metastasis of a murine melanoma model. It should be noted, however, that in human melanomas the cancer cells express large amounts of PAI-1 themselves *(126)*. In another study, primary tumor growth and metastasis were inhibited in athymic mice carrying a human prostate cancer cell line transfected with a human PAI-1 cDNA construct *(127)*. These results are in conflict with the results presented by Quax et al. *(128)*, demonstrating that PAI-1 is necessary for the metastasis of human melanoma in a nude mouse model. A study published by Tsuchiya et al. *(129)* shows that treatment of athymic nude mice with an antibody to human PAI-1 suppresses metastasis of the human fibrosarcoma cell line HT 1080, thus supporting the notion of a role for PAI-1 in promoting tumor progression.

At least 2 different roles for PAI-1 in cancer have been suggested:

1. PAI-1 mediates release of cells by displacing uPAR or integrins from vitronectin and thus facilitates the dissemination of cancer cells to distant tissue sites *(29,130)*. However, the experimental data are somewhat conflicting on this point, with in vitro experiments showing PAI-1 to inhibit cell migration *(130,131,132)* through its interaction with cell surface bound uPA:uPAR- complexes, integrins and vitronectin, while others have shown PAI-1 to stimulate cell migration on vitronectin *(133)*.
2. PAI-1 protects the tumor stroma from autodegradation by uPA catalyzed plasmin formation *(80)*. This hypothesis is mainly based on the *in situ* hybridization and immunohistochemical studies showing stromal localization of PAI-1 in many types of cancer, including breast cancer *(see above)*.

   One possible explanation for these conflicting results is the importance of the exact pericellular localization of PAI-1 in the cancer tissue. For example, if PAI-1 was in surplus at the trailing edge of the tumor cell, this could facilitate release of this edge from vitronectin, whereas a surplus of cell surface bound uPA:uPAR-complexes at the migratory leading edge of the cell *(134)* would facilitate formation of new adhesion sites and thus enhance migration.

5.5. PAI-2

In vitro assays have repeatedly shown that PAI-2 inhibits invasion of cancer cells through Matrigel *(135)* or human amniotic membranes *(136,137)*. The few in vivo studies conducted suggest that PAI-2 suppresses metastasis *(138,139)*.

6. CONCLUSION

The central role of the serine protease uPA, its cell-surface receptor and the specific inhibitors in facilitating breast cancer invasion and metastasis is well established. Immunohistochemical and *in situ* hybridzation data suggest a complex interaction between uPA, uPAR, PAI-1, and PAI-2, as some of the components are expressed by the epithelial carcinoma cells while others are expressed by stromal cells such as fibroblasts and endothelial cells. Quantitation by ELISA of the individual components of the uPA system has shown that the tumor tissue levels of these components are highly related to the prognosis of breast cancer patients. Future prospective studies will show as to which succes tumor and/or blood levels of these enzymes can be implicated in treatment decisions in the management of the individual breast cancer patients. Additionally, emerging experimental data has demonstrated the possibility of inhibiting invasion and metastatic tumor spread by chemical interference with the uPA system, and future investigations will focus on the clinical role of chemical uPA inhibitors and uPAR antagonists as anti-cancer drugs.

REFERENCES

1. Danø, K., P. A. Andreasen, J. Grøndahl-Hansen, P. Kristensen, L. S. Nielsen, and L. Skriver. 1985. Plasminogen activators, tissue degradation and cancer. *Adv. Cancer Res.* **44:** 139–266.
2. Danø, K., N. Behrendt, N. Brünner, V. Ellis, M. Plough, and C. Pyke. 1994. The urokinase receptor. Protein structure and role in plasminogen activation and cancer invasion. *Fibronolysis* **8:** 189–213.
3. Andreasen, P. A., L. Kjøller, L. Christensen, and M. J. Duffy. 1997. The urokinase-type plasminogen activator system in cancer metastasis: a review. *Int. J. Cancer* **72:** 1–22.
4. Stephens, R. W. and A. Vaheri. 1993. *Guidebook to the extracellular matrix and adhesion proteins.* Oxford University Press, Oxford.
5. Nielsen, L. S., J. G. Hansen, L. Skriver, E. L. Wilson, K. Kaltoft, J. Zeuthen, and K. Danø. 1982. Purification of zymogen to plasminogen activator from human glioblastoma cells by affinity chromatography with monoclonal antibody. *Biochemistry* **21:** 6410–6415.
6. Skriver, L., L. S. Nielsen, R. Stephens, and K. Danø. 1982. Plasminogen activator released as inactive proenzyme from murine cells transformed by sarcoma virus. *Eur. J. Biochem.* **124:** 409–414.
7. Petersen, L. C., L. R. Lund, L. S. Nielsen, K. Danø, and L. Skriver. 1988. One-chain urokinase-type plasminogen activator from human sarcoma cells is a proenzyme with little or no intrinsic activity. *J. Biol. Chem.* **263:** 11,189–11,195.
8. Stephens, R. W., J. Pöllänen, H. Tapiovaara, K. C. Leung, P. S. Sim, E. M. Salonen, E. Rønne, N. Behrendt, K. Danø, and A. Vaheri. 1989. Activation of pro-urokinase and plasminogen on human sarcoma cells: a proteolytic system with surface-bound reactants. *J. Cell Biol.* **108:** 1987–1995.
9. Liotta, L. A., R. H. Goldfarb, R. Brudage, G. P. Siegal, V. Terranova, and S. Garbisa. 1981. Effect of plasminogen activator (urokinase), plasmin, and thrombin on glycoprotein and collagenous components of basement membrane. *Cancer Res.* **41:** 4629–4636.
10. Werb, Z., C. L. Mainardi, C. A. Vater, and J. Harris (eds.). 1977. Endogenous activiation of latent collagenase by rheumatoid synovial cells. Evidence for a role of plasminogen activator. *N. Engl. J. Med.* **296:** 1017–1023.
11. DeClerck, Y. A. and W. E. Laug. 1996. Cooperation between matrix metalloproteinases and the plasminogen activator-plasmin system in tumor progression. *Enzyme Protein* **49:** 72–84.
12. Ploug, M., E. Rønne, N. Behrendt, A. L. Jensen, F. Blasi, and K. Danø. 1991. Cellular receptor for urokinase plasminogen activator. Carboxyl-terminal processing and membrane anchoring by glycosyl-phosphatidylinositol. *J. Biol. Chem.* **266:** 1926–1933.
13. Behrendt, N., M. Ploug, L. Patthy, G. Houen, F. Blasi, and K. Danø. 1991. The Ligand-binding Domain of the Cell Surface Receptor for Urokinase-type Plasminogen Activator. *J. Biol. Chem.* **266:** 7842–7847.
14. Wei, Y., D. A. Waltz, N. Rao, R. J. Drummond, S. Rosenberg, and H. A. Chapman. 1994. Identifica tion of the urokinase receptor as an adhesion receptor for vitronectin. *J. Biol. Chem.* **269:** 32,380–32,388.
15. Pöllänen, J., R. W. Stephens, and A. Vaheri. 1991. Directed plasminogen activation at the surface of normal and malignant cells. *Adv. Cancer Res.* **57:** 273–328.
16. Pedersen, N., M. Schmitt, E. Ronne, M. I. Nicoletti, G. Høyer-Hansen, M. Conese, R. Giavazzi, K. Dano, W. Kuhn, F. Janicke, and et al. 1993. A ligand-free, soluble urokinase receptor is present in the ascitic fluid from patients with ovarian cancer. *J. Clin. Invest.* **92:** 2160–2167.

17. Stephens, R. W., N. A. Pedersen, H. J. Nielsen, M. J. A. G. Hamers, G. Høyer-Hansen, E. Rønne, E. Dybkjær, K. Danø, and N. Brünner. 1997. ELISA determination of soluble urokinase receptor in blood from healthy donors and cancer patients. *Clin. Chem.* **43:** 1868–1876.

18. Høyer-Hansen, G., E. Rønne, H. Solberg, N. Behrendt, M. Ploug, L. R. Lund, V. Ellis, and K. Danø. 1992. Urokinase plasminogen activator cleaves its cell surface receptor releasing the ligand-binding domain. *J. Biol. Chem.* **267:** 18,224–18,229.

19. Solberg, H., J. Rømer, N. Brünner, A. Holm, N. Sidenius, K. Danø, and G. Høyer-Hansen. 1994. A cleaved form of the receptor for urokinase-type plasminogen activator in invasive transplanted human and murine tumors. *Int. J. Cancer* **58:** 877–881.

20. Miles, L. A. and E. F. Plow. 1988. Ubiquitous sites for cellular regulation of fibrinolysis. *Fibrinolysis* 61–71.

21. Lyons, R. M., J. Keski-Oja, and H. L. Moses. 1988. Proteolytic Activation of Latent Transforming Growth Factor-β from Fibroblast-conditioned Medium. *J. Cell Biol.* **106:** 1659–1665.

22. Ellis, V., M. F. Scully, and V. V. Kakkar. 1989. Plasminogen activation initiated by single-chain urokinase-type plasminogen activator. Potentiation by U937 monocytes. *J. Biol. Chem.* **264:** 2185–2188.

23. Myohanen, H. T., R. W. Stephens, K. Hedman, H. Tapiovaara, E. Rønne, G. Høyer-Hansen, K. Danø, and A. Vaheri. 1993. Distribution and Lateral Mobility of the Urokinase-Receptor Complex at the Cell Surface. *J. Histochem. Cytochem.* **41:** 1291–1301.

24. Lindahl, T. L., O. Sigurdardottir, and B. Wiman. 1989. Stability of plasminogen activator inhibitor 1 (PAI-1). *Thromb. Haemost.* **62:** 748–751.

25. Salonen, E. M., A. Vaheri, J. Pöllänen, R. Stephens, P. Andreasen, M. Mayer, K. Danø, J. Gailit, and E. Ruoslahti. 1989. Interaction of plasminogen activator inhibitor (PAI-1) with vitronectin. *J. Biol. Chem.* **264:** 6339–6343.

26. Cubellis, M. V., T. C. Wun, and F. Blasi. 1990. Receptor-mediated internalization and degradation of urokinase is caused by its specific inhibitor PAI-1. *EMBO J.* **9:** 1079–1085.

27. Nykjaer, A., M. Conese, E. I. Christensen, D. Olson, O. Cremona, J. Gliemann, and F. Blasi. 1997. Recycling of the urokinase receptor upon internalization of the uPA:serpin complexes. *EMBO J.* **16:** 2610–2620.

28. Stephens, R. W., H. Tapiovaara, T. Reisberg, J. Bizik, and A. Vaheri. 1991. Alpha 2-macroglobulin restricts plasminogen activation to the surface of RC2A leukemia cells. *Cell Regul.* **2:** 1057–1065.

29. Deng, G., S. A. Curriden, S. J. Wang, S. Rosenberg, and D. J. Loskutoff. 1996. Is plasminogen activator inhibitor-1 the molecular switch that governs urokinase receptor-mediated cell adhesion and release. *J. Cell Biol.* **134:** 1563–1571.

30. Alitalo, K. and A. Vaheri. 1982. Pericellular matrix in malignant transformation. *Adv. Cancer Res.* **37:** 111–158.

31. Nielsen, B. S., M. Sehested, S. Timshel, C. Pyke, and K. Danø. 1996. Messenger RNA for urokinase plasminogen activator is expressed in myofibroblasts adjacent to cancer cells in human breast cancer. *Lab. Invest.* **74:** 168–177.

32. Wolf, C., N. Rouyer, Y. Lutz, C. Adida, M. Loriot, J. P. Bellocq, P. Chambon, and P. Basset. 1993. Stromelysin 3 belongs to a subgroup of proteinases expressed in breast carcinoma fibroblastic cells and possibly implicated in tumor progression. *Proc. Natl. Acad. Sci. USA* **90:** 1843–1847.

33. Nielsen, B. S., M. Sehested, S. Dunn, F. Rank, S. Timshel, J. Rygaard, K. Danø. 1997. (Unpublished).

34. Majno, G., G. Gabbiani, B. J. Hirschel, G. B. Ryan, and P. R. Statkov. 1971. Contraction of granulation tissue in vitro: similarity to smooth muscle. *Science* **173:** 548–550.

35. Sappino, A. P., O. Skalli, B. Jackson, W. Schurch, and G. Gabbiani. 1988. Smooth-muscle differentiation in stromal cells of malignant and non malignant breast tissues. *Int. J. Cancer* **41**: 707–712.

36. Carriero, M. V., P. Franco, S. Del Vecchio, O. Massa, G. Botti, G. D'Aiuto, M. P. Stoppelli, and M. Salvatore. 1994. Tissue distribution of soluble and receptor-bound urokinase in human breast cancer using a panel of monoclonal antibodies. *Cancer Res.* **54**: 5445–5454.

37. Costantini, V., A. Sidoni, R. Deveglia, O. A. Cazzato, G. Bellezza, I. Ferri, E. Bucciarelli, and G. G. Nenci. 1996. Combined overexpression of urokinase, urokinase receptor, and plasminogen activator inhibitor-1 is associated with breast cancer progression: an immunohistochemical comparison of normal, benign, and malignant breast tissues. *Cancer* **77**: 1079–1088.

38. Costantini, V., L. R. Zacharski, V. A. Memoli, B. J. Kudryk, S. M. Rousseau, and D. C. Stump. 1991. Occurrence of components of fibrinolysis pathways in situ in neoplastic and nonneoplastic human breast tissue. *Cancer Res.* **51**: 354–358.

39. Damjanovich, L., C. Turzo, and R. Adany. 1994. Factors involved in the plasminogen activation system in human breast tumours. *Thromb. Haemost.* **71**: 684–691.

40. Del Vecchio, S., M. P. Stoppelli, M. V. Carriero, R. Fonti, O. Massa, P. Y. Li, G. Botti, M. Cerra, G. D'Aiuto, and G. Esposito. 1993. Human urokinase receptor concentration in malignant and benign breast tumors by in vitro quantitative autoradiography: comparison with urokinase levels. *Cancer Res.* **53**: 3198–3206.

41. Jankun, J., H. W. Merrick, and P. J. Goldblatt. 1993. Expression and localization of elements of the plasminogen activation system in benign breast disease and breast cancers. *J. Cell Biochem.* **53**: 135–144.

42. Jänicke, F., M. Schmitt, and H. Graeff. 1991. Clinical relevance of the urokinase-type and tissue-type plasminogen activators and of their type 1 inhibitor in breast cancer. *Semin. Thromb. Hemost.* **17**: 303- 312.

43. Sumiyoshi, K., S. Baba, S. Sakaguchi, T. Urano, Y. Takada, and A. Takada. 1991. Increase in levels of plasminogen activator and type-1 plasminogen activator inhibitor in human breast cancer: Possible roles in tumor progression and metastasis. *Thromb. Res.* **63**: 59–71.

44. Christensen, L., S. A. Wiborg, C. W. Heegaard, S. K. Moestrup, J. A. Andersen, and P. A. Andreasen. 1996. Immunohistochemical localization of urokinase-type plasminogen activator, type-1 plasminogen-activator inhibitor, urokinase receptor and alpha(2)-macroglobulin receptor in human breast carcinomas. *Int. J. Cancer* **66**: 441–452.

45. Pyke, C., N. Graem, E. Ralfkiaer, E. Rønne, G. Høyer-Hansen, N. Brunner, and K. Danø. 1993. Receptor for urokinase is present in tumor-associated macrophages in ductal breast carcinoma. *Cancer Res.* **53**: 1911–1915.

46. Bianchi, E., R. L. Cohen, A. T. Thor, R. F. Todd, I. F. Mizukami, D. A. Lawrence, B. M. Ljung, M. A. Shuman, and H. S. Smith. 1994. The urokinase receptor is expressed in invasive breast cancer but not in normal breast tissue. *Cancer Res.* **54**: 861–866.

47. Luther, T., V. Magdolen, S. Albrecht, M. Kasper, C. Riemer, H. Kessler, H. Graeff, M. Muller, and M. Schmitt. 1997. Epitope-mapped monoclonal antibodies as tools for functional and morphological analyses of the human urokinase receptor in tumor tissue. *Am. J. Pathol.* **150**: 1231–1244.

48. Bianchi, E., R. L. Cohen, A. Dai, A. T. Thor, M. A. Shuman, and H. S. Smith. 1995. immunohistochemical localization of the plasminogen activator inhibitor-1 in breast cancer. *Int. J. Cancer* **60**: 597–603.

49. Reilly, D., L. Christensen, M. Duch, N. Nolan, M. J. Duffy, and P. A. Andreasen. 1992. Type-1 plasminogen activator inhibitor in human breast carcinomas. *Int. J. Cancer* **50**: 208–214.

50. Pappot, H., H. Gardsvoll, J. Rømer, A. N. Pedersen, J. Grøndahl-Hansen, C. Pyke, and N. Brunner. 1995. Plasminogen activator inhibitor type 1 in cancer: therapeutic and prognostic implications. *Biol. Chem. Hoppe Seyler* **376:** 259–267.

51. McGuire, W. L. and G. M. Clark. 1992. Prognostic factors and treatment decisions in axillary-node- negative breast cancer. (Commentaries) *N. Engl. J. Med.* **326:** 1756–1761.

52. Duffy, M. J., P. O'Grady, D. Devaney, L. O'Siorain, J. J. Fennelly, and H. J. Lijnen. 1988. Urokinase- plasminogen activator, a marker for aggressive breast carcinomas. Preliminary report. *Cancer* **62:** 531–533.

53. Yamashita, J., M. Ogawa, K. Inada, S. Yamashita, Y. Nakashima, T. Saishoji, and K. Nomura. 1993. Breast cancer prognosis is poor when total plasminogen activator activity is low. *Br. J. Cancer* **67:** 374–378.

54. Duffy, M. J., D. Reilly, C. O'Sullivan, N. O'Higgins, J. J. Fennelly, and P. Andreasen. 1990. Urokinase-plasminogen activator, a new and independent prognostic marker in breast cancer. *Cancer Res.* **50:** 6827–6829.

55. Grøndahl-Hansen, J., I. J. Christensen, C. Rosenquist, N. Brünner, H. T. Mouridsen, K. Danø, and M. Blichert-Toft. 1993. High levels of urokinase-type plasminogen activator and its inhibitor PAI-1 in cytosolic extracts of breast carcinomas are associated with poor prognosis. *Cancer Res.* **53:** 2513–2521.

56. Jänicke, F., M. Schmitt, K. Ulm, W. Gossner, and H. Graeff. 1989. Urokinase-type plasminogen activator antigen and early relapse in breast cancer [letter]. *Lancet* **2:** 1049.

57. Benraad, T. J., J. Geurts-Moespot, J. Grøndahl-Hansen, M. Schmitt, J. J. Heuvel, W. J. de, J. A. Foekens, R. E. Leake, N. Brunner, and C. G. Sweep. 1996. Immunoassays (ELISA) of urokinase-type plasminogen activator (uPA): report of an EORTC/ BIOMED-1 workshop. *Eur. J. Cancer* **32A:**1371–1381.

58. von Tempelhoff, G., L. Heilmann, M. Dietrich, D. Schneider, F. Niemann, and G. Hommel. 1997. Plasmatic plasminogen activator inhibitor activity in patients with primary breast cancer [letter]. *Thromb. Haemost.* **77:** 606–608.

59. Foekens, J. A., M. Schmitt, W. L. van Putten, H. A. Peters, M. D. Kramer, F. Janicke, and J. G. Klijn. 1994. Plasminogen activator inhibitor-1 and prognosis in primary breast cancer. *J. Clin. Oncol.* **12:** 1648- 1658.

60. Ganesh, S., C. F. Sier, M. M. Heerding, K. J. van, G. Griffioen, K. Welvaart, van de Velde CJ, J. H. Verheijen, C. B. Lamers, and H. W. Verspaget. 1997. Contribution of plasminogen activators and their inhibitors to the survival prognosis of patients with Dukes' stage B and C colorectal cancer. *Br. J. Cancer* **75:** 1793–1801.

61. Jänicke, F., M. Schmitt, L. Pache, K. Ulm, N. Harbeck, H. Hofler, and H. Graeff. 1993. Urokinase (uPA) and its inhibitor PAI-1 are strong and independent prognostic factors in node-negative breast cancer. *Breast Cancer Res. Treat.* **24:** 195–208.

62. Sweep, F., J. Geurtmoespot, N. Grebenschikov, H. De Witte, J. J. T. M. Heuvel, M. Scmitt, M. J. Duffy, M. D. Kramer, J. A. Foekens, N. Brünner, A. N. Pedersen, T. J. Benraad. 1998. External quality assessment of trans European antigen determination (ELISA) of urokinase-type plasminogen activator (UPA) and its type-1 inhibitor (PAi-1) in human breast cancer tissue extracts. *Br. J. Cancer*, in press.

63. Bouchet, C., F. Spyratos, P. M. Martin, K. Hacene, A. Gentile, and J. Oglobine. 1994. Prognostic value of urokinase-type plasminogen activator (uPA) and plasminogen activator inhibitors PAI-1 and PAI-2 in breast carcinomas. *Br. J. Cancer* **69:** 398–405.

64. Fernö, M., P.-O. Bendahl, Å. Borg, J. Brundell, L. Hirschberg, H. Olsson, and D. Killander. 1996. Urokinase plasminogen activator, a strong independent prognostic factor in breast cancer, analysed in steroid receptor cytosols with a luminometric immunoassay. *Eur. J. Cancer* **32A:** 793–801.

65. Duggan, C., T. Maguire, E. McDermott, N. O'Higgins, J. J. Fennelly, and M. J. Duffy. 1995. Urokinase plasminogen activator and urokinase plasminogen activator receptor in breast cancer. *Int. J. Cancer* **61:** 597–600.

66. Rønne, E., G. Høyer-Hansen, N. Brünner, H. Pedersen, F. Rank, C. K. Osborne, G. M. Clark, K. Danø, and J. Grøndahl-Hansen. 1995. Urokinase receptor in breast cancer tissue extracts. Enzyme-linked immunosorbent assay with a combination of mono- and polyclonal antibodies. *Breast Cancer Res. Treat.* 199–207.

67. Grøndahl-Hansen, J., H. A. Peters, L. J. van Putten, M. P. Look, H. Pappot, E. Rønne, K. Danø, J. G. M. Klijn, N. Brünner, and J. A. Foekens. 1995. Prognostic significance of the receptor for urokinase plasminogen activator in breast cancer. *Clin. Cancer Res.* **1:** 1079–1087.

68. Grøndahl-Hansen, J., I. J. Christensen, P. Briand, H. Pappot, H. T. Mouridsen, M. Blichert-Toft, K. Danø, and N. Brünner. 1997. Plasminogen activator inhibitor type 1 in cytosolic tumor extracts predicts prognosis in low-risk breast cancer patients. Clinical *Cancer Res.* **3:** 233–239.

69. Jänicke, F., L. Pache, M. Schmitt, K. Ulm, C. Thomssen, A. Prechtl, and H. Graeff. 1994. Both the cytosols and detergent extracts of breast cancer tissues are suited to evaluate the prognostic impact of the urokinase-type plasminogen activator and its inhibitor, plasminogen activator inhibitor type 1. *Cancer Res.* **54:** 2527–2530.

70. Pedersen, A. N., H. G. Hoyer, N. Brunner, G. M. Clark, B. Larsen, H. S. Poulsen, K. Dano, and R. W. Stephens. 1997. The complex between urokinase plasminogen activator and its type–1 inhibitor in breast cancer extracts quantitated by ELISA. *J. Immunol. Methods* **203:** 55–65.

71. Foucre, D., C. Bouchet, K. Hacene, N. Pourreau-Schneider, A. Gentile, P. M. Martin, A. Desplaces, and J. Oglobine. 1991. Relationship between cathepsin D, urokinase, and plasminogen activator inhibitors in malignant vs benign breast tumours. *Br. J. Cancer* **64:** 926–932.

72. Hildenbrand, R., I. Dilger, A. Horlin, and H. J. Stutte. 1995. Urokinase plasminogen activator induces angiogenesis and tumor vessel invasion in breast cancer. *Pathol. Res. Pract.* **191:** 403–409.

73. Foekens, J. A., M. Schmitt, P. W. van, H. A. Peters, M. Bontenbal, F. Janicke, and J. G. Klijn. 1992. Prognostic value of urokinase-type plasminogen activator in 671 primary breast cancer patients. *Cancer Res.* **52:** 6101–6105.

74. Spyratos, F., P. M. Martin, K. Hacene, S. Romain, C. Andrieu, M. Ferrero-Pous, S. Deytieux, D. V. Le, M. Tubiana-Hulin, and M. Brunet. 1992. Multiparametric prognostic evaluation of biological factors in primary breast cancer. *J. Natl. Cancer Inst.* **84:** 1266–1272.

75. Duffy, M. J., D. Reilly, E. McDermott, N. O'Higgins, J. J. Fennelly, and P. A. Andreasen. 1994. Urokinase plasminogen activator as a prognostic marker in different subgroups of patients with breast cancer. *Cancer* **74:** 2276–2280.

76. Foekens, J. A., M. P. Look, H. A. Peters, P. W. van, H. Portengen, and J. G. Klijn. 1995. Urokinase- type plasminogen activator and its inhibitor PAI-1: predictors of poor response to tamoxifen therapy in recurrent breast cancer. *J. Natl. Cancer Inst.* **87:** 751–756.

77. Needham, G. K., G. V. Sherbet, J. R. Farndon, and A. L. Harris. 1987. Binding of urokinase to specific receptor sites on human breast cancer membranes. *Br. J. Cancer* **55:** 13–16.

78. Sumiyoshi, K., K. Serizawa, T. Urano, Y. Takada, A. Takada, and S. Baba. 1992. Plasminogen activator system in human breast cancer. *Int. J. Cancer* **50:** 345–348.

79. Kristensen, P., C. Pyke, L. R. Lund, P. A. Andreasen, and K. Danø. 1990. Plasminogen activator inhibitor-type 1 in Lewis lung carcinoma. Histochemistry **93:** 559–566.

80. Pyke, C., P. Kristensen, E. Ralfkiœr, J. Eriksen, and K. Danø. 1991. The plasminogen activation system in human colon cancer: messenger RNA for the inhibitor PAI-1 is located in endothelial cells in the tumor stroma. *Cancer Res.* **51:** 4067–4071.

81. Jänicke, F., C. Thomssen, L. Pache, M. Schmitt, and H. Graeff. 1994. Urokinase (uPA) and PAI-1 as selection criteria for adjuvant chemotherapy in axillary node-negative breast cancer patients, in Prospects in Diagnosis and Treatment of Breast Cancer (Scmitt, M., et al., eds.), Elsevier, Amsterdam, pp. 207–218.

82. Oka, T., T. Ishida, T. Nishino, and K. Sugimachi. 1991. Immunohistochemical evidence of urokinase-type plasminogen activator in primary and metastatic tumors of pulmonary adenocarcinoma. *Cancer Res.* **51:** 3522–3525.

83. Pedersen, H., N. Brünner, D. Francis, K. Østerlind, E. Rønne, H. H. Hansen, K. Danø, and J. Grøndahl-Hansen. 1994. Prognostic impact of urokinase, urokinase receptor, and type 1 plasminogen activator inhibitor in squamous and large cell lung cancer tissue. *Cancer Res.* **54:** 4671–4675.

84. Pedersen, H., J. Grøndahl-Hansen, D. Francis, K. Østerlind, H. H. Hansen, K. Danø, and N. Brünner. 1994. Urokinase and plasminogen activator inhibitor type 1 in pulmonary adenocarcinoma. *Cancer Res.* **54:** 120–123.

85. Mulcahy, H. E., M. J. Duffy, D. Gibbons, P. McCarthy, N. A. Parfrey, D. P. O'Donoghue, and K. Sheahan. 1994. Urokinase-type plasminogen activator and outcome in Dukes' B colorectal cancer. *Lancet* **344:** 583–584.

86. Heiss, M. M., H. Allgayer, K. U. Gruetzner, I. Funke, R. Babic, K. W. Jauch, and F. W. Schildberg. 1995. Individual development and uPA-receptor expression of disseminated tumour cells in bone marrow: a reference to early systemic disease in solid cancer. *Nat. Med.* **1:** 1035–1039.

87. Nekarda, H., M. Schmitt, K. Ulm, A. Wenninger, H. Vogelsang, K. Becker, J. D. Roder, U. Fink, and J. R. Siewert. 1994. Prognostic impact of urokinase-type plasminogen activator and its inhibitor PAI–1 in completely resected gastric cancer. *Cancer Res.* **54:** 2900–2907.

88. Plebani, M., L. Herszènyi, P. Carraro, M. D. Paoli, G. Roveroni, R. Cardin, Z. Tulassay, R. Naccarato, and F. Farinati. 1997. Urokinase-type plasminogen activator receptor in gastric cancer: tissue expression and prognostic role. *Clin. Exp. Metastasis* **15:** 418–425.

89. Kuhn, W., L. Pache, B. Schmalfeldt, P. Dettmar, M. Schmitt, F. Jänicke, and H. Graeff. 1994. Urokinase (uPA) and PAI–1 predict survival in advanced ovarian cancer patients (FIGO III) after radical surgery and platinum-based chemotherapy. *Gyn. Oncol.* 401–409.

90. Kobayashi, H., S. Fujishiro, and T. Terao. 1994. Impact of urokinase-type plasminogen activator and its inhibitor type 1 on prognosis in cervical cancer of the uterus. *Cancer Res.* **54:** 6539–6548.

91. Hofmann, R., A. Lehmer, M. Buresch, R. Hartung, and K. Ulm. 1996. Clinical relevance of urokinase plasminogen activator, its receptor, and its inhibitor in patients with renal cell carcinoma. *Cancer* **78:** 487–492.

92. Hasui, Y., K. Marutsuka, J. Suzumiya, S. Kitada, Y. Osada, and A. Sumiyoshi. 1992. The content of urokinase-type plasminogen activator antigen as a prognostic factor in urinary bladder cancer. *Int. J. Cancer* **50:** 871–873.

93. Hsu, D. W., J. T. Efird, and W. E. Hedley. 1995. Prognostic role of urokinase-type plasminogen activator in human gliomas. *Am. J. Pathol.* **147:** 114–123.

94. Witte, H. D., H. Pappot, N. Brünner, J. Grøndahl-Hansen, G. Høyer-Hansen, N. Behrendt, B. Guldhammer-Skov, F. Sweep, T. Benraad, and K. Danø. 1997. ELISA for complexes between urokinase-type plasminogen activator and its receptor in lung cancer tissue extracts. *Int. J. Cancer* **72:** 416-423.

95. Mignatti, P., E. Robbins, and D. B. Rifkin. 1986. Tumor invasion through the human amniotic membrane: Requirement for a proteinase cascade. *Cell* **47:** 487–498.

96. Meissauer, A., M. D. Kramer, M. Hofmann, L. J. Erkell, E. Jacob, V. Schirrmacher, and G. Brunner. 1991. Urokinase-type and tissue-type plasminogen activators are essential for in vitro invasion of human melanoma cells. *Exp. Cell Res.* **192:** 453–459.

97. Crowley, C. W., R. L. Cohen, B. K. Lucas, G. Liu, M. A. Shuman, and A. D. Levinson. 1993. Preven tion of metastasis by inhibition of the urokinase receptor. *Proc. Natl. Acad. Sci. USA* **90:** 5021–5025.

98. Kobayashi, H., H. Ohi, H. Shinohara, M. Sugimura, T. Fujii, T. Terao, M. Schmitt, L. Goretzki, N. Chucholowski, F. Janicke, and et al. 1993. Saturation of tumour cell surface

receptors for urokinase- type plasminogen activator by amino-terminal fragment and subsequent effect on reconstituted basement membranes invasion. *Br. J. Cancer* **67**: 537–544.

99. Quattrone, A., G. Fibbi, E. Anichini, M. Pucci, A. Zamperini, S. Capaccioli, and R. M. Del. 1995. Reversion of the invasive phenotype of transformed human fibroblasts by anti-messenger oligonucleotide inhibition of urokinase receptor gene expression. *Cancer Res.* **55**: 90–95.

100. Schlechte, W., M. Brattain, and D. Boyd. 1990. Invasion of extracellular matrix by cultured colon cancer cells: dependence on urokinase receptor display. *Cancer Commun.* **2**: 173–179.

101. Stonelake, P. S., C. E. Jones, J. P. Neoptolemos, and P. R. Baker. 1997. Proteinase inhibitors reduce basement membrane degradation by human breast cancer cell lines. *Br. J. Cancer* **75**: 951–959.

102. Lage, A., J. W. Diaz, and I. Gonzalez. 1978. Effect of proteinase inhibitor in experimental tumors. *Neoplasma* **25**: 257–259.

103. Ogawa, H., F. Sekiguchi, N. Tanaka, K. Ono, K. Tanaka, M. Kinjo, A. Iwakawa, and S. Naito. 1982. Effect of antifibrinolysis treatment on human cancer in nude mice. *Anticancer Res.* **2**: 339–344.

104. Ohkoshi, M. 1980. Effect of aprotinin on growth of 3-methylcholanthrene-induced squamous cell- carcinoma in mice. *Gann.* **71**: 246–250.

105. Ossowski, L. and E. Reich. 1983. Antibodies to plasminogen activator inhibit human tumor metastasis. *Cell* **35**: 611–619.

106. Ossowski, L., H. Russo-Payne, and E. L. Wilson. 1991. Inhibition of urokinase-type plasminogen activator by antibodies: The effect on dissemination of a human tumor in the nude mouse. *Cancer Res.* **51**: 274–281.

107. Wilhelm, O., M. Schmitt, S. Hohl, R. Senekowitsch, and H. Graeff. 1995. Antisense inhibition of urokinase reduces spread of human ovarian cancer in mice. *Clin. Exp. Metastasis* **13**: 296–302.

108. Yamamoto, T., K. Shiroshita, J. Kitawaki, and H. Okada. 1989. The inductive effects of pro gestogens on aromatase activity in stromal cells of human uterine endometrium. *J. End. Invest.* **12**: 201–204.

109. Holst-Hansen, C., B. Johannesen, G. Høyer-Hansen, J. Rømer, V. Ellis, and N. Brünner. 1996. Urokinase-type plasminogen activation in three human breast cancer cell lines correlates with their in vitro invasiveness. *Clin. Exp. Metastasis* **14**: 297–307

110. Pollanen, J., R. W. Stephens, and A. Vaheri. 1991. Directed plasminogen activation at the surface of normal and malignant cells. *Adv. Cancer Res.* **57**: 273–328.

111. Rønne, E., N. Behrendt, V. Ellis, M. Ploug, K. Danø, and G. Høyer-Hansen. 1991. Cell-induced potentiation of the plasminogen activation system is abolished by a monoclonal antibody that recognizes the NH-terminal domain of the urokinase receptor. *FEBS Lett.* **288**: 233–236.

112. Hoosein, N. M., D. D. Boyd, W. J. Hollas, A. Mazar, J. Henkin, and W. K. Chung. 1991. Involvement of urokinase and its receptor in the invasiveness of human prostatic carcinoma cell lines. *Cancer Commun.* **3**: 255–264.

113. Stahl, A. and B. M. Mueller. 1994a. Binding of urokinase to its receptor promotes migration and invasion of human melanoma cells in vitro. *Cancer Res.* **54**: 3066–3071.

114. Hollas, W., F. Blasi, and D. Boyd. 1991. Role of the urokinase receptor in facilitating extracellular matrix invasion by cultured colon cancer. *Cancer Res.* **51**: 3690–3695.

115. Kobayashi, H., J. Gotoh, H. Shinohara, N. Moniwa, and T. Terao. 1994. Inhibition of the metastasis of Lewis lung carcinoma by antibody against urokinase-type plasminogen activator in the experimental and spontaneous metastasis model. *Thromb. Haemost.* **71**: 474–480.

116. Lu, H., C. Mabilat, P. Yeh, J. D. Guitton, H. Li, M. Pouchelet, D. Shoevaert, Y. Legrand, J. Soria, and C. Soria. 1996. Blockage of urokinase receptor reduces in vitro the motility and the deformability of endothelial cells. *FEBS Lett.* **380:** 21–24.

117. Luparello, C. and R. M. Del. 1996. In vitro anti-proliferative and anti-invasive role of aminoterminal fragment of urokinase-type plasminogen activator on 8701-BC breast cancer cells. *Eur. J. Cancer* **32A:** 702–707.

118. Wilhelm, O., U. Weidle, S. Hohl, P. Rettenberger, M. Schmitt, and H. Graeff. 1994. Recombinant soluble urokinase receptor as a scavenger for urokinase-type plasminogen activator (uPA). Inhibition of proliferation and invasion of human ovarian cancer cells. *FEBS Lett.* **337:** 131–134.

119. Kobayashi, H., H. Shinohara, M. Fujie, J. Gotoh, M. Itoh, K. Takeuchi, and T. Terao. 1995. Inhibition of metastasis of Lewis lung carcinoma by urinary trypsin inhibitor in experimental and spontaneous metastasis models. *Int. J. Cancer* **63:** 455–462.

120. Mohanam, S., S. K. Chintala, Y. Go, A. Bhattacharya, B. Venkaiah, D. Boyd, Z. L. Gokaslan, R. Sawaya, and J. S. Rao. 1997. In vitro inhibition of human glioblastoma cell line invasiveness by antisense uPA receptor. *Oncogene* **14:** 1351–1359.

121. Kook, Y. H., J. Adamski, A. Zelent, and L. Ossowski. 1994. The effect of antisense inhibition of urokinase receptor in human squamous cell carcinoma on malignancy. *EMBO J.* **13:** 3983–3991.

122. Min, H. Y., L. V. Doyle, C. R. Vitt, C. L. Zandonella, J. R. Stratton Thomas, M. A. Shuman, and S. Rosenberg. 1996. Urokinase receptor antagonists inhibit angiogenesis and primary tumor growth in syngeneic mice. *Cancer Res.* **56:** 2428–2433.

123. Kobayashi, H., J. Gotoh, M. Fujie, H. Shinohara, N. Moniwa, and T. Terao. 1994. Inhibition of metastasis of Lewis lung carcinoma by a synthetic peptide within growth factor-like domain of urokinase in the experimental and spontaneous metastasis model. *Int. J. Cancer* **57:** 727–733.

124. Liu, G., M. A. Shuman, and R. L. Cohen. 1995. Co-expression of urokinase, urokinase receptor and PAI-1 is necessary for optimum invasiveness of cultured lung cancer cells. *Int. J. Cancer* **60:** 501–506.

125. Eitzman, D. T., J. C. Krauss, T. Shen, J. Cui, and Ginsburg. 1996. Lack of plasminogen activator inhibitor-1 effect in a transgenic mouse model of metastatic melanoma. *Blood* **87:** 4718–4722.

126. Delbaldo, C., I. Masouye, J. H. Saurat, J. D. Vassalli, and A. P. Sappino. 1994. Plasminogen activation in melanocytic neoplasia. *Cancer Res.* **54:** 4547–4552.

127. Soff, G. A., J. Sanderowitz, S. Gately, E. Verrusio, I. Weiss, S. Brem, and H. C. Kwaan. 1995. Expression of plasminogen activator inhibitor type 1 by human prostate carcinoma cells inhibits primary tumor growth, tumor-associated angiogenesis, and metastasis to lung and liver in an athymic mouse model. *J. Clin. Invest.* **96:** 2593–2600.

128. Quax, P. H., G. N. van Muijen, E. J. Weening Verhoeff, L. R. Lund, K. Dano, D. J. Ruiter, and J. H. Verheijen. 1991. Metastatic behavior of human melanoma cell lines in nude mice correlates with urokinase-type plasminogen activator, its type-1 inhibitor, and urokinase-mediated matrix degradation. *J. Cell Biol.* **115:** 191–199.

129. Tsuchiya, H., S. Katsuo, E. Matsuda, C. Sunayama, K. Tomita, Y. Ueda, and B. R. Binder. 1995. The antibody to plasminogen activator inhibitor-1 suppresses pulmonary metastases of human fibrosarcoma in athymic mice. *Gen. Diagn. Pathol.* **141:** 41–48.

130. Stefansson, S. and D. A. Lawrence. 1996. The serpin pai-1 inhibits cell migration by blocking integrin alpha(v)beta(3) binding to vitronectin. *Nature* **383:** 441–443.

131. Kjoller, L., S. M. Kanse, T. Kirkegaard, K. W. Rodenburg, E. Ronne, S. L. Goodman, K. T. Preissner, L. Ossowski, and P. A. Andreasen. 1997. Plasminogen activator inhibitor-1 represses integrin- and vitronectin-mediated cell migration independently of its function as an inhibitor of plasminogen activation. *Exp. Cell Res.* **232:** 420–429.

132. Petzelbauer, E., J. P. Springhorn, A. M. Tucker, and J. A. Madri. 1996. Role of plasminogen activator inhibitor in the reciprocal regulation of bovine aortic endothelial and smooth muscle cell migration by TGF-beta 1. *Am. J. Pathol.* **149:** 923–931.

133. Stahl, A. and B. M. Mueller. 1997. Melanoma cell migration on vitronectin: regulation by components of the plasminogen activation system. *Int. J. Cancer* **71:** 116–122.

134. Estreicher, A., J. Mühlhauser, J. L. Carpentier, L. Orci, and J. D. Vassalli. 1990. The receptor for urokinase type plasminogen activator polarizes expression of the protease to the leading edge of migrating monocytes and promotes degradation of enzyme inhibitor complexes. *J. Cell Biol.* **111:** 783–792.

135. Stahl, A. and B. M. Mueller. 1994b. Binding of urokinase to its receptor promotes migration and invasion of human melanoma cells in vitro. *Cancer Res.* **54:** 3066–3071.

136. Bruckner, A., A. E. Filderman, J. C. Kirchheimer, B. R. Binder, and H. G. Remold. 1992. Endogenous receptor-bound urokinase mediates tissue invasion of the human lung carcinoma cell lines A549 and Calu-1. *Cancer Res.* **52:** 3043–3047.

137. Kirchheimer, J. C., J. Wojta, G. Christ, and B. R. Binder. 1989. Functional inhibition of endoge nously produced urokinase decreases cell proliferation in a human melanoma cell line. *Proc. Natl. Acad. Sci. USA* **86:** 5424–5428.

138. Mueller, B. M., Y. B. Yu, and W. E. Laug. 1995. Overexpression of plasminogen activator inhibitor 2 in human melanoma cells inhibits spontaneous metastasis in scid/scid mice. *Proc. Natl. Acad. Sci. USA* **92:** 205–209.

139. Evans, D. M. and P. L. Lin. 1995. Suppression of pulmonary metastases of rat mammary cancer by recombinant urokinase plasminogen activator inhibitor. *Am. Surg.* **61:** 692–696.

140. Shapiro, R. L., J. G. Duquette, D. F. Roses, I. Nunes, M. N. Harris, H. Kamino, E. L. Wilson, and D. B. Rifkin. 1996. Induction of primary cutaneous melanocytic neoplasms in urokinase-type plasminogen activator (uPA)-deficient and wild-type mice: cellular blue nevi invade but do not progress to malignant melanoma in uPA-deficient animals. *Cancer Res.* **56:** 3597–3604.

16

Angiogenesis in Breast Cancer

Role in Biology, Tumor Progression, and Prognosis

Giampietro Gasparini

1. INTRODUCTION

The terminal ductal-lobular unit, which includes both a lobule and its most proximal ducts, is thought to be the structure of the mammary gland from which breast cancer develops. Tumorigenesis of mammary cells is likely to involve multistep, sequential, and coordinated molecular changes be accompanied by morphologically distinguishable alterations during the evolution from benign hyperplasia to atypical hyperplasia, and from *in situ* carcinoma to invasive cancer (reviewed in ref. *1*). At least four distinct characteristics are needed for a normal cell to progress to a neoplastic cell and to give rise to an invasive cancer. The first step is a deregulation of the cell cycle with consequent abnormal proliferation; the second step is the suppression of the pathways leading to apoptosis; the third, the acquisition of new characteristics able to induce alterations of the microenvironment where its growth potential can be realized; and the fourth step is that a tumor must also avoid destruction by the immune system (reviewed in ref. 32). Among the latter, the acquisition of the angiogenic phenotype is necessary for the passage from *in situ* to the invasive stage of breast cancer (reviewed in ref. *2*). Solid tumors are composed of tumor cells (parenchyma) and the surrounding extracellular matrix and stromal cells (stroma) *(4)*. Recent studies have shown that a mutual reciprocal stimulation may occur between tumor and stromal cells, which is mediated by several cytokines, growth factors acting via paracrine mechanisms *(5)*, and by adhesion molecules *(6)*.

Angiogenesis, i.e., the neoformation of microvessels from pre-existing blood vessels, is one of the essential conditions to create a permissive environment facilitating tumor growth beyond minimal dimensions *(7)* and it is also involved in the cascade of events permitting metastasis *(8)*.

There is evidence that most tumors are angiogenesis-dependent for their growth, even if a recent study undertaken in human non-small-cell lung cancer has identified a minority of lung-invasive cancers that seem capable to develop without evident neovascularization *(9)*.

From: Breast Cancer: Molecular Genetics, Pathogenesis, and Therapeutics
Edited by: A. M. Bowcock © Humana Press Inc., Totowa, NJ

2. STUDIES SUGGESTING
THAT BREAST CANCER IS ANGIOGENESIS-DEPENDENT

The exact mechanisms by which breast-cancer cells acquire the angiogenic pheno-type are not yet well-known *(3)*. However, it is presumed that neovascularization is the result of an altered balance between angiogenesis stimulation and inhibition *(10)* in favor of the first. Early studies by Brem et al. *(11,12)* and Jensen et al. *(13)* suggest that angiogenesis precedes the transformation of mammary hyperplasia to carcinoma in both chemically induced breast cancer in mice *(11)* and in human breast tissues *(12,13)*, respectively. Several more recent studies conducted on different experimental models found that up-regulation of angiogenic polypeptides is involved in breast-cancer tumor growth and metastasis (reviewed in ref. *14*). At present, two families of angiogenic factors, namely fibroblast growth factors (FGFs) and vascular endothelial growth factors (VEGFs) seem to play a major role in breast cancer angiogenesis. Table 1 summa-rizes the more relevant studies suggesting that angiogenesis is a necessary step for breast-cancer progression and metastasis.

The overexpression of angiogenic factors coupled with the abnormal expression of some stromal molecules such as integrin $\alpha6$ *(15)*, integrin $\alpha_v\beta_3$ *(16)* and tissue factor *(17,18)* induces altered interactions of tumor cells with the structural components of extracellular matrix which can facilitate tumor-cell invasiveness and neovascularization *(19–21)*. The results of a recent study shown that bFGF stimulates expression of the integrin $\alpha_v\beta_3$,which cooperates with the tissue metalloproteinase MMP-2 in the degra-dation of extracellular matrix *(22)*. Also, tenascin *(23)* and the 67Kda-laminin receptor *(24)* are overexpressed approximately in one-third and two-thirds of invasive breast cancers, respectively, and are associated with tumor progression.

In general, as recently suggested by Brooks *(6)*, during tumor progression and angiogenesis dynamic modifications of extracellular matrix occur. These alterations are mediated by the activation of several proteolytic enzymes that degrade structural proteins and by the new synthesis of abnormal amount of some molecules such as laminin, collagens, fibronectin, integrins, and immunoglobulin-like molecules, are per-missive for tumor growth and invasiveness.

A number of clinicopathologic studies have assessed the degree of vascularization of benign lesions, *in situ* and invasive carcinomas of the breast. Using markers specific for endothelial cells and immunohistochemical techniques, it is possible to obtain a static quantitative measure of angiogenesis that is presumed to be the result of the balance of angiogenic and angioinhibitory stimuli *(25)*.

Guinebretiere and colleagues *(26)* found that the more vascularized a fibrocystic lesion is, the higher the likelihood is of the patient developing an invasive breast can-cer. The seminal study of Weidner et al. *(25)* was the first to show a correlation of intratumoral microvessel density and metastasis in invasive breast cancer. The authors *(25)* also described the concomitant presence of both avascular and vascular ductal *in situ* carcinomas in areas adjacent to invasive cancer.

Subsequent studies by Guidi et al. *(27)*, Heffelfinger et al. *(28)*, Lee et al. *(29)*, and Engels et al. *(30)* confirmed, in larger series of patients with *in situ* carcinomas of the breast, the presence of both avascular and vascular lesions. Moreover, two characteris-tic patterns of neovascularization associated with *in situ* carcinomas have been identi-

Table 1
Studies Suggesting that Breast Carcinoma is Angiogenesis-Dependent

Author	Ref.	Study
Indirect Evidence		
Brem	*(11)*	In an invivo model of neovascularization in rabbit iris, it was shown that angiogenesis precedes transformation of mammary hyperplasia to carcinoma in chemically-induced neoplastic mouse mammary fragments.
Jensen	*(13)*	Angiogenesis preceeds transformation of normal cells to cancer cells in human breast tissue.
Liotta	*(32)*	Tumor vascularization is associated with hematogenous metastasis following tumor implantation.
McLeskey, Costa	*(86,87)*	FGFs induce tumor growth and favor metastasis in human breast-cancer cell lines in vitro and transplanted in mice in vivo.
Kurebayashi	*(44)*	Co-transfection with FGF4 and *Lac 2* induces rapid growth and metastasis in nude-mice transfectants of MCF-7.
Zhang	*(45)*	Transfection of cancer cells with $VEGF_{121}$ induces rapid tumor growth and rich vascularization in vivo.
Guinebretiere	*(26)*	The degree of intralesional vascularization of fibrocistyc disease is associated with the risk of patients of developing invasive cancer.
Weidner	*(25)*	The degree of intratumoral vascularization is associated with metastasis in invasive breast cancer.
Brooks	*(16)*	Integrin $\alpha_v\beta_3$, which is essential for angiogenesis, is involved in breast-cancer progression.
Contrino	*(17)*	Tussue factor is a marker of angiogenic phenotype and of malignancy in breast cancer.
Vrana	*(18)*	Expression of tissue factor correlates with progression to invasive cancer.
McCulloch	*(31)*	The degree of vascularization of primary breast cancer is associated with tumor cell shedding into venous blood during surgery.
Zajchowski	*(33)*	Thrombospondin-1 expression is often lost in tumors.
Weinstat-Saslow	*(39)*	Thrombospondin-1, an endogenous angiogenesis inhibitor, suppresses tumor growth and metastasis in vivo.
Volpert	*(35)*	Thrombospondin-1 production in response to wtp53 can switch breast-cancer cells to an antiangiogenic phenotype.
Direct Evidence		
Weinstat-Saslow	*(39)*	Transfection of breast cancer cells with thrombospondin 1 causes inhibition of angiogenesis, tumor growth, and metastasis in vivo.
Brooks	*(16)*	Systemic therapy with the antibody LM609 neutralizating integrin $\alpha_v\beta_3$ blocks angiogenesis and induces tumor regression in vivo.
O'Reilly	*(40)*	Systemic therapy with angiostatin inhibits angiogenesis, prolongs tumor dormancy, and prevents metastasis growth in vivo.

fied: the more frequent is the diffuse presence of microvessels within the stroma. The other pattern is a cuffing of tumor cells around microvessels in involved spaces. High diffuse stromal neovascularization is associated with comedo-type lesions, desmoplasia, elevated cell kinetics, and other markers of biological aggressiveness *(27–30)* (Table 2). Therefore, this pattern may be associated with a major risk of developing an invasive cancer. Prospective clinicopathologic studies are warranted to verify this finding.

The elegant study by McCulloch et al. *(31)* suggests a direct relationship of the degree of vascularization of primary breast-invasive tumors with the presence of tumor cell shedding into effluent venous blood during surgery. This observation coupled with the study by Liotta et al. *(32)* showing that the extent of tumor vascularization is associated with hematogenous metastasis following tumor implantation in experimental animal models, strongly suggest a relationship of angiogenesis with metastasis. Indirect evidence of the role of angiogenesis in breast-cancer growth, progression, and metastasis also emerges from the studies that assessed the biological effects of endogenous angiogenesis inhibitors. Among these, thrombospondin 1 (TSP-1) was up to now the more studied. Zajchowski et al. *(33)* found that overexpression of TSP-1 is associated with suppression of tumor-forming ability in MCF-7 human breast-cancer cells fused with immortal mammary epithelial cells.

The Bouck group first suggested that TSP-1 is regulated, in certain cells, by wild-type p53 *(34)*. For example, in the BT549 human breast-cancer cell line, reintroduction of wild-type p53 upregulated the expression of TSP-1 with a consequent loss of the angiogenic phenotype *(35)*.

However, TSP-1 may play a variety of biological roles in breast cancer. Incardona et al. *(36)* found that TSP-1 modulates adhesion of aggregates of breast-cancer cells to vascular endothelium in vitro. The authors suggested that these interactions may facilitate the hematogenous spread of tumor cells. Arnoletti et al. *(37)* showed that treatment of MDA-MB-231 breast cancer cells with either TSP-1 or transforming growth factor β_1 (TGF-β_1)caused increased secretion of urokinase-type plasminogen activator (uPA) and plasminogen activator inhibitor-1 with a concomitant decrease in plasmin activity. These authors *(37)* suggested that TSP-1 is an adhesive molecule that through activation of TGF-β1 may modulate cell-surface protease expression and promote metastasis by an uPA-mediated cell-invasion mechanism, although if this were true, one would expect more, not less, plasmin activation.

More recently, Bertin et al. *(35)* studied TSP-1 and -2 messenger RNA overexpression in normal, benign, and invasive breast cancer. They observed that both TSP-1 and -2 were overexpressed in invasive ductal breast carcinomas compared to normal and benign lesions. Moreover, expression of TSP-1 in invasive cancers did not significantly correlate with the conventional prognostic indicators, but it was higher in desmoplastic-rich stroma tumors as well as in highly vascularized cancers. Therefore, at present, it is difficult to conclude under which circumstances TSP-1 exerts antiangiogenic or pro-angiogenic activity in human breast cancer. As reported in table 1, three elegant published studies give direct evidence that breast cancer is an angiogenesis-dependent neoplasia. Weinstat-Saslow and colleagues *(39)* found that transfection of TSP-1 complementary DNA in the metastatic human cell line MDA-435 strongly inhibited in vivo neovascularization of the neoplastic lesions and reduced the

Table 2
Characteristics of Vascularization of In Situ Carcinomas

Author	Endothelial marker	Number of patients	Patterns of vascularization		Association of high vascularity with the other features
			Diffuse stromal microvessels (%)	Microvessels cuffing the involved spaces (%)	
Guidi (27)	fVIII-RA	55	62	38	Diffuse pattern of vascularization is associated with: Comedo-type lesions Marked desmoplasia c-erbB-2 expression High cell kinetics
Heffelfinger (28)	fVIII-RA	90	70	30	High vascularization is associated with: Coincidental invasion Proliferative breast disease Lobular-type lesions Comedo-type lesions
Lee (29)	fVIII-RA	41	58	42	High vascularization is associated with: Inflammation c-erbB-2 expression
Engels (30)	fVIII-RA	75	57	43	Vascularization is associated with: High-grade DCIS lesions

number of lung metastasis over the parental (control) tumor cell line. A second study by Brooks et al. *(16)* showed that systemic therapy with the LM609 monoclonal antibody (MAb)against $\alpha_v\beta_3$ integrin blocked angiogenesis and induced regression of transplanted human breast cancer in a severe combined immunodeficient (SCID) mouse/human chimera model in vivo.

Finally, Folkman's group *(40)* administered angiostatin, one of the more potent inhibitors of angiogenesis up to now sequenced and developed, to nude mice bearing MDA-MBV human breast cancer. The systemic administration of this endogenous angiosuppressive polypeptide induced the rapid inhibition of angiogenesis and regression of the volume of transplanted tumors.

Overall, the findings of the studies up to now performed on angiogenesis in breast cancer suggest that angiogenesis occurs as an early step during tumor progression *(3)*, that it is involved in the cascade of events permitting metastasis *(41)*, and that angiosuppression is a promising new therapeutic approach, worthy of clinical testing *(42)*.

3. ANGIOGENESIS AND HORMONE PATHWAYS IN THE CONTROL OF TUMOR GROWTH

Recently Kern and Lippman *(14)* suggested a model of tumorigenesis in breast cancer in which a combination of mitogenic (amplification of c-erbB-2 oncogene; overexpression of epidermal growth factor [EGF] and estrogens) and angiogenic stimuli cooperate in facilitating tumor growth and metastasis. In endocrine-related cancers, such as breast cancer, very complex relationships may develop involving hormone pathways, tumor growth factors, and their receptors that may act via autocrine and paracrine mechanisms as well as oncogenes and tumor-suppressor genes *(34,43)*. During the process of breast-cancer progression, stromal cells including endothelial cells, fibroblasts, mononuclear cells, mast cells, and so on, may play an active role by producing enzymes, diffusible growth factors, and cytokines, which stimulate the malignant epithelial component (parenchyma) to grow (reviewed in ref. *43*). However, our present knowledge of the pathways regulating hormone and angiogenesis in breast cancer suggests that endocrine factors and neovascularization act as separate growth-signaling pathways as reviewed by Gasparini *(2)*. This conclusion is mainly based on the experimental studies showing that members of the FGF family are able to induce tumor growth and metastasis without estrogen supplementation in MCF-7 breast-cancer cells *(44)*, and that upon transfection of MCF-7 cells with VEGF121, they acquire a growth advantage without any effect on their estrogen dependence or tamoxifen sensitivity *(45)*. Moreover, studies on the expression of several angiogenic polypeptides in human breast cancer did not find any relationship of VEGF *(46–48)*, thymidine phosphorylase *(49,50)*, or hepatocyte growth factor *(51)* with the estrogen receptor status. In addition, a large number of clinicopathologic studies investigating vascularization of invasive primary breast cancer as a prognostic tool do not find a significant relationship between the intratumoral microvessel density (IMD) and the expression of hormone receptors, independent of disease-stage, age, and menopausal status of the patients (reviewed in ref. *2*).

The studies by Macaulay et al. *(52)* and Gasparini et al. *(53)*, selectively performed in patients treated with adjuvant tamoxifen, found that high angiogenesis (i.e., microvessel counts) and lack of estrogen receptor are unfavorable independent prognostic factors. Thus the subgroup of patients with estrogen receptor-negative and weakly vascularized tumors had good prognosis and, perhaps, gained benefit from tamoxifen. Conversely, the subgroup of patients with estrogen receptor-positive and highly vascularized tumors had worse prognosis even if treated with tamoxifen *(53)*.

4. RELATIONSHIP OF ANGIOGENESIS WITH THE OTHER BIOLOGICAL PROGNOSTIC MARKERS IN INVASIVE BREAST CANCER

The main prerequisites for a new prognostic marker are:

1. It should be related to a well-defined biological mechanism involved in tumor growth and metastasis;
2. It needs to add useful prognostic information over conventional prognostic markers;
3. Its method of detection must be feasible and reproducible worldwide and, finally
4. Hopefully, it also may represent a surrogate marker of a target against which a new, selective, anticancer therapy may be developed *(54,55)*.

As far as human invasive breast cancer is concerned, several conventional prognostic indicators are currently in use and are employed to select subgroups of patients at different risk to be treated accordingly.

Among these, nodal status and estrogen-receptor status still represent the key prognostic factors for therapeutic decision in the adjuvant setting *(54)*. However, approx 20–30% of patients with node-negative disease do poorly and some with positive hormone receptors do not benefit from tamoxifen *(54)*. This clinical problem has justified the enormous efforts made in the last decade for the identification of new, biologically-related prognostic markers. Various measures of angiogenesis, mainly quantitation of microvessels within tumoral stroma, have been proposed *(56)*.

Most of the authors who determined intratumoral microvessel density in invasive breast carcinoma adopted the method suggested by Weidner et al. *(25)*. In brief, Weidner and associates *(25)* described a combined method based on the selection of paraffin-embedded blocks combining the invasive components of breast-cancer specimens by analyzing corresponding sections stained with hematoxylin and eosin. Using a conventional immunohistochemical technique, vessels were stained using the antibody to factor VIII-related antigen. Then the area of most vascularization ("vascular hot spot") was selected in each tumor by scanning the tumor section at low magnification (10–100×). Usually, vascular "hot spots" are encountered at the peripheral tumor margin and within this the microvessels are counted at higher magnification (400×) in order to be able to count each individual vessel.

Weidner et al. *(25,57)* suggested that the optimal field size for counting microvessel cells or cell clusters clearly separate from adjacent microvessels or tumor cells or other stromal elements, should be regarded as a single, evaluable microvessel. Presence of a lumen is not required and a cut-off caliber size was not defined.

Certain authors introduced some changes to the method proposed by Weidner et al. *(25)* mainly by the use of different panendothelial markers *(52,58–62)* or by more relevant methodological deviances in counting or evaluating the degree of vascularization *(63–65)*. A critical review on the methodological aspects of quantification of angiogenesis in solid tumors has been recently published *(42)*. The relationship of vascularization to the conventional prognostic factors varies widely, in particular regarding nodal status and grading as reported in Table 3. In contrast, data suggesting a lack of association of angiogenesis with other biological prognostic markers is more homogeneous. These markers include: tumor cell-proliferation indexes (S-phase-fraction by flow cytometry, Ki-67 labeling and others), expression of p53 protein and c-erbB-2 oncogene, DNA ploidy and, as previously described, with hormone-receptor status (Table 3).

Few studies have appropriately investigated, in a sufficiently large and homogeneous series, whether angiogenesis and other biological markers are independent prognostic factors. A study by Gasparini et al. *(66)* performed in more than 250 patients with node-negative breast cancer assessed the prognostic value of angiogenesis, p53, and c-erbB-2 and found that both microvessels count and p53 protein expression retained statistical significance in multivariate analysis. However, a subsequent study from the same group *(60)* suggested that angiogenesis retained prognostic value in both the patients with node-negative and node-positive disease, whereas the prognostic contribution of p53 seemed to be restricted to the subgroup of patients with node-negative breast cancer. However, the results of the majority of the studies reported in Table 3 are to be considered with caution owing to the small and heterogeneous groups of patients evaluated in each single study and the limited power of the statistical analysis.

5. CLINICAL SIGNIFICANCE OF THE DETERMINATION OF ANGIOGENESIS

5.1. Prognosis

5.1.1. Prognostic Value of Intratumoral Microvessel Count

Studies reporting on the prognostic value of the determination of IMD *(55,67)* or expression of angiogenic peptides *(68)* have been recently reviewed. An update of published studies, with emphasis on the characteristics of the patients enrolled, is presented here. "Mixed series" are those that included patients with both node-negative and node-positive breast cancers; studies on node-negative patients included only homogeneous series of patients without axillary-node involvement at the time of surgery; and finally, studies on node-positive patients included series of patients who received adjuvant therapy. The aforementioned sub-classification is clinically relevant because the aims and the end-points of studying a prognostic factor are different among these subgroup of patients. Overall, of the 32 studies considered here, 23 studies (72%) are positive (Table 4) regarding the prognostic value of IMD in series of operable breast cancers, and 9 are negative (Table 5).

5.1.2. Mixed Series

At least 21 studies have been published up to now on the prognostic value of vascularization in series including patients with both node-negative and node-positive invasive breast carcinoma (Tables 4, 5).

The main aims of these studies were to verify methodology, to study the association of vascularization with the other prognostic factors, and to demonstrate the prognostic value of IMD by univariate and multivariate statistical analyses. The most relevant

Table 3
Association of Intratumoral Vascularization of Invasive Cancers with the Clinicopathologic Features and Other Biological Markers

	Significant association	No association
Age/menopausal status		Gasparini (66) Morphopoulos (73), Toi (90), Obermair (89)
Tumor size	Weidner (57), Heimann (61)	Siitonen (90), Axelsson ((71), Morphopoulos (73), Toi (88), Obermair (89)
Nodal status	Horak (91), Bosari (92), Weidner (57), Toi (88)	Khanuja (62), Goulding (88), Axelsson (71), Morphopoulos (73)
Grading	Van Hoef (97), Weidner (57), Gasparini (66)	Siitonen (90), Costello (63), Axelsson ((71), Horak (91), Bosari (92), Obermair (89)
Cell kinetics	Kaldjian (95)	Weidner (57), Monschke (96), Vartanian (97), Fox (98), Siitonen (90), Bosari (92)
Venous blood tumor cell shedding	McCulloch (31)	
Macrophage infiltration	Leek (99)	
p53		Costello (63), Horak (91), Gasparini (66)
c-erbB-2	Toi (88)	Siitonen (90), Costello (63), Horak (91), Weidner (57)
DNA ploidy	—	Siitonen (90), Bosari (92), Weidner (57)
ER/PgR	Ogawa (80)	Siitonen (90), Costello (63), Axelsson ((71), Horak (91), Weidner (57), Toi (88), Obermair (89)

355

Table 4
Intratumoral Vascularization and Prognosis: Published Positive Studies.

Authors	Endothelial marker	Number of patients	Stage	Node-negative patients	Association with		Multivariate analysis		Median follow-up (years)
					RFS[b]	OS[c]	RFS	OS	
Mixed series									
Horak (90)	CD-31	103	I–II	64	ND[a]	0.006	ND	ND	2.5
Weidner (57)	fVIII-RA	165	I–II	83	<0.001	<0.001	<0.001	<0.001	4.0
Bosari (91)	fVIII-RA	180	I–II	151	<0.004	<0.008	<0.03	<0.03	9.0
Visscher (52)	Type IV collagenase	58	I–IV	28	0.001	ND	NS	ND	5.1
Obermair (100)	fVIII-RA	64	I–II	32	<0.001	ND	<0.01	ND	4.1
Ogawa (101)	fVIII-RA	155	I–II	91	<0.001	0.025	<0.002	<0.001	7.0
Fox (59)	CD-31	211	I–II	112	ND	0.02	ND	0.05	3.5
Toi (87)	fVIII-RA/CD-31	125	I–II	57	<0.01	ND	<0.01	ND	5.1
Macaulay (52)	CD-31	88	I–II	23	0.02	ND	ND	ND	2.5
Toi (102)	fVIII-RA	328	I–II	130	<0.001	ND	<0.0001	ND	4.6
Kato (103)	fVIII-RA	115	I–II	92	ND	0.008	ND	ND	5.0
Kato (104)	fVIII-RA	109	I–II	87	ND	0.03	ND	ND	14.0
Simpson (105)	fVIII-RA	178	I–II	87	0.003	0.047	0.002	0.016	6.0
Ravazoula (62)	CD-31	106	I–II	60	0.022	ND	ND	ND	ND
Gasparini (60)	CD-31	531	I–II	260	<0.001	<0.001	<0.001	<0.001	6.3
Node-negative patients									
Bevilacqua (58)	CD-31	211	I		<0.0001	0.018	<0.0001	0.044	6.6
Obermair (88)	fVIII-RA	230	I		<0.0001	<0.0001	ND	<0.001	4.6
Fox (106)	CD-31	109	I		0.01	0.028	0.04	0.01	2.0
Heimann (61)	CD-34	167	I		0.018	ND	0.04	ND	20.0
Barbareschi (107)	CD-31	91	I		0.035	ND	0.006	ND	5.5
Lee (108)	fVIII-RA	88	I		0.08	ND	ND	ND	7.8
Node-positive patients									
Gasparini (70)	CD-31	191	II		<0.01	<0.01	<0.01	<0.01	5.5
Gasparini (53)	CD-31	178	II		<0.01	<0.01	<0.01	<0.01	5.2

[a]ND, not done. [b]RFS, relapse-free survival. [c]OS, overall survival.

Table 5
Intratumoral Vascularization and Prognosis: Published Negative Studies

Authors	Number of patients	Stage	Node-negative patients	Endothelial marker	Association with RFS[b]	OS[c]	Multivariate analysis RFS	OS	Median follow-up (years)	Comments
Mixed series										
Hall (64)	87	I–II	50	fVIII-RA	NS[b]	ND[a]	NS	ND	9.5, 1.5	Not consecutive series
Khanuja (92)	164	I–II	125	fVIII-RA	NS	ND	ND	ND	8.0	Only small primary tumors (≥cm) included
Goulding (93)	165	I–II	ND	CD-34	NS	NS	ND	ND	12.0	Not consecutive series; nodal status not reported
Axelsson (71)	220	I–II	110	fVIII-RA	NS	NS	NS	NS	11.5	See ref. 72
Morphorpoulos (73)	160	I–II	46	fVIII-RA	NS	NS	ND	ND	5.1	Only infiltrating lobular cancers considered
Sterns (109)	50	I–II	31	fVIII-RA	NS	NS	ND	ND	Variable	Not consecutive series
Node-negative patients										
Van Hoef (65)	93	I	93	fVIII-RA	NS	NS	NS	NS	13.0	Evaluation in a too small area
Siitonen (94)	77	I	77	fVIII-RA CD-31 CD-34	NS	ND	ND	ND	8.0	Not consecutive series
Costello (63)	87	I	87	fVIII-RA	NS	NS	ND	ND	2.9	Evaluation in a too small area; short follow-up

[a]ND, not done. [b]NS, not significant. [c]RFS, relapse-free survival. [d]OS, overall survival.

end-point was to verify whether angiogenesis is an independent prognostic marker when nodal status is also evaluated in the analysis. Overall, 3363 patients were studied of whom 1719 with node-negative disease. Among these 21 studies, only 4 included more than 200 cases as a single series (Tables 4, 5) and with the exception of Visscher et al. *(69)*, all the authors stained endothelium using the antibodies fVIII-RA or anti-CD31. The median follow-up of these series varied considerably, from 1.5–12 yr. The results of the univariate analyses on relapse-free survival (RFS) and/or overall survival (OS) gave a positive, statistically significant, relationship of IMD with prognosis in 15 studies, whereas 6 studies were totally negative.

A multivariate analysis was performed only in 12 studies and in 10 of these the results suggested that IMD is an independent prognostic indicator when nodal status, as well as other conventional or biological variables, were considered in the statistical model.

5.1.3. Node-Negative Patients

Nine published studies have reported the results of the prognostic value of IMD in homogeneous series of node-negative invasive breast carcinoma (Tables 4,5). Overall, 1153 patients were included, but only in two studies were series of more than 200 cases enrolled. Of concern is the fact that 6 of these studies (Tables 4,5) included less than 100 cases. The endothelial markers used in these studies were the antibodies fVIII-RA, anti-CD31, and CD34. The median period of follow-up ranged from 2–20 yr.

Because the expected frequency of recurrence and death at 10 yr of follow-up in series of node-negative breast cancer are approximately 30 and 20%, respectively, it is evident that a study small in size or with a too-short follow-up (<3 yr) cannot give any relevant prognostic information in such a subset of patients *(54)*. It is under this context that the three negative studies reported in Table 5 should be considered. Finally, only six studies had multivariate analysis and five of these suggested that the determination of IMD is an independent prognostic indicator. Therefore, determination of IMD is emerging as an interesting prognostic indicator in node-negative disease and its prognostic value merits to be investigated in future prospective controlled clinical trials.

5.1.4. Node-Positive Patients

At present, only two studies performed by Gasparini et al. *(53,70)* assessed the prognostic value of the determination of IMD in homogeneous groups of patients with node-positive breast cancer. In both of these studies the antibody anti-CD31 was employed to stain microvessels and the median follow-up exceeded 5 yr. The first series *(70)* included 191 patients treated either with adjuvant chemotherapy (CMF schedule) or hormone therapy (tamoxifen). In both of the subgroups, IMD was a significant and independent prognostic indicator. The second study *(53)* included 178 patients treated with hormone adjuvant therapy alone (tamoxifen) and vascularization was assessed with the use of the Chalkley score, in collaboration with Harris and colleagues of the University of Oxford. Chalkley point counting is a technique developed in the attempt to simplify the measurement of angiogenic activity and to make the evaluation of the degree of vascularization more objective. This method still implies scanning of the tumor section at low magnification to identify the 3–5 areas of higher vascularization. Then, at a higher magnification (200–500×), instead of counting each individual microvessel, an eyepiece graticule with 25 randomly positioned dots is rotated so that the maximum number of points are on or within the vessels of the vascular "hot spot" *(53)*. The authors found that Chalkley score was a significant and independent prognostic indicator for both RFS and OS.

Of importance is that both the studies *(53,70)* suggested that the degree of vascularization and the number of involved axillary lymph nodes were the strongest prognostic factors in these series of patients treated with adjuvant therapy.

5.1.5. Some Considerations on the Studies Reporting

Negative results as shown in Table 5, nine studies did not find the determination of IMD to be of prognostic value in operable invasive breast cancer. These include six studies on patients with mixed node status and three studies on node-negative disease for a total of 1103 tumors (619 node-negative).

The major criticisms that can be raised on these studies can be summarized as follows: The three studies, conducted in a series of node-negative patients only, enrolled too few cases to reach an adequate statistical power. Only the study by Axelsson et al. *(71)* included more than 200 cases in the statistical analysis. Overall, in only three studies was a multivariate analysis performed, therefore the other six studies were unable to demonstrate whether angiogenesis, as well as the other markers tested, were independent prognostic markers.

Potential methodological biases included: deviations on the technique suggested by Weidner et al. *(25)*, enrollment of nonconsecutive or selected series, short follow-up and heterogeneous treatments *(55,67,72)*.

Of interest are, however, the results of the study by Morphopoulous et al. *(73)* suggesting that determination of IMD does not seem to be of prognostic relevance in the histological subset of infiltrating lobular cancers. This observation is of clinical importance, because it is based on a quite large series of patients followed for a median follow-up of 5 yr. Only 46 cases with node-negative disease were considered, so the results observed in this subset of patients with infiltrating lobular cancers of the breast will need to be confirmed in future studies with larger series of patients.

5.1.6. General Comments and Conclusions
on the Prognostic Relevance of Determination of Microvessel Density

Some guidelines to properly evaluate the new prognostic indicator in breast cancer have been previously suggested *(54)*. With regard to retrospective studies, once at least two independent studies suggest the prognostic relevance of a new prognostic indicator, further studies should be carried out to solve problems related to reproducibility and standardization of the technique of determination.

The prognostic value of the new marker in homogeneous groups of patients should also be evaluated. As far as node-negative breast cancer is concerned, the following points are to be borne in mind in order that a study may lead to some definitive conclusions:

1. Selection of the patients: a homogeneous series should involve patients with similar stages of disease (for example, T_1 vs T_2 primary tumors); who received the same therapy (for example only surgery versus a well-defined adjuvant treatment);
2. Size of the cohort of patients studied: it is suggested that at least 200 homogeneous cases are needed if the median length of the follow-up is of 5 yr;
3. Follow-up: well-defined criteria of the timing of the visit and on the schedule of laboratory or radiographic examinations should be prospectively defined.

The optimal median follow-up for evaluation of prognostic factors is approximately 10 yr and studies reporting results with periods of follow-up less than 5 yr should be considered as preliminary.

As far as patients with node-positive breast cancer are concerned, there are three critical points in evaluating a new prognostic marker.

1. The type of adjuvant therapy administered must be considered. Besides a prospective clinical trial, patients treated with different adjuvant treatments cannot be evaluated together, in order to avoid biases related to the different criteria of assignment of each treatment that are often based on the clinicopathologic characteristics of the patients.
2. The prediction of the efficacy of a specific adjuvant therapy requires a prospective randomized comparison in which the same marker is determined in a control group of patients who do not receive the therapy vs the treated group;
3. A well-balanced distribution of the known prognostic factors (tumor size, number of involved axillary lymph nodes, hormone receptors, and so on) among the different series is mandatory for a proper comparison and evaluation of the clinical relevance of the prognostic marker to be evaluated.

Taking into account the aforementioned methodological features, it is evident that definitive conclusions on meta-analyses performed on retrospective studies are subject to several potential biases.

Only the determination of microvessel counts within prospective controlled clinical trials in homogeneous groups of patients could give definitive results on the prognostic value of its determination in different subgroups of patients and in relation to adjuvant therapy *(54)*. However, the overview of the results of the retrospective studies that evaluated the prognostic value of IMD by applying multivariate statistical analysis, suggests that most of the studies found that this marker maintains prognostic significance in models that include in the analysis at least the conventional prognostic indicators (*see* Tables 4 and 5). These encouraging findings from retrospective studies need to be confirmed in future prospective clinical trials before determination of angiogenesis may be proposed as a routine prognostic marker in operable breast cancer.

5.1.7. Prognostic Value of Determination of Angiogenic Polypeptides

Ten studies (nine published) have reported on the prognostic value of the determination of angiogenic growth factors assessed by using different methods (Table 6). Up to now, the most studied is VEGF. Toi et al. *(48,68)* in two different series of patients with "mixed disease" studied expression of VEGF by immunocytochemistry. They found that about 50% of the tumors were VEGF-positive and that VEGF expression was associated with the degree of intratumoral vascularization. In both univariate and multivariate analysis, VEGF was a significant and independent prognostic factor for RFS.

Gasparini's group in a collaborative study with Toi and colleagues *(46)* assessed the prognostic value of cytosolic concentrations of VEGF using immunometric assays. One study *(46)* was conducted in a series of 260 patients with node-negative breast cancer, median follow-up exceeding 5 yr. The levels of VEGF did not correlate with any other prognostic marker and were of prognostic value in both univariate and multivariate analysis. A second analysis has been performed by the same group in this series of patients by adding the determination of p53 protein, cathepsin-D, and of thy-

Table 6
Expression or Levels of Angiogenic Polypeptides and Prognosis

Authors	Angiogenic factor	Number of patients	Stage	Method	Association with RFS[b]	Association with OS[c]	Multivariate analysis RFS	Multivariate analysis OS	Comments
Relf (47)	VEGF*; a-b FGF; TP; others	64	I–II	Rnase protection analysis	0.03*	ND[a]	ND	ND	VEGF associated with risk of recurrence
Gasparini (46)	VEGF	260	I	Immuno-metric	<0.001	<0.001	<0.001	<0.001	—
Toi (48)	VEGF	103	I–II	ICA[c]	<0.01	ND	0.039	ND	VEGF associated with IMD
Toi 68	VEGF	230	I–II	ICA	<0.01	ND	<0.01	ND	VEGF associated with IMD
Seymour (78)	PDGF	58	III–IV	ICA	ND	0.002	ND	ND	Advanced stages
Fox (74)	TP	328	I–II	ICA	0.02	0.02	NS	0.03	Prognostic in the CMF group
Fox (49)	TP	240	I–II	ICA	NS[b]	NS	NS	NS	No associated with IMD
Visscher (77)	bFGF	79	I–II	ICA	<0.05	ND	ND	ND	No associated with IMD
Yamashita (76)	HGF	258	I–II	Immuno-enzymatic	<0.01	<0.01	<0.01	<0.01	—
Gasparini (unpublished)	VEGF*; TP	353	II	Immuno-metric	<0.01*	<0.05*	<0.05*	<0.05*	—

[a]ND, not done. [b]NS, not significant. [c]ICA, immunocytochemical assay. [d]RFS, relapse-free survival. [e]OS, overall survival.
*VEGF, vascular endothelial growth factor.

midine phosphorylase (TP) assessed by immunometric assays. The concentrations of VEGF were not associated with p53 or TP, and the co-determination of VEGF and TP added prognostic information in the multivariate analysis *(50)*. A third study, still unpublished (Gasparini, Toi, et al., manuscript in preparation), was performed in a series of 353 patients with node-positive breast cancer and treated with radiation therapy (control group) or either with adjuvant chemotherapy or hormone therapy. In the cytosol of tumor tissue, the authors determined VEGF and TP with the same method previously adopted in the series of node-negative cases *(46,50)*. As a main result, VEGF concentrations were found to be of prognostic value in the overall series. A subanalysis of the prognostic value of the variables studied in the subgroups of patients who received different treatment is ongoing.

Recently, Relf et al. *(47)* adopted a RNase protection analysis to study the expression of VEGF, TP, acidic and basic FGF and pleiotropin in the primary tumor of 64 patients with breast cancer. Among the angiogenic factors studied, VEGF was the single angiogenic polypeptide most frequently expressed in invasive breast cancer and it was significantly associated with the risk of recurrence.

Two studies have been published by Harris' group *(49,74)* on the prognostic value of TP expression assessed by immunohistochemistry. The first study did not find any significant prognostic value *(49)*, whereas the second study *(74)* suggested that TP levels are predictive of good outcome in the subgroup of patients with node-positive disease treated with adjuvant chemotherapy. Taking into account that TP is a target enzyme for the activity of 5-fluorouracil and methotrexate (two of the three drugs of the CMF schedule) (reviewed in refs. *49,50,74*), the results of this latter study are supported by a strong pharmacological rationale.

A recent study by Lamszus and associates *(75)* suggests that hepatocyte growth factor (HGF, also known as scatter factor), may be a primary angiogenic factor in breast cancer. The authors *(75)* found that some HGF-positive clones of MDAMB231 human mammary carcinoma cells showed increased primary tumor volume and higher rates of axillary lymph-nodes metastasis in vivo as compared with two HGF-negative clones. The HGF-positive tumors also both had higher microvessels as compared to those HGF-negative. Overall, the findings of the study suggest that HGF promotes the orthotopic growth of human breast cancer, in part by stimulating tumor angiogenesis. Yamashita et al. (107) studied the prognostic relevance of HGF in a large series of patients with an immunoenzymatic assay and found that HGF levels were associated with prognosis in both univariate and multivariate analysis. Finally, Visscher et al. *(77)* and Seymour et al. *(78)* assessed the prognostic value of basic FGF (bFGF) and of platelet-derived cell growth factor (PDGF), respectively, by immunohistochemical methods. In small series of patients, the authors found that bFGF is associated with poor RFS *(77)*, whereas PDGF is associated with poor survival (in patients with advanced stages of disease) *(78)*.

5.1.8. Prognostic Value of Other Investigational Techniques to Assess Angiogenic Activity

5.1.8.1. ENDOTHELIAL-CELL ADHESION MOLECULES (ECAMs)

Recent studies have shown that ECAMs not only have a physiological role in immune and inflammatory response, but that they are also involved in angiogenesis, tumor invasiveness, and metastasis. Fox et al. *(79)* assessed the differentiating expression of platelet endothelial cell adhesion molecule (PECAM) (CD31), intercellular adhesion molecule (ICAMs), vascular cell adhesion molecule (VCAM-1), and P- and E-selectin in endothelium within normal breast tissue as compared to tumor-associated microvessels. The results suggested that activated endothelium within tumoral stroma expresses high levels of PECAM, ICAMs 1–3, and selectins resembling a pro-inflammatory phenotype, probably as a result of cytokine stimulation.

5.1.8.2. INTEGRINS

The expression of the integrin family may be different between normal breast epithelium and breast cancer *(80)*. Friedrichs et al. *(15)* found a high expression of α6 integrin in 50% of the human breast cancers tested. In univariate analysis the patients with grade IV expression of this integrin had a significantly worse overall survival when compared to those with lower grades of expression.

Brooks et al. *(16)* demonstrated in an elegant experimental study that integrin $\alpha_v\beta_3$ on endothelial cells is necessary for breast-cancer angiogenesis and that its neutralization is accompanied by reduced neovascularization and regression of transplanted human breast cancer in a SCID mouse/human chimeric model.

We investigated the expression of integrin $\alpha_v\beta_3$ in a large series of invasive breast cancers and found high levels of expression in invasive cancers as compared to normal breast tissues. In tumors, it is associated with proliferating endothelium, metastasis, and poor prognosis (Gasparini, Brooks et al., manuscript in preparation).

5.1.8.3. TENASCIN

This extracellular matrix glycoprotein is an important factor for modulation of reciprocal interactions between the epithelium and the mesenchyme during embryogenesis and is preferentially expressed in some human solid cancers (reviewed in ref. *23*). Ishihara et al. *(23)* studied tenascin expression in cancer cells and stroma of 210 human breast cancers. Approximately one-third of the tumors were tenascin-positive in the stroma, but in only 5.7% of the cancers a cytoplasmic staining of cancer cells was found. The subgroup of patients with tenascin expression in both stroma and cancer cells had the worse prognosis.

5.1.8.4. TISSUE FACTOR

The potent procoagulant, tissue factor, is expressed in both tumor cells and vascular endothelial cells of human breast cancer and may contribute to the production of thrombin, which can generate fibrin within the tumor. Fibrin is capable of increasing endothelial-cell mobility and potentiating angiogenesis may contribute to an increased risk of thrombosis in cancer patients (reviewed in ref. *(81)*). Contrino et al. *(17)* found that determination of tissue factor is a useful marker for the "switch to the angiogenic phenotype" in human breast disease, being preferably expressed in breast cancer. This interesting observation suggests the possibility that tissue factor may be of clinical usefulness in distinguishing preinvasive to invasive angiogenic lesions and as a prognostic marker. Further studies are needed to properly verify this hypothesis.

5.1.8.5. PROTEOLYTIC ENZYMES

Plasminogen activators and tissue matrix metalloproteinases play a pivotal role in tumor cell invasion and metastasis as well as in angiogenesis. uPA, often induced by angiogenic factors, stimulates the degradation of extracellular matrix and thereby the further release of angiogenic factors.

Harris' group demonstrated a significant relationship between highly vascularized tumors and uPA in human breast cancer and several studies have shown that elevated expression or levels of uPA are associated with poor prognosis (reviewed in ref. *82*). Also the expression of some tissue matrix metalloproteinases is associated with poor prognosis (M. Toi, personal communication) in series of breast cancer. This is clinically of interest because metalloproteinase inhibitors are already in clinical trial as new anticancer compounds *(83)*.

5.2. Therapeutic Target

Some retrospective studies have suggested that IMD may be useful in identifying subsets of patients responsive to conventional adjuvant therapy *(52,53,57,60,70)*. Those patients with highly vascularized tumors who have a poor outcome even if treated with postoperative chemotherapy or hormone therapy may benefit of angiosuppressive therapy. Determination of the vascularization of primary breast tumors as well as of the angiogenic factors present even in each single tumor might be useful in predicting response to specific antiangiogenic treatments and to monitoring their efficacy in time *(83)*.

Appropriate study-designs for the development of antiangiogenic drugs would include also the determination in tumoral tissue or serum and urine of the patients of markers of angiogenic activity. These surrogate markers may be useful to define the angiogenic activity of each tumor and for a proper monitoring of the pharmacological effect of angiogenesis inhibitors in each patient.

6. CONCLUSIONS AND FUTURE DIRECTIONS OF RESEARCH

There is now compelling experimental data suggesting that angiogenesis is necessary for breast cancer growth, progression and metastasis *(55,67,84)*. However, several questions on the biology of tumor angiogenesis in human breast cancer are still unanswered:

1. What are the mechanisms responsible for the angiogenic switch?
2. Which are the more relevant angiogenic polypeptides?
3. What is the clinical relevance of the assessment of the balance of angiogenic factors and inhibitors, and which are the more important endogenous angiogenesis inhibitors?

A central area of research, still in its infancy, is to clarify the role played by angiogenesis in the sequential, multistep molecular mechanisms involved in human breast-cancer growth *(42)*. A better understanding of the relationship of angiogenesis with the other biological pathways favoring or suppressing tumor progression will be the key for the identification of sequential targets against which selective new biologically-based coordinated therapeutic strategies may be developed in future years *(85)*.

Because clinicopathologic studies have suggested that angiogenic activity and expression of some other biological factors, for example p53, c-erbB-2 which can be therapeutically targeted, are independent prognostic factors in human breast cancer (Table 3), it seems appropriate to speculate that concurrent treatments with inhibitors of angiogenesis, neutralizing antibodies to c-erbB-2, and gene therapy, restoring wild-type p53, might produce synergic anticancer therapy.

As far as the clinical usefulness of the determination of angiogenic activity in human breast cancer is concerned, several methods are currently available and under evaluation. Up to now, the most common method to quantify angiogenesis is the immunohistochemical evaluation of microvessels count. Most of the retrospective studies published thus far have shown that IMD is of prognostic value, possibly with the exception of the lobular histologic type. Moreover, some authors who studied IMD in series of patients treated with conventional adjuvant therapy found that highly vascularized tumors are associated with poor outcome.

Future well-designed prospective clinical studies should be planned to verify the real value of determination of angiogenesis as a prognostic tool, as a predictive marker of efficacy of specific adjuvant treatment and as a method to monitor the efficacy of inhibitors of angiogenesis in each patient.

REFERENCES

1. Deng, G., Y. Lu, G. Zlotnikov, A. D. Thor, and H. S. Smith. 1996. Loss of heterozygosity in normal tissue adjacent to breast carcinomas. *Science* **274:** 2057–2059.
2. Gasparini, G. 1997. Angiogenesis in endocrine-related tumors. *Endocr. Rel. Cancers* **4:** 423–445.
3. Folkman, J. 1995. The influence of angiogenesis research on management of patients with breast cancer. *Breast Cancer Res. Treat.* **36:** 109–118.
4. Dvorak, H. F. 1986. Tumors: wounds that do not heal. Similarities between tumor stroma generation and wound healing. *N. Engl. J. Med.* **315:** 1650–1659.
5. Rak, J., J. Filmus, and R. S. Kerbel. 1996. Reciprocal paracrine interactions between tumour cells and endothelial cells: the 'angiogenesis progression' hypothesis. *Eur. J. Cancer* **32A:** 2451–2460.
6. Brooks, P. C. 1996. Role of integrins in angiogenesis. *Eur. J. Cancer* 32A: 2423–2429.
7. Folkman, J. 1995. Angiogenesis in cancer, vascular, rheumatoid and other disease. *Nature Med.* **1:** 27–31.
8. Fidler, I. J. and L. M. Ellis. 1994. The implications of angiogenesis for the biology and therapy of cancer metastasis. *Cell* **79:** 185–188.
9. Pezzella, F., U. Pastorino, E. Tagliabue, S. Andreola, G. Sozzi, G. Gasparini, S. Menard, K. C. Gatter, A. L. Harris, S. Fox, M. Buyse, S. Pilotti, M. Pierotti, and F. Rilke. 1997. Non-small cell lung carcinoma tumor-growth without neoangiogenesis. *Am. J. Pathol.* **151:** 1417–1423.
10. Hanahan, D. and J. Folkman. 1996. Patterns of emerging mechanisms of the angiogenic switch during tumorigenesis. *Cell* **86:** 353–364.
11. Brem, S. S., P. M. Gullino, and D. Medina. 1997. Angiogenesis: a marker for neoplastic transformation of mammary papillary hyperplasia. *Science* **195:** 880–881.
12. Brem, S. S., H. M. Jensen, and P. M. Gullino. 1978. Angiogenesis as a marker of preneoplastic lesions of the human breast. *Cancer* **41:** 239–244.
13. Jensen, H. M., I. Chen, M. R. DeValut, and A. E. Lewis. 1982. Angiogenesis induced by "normal" human breast tissue: a probable marker for precancer. *Science* **218:** 293–295.
14. Kern, F. G. and M. E. Lippman. 1996. The role of angiogenic growth factors in breast cancer progression. *Cancer Met. Rev.* **15:** 213–219.
15. Friedrichs, K., P. Ruiz, F. Franke, I. Gille, H. J. Terpe, and B. A. Imhof. 1995. High expression level of $\alpha 6$ integrin in human breast carcinoma is correlated with reduced survival. *Cancer Res.* **55:** 901–906.
16. Brooks, P. C., S. Stromblad, R. Klemke, D. Visscher, F. H. Sarkar, and D. A. Cheresh. 1995. Antiintegrin $\alpha_v\beta_3$ blocks human breast cancer growth and angiogenesis in human skin. *J. Clin. Invest.* **96:** 1815–1822.

17. Contrino, J., G. Hair, D. L. Kreutzer, and F. R. Rickles. 1996. In situ detection of tissue factor in vascular endothelial cells: correlation with the malignant phenotype of human breast disease. *Nature Med.* **2**: 209–215.
18. Vrana, J. A., M. T. Stang, J. P. Grande, and M. J. Getz. 1996. Expression of tissue factor in tumor stroma correlates with progression to invasive human breast cancer: paracrine regulation by carcinoma cell-derived members of the transforming growth factor β family. *Cancer Res.* **56**: 5063–5070.
19. Maemura, M. and R. B. Dickson. 1994. Are cellular adhesion molecules involved in the metastasis of breast cancer? *Breast Cancer Res. Treat.* **32**: 239–260.
20. Polverini, P. J. 1996. Cellular adhesion molecules. Newly identified mediators of angiogenesis. (commentary). *Am. J. Pathol.* **148**: 1023–1029.
21. Stetler-Stevenson, W. G., S. Aznavoorian, and L. A. Liotta. 1993. Tumor cell interactions with the extracellular matrix during invasion and metastasis. *Ann. Rev. Cell. Biol.* **9**: 541–573.
22. Brooks, P. C., S. Strömblad, L. C. Sanders, T. L. von Schalscha, R. T. Aimes, W. G. Stetler-Stevenson, J. P. Quigley, and D. A. Cheresh. 1996. Localization of matrix metalloproteinase MMP–2 to the surface of invasive cells by interaction with integrin $\alpha_v\beta_3$. *Cell* **85**: 683–693.
23. Ishihara, A., T. Yoshida, H. Tamaki, and T. Sakakura. 1995. Tenascin expression in cancer cells and stroma of human breast cancer and its prognostic significance. *Clin. Cancer Res.* **1**: 1035–1041.
24. Gasparini, G, M. Barbareschi, P. Boracchi, P. Bevilacqua, P. Verderio, P. Dalla Palma, and S. Menard. 1995. 67-Kda laminin-receptor expression adds prognostic information to intra-tumoral microvessel density in node-negative breast cancer. *Int. J. Cancer* **60**: 604–610.
25. Weidner, N., J. P. Semple, W. R. Welch, and J. Folkman. 1991. Tumor angiogenesis and metastasis—correlation in invasive breast carcinoma. *N. Engl. J. Med.* **324**: 1–8.
26. Guinebretiere, J. M., G. L. Monique, A. Gavoille, J. Bahi, and G. Contesso. 1994. Angiogenesis and risk of breast cancer in women with fibrocystic disease. *J. Natl. Cancer Inst.* **86**: 635–636.
27. Guidi, A. J., L. Fisher, J. R. Harris, and S. J. Schnitt. 1994. Microvessel density and distribution in ductal carcinoma in situ of the breast. *J. Natl. Cancer Inst.* **86**: 614–619.
28. Heffelfinger, S. C., R. Yassin, M. A. Miller, and E. Lower. 1996. Vascularity of proliferative breast disease and carcinoma in situ correlates with histological features. *Clin. Cancer Res.* **2**: 1873–1878.
29. Lee, A. H. S., L. C. Happerfield, L. G. Bobrow, and R. R. Millis. 1997. Angiogenesis and inflammation in ductal carcinoma in situ of the breast. *J. Pathol.* **181**: 200–206.
30. Engels, K., S. B. Fox, R. M. Whitehouse, K. C. Gatter, and A. L. Harris. 1997. Distinct angiogenic patterns are associated with high-grade in situ ductal carcinomas of the breast. *J. Pathol.* **181**: 207–212.
31. McCulloch, P., A. Choy, and L. Martin. 1995. Association between tumour angiogenesis and tumour cell shedding into effluent venous blood during breast cancer surgery. *Lancet* **346**: 1334–1335.
32. Liotta, L. A., J. Kleinerman, and G. M. Saidel. 1974. Quantitative relationships of intravascular tumor cells, tumor vessels, and pulmonary metastases following tumor implantation. *Cancer Res.* **34**: 997–1004.
33. Zajchowski, D. A., V. Band, D. K. Trask, D. Kling, J. L. Connolly, and R. Sager. 1990. Suppression of tumor-forming ability and related traits in MCF-7 human breast cancer cell by fusion with immortal mammary epithelial cells. *Proc. Natl. Acad. Sci. USA* **87**: 2314–2318.
34. Dameron, K. M., O. V. Volpert, M. A. Tainsky, and N. Bouck. 1994. Control of angiogenesis in fibroblasts by p53 regulation of thrombospondin-1. *Science* **265**: 1582–1585.

35. Volpert, O., V. Stellmach, and N. Bouck. 1995. The modulation of thrombospondin and other naturally occurring inhibitors of angiogenesis during tumor progression. *Breast Cancer Res. Treat.* **36:** 119–126.

36. Incardona, F., J. M. Leivalle, V. Morandi, S. Lambert, Y. Legrandl, J. M. Foidart, and C. Legrand. 1995. Thrombospondin modulates human breast adenocarcinoma cell adhesion to human vascular endothelial cells. *Cancer Res.* **55:** 166–173.

37. Arnoletti, J. P., D. Albo, M. S. Granick, M. P. Solomon, A. Castiglioni, V. L. Rothman, and G. P. Tuzynski. 1995. Thrombospondin and transforming growth-factor beta 1 increase expression of urokinase-type plasminogen activator and plasminogen activator inhibitor-1 in human MDA-MB-231 breast cancer cells. *Cancer* **76:** 998–1005.

38. Bertin, N., P. Clezardin, R. Kubiak, and L. Frappart. 1997. Thrombospondin-1 and -2 messanger RNA expression in normal, benign, and neoplastic human breast tissues: correlation with prognostic factors, tumor angiogenesis, and fibroblastic desmoplasia. *Cancer Res.* **57:** 396–399.

39. Weinstat-Saslow, D. L., V. S. Zabrenetzky, K. VanHoutte, W. A. Frazier, D. D. Roberts, and P. S. Steeg. 1994. Transfection of thrombospondin 1 complementary DNA into a human breast carcinoma cell line reduces primary tumor growth, metastatic potential, and angiogenesis. *Cancer Res.* **54:** 6504–6511.

40. O'Reilly, M. S., L. Holmgren, C. Chen, and J. Folkman. 1996. Angiostatin induces and sustains dormancy of human primary tumors. *Nature Med.* **2:** 689–692.

41. Ellis, L. M. and I. J. Fidler. 1995. Angiogenesis and breast cancer metastasis. *Lancet* **346:** 388–390.

42. Gasparini, G. 1996. Angiogenesis research up to 1996. A commentary on the state of art and suggestions for future studies. *Eur. J. Cancer* **32A:** 2379–2385.

43. Osborne, C. K. 1993. Regulation of breast cancer growth by steroid hormones and growth factors: clinical implications. *Cancer Bull.* **45:** 483–488.

44. Kurebayashi, J., S. W. McLeskey, M. D. Johnson, M. E. Lippman, R. B. Dickson, and F. G. Kern. 1993. Quantitative demonstration of spontaneous metastasis by MCF-7 human breast cancer cells cotransfected with fibroblast growth factor 4 and LacZ. *Cancer Res.* **53:** 2178–2187.

45. Zhang, H.-T., P. Craft, P. A. E. Scott, M. Ziche, H. A. Welch, A. L. Harris, and R. Bicknell. 1995. Enhancement of tumor growth and vascular density by transfection of vascular endothelial cell growth factor into MCF-7 human breast carcinoma cells. *J. Natl. Cancer Inst.* **87:** 213–219.

46. Gasparini, G., M. Toi, M. Gion, P. Verderio, R. Dittadi, M. Hanatani, I. Matsubara, O. Vinante, E. Bonoldi, P. Boracchi, C. Gatti, I. Suzuki, and T. Tominaga. 1997. Prognostic significance of vascular endothelial growth factor protein in node-negative breast carcinoma. *J. Natl. Cancer Inst.* **89:** 139–147.

47. Relf, M., S. LeJeune, P. A. E. Scott, S. Fox, K. Smith, R. Leek, A. Moghaddam, R. Whitehouse, R. Bicknell, and A. L. Harris. 1997. Expression of the angiogenic factors vascular endothelial cell growth factor, acidic and basic fibroblast growth factor, tumor growth factor β-1, platelet-derived endothelial cell growth factor, placenta growth factor, and pleiotrophin in human primary breast cancer and its relation to angiogenesis. *Cancer Res.* **57:** 963–969.

48. Toi, M., S. Hoshima, T. Takayanagi, and T. Tominaga. 1994. Association of vascular endothelial growth factor expression with tumor angiogenesis and with early relapse in primary breast cancer. *Jpn. J. Cancer Res.* **85:** 1045–1049.

49. Fox, S. B., M. Westwood, A. Moghaddam, M. Comley, H. Turley, R. M. Whitehouse, R. Bicknell, K. C. Gatter, and A. L. Harris. 1996. The angiogenic factor platelet-derived endothelial cell growth factor/thymidine phosphorylase is up-regulated in breast cancer epitehlium and endothelium. *Br. J. Cancer* **73:** 275–280.

50. Toi, M., M. Gion, E. Biganzoli, R. Dittadi, P. Boracchi, R. Miceli , S. Meli, K. Mori, T. Tominaga, and G. Gasparini. 1997. Co-determination of the angiogenic factors thymidine phosphorylase and vascular endothelial growth factor in node-negative breast cancer: prognostic implications. *Angiogenesis* **1:** 71–83.

51. Nagy, J., G. W. Curry, K. J. Hillan, E. Mallon, A. D. Purushotham, and W. D. George. 1996. Hepatocyte growth factor/scatter factor, angiogenesis and tumour cell proliferation in primary breast cancer. *Breast* **5:** 105–109.

52. Macaulay, V. M., S. B. Fox, H. Zhang, R. M. Whitehouse, R. D. Leek, K. C. Gatter, R. Bicknell, and A. L. Harris. 1995. Breast cancer angiogenesis and tamoxifen resistance. *Endocr. Rel. Cancer* **2:** 97–103.

53. Gasparini G, Fox SB, Verderio P, Bonoldi E, Bevilacqua P, Boracchi P, Dante S, Marubini E and Harris AL. 1996. Determination of angiogenesis adds information to estrogen receptor status in predicting the efficacy of adjuvant tamoxifen in node-positive breast cancer patients. *Clin. Cancer Res.* **2:** 1191–1198.

54. Gasparini, G., F. Pozza, and A. L. Harris. 1993. Evaluating the potential usefulness of new prognostic and predictive indicators in node-negative breast cancer patients. *J. Natl. Cancer Inst.* **85:** 1206–1219.

55. Gasparini, G. and A. L. Harris. 1995. Clinical importance of the determination of tumor angiogenesis in breast carcinoma: much more than a new prognostic tool. *J. Clin. Oncol.* **13:** 765–782.

56. Vermeulen, P. B., G. Gasparini, S. B. Fox, M. Toi, L. Martin, P. McCulloch, F. Pezzella, G. Viale, N. Weidner, A. L. Harris, and L. Y. Dirix. 1996. Quantification of angiogenesis in dolid human tumours: an international consensus on the methodology and criteria of evaluation. *Eur. J. Cancer* **32A:** 2474–2484.

57. Weidner, N., J. Folkman, F. Pozza, P. Bevilacqua, E. N. Allred, D. H. Moore, S. Meli, and G. Gasparini. 1992. Tumor angiogenesis: a new significant and independent prognostic indicator in early-stage breast carcinoma. *J. Natl. Cancer Inst.* **84:** 1875–1887.

58. Bevilacqua, P., M. Barbareschi, P. Verderio, P. Boracchi, O. Caffo, P. Dalla Palma, S. Meli, N. Weidner, and G. Gasparini. 1995. Prognostic value of intratumoral microvessel density, a measure of tumor angiogenesis, in node-negative breast carcinoma. Results of a multiparametric study. *Breast Cancer Res. Treat.* **36:** 205–217.

59. Fox, S. B., G. D. H. Turner, R. D. Leek, R. M. Whitehouse, K. C. Gatter, and A. L. Harris. 1996. The prognostic value of quantitative angiogenesis in breast cancer and role of adhesion molecule expression in tumor endothelium. *Breast Cancer Res. Treat.* **36:** 219–226.

60. Gasparini, G., M. Toi, P. Verderio, M. Barbareschi, S. Dante, P. Boracchi, P. Dalla Palma, and T. Tominaga. 1997. Prognostic significance of p53, angiogenesis, and other conventional features in operable breast cancer. Subanalysis in node-positive and node-negative patients. *J. Exp. Ther. Oncol.* **2:** 1–9.

61. Heimann, R., D. Ferguson, C. Powers, W. M. Recant , R. R. Wichselbaum, and S. Hellman. 1996. Angiogenesis as a predictor of long-term survival for patients with node-negative breast cancer. *J. Natl. Cancer Inst.* **88:** 1764–1769.

62. Ravazoula, P., O. Hatjikondi, D. Kardamakis, M. Maragoudalkis, and D. Bonikos D. 1996. Angiogenesis and metastatic potential in breast carcinoma. *Breast* **5:** 418–421.

63. Costello, P., A. McCann, D. N. Carney, and P. A. Dervan. 1995. Prognostic significance of microvessel density in lymph node negative breast carcinoma. *Human Pathol.* **26:** 1181–1184.

64. Hall, N. R., D. E. Fish, N. Hunt, R. D. Goldin, P. J. Gullino, J. R. T. Monson. 1992. Is the relationship between angiogenesis and metastasis in breast cancer real? *Surg. Oncol.* **1:** 223–229.

65. Van Hoef, M. E. H. N., W. F. Knox, S. S. Dhesi, A. Howell, and A. M. Schor. 1996. Assessment of tumour vascularity as a prognostic factor in lymph node negative invasive breast cancer. *Eur. J. Cancer* **29A**: 1141–1145.

66. Gasparini, G., N. Weidner, P. Bevilacqua, P. Dalla Palma, O. Caffo, M. Barbareschi, P. Boracchi, E. Marubini, and F. Pozza. 1994. Tumor microvessel density, p53 expression, tumor size and peritumoral lymphatic vessel invasion are relevant prognostic markers in node-negative breast carcinoma. *J. Clin. Oncol.* **12**: 454–466.

67. Gasparini, G. 1996. Clinical significance of the determination of angiogenesis in human breast cancer: update of the biological background and overview of the Vicenza studies. *Eur. J. Cancer* **32A**: 2485–2493.

68. Toi, M., T. Taniguchi, Y. Yamamoto, T. Kurisaki, H. Suzuki, and T. Tominaga. 1996. Clinical significance of the determination of angiogenic factors. *Eur. J. Cancer* **32A**: 2513–2519.

69. Visscher, D. W., S. Smilanetz, S. Drozdowicz, and S. M. Wykes. 1993. Prognostic significance of image morphometric microvessel enumeration in breast carcinoma. *Anal. Quant. Cytol. Histol.* **15**: 88–92.

70. Gasparini, G., M. Barbareschi, P. Boracchi, P. Verderio, O. Caffo, S. Meli, P. Dalla Palma, E. Marubini, and P. Bevilacqua. 1995. Tumor angiogenesis predicts clinical outcome of node-positive breast cancer patients treated with adjuvant hormone therapy or chemotherapy. *Cancer J. Sci. Am.* **1**: 131–141.

71. Axelsson K, Ljung B-ME, More II DH, Thor AD, Chew KL, Edgerton SM, Smith HS, Mayall BH. 1995. Tumor angiogenesis as a prognostic assay for invasive ductal breast carcinoma. *J. Natl. Cancer Inst.* **87**: 997–1008.

72. Gasparini, G. 1995. Tumor angiogenesis as a prognostic assay for invasive ductal breast carcinoma (letter). *J. Natl. Cancer Inst.* **87**: 1799–1801.

73. Morphopoulos, G., M. Pearson, W. D. J. Ryder, A. Howell, and M. Harris. 1996. Tumour angiogenesis as a prognostic marker in infiltrating lobular carcinoma of the breast. *J. Pathol.* **180**: 44–49.

74. Fox, S. B., K. Engels, M. Comley, R. M. Whitehouse, H. Turley, K. C. Gatter, and A. L. Harris. 1997. Relationship of elevated tumour thymidine phosphorylase in node-positive breast carcinomas to the effects of adjuvant CMF. *Ann. Oncol.* **8**: 271–275.

75. Lamszus, K., L. Jin, A. Fuchs, E. Shi, S. Chowdhury, Y. Yao, P. J. Polverini, J. Laterra, I. D. Goldberg, and E. M. Rosen. 1997. Scatter factor stimulates tumor growth and tumor angiogenesis in human breast cancers in the mammary fat pads of nude mice. *Lab. Invest.* **76**: 339–353.

76. Yamashita, J., M. Ogawa, S. Jamashita, K. Nomura, M. Kuramoto, T. Saishoji, and S. Shin. 1994. Immunoreactive hepatocyte growth factor is a strong and independent predictor of recurrence and survival in human breast cancer. *Cancer Res.* **54**: 1630–1633.

77. Visscher, D. W., F. De Mattia, S. Ottosen, F. H. Sarkar, and J. D. Crissman. 1995. Biologic and clinical significance of basic fibroblast growth factor immunostaining in breast carcinoma. *Modern Pathol.* **8**: 665–670.

78. Seymour, L. and W. R. Bezwoda. 1994. Positive immunostaining for platelet derived growth factor (PDGF) is an adverse prognostic factor in patients with advanced breast cancer. *Breast Cancer Res. Treat.* **32**: 229–233.

79. Fox, S. B., R. D. Leek, M. P. Weekes, R. M. Whitehouse, K. C. Gatter, and A. L. Harris. 1995. Quantitation and prognostic value of breast cancer angiogenesis: comparison of microvessel density, Chalkley count and computer image analysis. *J. Pathol.* **177**: 275–283.

80. Howlett, A. R., N. Bailey, C. Damsky, O. W. Petersen, and M. J. Bissell. 1995. Cellular growth and survival are mediated by β1 integrins in normal human breast epithelium but not in breast carcinoma. *J. Cell Sci.* **108**: 1945–1957.

81. Folkman, J. 1996. Tumor angiogenesis and tissue factor. *Nature Med.* **2:** 167–168.

82. Fox, S. B. and A. L. Harris. 1997. Markers of tumor angiogenesis: clinical applications in prognosis and anti-angiogenic therapy. *Invest. New Drugs* **15:** 15–28.

83. Gasparini, G. 1997. Antiangiogenic drugs as a novel anticancer therapeutic strategy. Which are the more promising agents? Which are the clinical developments and indications? *Crit Rev. Oncol Hematol.* **26:** 147–162.

84. Gasparini, G. 1995. Biological and clinical role of angiogenesis in breast carcinoma. *Breast Cancer Res. Treat.* **36:** 103–107.

85. Marx, J. 1993. Cellular changes on the route to metastasis. *Science* **259:** 626–629.

86. McLeskey, S. W., J. Kurebayashi, S. F. Honig, J. Zwiebel, M. E. Lippman, R. B. Dickson, and F. G. Kern. 1993. Fibroblast growth factor 4 transfection of MCF-7 cells produces cell lines that are tumorigenic and metastatic in ovariectomized or tamoxifen-treated athymic nude mice. *Cancer Res.* **53:** 2168–2177.

87. Costa, M., R. Danesi, C. Agen, A. Di Paolo, F. Basolo, S. Del Bianchi, and M. Del Tacca. 1994. MCF-10A cells infected with the int-2 oncogene induce angiogenesis in the chick choriollantoic membrane and in the rat mesentary. *Cancer Res.* **54:** 9–11.

88. Toi, M., J. Kashitani, and T. Tominaga. 1993. Tumor angiogenesis is an independent prognostic indicator in primary breast carcinoma. *Int. J. Cancer* **55:** 371–374.

89. Obermair, A., C. Kurz, K. Czerwenka, M. Tholma, A. Kaider, T. Wagner, G. Gitsch, and P. Sevelda. 1995. Microvessel density and vessel invasion in lymph-node-negative breast cancer: effect on recurrence-free survival. *Int. J. Cancer* **62:** 126–131.

90. Siitonen, S. M., H. K. Haapasalo, I. S. Rantala, H. J. Helin, and J. J. Isola. 1995. Comparison of different immunohistochemical methods in the assessment of angiogenesis: lack of prognostic value in a group of 77 selected node-negative breast carcinomas. *Modern Pathol.* **8:** 745–752.

91. Horak, E. R., R. Leek, N. Klenk, S. LeJeune, K. Smith , N. Stuart, M. Greenall, K. Stepniewska, and A. L. Harris. 1992. Angiogenesis, assessed by platelet/endothelial cell adhesion molecule antibodies, as indicator of node metastases and survival in breast cancer. *Lancet* **340:** 1120–1124.

92. Bosari, S., A. K. C. Lee, R. A. DeLellis, B. D. Wiley, G. J. Heatley, and M. L. Silverman. 1992. Microvessel quantification and prognosis in invasive breast carcinoma. *Human Pathol.* **23:** 755–761.

93. Khanuja, P. S., P. Gimotty, T. Fregene, J. George, and K. J. Pienta. 1993. Angiogenesis quantitation as a prognostic factor for primary breast carcinoma 2 cms or less, in *Adjuvant Therapy of Cancer VII* (Salmon, S. E., ed.), Lippincott, Philadelphia, PA, pp. 226–232.

94. Goulding, H., N. F. Nik Abdul Rashid, F. Robertson, J. A. Bell, C. W. Elston, R. W. Blamey, and I. O. Ellis. 1995. Assessment of angiogenesis in breast carcinoma: An important factor in prognosis? *Human Pathol.* **26:** 1196–1200.

95. Kaldjian, E. P., L. Jin, R. D. Davenport, and R. V. Lloyd. 1993. Immunohistochemical analysis of hormone receptors, tumor vascularity, and proliferative activity in paraffin-embedded sections of breast carcinoma tissues. *Appl. Immunoistochem.* **1:** 31–38.

96. Monschke, F., W. U. Muller, U. Winkler, and C. Streffer. 1991. Cell proliferation and vascularization in human breast carcinomas. *Int. J. Cancer* **49:** 812–815.

97. Vartanian, R. K. and N. Weidner. 1994. Correlation of intratumoral endothelial cell proliferation with microvessel density (tumor angiogenesis) and tumor cell proliferation in breast carcinoma. *Am. J. Pathol.* **144:** 1188–1194.

98. Fox, S. B., C. Gatter, R. Bicknell, J. J. Going, P. Stanton, T. G. Cooke, and A. L. Harris. 1993. Relationship of endothelial cell proliferation to tumor vascularity in human breast cancer. *Cancer Res.* **53:** 4161–4163.

99. Leek, R. D., C. E. Lewis, R. Whitehouse, M. Greenall, J. Clarke, and A. L. Harris. 1996. Association of macrophage infiltration with angiogenesis and prognosis in invasive breast carcinoma. *Cancer Res.* **56:** 4625–4629.

100. Obermair, A., K. Czerwenka, C. Kurz, P. Buxhaum, M. Schemper, and P. Sevelda. 1994. Influence of tumoral microvessel density on the recurrence-free survival in human breast cancer: preliminary results. *Onkologie* **17**: 44–49.

101. Ogawa, Y., Y.-S. Chung, B. Nakata, S. Takasuka, K. Maeda, T. Sawada, Y. Kato, K. Yoshikawa, M. Sakurai, and M. Sowa. 1995. Microvessel quantitation in invasive breast cancer by staining for factor VIII-related antigen. *Br. J. Cancer* **71**: 1297–1301.

102. Toi, M., K. Inada. H. Suzuki, and T. Tominaga. 1995. Tumor angiogenesis in breast cancer: its importance as a prognostic indicator and the association with vascular endothelial growth factor expression. *Breast Cancer Res. Treat.* **36**: 193–204.

103. Kato, T., T. Kimura, H. Muraki, T. Kamio, A. Fujii, K. Yamamoto, and K. Hamano. 1992. A study on angiogenesis in breast cancer with factor VIII-related antigen staining. *J. Jpn. Soc. Cancer Ther* **27**: 1819–1828.

104. Kato, T., T. Kimura, H. Muraki, T. Kamio, A. Fujii, K. Yamamoto, and K. Hamano. 1995. A clinicopathological study of angiogenesis in breast cancer. *J. Jpn. Surg. Soc.* **28**: 709–718.

105. Simpson, J. F., C. Ahn, H. Battifora, and J. M. Esteban. 1996. Endothelial area as a prognostic indicator for invasive breast carcinoma. *Cancer* **77**: 2077–2085.

106. Fox, S. B., R. D. Leek, K. Smith, J. Hollyer, M. Greenall, and A. L. Harris. 1994. Tumor angiogenesis in node-negative breast carcinomas: relationship with epidermal growth factor receptor, estrogen receptor, and survival. *Breast Cancer Res. Treat.* **29**: 109–116.

107. Barbareschi, M., N. Weidner, G. Gasparini, L. Morelli, S. Forti, C. Eccher, P. Fina, E. Leonardi, F. Mauri, P. Bevilacqua, and P. Dalla Palma. 1995. Microvessel density quantification in breast carcinomas: Assessment by light microscopy vs. a computer-aided image analysis system. *Appl. Immunoistochem.* **3**: 75–84.

108. Lee, A. K. C., M. Loda, G. Mackarem, S. Bosari, R. A. DeLellis, G. J. Heatley, and K. Hughes. 1997. Lymph node negative invasive breast carcinoma 1 centimeter or less in size (T1a,bNoMo): clinicopathologic features and outcome. *Cancer* **79**: 761–771.

109. Sterns, E. E., S. SenGupta, and B. Zee. 1997. Macromolecular interstitital clearance, tumour vascularity, other prognostic factors and breast cancer survival. *Breast Cancer Res. Treat.* **42**: 113–120.

III
Therapeutics and Diagnostics
Diagnosis

17

Cytogenetic Approaches to Breast Cancer

Sverre Heim, Manuel R. Teixeira, and Nikos Pandis

1. INTRODUCTION

According to the somatic mutation theory of cancer, stable changes of the hereditary material may bring about neoplastic transformation of the target cells harboring them, i.e., unleash the tumorous phenotype. Such somatic cell mutations may be studied at different resolution levels, corresponding to the complex modes and manners in which genetic information is packed and organized: as cytological examination of whole cells, as measurements of total cellular DNA content by flow cytometry, by microscopic investigation of the cells' chromosome complement, and, biochemically, by the study of individual genes and base pairs. Although the information obtained via these approaches to some extent overlaps, each has its inherent methodological and epistemological advantages and disadvantages (1), and none can today be supplanted by any other without significant loss of investigative power. The main advantages of the cytogenetic approach, compared with the currently more popular molecular genetic one, are twofold: First, chromosome banding analysis is a screening method that gives an overview of the entire genome at the chosen level of investigation. The information obtained is therefore not limited by the initial choice of a specific, limited set of probes, as has been the case with most molecular approaches available until now, a choice that of necessity must always contain an element of arbitrariness, and, hence, may not always include the means to detect the pathogenetically most important changes. Second, since cytogenetics is a cytological technique, it provides information about the characteristics of individual cells, and not of any theoretical mean within the sampled tissue. Only if no intratumor genomic heterogeneity exists will the importance of the latter point be negligible.

Although the present review focuses almost exclusively on the chromosome banding appearance of breast cancer cells, it may at this juncture be pertinent to mention also some recent methodological improvements that lie at the interface of what has traditionally been perceived as classic cytogenetic and classic molecular genetic techniques, and which promise to eventually bridge the investigative gap between the two resolution levels. Fluorescence *in situ* hybridization (FISH) with chromosome-specific DNA probes (2) can identify rearrangements too subtle or too complex to be disclosed by chromosome banding. On the negative side, FISH only reveals those aberrations one tests for, and is therefore better suited for the final characterization of marker

From: Breast Cancer: Molecular Genetics, Pathogenesis, and Therapeutics
Edited by: A. M. Bowcock © Humana Press Inc., Totowa, NJ

chromosomes whose identity could not be fully determined by banding, than for initial tumor screening. Comparative genomic hybridization (CGH), on the other hand, which uses tumor genomic DNA and normal DNA as competing probes and normal metaphases as templates, is a genuine screening method that detects copy-number changes *(3,4)*. CGH does not detect balanced rearrangements, however, nor does it detect differences among cells. A new FISH technology called multicolor spectral karyotyping *(5)* or multiplex-fluorescence hybridization *(6)* uses a pool of chromosome painting probes, each of which is labeled with a different fluorochrome combination. This powerful technique has wider specificity than the original FISH methods, and is particularly promising in the characterization of complex interchromosomal rearrangements and changes involving chromosome segments too small or too similarly banded to be adequately described by banding. It does not detect intrachromosomal changes, however, and breakpoint assignment is unreliable. Chromosome banding analysis, therefore, remains the best initial screening method, because it enables the detection of previously unsuspected rearrangements in tumor cells and at the same time allows an evaluation of genetic heterogeneity within the neoplastic parenchyma.

Whereas research on the cytogenetic abnormalities that characterize hematologic malignancies has proceeded actively for nearly three decades and has led to the accumulation of data on nearly 20,000 cases, comparable studies on solid tumors lag some 20 yr behind *(7)*. Despite this, typical karyotypic aberration patterns have now been found also in many benign and malignant epithelial and, especially, nonepithelial tumors *(8–10)*. Since different tumor types are characterized by different chromosomal anomalies, the karyotype can often be used diagnostically, either to establish that a sampled lesion is indeed neoplastic, to decide whether a tumor is benign or malignant, or to arrive at specific diagnoses. Good clinical use may also be made of the prognostic information carried by particular aberration patterns, which often seems to be independent of other phenotypic disease characteristics *(7,9)*. From the research point of view, finally, the karyotypic data can be used to draw conclusions about the pathogenetic mechanisms that are operative, both regarding which genes are involved and how, and as a key to the proliferating target cells' clonal evolution during multistage tumorigenesis.

2. CHROMOSOME ABERRATIONS IN SPORADIC BREAST CARCINOMAS

About 500 breast carcinomas studied with chromosome banding techniques and found to carry clonal abnormalities have been scientifically reported *(8,* updated*)*. Whereas some investigators have harvested the tumor cells directly or after only a few hours in vitro incubation, thus in effect examining only cells that were dividing already in vivo *(11–13)*, others have used short-term culturing prior to cytogenetic analysis *(14,15)*. Although, both theoretically and in practice, this may lead to different pictures of the tumors' chromosomal constitution *(16,17)* (e.g., the direct technique yields a much higher incidence of cytogenetically normal carcinomas, but also, on average, more complex karyotypes in those that are found to be abnormal), by and large the information obtained by the two approaches shows good correspondence. In addition to the banding information, several studies of breast cancers characterized by CGH

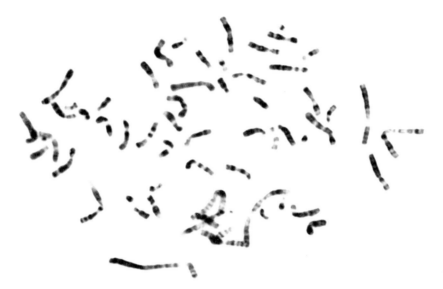

Fig. 1. Complex metaphase plate from a breast carcinoma with numerous numerical and structural chromosome abnormalities.

have also been published recently *(18–22)*. It is not the purpose of this review to present the CGH picture of breast carcinogenesis, but in general it seems to corroborate what was already known from more traditional cytogenetic analyses.

The main conclusion to emerge is that although nonneoplastic breast tissue is karyo-typically normal *(23)*, nonrandom acquired clonal chromosome aberrations character-ize breast tumors *(8,11–13,17,23–29)*. In studies utilizing short-term in vitro culturing *(27,30)*, nearly 50% of all breast carcinomas are found to have only a single aberration per cell, which fits well with the fact that 40% are flow cytometrically diploid *(31)*. Other tumors, perhaps especially ductal and comedo type carcinomas *(30)*, may carry moderately to extremely complex karyotypic changes (Fig. 1).

At least 11 chromosomal aberrations have been found repeatedly, both as the only change and as part of more complex karyotypes, thus meeting the requirements for a primary cancer-associated cytogenetic anomaly. They are the structural rearrangements der(1;16)(q10;p10), i(1)(q10), del(1)(q11–12), del(1)(q42), del(3)(p12–13p14–21), and del(6)(q21–22) (Fig. 2), and the numerical changes +7, +8, +12, +18, and +20. The most common chromosomal imbalances encountered are gains of chromosomes and chromosome arms 1q, 7, 8, 18, and 20, and losses of X, 1p, 1q, 3p, 6q, 8p, 11p, 11q, 13q, 16q, 17p, 19p, 19q, and 22, which is in good accord with data stemming from molecular genetic investigations based on the loss of heterozygosity principle *(32)*, as well as with information obtained by various fluorescence hybridization techniques, including comparative genomic hybridization *(33,34)*. The breakpoints preferentially involved in structural chromosome rearrangements are 1p36, 1p22, 1q11–12, 1q21, 3p21, 3p12–14, 3q29, 4q21, 5p15, 6q21, 7p22, 7q11, 8p21, 11p15, 11q13, 13q12, 15cen, 16p13, 16cen, 16q22, and 19q13. These bands are likely to harbor genes impor-tant in mammary carcinogenesis.

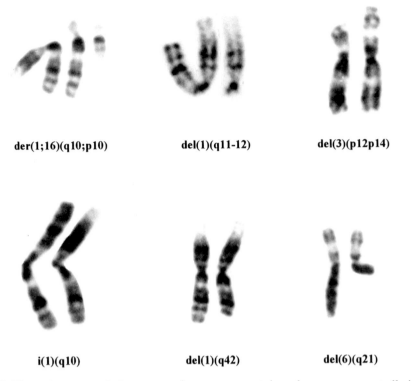

der(1;16)(q10;p10)   del(1)(q11-12)   del(3)(p12p14)

i(1)(q10)   del(1)(q42)   del(6)(q21)

Fig. 2. These six structural chromosomal rearrangements have been seen repeatedly in breast carcinomas, both as the only change and as part of complex karyotypes. They are likely to represent pathogenetically important primary abnormalities in mammary carcinogenesis.

3. CHROMOSOME ABERRATIONS IN CANCER-PRONE BREASTS

About 20% of breast cancer patients have a positive family history, and, in perhaps one-fourth of these cases, the segregation pattern of the disease among family members indicates that the predisposition is inherited as an autosomal dominant trait *(35,36)*. Such hereditary breast cancer is relatively often bilateral and has a tendency to occur in younger women. It may be site-specific, in which case it may also be associated with an increased frequency of ovarian cancer, or, more rarely, it may occur as part of complex phenotypic pictures in the Li-Fraumeni syndrome, ataxia telangiectasia, Lynch syndrome type II, Peutz-Jegher syndrome, Klinefelter syndrome, Reifenstein syndrome, and Cowden's disease *(37,38)*.

At present, two quantitatively important genes predisposing to breast cancer have been identified, the BRCA1 in 17q21 and the BRCA2 in 13q12–13 *(39,40)*; taken together, germ-line mutations of these genes probably account for some two-thirds of all hereditary site-specific breast cancers. Loss of heterozygosity and linkage analysis data point to the presence of a third susceptibility gene in 8p *(41,42)*, and the existence of yet others is by no means ruled out.

Although some chromosome abnormalities have been seen that involve bands harboring known breast cancer susceptibility genes, most aberrations affect other genomic regions, and their pathogenetic effect must hence have been achieved via other mechanisms. It should be underscored that the data behind this conclusion stem almost exclusively from investigations of sporadic tumors; for familial breast cancer, practically no cytogenetic information exists, because only two relatively small studies have utilized chromosome-banding technique to study the genetic aberrations acquired by hereditarily predisposed breast cells during carcinogenesis. Teixeira et al. *(43)* examined samples from three bilateral prophylactic mastectomies and one *in situ* ductal carcinoma from four women belonging to a family with hereditary breast cancer. Clonal chromosome aberrations were found in five of the six prophylactically removed breasts, all of which had the histologic diagnosis epithelial hyperplasia without atypia, and in the *in situ* carcinoma. The same karyotypic imbalance, a loss of 3p12–14 (Fig. 2), was detected in the *in situ* carcinoma as well as in one of the hyperplasias. Also, Petersson et al. *(44)* detected clonal karyotypic changes in five of eight prophylactically removed breasts from five unrelated women who belonged to families with a known hereditary predisposition to breast cancer; that study did not include examination of any actual tumors. Finally, Lindblom et al. *(45)* examined polymorphic markers at 45 loci for loss of heterozygosity in an allelotyping study of 82 familial breast carcinomas. The most frequently involved chromosome arms were 8p, 16q, 17p, 17q, and 19p. At present, therefore, there is nothing to indicate that the pattern of acquired genomic changes in hereditary breast cancer differs from that in sporadic carcinomas, but it must be emphasized again that the data are extremely rudimentary, and that the situation may well turn out to be one in which absence of evidence should not be taken to mean evidence of absence.

4. MALIGNANT VS BENIGN BREAST TUMORS

As mentioned under the preceding subheading, clonal chromosome aberrations have, in women belonging to breast cancer families, been detected in nontumorous mammary epithelium that, though hyperplastic, did not show signs of atypia. Several studies of benign mammary lesions from women at no increased hereditary risk have confirmed that, in the breast, as indeed in all other organs and tissues, acquired chromosome abnormalities are a feature of neoplastically transformed cells generally, not only of malignant ones.

Abnormal karyotypes have been described in more than 30 fibroadenomas, benign breast tumors of biphasic origin *(46–55)*. Some fibroadenomas have been demonstrated to contain more than one abnormal clone, which is indicative of polyclonal tumorigenesis. Attempts have been made by differential sedimentation and culturing *(52)*, as well as by immunological methods *(47,49)*, to determine the cellular origin of the clones. Both the mesenchymal and epithelial tumor components carry acquired abnormalities, as would be expected of truly biphasic tumors. The impression is that whereas one clone only is found corresponding to the mesenchymal component, several clones may exist among the epithelial cells *(52)*.

The chromosomal arms that have been repeatedly found to be involved in aberrations in fibroadenomas are 1q, 2q, 3p, 4q, 5q, 6p, 6q, 8q, 9p, 9q, 12p, 12q, 14q, 15q, and 16q. Recurrent numerical changes have included gain of chromosomes 4, 5, 7, 11, 18, and 20, and loss of chromosomes 6 and 17. Some of the aberrations, in particular der(1;16), del(3p), and del(6q), are among those consistently associated also with breast carcinomas (Fig. 2). Presumably, the cells of carcinomas are primed for malignant behavior in some additional, unknown way, perhaps by carrying submicroscopic additional acquired genomic anomalies, or subtle differences in target cell differentiation may account for the variable response to seemingly identical genetic injuries.

Also another biphasic neoplasm of the breast, phyllodes tumor, has been examined cytogenetically (56–60). Again, both the mesenchymal and epithelial tumor components have been shown to harbor clonal chromosome abnormalities, and again several cytogenetically unrelated clones are sometimes found. Among the aberrations detected, in particular from cells belonging to the epithelial tumor fraction, are also changes that have been seen repeatedly in cells from breast carcinomas, e.g., i(1q) and del(3p). Whereas benign and borderline phyllodes tumors seem to have relatively small deviations from the normal diploid karyotype, the malignant ones have had massive numerical and structural chromosomal aberrations (58,59). In contrast to phyllodes tumors and fibroadenomas, adenolipomas of the breast seem to carry chromosome abnormalities only in cells belonging to the connective tissue component, indicating that the concomitant proliferation of glandular elements seen in these tumors is nonneoplastic (61).

Other benign tumors and proliferative disturbances of the breast that have been subjected to cytogenetic investigation are hamartoma, papilloma, and hyperproliferative (fibrocystic) breast disease with or without concomitant cellular atypia. Both hamartomas studied by Dietrich et al. (62) were karyotypically abnormal, testifying to the neoplastic nature of these lesions. Rearrangements of 3p13–14 were seen in both tumors; in one of them, this led to obvious loss of material. Dietrich et al. (52) described clonal chromosome abnormalities in four of five papillomas. In two of them, the aberrations included 3p deletions. Finally, clonal chromosome aberrations have also been detected in benign hyperproliferative breast disorders (43,52,63), indicating that although no macroscopic tumorous lesions exist, the target cells have acquired mutations upsetting normal growth regulation, i.e., they have become neoplastic. Again, we are faced with evidence that some of the cancer-associated lesions, including der(1;16)(q10;p10), del(1)(q12), and del(3)(p12p14), by themselves may not be sufficient to unleash the full malignant phenotype in all breast cells at all times and at all stages of development and differentiation.

5. INTRATUMOR HETEROGENEITY

Breast cancer is an extremely heterogeneous malignancy, both regarding its clinical course and the tumor histology (64,65). One factor that might contribute to the heterogeneity is genetic differences among cells belonging to the tumor parenchyma; after all, striking genotype–phenotype parallels are no less common among neoplasms than among organisms. The cytological nature of chromosome banding analysis makes it ideally suited to assess such cell-to-cell differences, and also to find out whether the genetically different subpopulations, alluded to repeatedly above, are uniformly distributed within the tumor or occupy separate topological domains.

Teixeira et al. (23,66) performed an in-depth study of intratumor cytogenetic heterogeneity, analyzing the chromosome banding pattern of 5,096 metaphases from 73 samples taken from 10 breast cancer cases (from nine women; one had bilateral disease). From each case, one sample from each tumor quadrant (success rate, 90%), as well as four samples from the surrounding, macroscopically normal-looking breast tis-

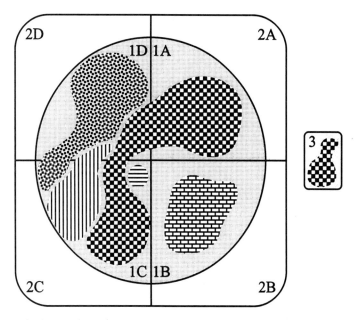

Fig. 3. Schematic illustration of a breast cancer case in which four tumor quadrants (1A–D), their corresponding areas of surrounding, normal-looking breast (2A–D), and a subcutaneous metastasis (3) were cytogenetically analyzed. The five different texture patterns in irregular areas within 1A–D represent the five cytogenetically unrelated, karyotypically abnormal clones that were found; the size of each area reflects the number of cells making up that particular clone. Although no clonal abnormalities were found in the histologically normal breast tissue of 2A–D, cells with a del(3)(p13p14) as the only change were found in the subcutaneous metastasis, 3. Cells with the same chromosome anomaly were also found in carcinoma quadrants 1A, 1C, and 1D, but then as part of a polyclonal primary tumor karyotype.

sue (success rate, 94%), were cultured and processed for analysis. When the cases included metastases, attempts were made to examine them, too.

All 10 breast carcinomas were shown to contain clonal chromosome abnormalities in 89% of the tumor samples (32 of 36). Multiple clones (two to nine) were detected in seven of the 10, and were always unevenly distributed within the tumor mass (Fig. 3). This demonstration of genomic variability, corresponding to macroscopic tumor domains, strengthens the likelihood that at least part of breast cancer phenotypic heterogeneity may be accounted for by reference to intratumor differences in the patterns of acquired genomic aberrations. In addition, and no less important regarding the reliability and completeness of studies assessing breast cancer-associated changes, it is clear that sampling of multiple tumor sites is necessary if one wants to obtain an as complete as possible, balanced picture of the whole tumor's genetic characteristics. Similar conclusions have also been reached via other investigative approaches. Beerman et al. *(67)* showed that at least four breast carcinoma samples are necessary to detect all stemlines by flow cytometry with a larger than 90% probability. Barranco et al. *(68)* reported that the DNA index intersample variability was so great that there was only a 61% chance of identifying an aneuploid tumor clone (when present), if only a single site was analyzed; the authors made the point that this intratumor variability could be the cause of conflicting estimates of patient survival and response to therapy. The existence of intratumor genetic heterogeneity has also been suggested by the results of loss of heterozygosity *(69)* and gene amplification *(70,71)* studies. It seems clear that analyses of the genomic constitution of breast carcinomas (be it at the total DNA, chromosomal, or genic level) that do not take this into consideration should be interpreted with caution.

The analysis of samples taken outside the tumors sometimes revealed chromosomal aberrations similar to those found in the carcinoma, but then the microscopic examination of neighboring sections always showed that detectable disease spreading had taken place. Histologically normal breast tissue was found to be cytogenetically normal.

6. MULTIFOCAL AND MULTICENTRIC BREAST CARCINOMAS

Several histopathologic studies have shown that between one-fourth and one-half of all patients with breast cancer have another carcinoma focus in the same breast in addition to the index tumor *(72–75)*. Because the majority of malignant breast tumors are ductal carcinomas of no special type, histological examination in most instances cannot discriminate between multifocal carcinomas (in which case intramammary spreading from a single primary tumor has occurred) and multicentric carcinomas (more than one primary tumor exists within the breast). Other parameters, such as the location of the foci in different quadrants and the presence of *in situ* components in each lesion, have therefore been relied on to diagnose multicentricity *(75)*, but the actual ability of these features to differentiate between the two pathogenetically different entities remains uncertain.

Because even the most common breast cancer-associated chromosome abnormalities occur in no more than 10% of the tumors in the largest studies relying on the same technique *(27)*, cytogenetics can be used to determine whether the tumor cell populations of two macroscopically distinct lesions within the same breast are clonally related. Teixeira et al. *(76,77)* and Pandis et al. *(78)* addressed this question, examining 37 tumorous lesions from 17 patients. Clonal chromosome abnormalities were found in 27 lesions. The overall karyotypic pattern did not differ from that of solitary sporadic breast carcinomas, inasmuch as cytogenetic polyclonality with near- or pseudo-diploid clones and many of the common breast cancer-associated rearrangements, including del(3p), der(1;16), and i(1q) (Fig. 2), were seen. At least two macroscopically distinct carcinoma foci were karyotypically abnormal in each of 12 patients, making them informative regarding the clonal relationship among the breast tumors. Nine of these cases had an evolutionarily related, cytogenetically abnormal clone in the different tumor lesions from the same breast, strongly indicating that the dominant mechanism for the origin of multiple, ipsilateral breast carcinomas is intramammary spreading from a single tumor, i.e., these carcinomas were multifocal. In the remaining three informative patients, no one clonal aberration was common to the foci, indicating that the synchronous lesions arose by pathogenetically independent processes within the same breast, although the possibility that the karyotypically unique foci may have been related through some shared submicroscopic mutation cannot be completely disregarded.

Of particular interest was the observation that some foci that, by virtue of their karyotypic similarities, must have been part of the same clonal neoplastic process, nevertheless harbored carcinoma *in situ* areas; evidently, this is not a good marker of multicentricity. On the other hand, and with the caveat that the numbers involved are small, the available data do indicate that the distance between tumors may be informative regarding whether they are clonally related or not; tumors far apart are more likely to be multicentric than are those close to one another.

7. BILATERAL BREAST CARCINOMAS

Bilateral breast cancer may be synchronous or metachronous. The risk of developing a carcinoma in the contralateral breast in the decade following treatment for a first tumor has been estimated at 5–10% *(79,80)*. The principal question is the same as for multiple ipsilateral lesions: Are the tumors clonally related or not?

We have examined cytogenetically 19 carcinomas from 10 women with bilateral disease (only the left-sided tumor was available in one of the cases) *(23,43,78)*. Seven of the cases were informative regarding the clonal relationship between the two lesions, with the cytogenetic findings in five supporting the notion that each carcinoma arose independently as a genuinely new tumor; the remaining two cases had cytogenetic similarities, indicating that spreading had occurred from one side to the other. In bilateral carcinomas, too, areas showing *in situ* carcinoma could be detected in what, based on the cytogenetic evolution pattern, must surely have been a metastasis, underscoring again that this is an insufficient criterion to deem any lesion primary.

8. PRIMARY TUMORS AND THEIR METASTASES

For all common malignant diseases, surprisingly little is known about the genetic, let alone cytogenetic, relationship between the primary tumors and their metastases *(9)*. Regarding the breast cancer situation specifically, the most pertinent questions are the following: Do lymph node metastases exhibit the same chromosomal aberrations that are found in primary breast carcinomas? Is cytogenetic heterogeneity, including polyclonality, an equally prominent feature of lymph node metastases as of primary breast tumors? Are there some aberrations that particularly facilitate the metastatic process and which, as a consequence, are found more often in metastatic lesions?

It is now clear that some breast cancer metastases are karyotypically simple *(8,23,81–84)*, as had already been surmised based on flow cytometric findings *(85,86)*. Among simple chromosomal abnormalities that have been found both in primary tumors and metastases are del(3p), del(1q), and der(1;16) *(23,82,83)*, i.e., the very changes that are found most frequently as sole aberrations in sporadic carcinomas (Fig. 2). The finding of simple chromosomal changes in breast cancer metastases is of interest from several perspectives. Most important is that it constitutes strong evidence that the cells carrying these abnormalities really belong to the neoplastic parenchyma, despite the fact that seemingly identical aberrations may also be detected in benign breast lesions. Especially in cases in which karyotypically complex clones are found alongside others with only simple abnormalities, doubt has lingered about the importance of the latter; is it not more likely that they reflect secondary changes taking place in the tumor stroma? The demonstration now of the same simple abnormalities in both the primary tumor and its lymph node metastasis disproves this view, and shows that karyotypic complexity is an insufficient criterion by which to judge the malignant capacity of cells. Second, the karyotypic simplicity of some of the metastatic clones

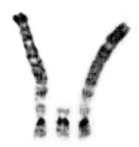

Fig. 4. Homogeneously staining regions (hsr) were present on the short arm of two of the three copies of chromosome 16 present in this cell from a lymph node breast cancer metastasis. Such regions, which are the cytogenetic evidence of high-grade gene amplification, seem to be more common in metastatic than in primary breast carcinomas.

indicates that spreading of the disease must have taken place at a relatively early stage in the tumor's life. It is, of course, possible that cells with simple karyotypic changes may also carry submicroscopic mutations, and our findings therefore do not constitute any conclusive counterargument to the view that metastatic lesions represent the genetically complex end-stage of multistep neoplastic processes. This is especially so since a higher percentage of the lymph node metastases (9 of 12 with an abnormal karyotype) than that found in primary tumors had a relatively complex karyotype (23,83). The data are few and exceptions unquestionably exist, but by and large it seems that metastatic cases tend to be karyotypically more complex than primary breast carcinomas in the sense that the average clone has more extensive changes, but less complex in the sense that cytogenetic polyclonality is rarer (Fig. 3).

Except for the overall karyotypic complexity, does the available information provide any clues as to which aberrations may be more characteristic of metastatic breast cancer than of primary tumors? The data are very limited, but homogeneously staining regions (hsr) have been found in as many as one-third of all metastatic cases (Fig. 4); the amplified genes are unknown, though. Other aberrations seen more frequently in metastases are –17 and loss of all or parts of chromosome 22. Again, the gene changes this might correspond to are unknown.

9. IS THERE A CLINICAL ROLE
FOR BREAST CANCER CYTOGENETICS?

Cancer cytogenetics is not only a research endeavor but has increasingly become incorporated into state-of-the-art clinical management of oncological patients (7,9). The clinical usefulness of the neoplastic karyotype was first demonstrated for hematologic disorders, but in recent years some types of solid tumor cytogenetics, especially the analysis of sarcomas and childhood tumors, have found their way into clinical practice. Can breast cancer cytogenetics be expected to play a similar role?

Although the pattern of acquired chromosomal aberrations in breast cancer is unquestionably nonrandom, no single aberration has been so unambiguously associated with breast cancer in general, or with any of the histological subgroups in particular, as to be diagnostically useful. Some of the changes consistently found in carcinomas have also occasionally been found in the epithelial component of benign breast proliferations, usually atypically epithelial hyperplasias, indicating that these chromosomal changes confer upon the cells harboring them a proliferative advantage over their neighbors but not a malignant phenotype per se *(43,44,52,63)*. A future diagnostic role for cytogenetics in the management of breast tumor patients is therefore more likely to be based on the degree and pattern of karyotypic complexity than on the presence of any particular chromosome abnormality. Cytogenetic investigations have revealed that benign phyllodes tumors have simple chromosome aberrations whereas the malignant ones are karyotypically complex *(58,59)*. Because grading individual phyllodes tumors, based solely on their histopathologic features, can be difficult, karyotypic complexity may become an important parameter for the correct diagnosis.

A second possible clinical role for cytogenetic investigations of breast tumors in the future may be to ascertain whether patients with multiple ipsilateral or bilateral carcinomas have pathogenetically independent neoplasms or if the separate tumors arose by spreading of a single neoplastic process. Knowledge about the biological relationship among multiple breast tumors may help classify individual patients within families with a hereditary predisposition to breast cancer, may turn out to have prognostic value, and may in general influence future therapeutic choices (for instance, the extent of local resection or the need and type of adjuvant therapy). With the emergence of conservative surgical management (e.g., lumpectomy) as a major therapeutic modality, knowledge as to whether a breast carcinoma after treatment for a previous tumor represents a recurrence or a second primary originating in the remaining breast tissue, is likely to become more important. This type of information may be obtained by comparing the karyotypes of the original and the new tumor.

A third possible clinical use for karyotypic data on breast tumors relates to the prognostic information the presence of particular cytogenetic aberrations may carry. The available database is still too small to allow reliable correlation analyses, but the following questions should be addressed in the future: Does a patient's risk of developing invasive breast carcinoma from a benign hyperproliferative lesion or an *in situ* carcinoma depend on which chromosome aberration(s) the premalignant lesion contains (particularly suspicious seem those chromosomal aberrations that have been identified as primary changes in breast carcinoma)? Does the prognosis of a patient diagnosed with breast cancer depend on the type and extent of the karyotypic aberrations present in the primary tumor? Some preliminary findings indicate that informative correlations may exist. Zafrani et al. *(87)* reported that patients considered to have a poor prognosis by conventional factors, e.g., young age, high histologic grade, metastatic disease, and loss of hormonal receptors, more often had homogeneously staining regions in the tumor's karyotype. Presumably because the number of cases was too low, the observed skewness did not reach statistical significance, however. Steinarsdóttir et al. *(17)* reported that survival at 36 mo was lower (63%) for the patient group whose tumors had complex clonal chromosome abnormalities, compared with the ones with only simple changes or a normal karyotype (92%). Finally, Pandis et al. *(30)* found associations between the chromosome number and mitotic activity in vivo, and between cytogenetic polyclonality and tumor grade; both differences turned out to be statistically significant in multivariate models.

REFERENCES

1. Heim, S. 1992. Is cancer cytogenetics reducible to the molecular genetics of cancer cells? *Genes Chromosom. Cancer* **5:** 188–196.
2. Lichter, P. and T. Cremer. 1992. Chromosome analysis by nonisotopic in situ hybridization, in *Human Cytogenetics: A Practical Approach,* vol. 1, *Constitutional Analysis,* 2nd ed. (Rooney, D. E. and B. H. Czepulkowski, eds.), IRL, Oxford, pp. 157–192.
3. Kallioniemi, A., O. P. Kallioniemi, D. Sudar, D. Rutovitz, J. W. Gray, F. Waldman, and D. Pinkel. 1992. Comparative genomic hybridization for molecular cytogenetic analysis of solid tumors. *Science* **258:** 818–821.
4. du Manoir, S., M. R. Speicher, S. Joos, E. Schröck, S. Popp, H. Döhner, et al. 1993. Detection of complete and partial chromosome gains and losses by comparative genomic hybridization. *Hum. Genet.* **90:** 590–610.
5. Schröck, E., S. du Manoir, T. Veldman, B. Schoell, J. Wienberg, M. A. Ferguson-Smith, et al. 1996. Multicolor spectral karyotyping of human chromosomes. *Science* **273:** 494–497.
6. Speicher, M. R., S. Gwyn Ballard, and D. C. Ward. 1996. Karyotyping human chromosomes by combinatorial multi-fluor FISH. *Nature Genet.* **12:** 368–375.
7. Mitelman, F., B. Johansson, N. Mandahl, and F. Mertens. 1997. Clinical significance of cytogenetic findings in solid tumors. *Cancer Genet. Cytogenet.* **95:** 1–8.
8. Mitelman, F. 1994. *Catalog of Chromosome Aberrations in Cancer,* 5th ed., Wiley-Liss, New York.
9. Heim, S. and F. Mitelman. 1995. *Cancer Cytogenetics*, 2nd ed., Wiley-Liss, New York.
10. Mitelman, F., F. Mertens, and B. Johansson. 1997. A breakpoint map of recurrent chromosomal rearrangements in human neoplasia. *Nature Genet.* **15:** 417–474.
11. Dutrillaux, B., M. Gerbault-Seureau, and B. Zafrani. 1990. Characterization of chromosomal anomalies in human breast cancer. A comparison of 30 paradiploid cases with few chromosome changes. *Cancer Genet. Cytogenet.* **49:** 203–217.
12. Hainsworth, P. J., K. L. Raphael, R. G. Stillwell, R. C. Bennett, and O. M. Garson. 1991. Cytogenetic features of twenty-six primary breast cancers. *Cancer Genet. Cytogenet.* **53:** 205–218.
13. Lu, Y. J., S. Xiao, Y. S. Yan, S. B. Fu, Q. Z. Liu, and P. Li. 1993. Direct chromosome analysis of 50 primary breast carcinomas. *Cancer Genet. Cytogenet.* **69:** 91–99.
14. Limon, J., P. Dal Cin, and A. A. Sandberg. 1986. Application of long-term collagenase disaggregation for the cytogenetic analysis of human solid tumors. *Cancer Genet. Cytogenet.* **23:** 305–313.
15. Pandis, N., S. Heim, G. Bardi, J. Limon, N. Mandahl, and F. Mitelman. 1992. Improved technique for short-term culture and cytogenetic analysis of human breast cancer. *Genes Chromosom. Cancer* **5:** 14–20.
16. Pandis, N., G. Bardi, and S. Heim. 1994. Interrelationship between methodological choices and conceptual models in solid tumor cytogenetics. *Cancer Genet. Cytogenet.* **76:** 77–84.
17. Steinarsdóttir, M., I. Pétursdóttir, S. Snorradóttir, J. E. Eyfjörd, and H. M. Ögmundsdóttir. 1995. Cytogenetic studies of breast carcinomas: different karyotypic profiles detected by direct harvesting and short-term culture. *Genes Chromosom. Cancer* **13:** 239–248.
18. Courjal, F. and C. Theillet. 1997. Comparative genomic hybridization analysis of breast tumors with predetermined profiles of DNA amplification. *Cancer Res.* **57:** 4368–4377.
19. James, L. A., E. L. D. Mitchell, L. Menasce, and J. M. Varley. 1997. Comparative genomic hybridisation of ductal carcinoma in situ of the breast: identification of regions of DNA amplification and deletion common with invasive breast carcinoma. *Oncogene* **14:** 1059–1065.
20. Kuukasjärvi, T., R. Karhu, M. Tanner, M. Kähkönen, A. Schäffer, N. Nupponen, et al. 1997. Genetic heterogeneity and clonal evolution underlying development of asynchronous metastasis in human breast cancer. *Cancer Res.* **57:** 1597–1604.

21. Lu, Y. J., S. Birdsall, P. Osin, B. Gusterson, and J. Shipley. 1997. Phyllodes tumors of the breast analyzed by comparative genomic hybridization and association of increased 1q copy number with stromal overgrowth and recurrence. *Genes Chromosom. Cancer* **20:** 275–281.

22. Nishizaki, T., S. DeVries, K. Chew, W. H. Goodson III, B.-M. Ljung, A. Thor, and F. M. Waldman. 1997. Genetic alterations in primary breast cancers and their metastases: direct comparison using modified comparative genomic hybridization. *Genes Chromosom. Cancer* **19:** 267–272.

23. Teixeira, M. R., N. Pandis, G. Bardi, J. A. Andersen, and S. Heim. 1996. Karyotypic comparisons of multiple tumorous and normal tissue samples from patients with breast cancer. *Cancer Res.* **56:** 855–859.

24. Pandis, N., S. Heim, G. Bardi, I. Idvall, N. Mandahl, and F. Mitelman. 1992. Whole-arm t(1;16) and i(1q) as sole anomalies identify gain of 1q as a primary chromosomal abnormality in breast cancer. *Genes Chromosom. Cancer* **5:** 235–238.

25. Pandis, N., S. Heim, G. Bardi, I. Idvall, N. Mandahl, and F. Mitelman. 1993. Chromosome analysis of 20 breast carcinomas: cytogenetic multiclonality and karyotypic-pathologic correlations. *Genes Chromosom. Cancer* **6:** 51–57.

26. Pandis, N., Y. Jin, J. Limon, G. Bardi, I. Idvall, N. Mandahl, F. Mitelman, and S. Heim. 1993. Interstitial deletion of the short arm of chromosome 3 as a primary chromosome abnormality in carcinomas of the breast. *Genes Chromosom. Cancer* **6:** 151–155.

27. Pandis, N., Y. Jin, L. Gorunova, C. Petersson, G. Bardi, I. Idvall, et al. 1995. Chromosome analysis of 97 primary breast carcinomas: identification of eight karyotypic subgroups. *Genes Chromosom. Cancer* **12:** 173–185.

28. Thompson, F., J. Emerson, W. Dalton, J. M. Yang, D. McGee, H. Villar, et al. 1993. Clonal chromosome abnormalities in human breast carcinomas. I. Twenty-eight cases with primary disease. *Genes Chromosom. Cancer* **7:** 185–193.

29. Rohen, C., K. Meyer-Bolte, U. Bonk, T. Ebel, B. Staats, E. Leuschner, et al. 1995. Trisomy 8 and 18 as frequent clonal and single-cell aberrations in 185 primary breast carcinomas. *Cancer Genet. Cytogenet.* **80:** 33–39.

30. Pandis, N., I. Idvall, G. Bardi, Y. Jin, L. Gorunova, F. Mertens, et al. 1996. Correlation between karyotypic pattern and clincopathologic features in 125 breast cancer cases. *Int. J. Cancer* **66:** 191–196.

31. Wenger, C. R., S. Beardsiee, M. A. Owens, G. Pounds, T. Oldaker, P. Vendely, et al. 1993. DNA ploidy, S-phase, and steroid receptors in more than 127,000 breast cancer patients. *Breast Cancer Res. Treatment* **28:** 9–20.

32. Devilee, P. and C. J. Cornelisse. 1994. Somatic genetic changes in human breast cancer. *Biochim. Biophys. Acta* **1198:** 113–130.

33. Kallioniemi, A., O. P. Kallioniemi, J. Piper, M. Tanner, T. Stokke, L. Chen, et al. 1994. Detection and mapping of amplified DNA sequences in breast cancer by comparative genomic hybridization. *Proc. Natl. Acad. Sci. USA* **91:** 2156–2160.

34. Ried, T., K. E. Just, H. Holtgreve-Grez, S. du Manoir, M. R. Speicher, E. Schröck, et al. 1995. Comparative genomic hybridization of formalin-fixed, paraffin-embedded breast tumors reveals different patterns of chromosomal gains and losses in fibroadenomas and diploid and aneuploid carcinomas. *Cancer Res.* **55:** 5415–5423.

35. Evans, D. G., I. S. Fentiman, K. McPherson, D. Asbury, B. A. Ponder, and A. Howell. 1994. Familial breast cancer. *Br. Med. J.* **308:** 183–187.

36. Ford, D. and D. F. Easton. 1995. The genetics of breast and ovarian cancer. *Br. J. Cancer* **72:** 805–812.

37. Hodgson, S. V. and E. R. Maher. 1993. Genetics of human cancers by site of origin. Reproductive system: Breast, in *A Practical Guide to Human Cancer Genetics,* Cambridge University Press, Cambridge, UK, pp. 58–63.

38. Andersen, T. I. 1996. Genetic heterogeneity in breast cancer susceptibility. *Acta Oncol.* **35:** 407–410.

39. Miki, Y., J. Swensen, D. Shattuck-Eidens, P. A. Futreal, K. Harshman, S. Tavtigian, et al. 1994. A strong candidate for the breast and ovarian cancer susceptibility gene BRCA1. *Science* **266:** 66–71.

40. Wooster, R., G. Bignell, J. Lancaster, S. Swift, S. Seal, J. Mangion, et al. 1995. Identification of the breast cancer susceptibility gene BRCA2. *Nature* **378:** 789–792.

41. Kerangueven, F., L. Essioux, A. Dib, T. Noguchi, F. Allione, J. Geneix, et al. 1995. Loss of heterozygosity and linkage analysis in breast carcinoma: indication for a putative third susceptibility gene on the short arm of chromosome 8. *Oncogene* **10:** 1023–1026.

42. Seitz, S., K. Rohde, E. Bender, A. Nothnagel, K. Kölble, P. M. Schlag, and S. Scherneck. 1997. Strong indication for a breast cancer susceptibility gene on chromosome 8p12–p22: linkage analysis in German breast cancer families. *Oncogene* **14:** 741–743.

43. Teixeira, M. R., N. Pandis, A.-M. Gerdes, C. U. Dietrich, G. Bardi, J. A. Andersen, et al. 1996. Cytogenetic abnormalities in an in situ breast carcinoma and five prophylactically removed breasts from members of a family with hereditary breast cancer. *Breast Cancer Res. Treatment* **38:** 177–182.

44. Petersson, C., N. Pandis, F. Mertens, A. Adeyinka, C. Ingvar, A. Ringberg, et al. 1996. Chromosome aberrations in prophylactic mastectomies from women belonging to breast cancer families. *Genes Chromosom. Cancer* **16:** 185–188.

45. Lindblom, A., L. Skoog, S. Rotstein, B. Werelius, C. Larsson, and M. Nordenskjöld. 1993. Loss of heterozygosity in familial breast carcinomas. *Cancer Res.* **53:** 4356–4361.

46. Calabrese, G., C. Di Virgilio, E. Cianchetti, P. G. Franchi, L. Stuppia, G. Parruti, P. G. Bianchi, and G. Palka. 1991. Chromosome abnormalities in breast fibroadenomas. *Genes Chromosom. Cancer* **3:** 202–204.

47. Fletcher, J. A., G. S. Pinkus, N. Weidner, and C. C. Morton. 1991. Lineage-restricted clonality in biphasic solid tumors. *Am. J. Pathol.* **138:** 1199–1207.

48. Stephenson, C. F., R. I. Davis, G. E. Moore, and A. A. Sandberg. 1992. Cytogenetic and fluorescence in situ hybridization analysis of breast fibroadenomas. *Cancer Genet. Cytogenet.* **63:** 32–36.

49. Belda, F., S. C. Lester, J. L. Pinkus, G. S. Pinkus, and J. A. Fletcher. 1993. Lineage-restricted chromosome translocation in a benign fibrous tumor of the breast. *Hum. Pathol.* **24:** 923–927.

50. Leuschner, E., K. Meyer-Bolte, J. Caselitz, S. Bartnitzke, and J. Bullerdiek. 1994. Fibroadenoma of the breast showing a translocation (6;14), a ring chromosome and two markers involving parts of chromosome 11. *Cancer Genet. Cytogenet.* **76:** 145–147.

51. Ozisik, Y. Y., A. M. Meloni, C. F. Stephenson, A. Peier, G. E. Moore, and A. A. Sandberg. 1994. Chromosome abnormalities in breast fibroadenomas. *Cancer Genet. Cytogenet.* **77:** 125–128.

52. Dietrich, C. U., N. Pandis, M. R. Teixeira, G. Bardi, A. M. Gerdes, J. A. Andersen, and S. Heim. 1995. Chromosome abnormalities in benign hyperproliferative disorders of epithelial and stromal breast tissue. *Int. J. Cancer* **60:** 49–53.

53. Rohen, C., B. Staats, U. Bonk, S. Bartnitzke, and J. Bullerdiek. 1996. Significance of clonal chromosome aberrations in breast fibroadenomas. *Cancer Genet. Cytogenet.* **87:** 152–155.

54. Staats, B., U. Bonk, S. Wanschura, P. Hanisch, E. F. Schoenmakers, W. J. Van de Ven, S. Bartnitzke, and J. Bullerdiek. 1996. A fibroadenoma with a t(4;12)(q27;q15) affecting the HMG1-C gene, a member of the high mobility group protein gene family. *Breast Cancer Res. Treatment* **38:** 299–303.

55. Petersson, C., N. Pandis, H. Rizou, F. Mertens, C. U. Dietrich, A. Adeyinka, et al. 1997. Karyotypic abnormalities in fibroadenomas of the breast. *Int. J. Cancer* **70:** 282–286.

56. Birdsall, S. H., K. A. MacLennan, and B. A. Gusterson. 1992. t(6;12)(q23;q13) and t(10;16)(q22;p11) in a phyllodes tumor of breast. *Cancer Genet. Cytogenet.* **60:** 74–77.

57. Birdsall, S. H., B. M. Summersgill, M. Egan, I. S. Fentiman, B. A. Gusterson, and J. M. Shipley. 1995. Additional copies of 1q in sequential samples from a phyllodes tumor of the breast. *Cancer Genet. Cytogenet.* **83:** 111–114.

58. Dietrich, C. U., N. Pandis, G. Bardi, M. R. Teixeira, T. Soukhikh, C. Petersson, J. A. Andersen, and S. Heim. 1994. Karyotypic changes in phyllodes tumors of the breast. *Cancer Genet. Cytogenet.* **78:** 200–206.

59. Dietrich, C. U., N. Pandis, H. Rizou, C. Petersson, G. Bardi, H. Qvist, et al. 1997. Cytogenetic findings in phyllodes tumors of the breast: karyotypic complexity differentiates between malignant and benign tumors. *Hum. Pathol.* **28:** 1379–1382.

60. Dal Cin, P., P. Moreman, I. De Wever, H. Van den Berghe. 1995. Is i(1)(q10) a chromosome marker in phyllodes tumor of the breast? *Cancer Genet. Cytogenet.* **83:** 174–175.

61. Dietrich, C. U., N. Pandis, J. A. Andersen, and S. Heim. 1994. Chromosome abnormalities in adenolipomas of the breast: karyotypic evidence that the mesenchymal component constitutes the neoplastic parenchyma. *Cancer Genet. Cytogenet.* **72:** 146–150.

62. Dietrich, C. U., N. Pandis, G. Bardi, I. Hägerstrand, J. A. Andersen, F. Mitelman, and S. Heim. 1995. Rearrangement of chromosomal bands 3p13–14 in two hamartomas of the breast. *Int. J. Oncol.* **6:** 559–561.

63. Petersson, C., B. Johansson, N. Pandis, L. Gorunova, C. Ingvar, I. Idvall, N. Mandahl, and F. Mitelman. 1994. Clonal chromosome aberrations in fibrocystic breast disease associated with increased risk of cancer. *Int. J. Oncol.* **5:** 1207–1210.

64. Harris, J. R., M. E. Lippman, U. Veronesi, and W. Willett. 1992. Breast cancer. *N. Engl. J. Med.* **327:** 319–328.

65. Wolman, S. R. and G. H. Heppner. 1992. Genetic heterogeneity in breast cancer. *J. Natl. Cancer Inst.* **84:** 469–470.

66. Teixeira, M. R., N. Pandis, G. Bardi, J. A. Andersen, F. Mitelman, and S. Heim. 1995. Clonal heterogeneity in breast cancer: karyotypic comparisons of multiple intra- and extratumorous samples from three patients. *Int. J. Cancer* **63:** 63–68.

67. Beerman, H., V. T. Smit, P. M. Kluin, B. A. Bonsing, J. Hermans, and C. J. Cornelisse. 1991. Flow cytometric analysis of DNA stemline heterogeneity in primary and metastatic breast cancer. *Cytometry* **12:** 147–154.

68. Barranco, S. C., R. R. Perry, M. E. Durm, A. L. Werner, S. G. Gregorcyk, W. E. Bolton, P. Kolm, and C. M. Townsend, Jr. 1994. Intratumor variability in prognostic indicators may be the cause of conflicting estimates of patient survival and response to therapy. *Cancer Res.* **54:** 5351–5356.

69. Chen, L. C., W. Kurisu, B. M. Ljung, E. S. Goldman, D. Moore, and H. S. Smith. 1992. Heterogeneity for allelic loss in human breast cancer. *J. Natl. Cancer Inst.* **84:** 506–510.

70. Lönn, U., S. Lönn, B. Nilsson, and B. Stenkvist. 1994. Intratumoral heterogeneity for amplified genes in human breast carcinoma. *Int. J. Cancer* **58:** 40–45.

71. Szöllösi, J., M. Balazs, B. G. Feuerstein, C. C. Benz, and F. M. Waldman. 1995. ERBB-2 (HER2/neu) gene copy number, p185HER-2 overexpression, and intratumor heterogeneity in human breast cancer. *Cancer Res.* **55:** 5400–5407.

72. Schwartz, G. F., A. S. Patchesfsky, S. A. Feig, G. S. Shaber, and A. B. Schwartz. 1980. Multicentricity of non-palpable breast cancer. *Cancer* **45:** 2913–2916.

73. Holland, R., S. H. Veling, M. Mravunac, and J. H. Hendriks. 1985. Histologic multifocality of Tis, T1-2 breast carcinomas. Implications for clinical trials of breast-conserving surgery. *Cancer* **56:** 979–990.

74. Gump, F. E., S. Shikora, D. V. Habif, S. Kister, P. Logerfo, and A. Estabrook. 1986. The extent and distribution of cancer in breasts with palpable primary tumors. *Ann. Surg.* **204:** 384–390.

75. Dawson, P. J. 1993. What is new in our understanding of multifocal breast cancer. *Pathol. Res. Pract.* **189:** 111–116.

76. Teixeira, M. R., N. Pandis, G. Bardi, J. A. Andersen, N. Mandahl, F. Mitelman, and S. Heim. 1994. Cytogenetic analysis of multifocal breast carcinomas: detection of karyotypically unrelated clones as well as clonal similarities between tumour foci. *Br. J. Cancer* **70:** 922–927.

77. Teixeira, M. R., N. Pandis, G. Bardi, J. A. Andersen, P. J. Bøhler, H. Qvist, and S. Heim. 1997. Discrimination between multicentric and multifocal breast carcinoma by cytogenetic investigation of macroscopically distinct ipsilateral lesions. *Genes Chromosom. Cancer* **18:** 170–174.

78. Pandis, N., M. R. Teixeira, A.-M. Gerdes, J. Limon, G. Bardi, J. A. Andersen, et al. 1995. Chromosome abnormalities in bilateral breast carcinomas: cytogenetic evaluation of the clonal origin of multiple primary tumors. *Cancer* **76:** 250–258.

79. Healey, E. A., E. F. Cook, E. J. Orav, S. J. Schnitt, J. L. Connolly, and J. R. Harris. 1993. Contralateral breast cancer: clinical characteristics and impact on prognosis. *J. Clin. Oncol.* **11:** 1545–1552.

80. Broët, P., A. de la Rochefordière, S. M. Scholl, A. Fourquet, V. Mosseri, J. C. Durand, P. Pouillart, and B. Asselain. 1995. Contralateral breast cancer: annual incidence and risk parameters. *J. Clin. Oncol.* **13:** 1578–1583.

81. Trent, J., J. M. Yang, J. Emerson, W. Dalton, D. McGee, K. Massey, F. Thompson, and H. Villar. 1993. Clonal chromosome abnormalities in human breast carcinomas. II. Thirty-four cases with metastatic disease. *Genes Chromosom. Cancer* **7:** 194–203.

82. Pandis, N., G. Bardi, Y. Jin, C. Dietrich, B. Johansson, J. Andersen, et al. 1994. Unbalanced t(1;16) as the sole karyotypic abnormality in a breast carcinoma and its lymph node metastasis. *Cancer Genet. Cytogenet.* **75:** 158–159.

83. Pandis, N., M. R. Teixeira, A. Adeyinka, H. Rizou, G. Bardi, F. Mertens, et al. 1998. Cytogenetic comparisons of primary tumors and lymph node metastases in breast cancer patients. *Genes Chromosom. Cancer* **22:** 122–129.

84. Adeyinka, A., N. Pandis, J. Nilsson, I. Idvall, F. Mertens, C. Petersson, S. Heim, and F. Mitelman. 1996. Different cytogenetic patterns in skeletal breast cancer metastases. *Genes Chromosom. Cancer* **16:** 72–74.

85. Bonsing, B. A., H. Beerman, N. Kuipers-Dijkshoorn, G. J. Fleuren, and C. J. Cornelisse. 1993. High levels of DNA index heterogeneity in advanced breast carcinomas. Evidence for DNA ploidy differences between lymphatic and hematogenous metastases. *Cancer* **71:** 382–391.

86. Symmans, W. F., J. Liu, D. M. Knowles, and G. Inghirami. 1995. Breast cancer heterogeneity: evaluation of clonality in primary and metastatic lesions. *Hum. Pathol.* **26:** 210–216.

87. Zafrani, B., M. Gerbault Seureau, V. Mosseri, and B. Dutrillaux. 1992. Cytogenetic study of breast cancer: clinicopathologic significance of homogeneously staining regions in 84 patients. *Hum. Pathol.* **23:** 542–547.

III

Therapeutics and Diagnostics

Therapeutics and Drug Resistance

18

Current and Future Directions in Surgical and Chemotherapeutic Approaches to Breast Cancer Treatment

George N. Peters

1. INTRODUCTION

Until the mid-1970s, the surgical treatment of breast cancer had been totally influenced and dominated by the teachings of William S. Halsted. After reporting his experience with the radical mastectomy in 1894, the effects of the Halsted radical mastectomy on the outcome of breast carcinoma were immediate and dramatic *(1)*. The first description of treatment for "bulging tumors of the breast" came from a papyrus of Edwin Smith, Egyptologist, that was written in Egypt approx 5000 yr ago, when the only treatment was cauterization, or no treatment *(2)*. Although Hippocrates wrote little about cancer in general, and almost nothing about breast cancer, he did write, "It is better to omit treatment altogether; for, if treated, the patient soon dies, whereas if left alone, they may last a long time" *(3)*. What is known about the concept of cancer in the Greco-Roman era is derived from the writings of Aulus Cornelius Celsus, a Roman scholar of the first century A.D. He observed, "There is not so great a danger of a cancer, unless it be irritated by the imprudence of the physician" *(3)*. He noted that medicines were of no effect, cauterizing quickened cancer's progress, and, in excision, the cancer notwithstanding returned and caused death. He said, "The more violent the operations are, the more angry they grow" *(3)*. It is unlikely that any attempts at treatment in ancient times effected cures.

Prior to listerism, the danger of sepsis in a large wound was so great that surgeons performed as limited an operation as possible. Surgery proved ineffective, because it only encompassed removal of the part of the breast containing the tumor, and the axilla was only entered when it contained enlarged lymph nodes. In the preantiseptic era, many surgeons advised against operations for breast cancer, because there was only limited or no chance for success. In the two leading textbooks of the day, written by Adolf Burdeleben of Greifswald (published in 1865) and by Sir James Paget of London (published in 1870), it was written that breast cancer would not be cured by surgery. Surgeons were reluctant to operate on cancer, because it was felt from the beginning that cancer was a generalized and multicentric disease. In 1865, Carl Thiersch, a German surgeon, proved that skin cancer begins as a primary focus, and that metastases

From: Breast Cancer: *Molecular Genetics, Pathogenesis, and Therapeutics*
Edited by: *A. M. Bowcock* © *Humana Press Inc., Totowa, NJ*

result from lymphatic and vascular dissemination. In 1872, Wilhelm Waldeyer, a German anatomist, confirmed that this was true for all types of cancer, including breast cancer. Because of this new concept that breast cancer was a localized disease, in 1867, Charles H. Moore, of the Middlesex Hospital in London, advocated removal of the whole breast in continuity with the axillary tissues, only if lymph nodes appeared to be involved. Although this procedure received little acceptance in England, it became the standard operation in German and Austrian clinics after Richard von Volkmann introduced a similar operation in 1873. For the first time, cures, although few, were reported. In Volkmann's clinic, between 1874 and 1878, 11% of 200 patients treated were alive 3 yr later. In the United States, Samuel W. Gross of Philadelphia extended Moore's principles by performing axillary dissections in every case. All of this served as a prelude, when, in 1889, William S. Halsted began to perform the radical mastectomy. At once, Halsted obtained results that far exceeded any that had been obtained by his predecessors *(4)*.

2. ERA OF THE HALSTED RADICAL MASTECTOMY

"The convictions are steadily gaining ground that carcinoma of the breast is curable, and it is primarily a local affliction, and not the expression of a constitutional taint, dyscrasia, or diathesis" *(5)*. Gross maintained that this view was supported by such respected physicians as Virchow, Volkmann, Billroth, Moore, and McGraw *(5)*. Halsted mastered the problems of sepsis and hemorrhage, and developed an operation that was far more extensive than had been attempted before. Using meticulous technique, Halsted excised a large area of skin, the subcutaneous tissues and fascia over a wide area, the entire breast, both of the pectoral muscles, and all of the lymph nodes of the axilla. Skin grafts were essential for closure of the chest-wall defect. Dissemination of disease was attributed to lymphatic involvement. Halsted wrote that the ultimate outcome of surgery was dependent on the variety of the cancer, the time elapsed since its appearance, the degree of outlying involvement, and the thoroughness of the operation. In an era when malignancies were extensive and advanced, and there were no criteria for operability, Halsted's results were truly impressive. When Halsted presented his series of 133 patients to the American Surgical Association in 1898, the 3-yr survival rate was 53%, with a local recurrence of 9%. His impressive results would totally revolutionize the surgical approach to breast cancer, and influence treatment for three-quarters of a century *(6,7)*. During the same period, Willie Meyer of New York independently developed his surgical approach, with a radical operation similar to Halsted's, and confirmed Halsted's impressive results with this operation *(8)*.

In future decades, reports from Butcher, Finney, Anglem, Haagensen, and others would confirm and improve on the results of the Halsted radical mastectomy *(9-12)*. Ultimately, C. D. Haagensen and Arthur Purdy Stout, of the College of Physicians and Surgeons at Columbia University, would correlate the clinical features of advanced breast carcinoma, and develop the Columbia Criteria of Operability to determine which patients would benefit from surgery. Edema of the skin over the breast, satellite nodules of the skin, solid fixation of the tumor to the chest wall, axillary lymph nodes 2.5 cm or more in diameter, fixation of axillary nodes to the overlying skin or underlying chest wall, supraclavicular metastases, and inflammatory carcinoma were determined to be important clinical features that predicted poor results from surgery. This initial staging of breast cancer was an attempt at thorough patient selection, to determine which patients could be cured by surgery *(13)*. Haagensen reported the most extensive follow-up of patients treated with radical mastectomy. After a 47-yr follow-up of 591 patients, cumulative survival at 35 yr was 63% for stage A, with an overall local recurrence rate of 4.3% *(12)*.

To obtain better results, the extended radical mastectomy, which included removal of the internal mammary lymph nodes, was developed under the hypothesis that a more thorough operation would produce better survival benefits. In subgroups of patients with central or medial tumors greater than 2 cm in size, a significant improvement in overall survival was documented, especially with axillary involvement *(14,15)*. Pioneers such as Urban, Caceres, and Veronesi studied the procedure extensively. With the advent of systemic chemotherapy, and because of poor outcome, complexity of the surgery, and substantial morbidity, this procedure was ultimately abandoned by surgeons *(16-18)*.

3. MODIFIED RADICAL MASTECTOMY

Throughout the 1970s, there was a continued shift by surgeons toward using the modified radical mastectomy, although there had been no randomized prospective studies to compare the two procedures. In 1948, Patey reported on the use of modified radical mastectomy as appropriate therapy for T1 and T2 lesions that were not fixed to the pectoralis major muscle, and thus the muscle was preserved *(19)*. Surgeons initially were reluctant to convert to less radical surgery, for fear of increasing local recurrence and decreasing survival rates. Auchincloss, in a 1963 speculative report of 201 patients, concluded that modified radical mastectomy would have given equivalent results to radical mastectomy in all cases, except in four *(20)*. Over the next two decades, data from various retrospective studies began to accumulate, and demonstrated equivalence between the two procedures *(20-24)*. Nemoto further proved that an axillary dissection in a modified radical mastectomy is as complete as that in the Halsted radical mastectomy *(25)*. Between 1969 and 1976, in Manchester, England, 278 patients were treated with the Halsted radical mastectomy and 256 patients with the modified radical mastectomy, in a randomized prospective study. At a median follow-up of 5 yr, no statistical differences were observed regarding local recurrence, distant metastases, or disease-free or overall survival for stage I and stage II cancers between the two treatment groups *(26)*. In Alabama, between 1975 and 1978, a prospective randomized trial, comparing the Halsted radical mastectomy with the modified radical mastectomy, enrolled 311 patients. Patients with positive nodes were then randomized to receive melphalan or CMF (cyclophosphamide, methotrexate, and 5-fluorouracil) chemotherapy. There were 136 women in the radical mastectomy group, and 175 women in the modified radical mastectomy group. After a median follow-up of 5.5 yr, there was no significant difference in disease-free survival or overall survival. There was an increased incidence of local recurrence in patients undergoing a modified radical mastectomy (10 vs 3%), but there was no significant statistical difference *(27)*. Martin et al. concluded that, because 10-yr survivals after radical mastectomy (74.5%) and modified radical mastectomy (74.2%) were almost identical, the benefits derived from the less radical procedure justified the shift toward the modified radical. The authors also concluded that the advantages obtained from the modified radical were better functional result, lower incidence of lymphedema, improved cosmetic appearance, and ease of subsequent breast reconstruction with a submuscular implant *(24)*. Modified radical mastectomy was performed more frequently as surgeons realized the benefits of the less extensive procedure, and that survival was impacted by the stage of disease, rather than by the extent of surgery. By 1981, modified radical mastectomy was performed in 78.1% of cases of diagnosed breast cancer, and the use of radical mastectomy had decreased to 3.4% *(28,29)*.

4. BREAST RECONSTRUCTION

After modified radical mastectomy, approx 25% of women experienced some significant anxiety, depressed mood, and sexual problems *(30,31)*. At first, post-mastectomy reconstruction began to gain acceptance in those patients with early disease. It was felt that reconstruction should be delayed for 2 yr after mastectomy, because over 80% of recurrences are diagnosed during this period. Immediate reconstruction remained a matter of controversy, because surgeons were concerned with the possibility of masking a recurrence, and interfering with postmastectomy adjuvant therapy. Acceptance of breast reconstruction evolved after reports showed therapeutic and positive benefits in psychological, social, and sexual adaptation in women. Reconstruction appeared to reverse the negative effects of mastectomy *(32)*.

By 1984, the American Society of Plastic and Reconstructive Surgeons estimated that 98,000 reconstructions had been performed in 1 yr. Major changes in attitudes toward breast reconstruction in the past decade, which affected the numbers of women electing this procedure, included support and endorsement from physicians, no substantive evidence that implants cause or hide disease, impressive aesthetic outcome, availability of multiple surgical options, marked appreciation for the quality of life, third-party reimbursement, and public and media disclosure. Studies unexpectedly demonstrated that women who were in search of restitution for their surgically altered bodies were exhibiting positive coping and assertive problem solving, not neurotic compensation for an unresolved, narcissistic injury. Improved body image is the strongest impact of breast reconstruction. Specific reasons given by women who want breast reconstruction include the desire to be rid of the external prosthesis, which is irritating and distracting; the wish to feel more like their former selves and more like other women; the need to be less constricted in their choice of clothing and attire; the wish to feel less self-conscious and inhibited sexually; and the desire to be less preoccupied with the reason for having lost a breast. Variables that may influence a decision not to have reconstruction after mastectomy include the fear that something foreign in the body may contribute to disease or mask detection of recurrence, concern that the results do not justify the effect, concern that there is too much cultural pressure for women to live up to an idealized image of beauty and sexual attractiveness that is centered in large breasts, and a faulty assumption that reconstruction is equated with youth and being sexually active *(33)*.

As experience with delayed reconstruction showed that surgeons' concerns were unfounded, attention turned to immediate reconstruction. Patients with immediate reconstruction, or with reconstruction within 1 yr of mastectomy, were observed to experience less recalled distress about the mastectomy than patients with reconstruction after 1 yr *(34)*. Multiple studies on immediate reconstruction confirmed that this

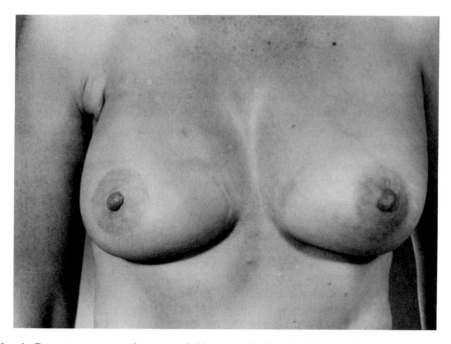

Fig. 1. Breast reconstruction can yield cosmetically pleasing results after mastectomy. Example of right TRAM flap reconstruction.

procedure can be done with excellent cosmesis, acceptable morbidity, and with no compromise of cancer therapy. Local recurrence ranged from 2 to 7%, no local recurrence was concealed by the reconstruction, and the reconstruction did not interfere with subsequent adjuvant radiation therapy or chemotherapy *(35–39)*. Reconstruction can be achieved with subpectoral saline implants, tissue expanders, latissimus dorsi flap reconstruction with an implant, transverse rectus abdominus myocutaneous reconstruction (TRAM), and microvascular myocutaneous free flaps. The TRAM and microvascular myocutaneous free flaps are technically demanding procedures, but offer the most elegant contour restoration of the breast. Replication of the form and consistency of the normal breast is the desired goal *(40)*. Immediate reconstruction is desired by patients, surgical oncologists, and plastic surgeons, whenever there is no contraindication (Fig. 1.). The type of reconstruction is determined by patients' expectations of aesthetics and outcome, extent of ablative surgery that is needed, body habitus, and technical difficulties involved with each procedure. Since the advent of the controversies involving implants, the TRAM has increased in popularity, because it does not require an implant, provides excellent aesthetic results, and also results in a "tummy tuck." Immediate reconstruction has the advantage of decreasing the number of surgical procedures required to obtain a cosmetically pleasing breast. The concern with blood-bank transfusions has been eliminated with the use of autologous blood. With meticulous hemostasis during mastectomy and reconstruction, it is more common not to even need a transfusion. An increased incidence of complications is only noted in patients with a history of smoking, diabetes, or a prior history of chest wall irradiation.

5. EARLY HISTORY OF BREAST CONSERVATION

During the 1950s and 1960s, radical mastectomy was the standard of care for treatment of breast cancer. Beginning in 1954, reports of experience with conservative treatment claimed that radical mastectomy was not necessary to control early disease *(41–46)*. The first to conduct a controlled clinical trial was Sir Hedley Atkins and his group at Guy's Hospital in London. In patients over the age of 50, no survival differences were noted up to 10 yr, in patients with uninvolved lymph nodes, although there was a high incidence of local recurrence in wide excisions, compared with radical mastectomies. Both local and distant recurrence rates were higher, and survival was less, in those patients with clinically involved lymph nodes *(47)*. Most of the reports concluded that local recurrences could be treated with salvage mastectomy, and that no overall survival differences were noted when compared with radical mastectomy. Vera Peters concluded that "mastectomy in early breast cancer may become as old-fashioned as blood letting" *(43)*. During this period, many patients underwent breast conservation, because of their refusal to undergo radical mastectomy. In these initial series, there was a lack of consensus on eligibility criteria, surgical technique, and whether radiation should be part of the treatment.

Single-institution experiences with breast conservation, especially from Britain and France, predominated in the published literature during the 1970s and early 1980s. Calle, from the Foundation Curie, reported on 514 stage I–III patients treated conservatively with surgery and radiation in 25% of the patients, and radiation exclusively in the other 75%. Although only two-thirds of the patients had a preserved breast at 5 yr, 5- and 10-yr survival rates were comparable to those resulting from radical surgery *(48)*. In the series from the Marseilles Cancer Institute, twenty-four percent of their patients were stage III, and were treated with radical radiation alone; stage I and II patients were treated with local excision and radiation. Locoregional recurrence rates with excision were 10.5% for stage I (T1,2 N0), and 25% for stage II (T1,2 N1). For patients treated without prior excision, locoregional failure rate was 34% at 10 yr. Ten-yr survival was equivalent to survival with radical mastectomy *(49)*. Although these studies demonstrated that equivalent survival rates could be obtained with breast conservation when compared with radical surgery, local recurrence rates were unacceptable, unless local excision would be combined with radiation. Osborne, in reviewing the Marsden experience, cautioned that 50% of locoregional relapses occur at least 5 yr after treatment, in contrast with early locoregional relapse after mastectomy *(50)*. Locoregional relapse occurred in 22% of patients with T1T2N0N1a tumors at 10 yr after surgery, and a continued decrease in survival was documented in these patients after 10 yr. This contrasted with the patterns of survival after mastectomy, in which the survival curve flattens at 10 yr. Salvage mastectomy provided a 42% relapse-free survival at 5 yr. Osborne concluded that the long-term results of clinical studies of conservative treatment, using modern methods of radiation should be evaluated before abandoning mastectomy for early-stage breast cancer; yet patients should be informed of the therapeutic options prior to making a decision concerning treatment. Others maintained that survival rates comparable to those for mastectomy could be obtained with low local recurrences ranging from 6.6% to 10% *(51–53)*. With conflicting data from various published reports comparing breast conservation to mastectomy, a more scientific approach was needed to better resolve the issue.

6. RANDOMIZED TRIALS AND THE EMERGENCE OF BREAST CONSERVATION

Because the early reports of breast conservation did not clearly define the merits of this procedure by direct comparison with mastectomy, many important issues remained that prevented the universal acceptance of a more conservative approach to breast cancer therapy. The Halstedian approach emphasized that curability in breast cancer could be achieved more effectively by more extensive en bloc dissection. Fisher developed an alternate hypothesis in which cancer was viewed as a systemic disease involving a complex spectrum of host–tumor interrelationships. Variations in locoregional therapy were unlikely to affect survival. The prospective, randomized, and controlled clinical trial was introduced, and became the primary mechanism for hypothesis testing to evaluate the worth of a particular therapy in comparison with other treatments *(54)*. In 1971, the National Surgical Adjuvant Breast and Bowel Project (NSABP) and 34 collaborating institutions introduced Protocol B-04 to test the Fisher hypothesis, and to evaluate the impact of different surgical approaches in the management of breast cancer. In this protocol, 1665 women with primary breast cancer and similar clinical nodal status and tumor location were prospectively randomized to receive radical mastectomy, total mastectomy followed by regional radiation, or a total mastectomy alone with subsequent removal of axillary nodes, if they became positive. Patients with clinically positive axillary nodes were treated by radical mastectomy or total mastectomy with radiation. After 10 yr of follow-up of both the clinically node-negative and node-positive patients, no differences were noted in respect to disease-free survival, distant-disease–free survival, or overall survival. Since 40% of patients in the clinically node-negative groups had histologically positive nodes in the removed axillary contents with radical mastectomy, it would be expected that 40% of women subjected to total mastectomy alone also had positive axillary nodes that were not removed and untreated. Based on the Halstedian hypothesis, these nodes should have served as a source of further tumor dissemination, resulting in an increase in distant treatment failure and mortality in the total mastectomy patients. Because such findings did not materialize, and locoregional recurrence did not adversely affect survival, the NSABP concluded that it was scientifically justifiable to proceed with a new study to establish the worth of breast conservation by local tumor excision, with or without radiation therapy *(55,56)*.

In 1973, only 2 yr after the NSABP had begun Protocol B-04, the National Cancer Institute in Milan began accrual in a randomized study directly comparing the Halsted radical mastectomy with breast conservation. Breast conservation consisted of resection of a breast quadrant, an axillary lymph node dissection, and radiotherapy. By 1980, 701 patients with breast cancer measuring less than 2 cm in diameter, and with no palpable axillary lymph nodes, had been randomized to the two treatment arms. The two patient groups were comparable in age distribution, size and site of the primary tumor, menopausal status, and frequency of axillary metastases. There was one local recurrence in the quadrantectomy group, and there were three in the Halsted group. Actuarial disease-free and overall survivals were equal in each group (Fig. 2.). At 13 yr follow-up, the data continued to show equal recurrence rates between the two groups, survival rates equal if not superior in breast conservation when compared with the radical procedure, and new primary cancers in the irradiated breast that were less than

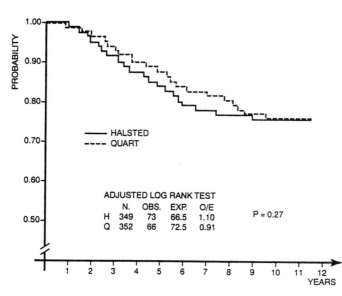

Fig. 2. Results from the Milan trial, indicating disease-free survival in patients treated with quadrantectomy with axillary dissection and radiotherapy (QUART), and with Halsted mastectomy. (Reproduced with permission from ref. *57.)*

the number of contralateral breast cancers. Because quadrantectomy involved the removal of a substantial amount of breast, its major disadvantage involved less-than-optimal cosmesis. The study did confirm that breast conservation provided results equal to the Halsted radical mastectomy in patients who had breast cancer less than 2 cm in diameter, and no palpable axillary lymph nodes *(57,58).* Veronesi et al. reconfirmed the safety of integrated radiosurgical conservative treatments in 1232 women with breast cancer. The survival curves of 352 cases of breast cancer lesions measuring less than 2 cm in diameter, treated in a randomized trial, and 880 similar cases routinely treated with an equivalent procedure outside of the study, were superimposable. Local recurrences and new ipsilateral tumors were 2.8 and 1.6% in each respective group. Overall survival at 5 and 10 yr was 91 and 78%, respectively *(59).*

Because of the increasing practice of breast conservation despite the paucity of information available from clinical trials to determine its efficacy, in 1976 the NSABP began Protocol B-06, to evaluate whether local excision, with or without radiation therapy, in a randomized study, would provide equivalent results to the modified radical mastectomy. Completely abandoning conventional concepts of cancer surgery, segmental mastectomy removed only sufficient tissue to ensure that margins were free of tumor. The specimens were then examined histologically to confirm that margins were free of tumor. Women with stage I and stage II breast cancer <4 cm in size were randomized to total mastectomy, segmental mastectomy alone, or segmental mastectomy followed by breast irradiation. All patients had axillary dissections, and patients with positive nodes received chemotherapy. The study was designed to determine the effectiveness of segmental mastectomy, whether radiation therapy reduces the incidence of tumor recurrence in the ipsilateral breast after segmental mastectomy, whether breast conservation results in a higher risk of distant disease and death than

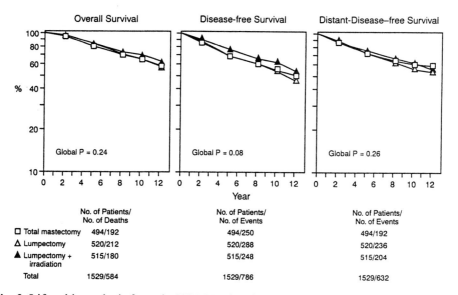

Fig. 3. Life-table analysis from the NSABP, showing overall survival, disease-free survival, and distant-disease–free survival among patients who were treated by total mastectomy, lumpectomy, or lumpectomy and breast irradiation, excluding patients from St. Luc Hospital. The number of deaths and events includes those occurring after the 12-year follow-up period. (Reproduced with permission from ref. *63*.)

does mastectomy, and the clinical importance of tumor multicentricity. The breast had to be of sufficient size, and the tumor located so that the cosmetic result after removal of the tumor would be acceptable.

In 1985, the NSABP first reported life-table estimates based on data from 1843 women. Treatment by segmental mastectomy, with or without breast irradiation, resulted in disease-free, distant-disease–free, and overall survival that was no worse than that after total breast removal. Of the 1257 patients treated by segmental resection, 10% were found to have tumor at the margins of resection, and subsequently had a total mastectomy. At 5 yr, only 7.7% of patients receiving radiation therapy had an ipsilateral breast recurrence, in contrast to 27.9% of patients treated by segmental resection without irradiation. The advantage associated with the use of breast irradiation was observed in patients with both negative and positive nodes. In the patient group with positive nodes, only 2.1% of patients who were irradiated had an ipsilateral breast recurrence, compared with 36.2% of patients who did not undergo breast irradiation. All positive-node patients in both groups received chemotherapy. The NSABP concluded that segmental mastectomy with breast irradiation in all patients was appropriate therapy for breast cancers that are no larger than 4 cm, if local excision yielded tumor-free margins and satisfactory cosmesis, and patients with positive nodes also received adjuvant chemotherapy *(60)*. Follow-up at 8, 10, and 12 yr continued to justify the use of segmental mastectomy (lumpectomy) and breast irradiation for the treatment of invasive breast cancer (Fig. 3.). At 12 yr of follow-up, the cumulative incidence of ipsilateral breast recurrence was 35% in the group treated by lumpectomy alone, and 10% in the group treated by lumpectomy and breast irradiation. In patients with node-negative cancer, the incidence was 32 and 12%, respectively. The decrease in ipsilateral breast recurrence was more evident after lumpectomy and breast irradiation than after lumpectomy alone (5 vs 41%), in patients with node-positive cancer who had received chemotherapy. At 12-yr follow-up, patients treated by lumpectomy with radiation resulted in disease-free survival, distant-disease–free survival, and overall survival rates that were not statistically different from those from total mastectomy. Observations at 12 yr continue to indicate that lumpectomy followed by breast irradiation is appropriate therapy for women with stage I and stage II breast cancer *(61–63)*.

After revelations that a single member institution of the NSABP falsified data entered into Protocol B-06, concerns arose about the findings from this protocol. Reanalysis by the NSABP showed no adverse effect in the outcome of the original Protocol B-06 conclusions *(63)*. An independent reanalysis by the EMMES Corporation in 1994, in which 354 patients from St. Luc Hospital, Montreal, Quebec, were excluded, further varified the validity of the original NSABP findings that breast conservation is equivalent to mastectomy for the surgical treatment of breast cancer *(64)*. The safeguards incorporated into the design of the NSABP study prevented the actions of one person from affecting the ultimate results. Both reanalysis by the NSABP and the National Cancer Institute should restore the confidence of patients and physicians in the Protocol B-06 findings.

A randomized study of 237 patients conducted by the National Cancer Institute between 1979 and 1987, at 10-yr follow-up, showed an overall survival rate of 75% for the patients assigned to mastectomy, and 77% for these assigned to lumpectomy plus radiation. Disease-free survival at 10 yr was 69 and 72%, respectively. No statistical difference was documented between the two treatment groups. Locoregional recurrence was 10% after mastectomy, and 5% after lumpectomy plus radiation. The projected 10-yr disease-free survival for patients undergoing salvage mastectomy is 67%. Similar results have been found in randomized trials from the Institut Gustave-Roussy, European Organization for Research and Treatment of Cancer (EORTC), the Danish Breast Care Group, and other retrospective and prospective studies *(65–70)*. After exhaustive trials comparing breast conservation with mastectomy, breast conservation is now well established as a safe alternative to mastectomy, and can provide equal results. Whole-breast irradiation, which is delivered at a dose of 4500–5000 cGy at 180–200 cGy per fraction, is essential in decreasing local recurrence. When a boost is needed, total dosage to the primary site is increased to 6000–6600 cGy.

7. STANDARDS FOR BREAST CONSERVATION TREATMENT

In 1992, the American College of Radiology, the American College of Surgeons, the American College of Pathology, and the Society of Surgical Oncology established standards of care in breast conservation. Because of the availability of multiple options for the surgical treatment of breast cancer, a thorough preoperative evaluation involving the multidisciplinary team is essential to provide careful patient selection. Education of the patient should include an unbiased review of the benefits of each treatment. Four crucial components in patient selection include a thorough history and physical examination, mammography, histologic assessment of the resected breast specimen, and assessment of the patient's needs and expectations.

A detailed history could reveal medical contraindications for radiation, such as collagen vascular disease. In reconstruction, a history of smoking or diabetes might influence the plastic surgeon to recommend delayed reconstruction. Physical examination provides necessary information to assess the potential cosmetic results of breast conservation vs mastectomy with reconstruction, whether one type of reconstruction might provide benefits over another, and whether adequate radiation can be delivered to the breast. Preoperative mammography is necessary to determine a patient's eligibility for breast conservation, because it defines the extent of the disease, and helps detect multicentricity in the ipsilateral breast and further unsuspected disease in the contralateral breast. Magnification and spot-impression views better evaluate microcalcifications, as well as defining the margins of masses. A post-stereotactic mammogram evaluates the extent of residual disease to be excised, and, if needle localization is used, a specimen radiograph is obtained to confirm removal of the mammographic abnormality. In a two-stage procedure for a carcinoma detected by mammographic microcalcifications, a postbiopsy, presurgical mammogram is obtained to document thoroughness of excision.

Excised tissue should be submitted for pathologic examination, with appropriate clinical history and proper orientation of the specimen. Meticulous gross and microscopic examination should document the amount of tissue removed, size of the carcinoma, and the distance from the tumor to all six margins. Certain particular pathologic findings that have an impact on local recurrence (i.e., extensive intraductal carcinoma, lymphatic invasion, invasive lobular carcinoma, and margin involvement) should be documented to provide necessary information for better decision-making. Prior to definitive surgery, it is essential that the patient and her physician discuss the benefits and risks of all options, as they pertain to her particular case. Having patients who have already undergone various treatments talk to a patient preoperatively helps to allay some fears and concerns. Each woman needs to consider how her choice of treatment will affect her sense of disease control, self-esteem, sexuality, physical functioning, and overall quality of life. Addressing fear of radiation, fear of disease, and fear of recurrence helps the patient to make a better and more appropriate decision. Patient discussion should include results of long-term survival; treatment options after local recurrence; the consequences of local recurrence; guidelines, effectiveness, and cost of follow-up; and psychological adjustment.

Absolute and relative contraindications to breast conservation in patient selection have been formulated:

1. First- and second-trimester pregnancies are an absolute contraindication to the use of breast irradiation. It is possible to perform breast conservation in the third trimester, if radiation can be delayed until after delivery.
2. Patients with two or more gross malignancies in separate quadrants of the breast, or with different malignant or indeterminate microcalcifications, are not candidates for breast conservation.
3. A history of prior irradiation of the involved breast, which would require retreatment to an excessively high total radiation because of a significant breast volume, is an absolute contraindication.
4. A history of collagen-vascular disease is a relative contraindication, because these patients do not tolerate irradiation well.

5. Tumor size over 5 cm without preoperative chemotherapy is a relative contraindication, because of the lack of published data concerning breast conservation in tumors larger than this size. Excision of a large tumor in a small breast, without preoperative chemotherapy, is a relative contraindication, if this procedure results in a significant cosmetic defect.

6. Large, pendulous breasts can be a relative contraindication, unless there is sufficient expertise to ensure reproducibility of patient setup, and availability of greater than 6-MeV photon-beam irradiation to obtain adequate dose homogeneity.

7. Tumor directly beneath the nipple may be a consideration in the choice of local treatment, when removal of all or part of the nipple areolar complex is necessary. Excellent cosmetic results have been reported after delayed nipple-areolar reconstruction.

After the report from NSABP Protocol B-06 showed the importance of margins, there has been an emphasis to obtain clear margins in breast conservation. Recent analysis suggests that a combination of margin status and histology is the critical factor in assessing risk of recurrence in breast conservation and radiation. A focally positive margin is defined as tumor at the margin encompassed by 1–3 low-power fields. The crude 5-yr rate of local recurrence of tumors with focally positive margins, and without extensive intraductal carcinoma (EIC), is 9%; in focally positive margins with EIC, recurrence is 7%. In contrast, recurrence of EIC-negative tumors with extensively positive margins is 19%, and, in EIC-positive tumors, is 42%. Patients should be informed of such findings before they are denied breast conservation because of margin involvement *(71,72)*.

8. OPTIMAL SURGICAL TECHNIQUE IN BREAST CONSERVATION

8.1. Segmental Resection

Many terms are used to describe the surgical procedure of lumpectomy, including segmental or partial mastectomy, lumpectomy, wide local excision, and tylectomy. The actual procedure may vary from surgeon to surgeon. The NSABP has always advocated a careful and specific approach in which surgical and pathologic techniques are more precisely controlled. The two major treatment objectives are complete excision of the tumor, with resection margins clear of tumor, and good cosmesis (Fig. 4.). These two basic treatment criteria should always be considered when contemplating a diagnostic biopsy or definitive excision for breast conservation. Curvilinear skin incisions, following Langer's lines, result in the best cosmetic results, although radial incisions at the 3:00 and 9:00 positions should be considered, to allow incorporation within a mastectomy incision without sacrifice of excess skin, if this should become necessary. The incision should always be placed over the tumor mass, and circumareolar incisions should be reserved for subareolar lesions. With tunneling from a distant incision, it is difficult to obtain clear margins around a tumor, and there is tracking of tumor cells. A narrow (<5 mm) ellipse of skin may be taken over the center of the specimen containing the tumor, for orientation and histologic examination for dermal lymphatics, but this is not essential. Pectoral fascia is not removed, unless tumor rests adjacent to the fascia, at which point the fascia and some muscle can be removed directly below the tumor. Hemostasis should be meticulously obtained to avoid both hematoma formation (which would make subsequent examination more difficult) and drains in the breast.

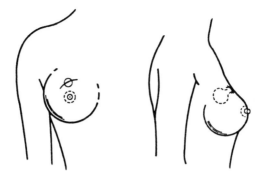

Fig. 4. The lumpectomy incision should always be placed over the tumor mass. Enough tissue is removed to achieve margins that are grossly free of tumor. No breast drain is used.

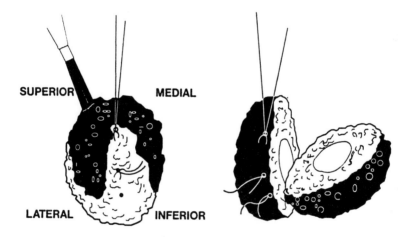

Fig. 5. The orientation of lumpectomy specimens is indicated by the surgeon. Margins should be inked and examined by the pathologist before the specimen is sectioned.

It is essential that the surgeon and pathologist work closely together. The surgeon should orient the specimen of tissue removed for pathological examination by using sutures or clips, or by marking the margins on the towel where the specimen is placed after excision. The specimen should not be sectioned before all margins are inked and inspected by the pathologist for gross tumor involvement (Fig. 5.). If there is evidence that the tumor has been transected, the surgeon should be informed, in order to re-excise an involved margin prior to closure. Because margins of resection primarily are comprised of adipose tissue, frozen section is to be avoided, to allow meticulous microscopic evaluation of the margins on permanent sections. In excision of the tumor, electrocautery should be used sparingly, because thermal injury may affect hormone receptor assays, and cause tissue artifacts that complicate pathologic interpretation of margins. Metal clips (the authors prefer titanium clips that do not compromise future breast examinations by magnetic resonance imaging) are placed at the base of the excisional site to aid the radiation oncologist in planning treatment, espe-

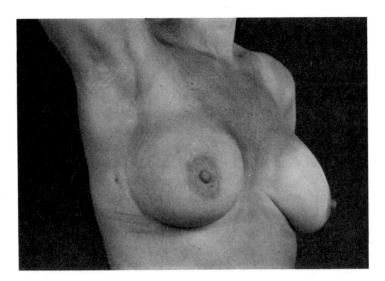

Fig. 6. Example of partial mastectomy and axillary dissection after radiation therapy.

cially when boosts are necessary. The cavity is closed in layers (to avoid chronic seroma formation) with interrupted 3-0 Vicryl suture. Closure is accomplished to obtain optimal cosmetic results, using running 4-0 Dexon in the subdermal area; skin is closed with either a 4-0 Prolene or Dexon continuous subcuticular running suture (*72–74*; Fig. 6.).

8.2. Axillary Dissection

Axillary dissection provides valuable information concerning patient prognosis and the need for chemotherapy and aids in locoregional control. The NSABP recommends a separate axillary incision from the breast incision, because a single incision results in poor cosmetic results. Axillary sampling is a procedure that should be condemned and abandoned, because there is a higher incidence of axillary recurrence in patients undergoing sampling rather than dissection, and a complete dissection is necessary for accurate determination of true nodal involvement *(39,75)*. Although either a longitudinal or transverse incision provides equal exposure to the axilla, the authors prefer a slow-S transverse incision in the axilla, extending from the lateral edge of the pectoralis muscle to the superior edge of the latissimus dorsi muscle, because it produces an excellent cosmetic result, and is not as prominent as the longitudinal incision. Level I and II axillary node removal is advised for invasive carcinomas. Axillary dissection extends from the Tail of Spence inferiorly, to the axillary vein superiorly, to the latissimus dorsi muscle laterally, and to the medial edge of the pectoralis minor muscle medially. The pectoralis minor muscle is neither cut nor removed. The thoracodorsal neurovascular bundle, the long thoracic nerve, the intercostobrachial nerve, and the medial pectoral nerve should be preserved, unless they are involved with grossly positive or suspicious nodes (Fig. 7.). Level I and II axillary dissection is optimal for clinically node-negative patients, because only 1.6% of

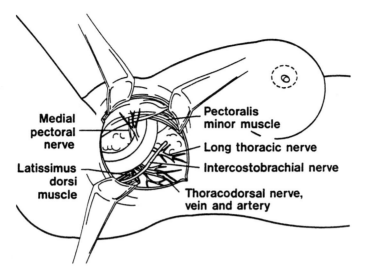

Fig. 7. Axillary dissection with preservation of nerves.

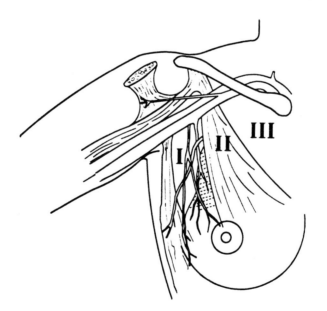

Fig. 8. Levels of axillary dissection. Levels I and II axillary dissection is optimal for node-negative patients, because less than 2% of these patients demonstrate skip metastases to level III.

these patients demonstrate skip metastases to level III. Additional level III dissection is necessary in the presence of obvious nodal disease (*76–79*; Fig. 8.). Closed suction drainage after axillary dissection is used until drainage volume is 25–30 cc/24 h (*72*; Fig. 9.).

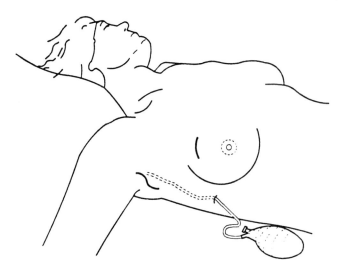

Fig. 9. After axillary dissection, closed suction drainage should be left in place until the drainage decreases to 25–30 cc/24 h.

9. THE CONTROVERSY OVER AXILLARY DISSECTION

It has been well established that axillary dissection provides valuable information relative to lymph node involvement with tumor, to determine patient prognosis, the need for chemotherapy, and locoregional control. The issue that axillary dissection provides survival benefit continues to be controversial. Fisher eloquently proposes that lymph node involvement is an indicator, rather than an instigator, of potential tumor dissemination *(75)*. Recht maintains that the initial use of effective axillary treatment may result in a small improvement in long-term outcome in some patient subgroups *(80)*. Ruffin reviewed five studies comparing axillary dissection to radiation or no treatment to the axilla. In each of these studies, the group receiving axillary surgical treatment had significantly improved survival rates, compared with the group receiving no treatment or axillary radiation. Overall, there is a theoretical minimal rate advantage of 10%; however, actual data are conflicting. Definitive conclusions regarding survival benefit are not possible at present *(81)*.

Axillary failure occurs in 16–28% of patients without axillary dissection, and without regional irradiation *(55,82,83)*. With complete axillary dissection, the incidence of failure is low, between 0 and 3%. Axillary radiation resulted in axillary failure rates of 2–5%. Because the time to develop clinical axillary failure after radiotherapy may be prolonged, higher failure rates may be recorded with further follow-up; therefore, the effectiveness of axillary irradiation cannot be fully determined at this time. Locoregional control of the axilla is critical, because failure in the untreated axilla, despite salvage treatment, may result in uncontrollable axillary recurrence in 11% of patients *(80)*. A complete axillary dissection is required for accurate determination of the number of lymph nodes involved with tumor. Although various protocols have shown benefit when adjuvant therapy is used in both negative and positive lymph nodes, prognosis and intensity of adjuvant therapy are related to the number of positive lymph nodes. Prognostic differences are noted with no nodal involvement, 1–3 positive lymph nodes, 4–9 positive lymph nodes, or 10 or more positive lymph nodes. Treatment decisions are made accordingly.

Present studies are concentrating on which subgroups of invasive breast cancer can be treated without an axillary dissection. It is universally accepted that axillary dissection should be omitted in ductal carcinoma *in situ*. Silverstein, from Van Nuys, reported that risk of nodal involvement for patients with nonpalpable tumors was 4% for T1 and 7% for T1b lesions; for palpable tumors, the risk was 6% for T1a and 23% for T1b lesions *(84)*. Tumors with ductal carcinoma *in situ*, and microinvasion, have a reported incidence of nodal involvement of only 0–3% *(85,86)*. A report combining single-institution data showed a 3.9% incidence of axillary lymph node metastases, compared with Surveillance, Epidemiology and End Results (SEER) of the National Cancer Institute data, showing an 11% metastatic rate. The report concluded that single-institution data better reflect metastases in T1a lesions than SEER data that are flawed *(87)*. Reviews of tumor registries consistently show higher lymph node involvement than single-institution reports *(88,89)*. Because of the inconsistency of various studies, conflicting recommendations have been made on whether axillary dissection should be undertaken for T1a lesions. Sentinel-node biopsy may soon resolve this dilemma. The sentinel lymph node is defined as the first node in the lymphatic basin that receives primary lymph flow. Intraoperative lymphatic mapping, using a vital blue dye and/or filtered technetium-labeled sulfur colloid, and sentinel node biopsy, in women with invasive breast cancer, successfully samples the axilla and provides full nodal status. When the sentinel node is isolated and biopsied, if it is negative for metastatic disease, a full axillary dissection can be avoided. If it is positive, a full axillary dissection should be completed. The procedure is operator-dependent, and there is a definite learning curve. The technique would enhance staging accuracy, and, with further refinements and experience, might alter the role of axillary node dissection *(90–92)*.

10. FUTURE SURGICAL DIRECTIONS

In June 1990, the National Institutes of Health convened a Consensus Development Conference concerning the treatment of early-stage breast cancer. Based on the results of multicenter trials, the consensus panel concluded that "breast conservation treatment is an appropriate method of primary therapy for the majority of women with stage I and II breast cancer and is preferable because it provides survival equivalent to total mastectomy and axillary dissection while preserving the breast" *(93)*. In 1991, a national survey by the Commission on Cancer reported that, although radical and extended radical mastectomies had almost disappeared by 1990, modified radical mastectomy (65.8%) was the most common surgery performed for breast cancer, and partial mastectomy had increased from 13.1% in 1983 to 25.4% in 1990 *(94)*. Although the use of breast conservation had increased, overall, to 49.2% in 1992, the increase was regional, ranging from 61.5% in the Northeast to 37.8% in the South *(95;* Fig. 10.). Tarbox et al. observed that, in 5 yr, from 1986 to 1990, in Colorado, the majority of women with T1 breast cancer lesions were treated by modified radical mastectomy. To understand the reason for this, 175 general surgeons were surveyed to evaluate how prospective treatment options were presented to patients. In the survey, 22% of surgeons did not think that treatment options were equivalent; 34% believed the two treatment options were equivalent, but felt the modified radical was the "gold standard,"

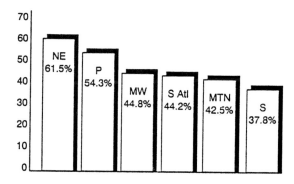

Fig. 10. Use of lumpectomy varies by region. (Reproduced with permission from ref. *95*.)

because of longer follow-up, and questioned the cosmetic results after radiation in breast conservation; and 44% believed the two treatment options were equivalent, and presented them in an unbiased approach. Their attitudes influenced whether breast conservation was preferred in each of these groups: 36, 40, and 55%, respectively *(96)*. Several studies have also looked at other factors that influence the use of breast conservation in breast cancer treatment. Lower use of breast conservation is seen in older patients, especially over the age of 70; patients with tumor size of ≥2 cm; higher stages of disease and positive lymph nodes; certain geographic locations (south, central, or non–New England regions); patients without a college degree or with lower income levels; patients without private insurance; and patients treated in smaller hospitals by older surgeons. In Connecticut, attitudes and practices of local physicians were believed to be important factors in explaining lower breast conservation rates for that state. Twelve yr after the initial report of the NSABP using Protocol B-06, this trend has to be reversed, to increase breast conservation. Future emphasis is imperative for increasing breast conservation through widespread education of surgeons, other health care providers, policy makers, and the public *(97–99)*.

In major breast centers, work continues to focus on even less invasive procedures for the treatment of breast cancer. Multicenter studies have demonstrated the effectiveness of stereotactic core needle biopsy in accurately obtaining diagnosis of nonpalpable mammographic lesions, therefore decreasing the need for open surgical biopsies. An added benefit is a reduction in cost of obtaining a diagnosis *(100–102)*. With the introduction of Mammotome (Biopsys Med, Irvine, CA), complete removal of mammographic lesions has been achieved with increasing frequency. The Mammotome obtains multiple, contiguous tissue cores using an 11-gage rotary needle with a vacuum system. A pilot study designed to assess the ability of the Mammotome to obtain a percutaneous lumpectomy is to be initiated at NSABP headquarters in Pittsburgh. In the future, stereotactic technology may be used for excision of breast cancers (≤1 cm) *(103)*. Others have initiated trials to determine the efficacy of tumor ablation by either laser or cryosurgery. Staren et al. have demonstrated that *in situ* breast cryosurgery is feasible and effective in small- and larger-animal studies, and has been successfully performed in one patient with breast cancer. In England, 27 cancers in 20 patients were treated with interstitial laser photocoagulation, and laser-induced necrosis was monitored by gadolinium-enhanced magnetic resonance imaging. Dowlatshahi, at Rush-Presbyterian in Chicago, is obtaining breast tumor ablation through laser technology in an investigational protocol *(104–107)*. In the foreseeable future, patients with breast cancer may undergo percutaneous ablation of their tumors by Mammotome, cryotherapy, or laser, and axillary dissection may be supplanted by sentinel node biopsy.

Many other issues remain to be fully addressed by surgeons. Will education of patients and surgeons increase the use of breast conservation? Should induction chemotherapy be given to all patients to make more patients eligible for breast conservation with improved cosmesis after downstaging? Can subgroups of patients with invasive cancer be selected who will not require irradiation? Are microscopically clear surgical margins essential? What are the criteria for optimal cosmesis with breast conservation, and when would mastectomy with primary reconstruction provide better results? Many challenges still confront surgeons in the treatment of breast cancer. The emphasis continues on less extensive surgery with less morbidity, to provide patients with more effective therapies.

11. ADJUVANT THERAPY

11.1. Chemotherapy

As early as 1865, Thiersch hypothesized that metastases from cancer result because of lymphatic and vascular dissemination *(4)*, but there was no significant interest in this theory until the mid-1950s. In 1958, the NSABP, under the direction of Bernard Fisher, initiated Protocol B-01. The goal was to determine whether perioperative chemotherapy, combined with the Halsted radical mastectomy, would have an impact on disease-free survival and overall survival, by destroying tumor cells disseminated at the time of surgery. Randomizing patients to thiotepa or placebo, no difference was noted in the overall patient group. In premenopausal patients with four or more positive lymph nodes, a difference in survival was noted at 5 and 10 yr in the treatment group. For the first time, this study demonstrated that the natural history of breast cancer could be altered by systemic therapy in at least a subgroup of patients with breast cancer *(108)*. In 1976, Bonadonna reported an advantage in disease-free survival and overall survival in premenopausal women with breast cancer and positive lymph nodes, who had been randomized to 12 cycles of cyclophosphamide, methotrexate, and 5-fluorouracil. After a median follow-up of 19.4 yr, benefit in disease-free survival and overall survival still persists in all subgroups of node-positive breast cancer patients, with the exception of postmenopausal women *(109,110*; Fig. 11.). Over the past two decades, a substantial effort in breast cancer research has been focused on adjuvant and chemotherapeutic therapy to provide a positive impact on the survival of breast cancer patients.

As early as 1977, it was demonstrated that adriamycin-containing regimens of chemotherapy achieved superior results, compared with methotrexate-containing regimens. Benefit was most notable in patients with 4–9 positive nodes, and especially in patients with 10 or more positive nodes. Although a combination of cyclophosphamide, methotrexate, and 5-fluorouracil (CMF) has been used more frequently in adjuvant therapy overall, a combination of 5-fluorouracil, adriamycin, and cyclophosphamide (FAC) is used in many institutions for more advanced lesions (stage IIB to IIIB), and an adriamycin regimen is used at M. D. Anderson Cancer Center for all adjuvant

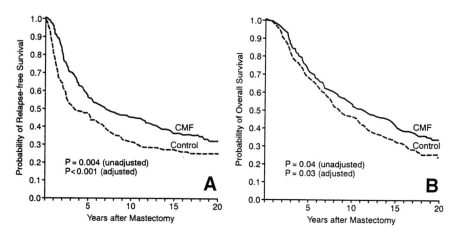

Fig. 11. Relapse-free survival **(A)** and overall survival **(B)**, according to treatment group. With respect to relapse-free survival, 48 of 179 patients in the control group were disease-free at 20 yr, compared with 74 of 207 patients in the CMF group. With respect to overall survival, 44 of 179 patients in the control group were alive at 20 yr, compared with 70 of 207 patients in the CMF group. (Reproduced with permission from ref. *110.*)

therapy. In inflammatory carcinoma, response rates of 100% have been reported with an adriamycin-containing regimen vs 57% with a methotrexate-containing regimen *(111,112).*

11.2. Hormonal Therapy

Since the end of the nineteenth century, it has been recognized that some breast cancers are influenced by endogenous hormones. Therefore, remissions were achieved by withdrawing systemic estrogens from breast cancers by performing oophorectomies. In the 1960s, specific intracellular receptors for estrogens were discovered. These receptors were associated with response to hormonal therapy.

The advent of tamoxifen, a nonsteroidal estrogen antagonist, offered a new form of adjuvant therapy for metastatic breast cancers that were estrogen receptor (ER)–positive. Prospective randomized trials of adjuvant tamoxifen were shown to improve both relapse-free and overall survival *(113).* Peto et al., at the St. Gallen Conference of 1992, reviewed the data from the Early Breast Cancer Trialists Collaborative Group. This study included 10-yr data for 75,000 women randomly assigned in 133 clinical trials. Specific positive findings were based on 30,000 women in tamoxifen trials, 1800 women below age 50 in ovarian ablation trials, and 11,000 women in combination chemotherapy trials *(114,115).* Peto concluded that the benefit of decreased mortality was seen between yr 5 and 9 with the addition of tamoxifen; ovarian ablation in patients under age 50 yr produced similar effects in the reduction of recurrence and mortality to those with combination chemotherapy; tamoxifen was effective for improving both relapse-free survival and overall survival for women older than age 50 yr, including those with tumors classified as ER-poor; there was a definite reduction in mortality from hormonal treatment in node-negative patients; and the administration of tamoxifen significantly reduced the incidence of contralateral breast cancers. The overview data indicated a highly significant trend toward a greater therapeutic effect for longer-term use (at least 2 yr) of tamoxifen. A clinical announcement by the National Cancer Insti-

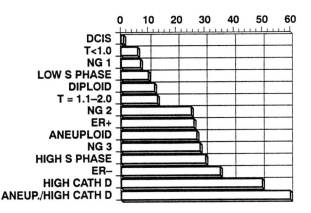

Fig. 12. The probability of recurrence at 5 yr, based on tumor characteristics in axillary node-negative breast cancer. Values were derived from published data, or were estimated by the authors. (Adapted with permission from ref. *119*.)

tute on November 30, 1995, showed results from the NSABP Protocol B-14 (evaluating 5 vs 10 yr of adjuvant tamoxifen for early breast cancer), which indicated no advantage for continuation of tamoxifen beyond 5 yr in women with node-negative, ER–positive breast cancers *(116)*. Through 10 yr of follow-up, a significant advantage in disease-free survival (75 vs 67%) and survival (80 vs 76%) was found in patients receiving tamoxifen for 5 yr vs the placebo group. The survival benefit extended to those 49 yr of age or younger and 50 yr of age or older. No additional advantage was obtained from continuing tamoxifen therapy for more than 5 yr *(117)*. The risk of endometrial carcinoma with tamoxifen use is low (0.5%), compared with its benefits to breast cancer patients *(118)*.

11.3. Prognostic Factors

Participants in the Fourth International Conference on Adjuvant Therapy of Primary Breast Cancer, held in St. Gallen, Switzerland, in 1992, concluded that, despite the proliferation of new prognostic factors, axillary lymph node status, the number of lymph nodes involved, tumor size, age or menopausal status, histopathology, and hormone receptor status are important prognostic factors that should be used to determine the use of adjuvant therapy *(115)*. In node-negative patients, McGuire et al. reviewed the literature, and formulated a framework for using prognostic factor information in making decisions concerning adjuvant therapy. Parameters evaluated included tumor size, nuclear grade, ER, proliferative rate, ploidy, Her-2 oncogene, and cathepsin D (Fig. 12.). In axillary node-negative patients, recurrence at 20 yr was only 14% in patients with tumors of 1 cm or less, but was 31% in those with tumors 1.1–2.0 cm. Nuclear grade 1 and 2 node-negative patients have a good prognosis, but grade 3 patients have a poorer prognosis. The difference in 5-yr disease-free survivals for patients whose tumors were ER–positive vs ER–negative was significant, but the magnitude of the difference was only 8–9%. Combining ER status with tumor size and oncogene expression provides useful information. The probability of recurrence within 5 yr was 12% in patients with diploid tumors, and 26% in those with aneuploid tumors.

The probability of recurrence with diploid tumors and low-percentage S-phase was 10% at 5 yr, compared with 29% with diploid tumors and high-percentage S-phase. In the aneuploid tumor group, the percent S-phase can further discriminate between high and low probability of relapse. In node-negative patients, an association has been found between Her-2/neu overexpression and decreased survival in women with tumors of good nuclear grade. Patients with high cathepsin D levels had a shorter disease-free survival, and a trend toward a shorter survival. A problem arises in assessing patient prognosis when there are multiple prognostic variables providing conflicting information *(119)*. Proliferative rate, ploidy, Her-2/neu oncogene, and cathepsin D were not included as predictive factors at the Fifth International Conference on Adjuvant Therapy of Primary Breast Cancer held in St. Gallen, Switzerland, in 1995 *(120)*.

11.4. Adjuvant Therapy Recommendations

In 1985 and 1990, the National Institutes of Health Consensus Development Conference presented data indicating that adjuvant chemotherapy and hormonal therapy are effective treatments for breast cancer patients with positive and negative lymph node involvement *(93,121)*. After review of world data available at the 1992 and 1995 St. Gallen conferences, treatment recommendations were made regarding adjuvant therapy for both node-negative and node-positive patients. The node-negative patients were divided into minimal/low-risk, good-risk, and high-risk, and treated accordingly (Table 1). The minimal/low-risk patients included noninvasive tumors (ductal carcinoma *in situ*), and incidentally discovered small (≤1 cm) invasive tumors detected by mammography, or by microscopic examination of tissue removed because of benign breast disease or *in situ* breast carcinoma. Patients with tubular, colloid (mucinous), and papillary tumors under 2 cm also were included in this subgroup. Observation without treatment is the current recommendation, and any benefits remain to be determined by ongoing trials. Chemotherapy should at least be discussed with the patient who has a breast tumor (<1 cm) that is ER–negative and has a high histologic and nuclear grade. A good-risk subgroup was defined as having an approx 85–90% chance of remaining disease-free at 5 yr. This includes patients with ER–positive tumors (>1 cm but ≤2 cm), and with low histologic and nuclear grade. It was recommended that both premenopausal and postmenopausal patients, including the elderly, be treated with tamoxifen. The high-risk group includes patients with ER–negative tumors (≥1 cm), ER–positive tumors (>2 cm), and nuclear grade III tumors. A high percentage of cells in S-phase, determined by flow cytometry, also is considered in evaluating high-risk patients. The presence of any one of these unfavorable prognostic indicators justifies the use of adjuvant therapy outside of a clinical trial.

The recommendations for node-negative, high-risk patients are as follows:

1. All premenopausal, node-negative, high-risk patients should receive adjuvant chemotherapy, regardless of ER status. Tamoxifen could be added to ER–positive patient therapy.
2. For postmenopausal, node-negative, high-risk patients, primary adjuvant therapy depends on ER status. Tamoxifen is the mainstay in this group, but tamoxifen with chemotherapy is a reasonable alternative. Adjuvant chemotherapy is indicated for postmenopausal, ER–negative patients.
3. For the elderly patient (>70 yr of age) in the high-risk, node-negative group, tamoxifen is beneficial irrespective of ER status. Elderly patients in good general medical condition, who are at high risk, may benefit from chemotherapy.

Table 1
Adjuvant Treatment for Patients with Lymph Node-Negative Breast Cancer[a]

Patient group	Minimal risk–low risk	Good risk	High risk
Premenopausal			
ER-positive	No adjuvant treatment vs tamoxifen[b]	**Tamoxifen** Oophorectomy[b] Chemotherapy[b] Gonadotropin-releasing hormone analog[b]	**Chemotherapy** ± tamoxifen[b] Oophorectomy[b] Gonadotropin-releasing hormone analog[b]
ER-negative	Not applicable	Not applicable	**Chemotherapy**
Postmenopausal			
ER-positive	No adjuvant treatment vs tamoxifen[b]	**Tamoxifen**	**Tamoxifen** ± chemotherapy[b]
ER-negative	Not applicable	Not applicable	**Chemotherapy** ± tamoxifen[b]
Elderly	No adjuvant treatment vs tamoxifen[b]	**Tamoxifen**	**Tamoxifen**; if ER-negative: **chemotherapy** ± tamoxifen[b]

[a]Bold entries are treatments accepted for routine use or base line in clinical trials. ER = estrogen receptor.
[b]Treatments still being tested in randomized clinical trials.
(Reproduced with permission from ref. *120*.)

Table 2
Adjuvant Treatment for Patients with Lymph Node-Positive Breast Cancer[a]

Patient group	Treatment
Premenopausal	
ER-positive	**Chemotherapy** ± tamoxifen[b] **Ovarian ablation** ± tamoxifen[b] Gonadotropin-releasing hormone analog[b] **Chemotherapy** ± ovarian ablation (gonadotropin-releasing hormone analog) ± tamoxifen[b]
ER-negative	**Chemotherapy**
Postmenopausal	
ER-positive	**Tamoxifen** ± chemotherapy[b]
ER-negative	**Chemotherapy** ± tamoxifen[b]
Elderly	**Tamoxifen**; if ER-negative: **chemotherapy** ± tamoxifen[b]

[a]Bold entries are treatments accepted for routine use or baseline in clinical trials. ER = estrogen receptor.
[b]Treatments still being tested in randomized clinical trials.
(Reproduced with permission from ref. *120*.)

Patients with node-positive breast cancer should receive some form of adjuvant therapy (Table 2). Recommendations from the 1995 St. Gallen conference are as follows:

1. For premenopausal, node-positive, hormone receptor–positive or –negative patients, chemotherapy should be administered. Tamoxifen remains an option in ER–positive patients.

2. For postmenopausal, node-positive, hormone receptor–positive patients, tamoxifen remains the accepted treatment, although there is increasing evidence of benefit by adding chemotherapy.
3. For postmenopausal, node-positive, hormone receptor–negative patients, adjuvant chemotherapy should be administered. Tamoxifen may add some benefit in disease-free and overall survival, in conjunction with chemotherapy.
4. For elderly (>70 yr of age) patients who are node-positive and hormone receptor–positive, the standard of care is tamoxifen. However, chemotherapy should be considered for patients who are receptor-negative and in generally good medical condition.

12. FUTURE TREATMENT DIRECTIONS

Recent studies have been undertaken to determine whether preoperative chemotherapy may permit more breast conservation and decrease the incidence of positive nodes in all stages of breast cancer. Breast tumor reduction is seen in 80% of patients, with an increase in breast conservation, and a 37% increase in the incidence of pathologically negative nodes. It is too early to determine whether there is a survival benefit in early breast cancers. Future application of preoperative chemotherapy will be better defined by NSABP protocol B-27 *(122–125)*. Studies of high-dose chemotherapy, with autologous stem-cell support, have shown better 3-yr survival, but the ultimate benefit still needs to be determined by randomized studies *(126)*.

Paclitaxel is the newest addition to chemotherapeutic agents used in advanced breast cancer. It is a drug with single-agent activity that parallels polychemotherapy regimens. Patients with minimal prior chemotherapy have a >50% response rate to paclitaxel, and a 23% response rate in a salvage setting, even when extensive prior chemotherapy has been administered. A second taxane in clinical development is docetaxel *(127)*. A new era in the treatment of breast cancer will witness the use of agents designed from the study of tumor biology. Agents will be developed that will interfere with tumor growth mechanisms, tumor invasive capacity, and tumor angiogenesis. The future of adjuvant therapy will involve the use of agents that block the progression of tumors from micrometastasis to overt metastatic disease, rather than killing all micrometastatic cells *(113)*.

REFERENCES

1. Haagensen, C. D. 1986. Diseases of the breast, 3rd ed., chapter 54. W.B. Saunders, Philadelphia, PA.
2. Breasted, J. H. 1930. The Edwin Smith surgical papyrus, p. 363–463. University of Chicago Press, Chicago, IL.
3. Robbins, G. F. 1981. Silvergirl's surgery: the breast, p. 15–17. Silvergirl, Austin, TX.
4. Haagensen, C. D. and W. E. Lloyd. 1943. A Hundred Years of Medicine, p. 266–269. Sheridan House, Inc., New York, NY.
5. Gross, W. S. 1880. A practical treatise on tumors of the mammary gland. New York.
6. Halsted, W. S. 1898. A clinical and histological study of certain adenocarcinomata of the breast. *Trans. Am. Surg. Assoc.* **16:** 144–181.
7. Halsted, W. S. 1907. The results of radical operations for the cure of carcinoma of the breast. *Ann. Surg.* **46:** 1–19.
8. Meyer, W. 1894. An improved method of the radical operation for carcinoma of the breast. *M. Rec.* **46:** 746.
9. Anglem, T. J. and R. E. Leber. 1971. Characteristics of ten year survivors after radical mastectomy for cancer of the breast. *Am. J. Surg.* **121:** 363–367.

10. Butcher, H. E., Jr. 1969. Radical mastectomy for mammary carcinoma. *Ann. Surg.* **170:** 883–884.

11. Finney, G. G., Sr., G. G. Finney, Jr., and E. L. Diamond. 1970. A rational approach to the treatment of carcinoma of the breast. *Ann. Surg.* **171:** 859–863.

12. Haagensen, C. D. and C. Bodian. 1984. A personal experience with Halsted's radical mastectomy. *Ann. Surg.* **199:** 143–150.

13. Haagensen, C. D. and A. P. Stout. 1943. Carcinoma of the breast: criteria of operability. *Ann. Surg.* **118:** 859-891.

14. Lacour, J., P. Bucalossi, E. Cacers, G. Jacobelli, T. Koszarowski, M. Le, C. Rumeau-Rouquette, and U. Veronesi. 1976. Radical mastectomy versus radical mastectomy plus internal mammary dissection. Five-year results of an international cooperative study. *Cancer* **37:** 206–214.

15. Li, K. Y. and Z. Z. Shen. 1984. An analysis of 1242 cases of extended radical mastectomy. *Breast* **10:** 10–19.

16. Urban, J. A. 1951. Local excision of the chest wall for mammary cancer. *Cancer* **4:** 1263–1285.

17. Urban, J. A. 1978. Management of operable breast cancer: the surgeon's view. *Cancer* **42:** 2066–2077.

18. Veronesi, U. and P. Valagussa. 1981. Inefficacy of internal mammary nodes dissection in breast cancer surgery. *Cancer* **47:** 170–175.

19. Patey, D. H. and W. H. Dysen. 1948. The prognosis of carcinoma of the breast in relation to the type of operation performed. *Br. J. Cancer* **2:** 7–13.

20. Auchincloss, H. 1963. Significance of location and number of axillary metastases in carcinoma of the breast: a justification for a conservative operation. *Ann. Surg.* **158:** 37–46.

21. Handley, R. S. and A. C. Thackray. 1969. Conservative radical mastectomy (Patey's operation). *Ann. Surg.* **170:** 880–882.

22. Henderson, I. C. and G. P. Canellos. 1980. Cancer of the Breast: the past decade. *N. Engl. J. Med.* **302:** 17–30.

23. Madden, J. L. 1965. Modified radical mastectomy. *Surg. Gynecol. Obstet.* **121:** 1221–1230.

24. Martin, J. K., Jr., J. A. van Heerden, W. F. Taylor, and T. A. Gaffey. 1986. Is modified radical mastectomy really equivalent to radical mastectomy in treatment of carcinoma of the breast? *Cancer* **57:** 510–518.

25. Nemoto, T. and T. L. Dao. 1975. Is modified radical mastectomy adequate for axillary lymph node dissection? *Ann. Surg.* **182:** 722–723.

26. Turner, L., R. Swindell, W. G. Bell, R. C. Hartley, J. H. Tasker, W. W. Wilson, M. R. Alderson, and I. M. Leck. 1981. Radical versus modified radical mastectomy for breast cancer. *Ann. R. Coll. Surg. Engl.* **63:** 239–243.

27. Maddox, W. A., J. T. Carpenter, Jr., H. L. Laws, S. J. Soong, G. Cloud, M. M. Urist, and C. M. Balch. 1983. A randomized prospective trial of radical (Halsted) mastectomy versus modified radical mastectomy in 311 breast cancer patients. *Ann. Surg.* **198:** 207–212.

28. Vana, J., R. Bedwani, C. Mettlin, and G. P. Murphy. 1981. Trends in diagnosis and management of breast cancer in the U.S.: from the surveys of the American College of Surgeons. *Cancer* **48:** 1043–1052.

29. Wilson, R. E., W. L. Donegan, C. Mettlin, N. Natarajan, C. R. Smart, and G. P. Murphy. 1984. The 1982 national survey of carcinoma of the breast in the United States by the American College of Surgeons. *Surg. Gynecol. Obstet.* **159:** 309–318.

30. Schain, W. S. 1988. The sexual and intimate consequences of breast cancer treatment. *CA Cancer J. Clin.* **38:** 154–161.

31. Maguire, P. 1989. Breast conservation versus mastectomy: psychological considerations. *Semin. Surg. Oncol.* **5:** 137–144.

32. Teimourian, B. and M. N. Adham. 1982. Survey of patients' responses to breast reconstruction. *Ann. Plast. Surg.* **9:** 321–325.

33. Schain, W. S. 1991. Breast reconstruction. Update of psychosocial and pragmatic concerns. *Cancer* **68:** 1170–1175.

34. Schain, W. S., D. K. Wellisch, R. O. Pasnau, and J. Landsverk. 1985. The sooner the better: a study of psychological factors in women undergoing immediate versus delayed breast reconstruction. *Am. J. Psychiatry* **142:** 40–46.

35. Frazier, T. G. and R. B. Noone. 1985. An objective analysis of immediate simultaneous reconstruction in the treatment of primary carcinoma of the breast. *Cancer* **55:** 1202–1205.

36. Georgiade, G. S., N. G. Georgiade, K. S. McCarty, Jr., B. J. Ferguson, and H. F. Seigler. 1981. Modified radical mastectomy with immediate reconstruction for carcinoma of the breast. *Ann. Surg.* **193:** 565–573.

37. Hartrampf, C. R., Jr., and G. K. Bennett. 1987. Autogenous tissue reconstruction in the mastectomy patient. A critical review of 300 patients. *Ann. Surg.* **205:** 508–519.

38. Webster, D. J., R. E. Mansel, and L. E. Hughes. 1984. Immediate reconstruction of the breast after mastectomy. Is it safe? *Cancer* **53:** 1416–1419.

39. Benson, E. A. and J. Thorogood. 1986. The effect of surgical technique on local recurrence rates following mastectomy. *Eur. J. Surg. Oncol.* **12:** 267–271.

40. Bland, K. I. and E. M. Copeland III. 1991. The breast: comprehensive management of benign and malignant diseases. Saunders, Philadelphia, PA.

41. Crile, G., Jr., C. B. Esselstyn, R. E. Hermann, and S. O. Hoerr. 1973. Partial mastectomy for carcinoma of the breast. *Surg. Gynecol. Obstet.* **136:** 929–933.

42. Mustakallio, S. 1954. Treatment of breast cancer by tumor extirpation and roentgen therapy instead of radical operation. *J. Fac. Radiol.* **6:** 23–26.

43. Peters, M. V. 1977. Wedge resection with or without radiation in early breast cancer. *Int. J. Radiat. Oncol. Biol. Phys.* **2:** 1151–1156.

44. Porritt, A. 1964. Early carcinoma of the breast. *Br. J. Surg.* **51:** 214–216.

45. Taylor, H., R. Baker, R. W. Fortt, and J. Hermon-Taylor. 1971. Sector mastectomy in selected cases of breast cancer. *Br. J. Surg.* **58:** 161–163.

46. Wise, L., A. Y. Mason, and L. V. Ackerman. 1971. Local excision and irradiation: an alternative method for the treatment of early mammary cancer. *Ann. Surg.* **174:** 392–401.

47. Atkins, H., J. L. Hayward, D. J. Klugman, and A. B. Wayte. 1972. Treatment of early breast cancer: a report after ten years of a clinical trial. *Br. Med. J.* **2:** 423–429.

48. Calle, R., J. P. Pilleron, P. Schlienger, and J. R. Vilcoq. 1978. Conservative management of operable breast cancer: ten years experience at the Foundation Curie. *Cancer* **42:** 2045–2053.

49. Amalric, R., F. Santamaria, F. Robert, J. Seigle, C. Altschuler, J. M. Kurtz, et al. 1982. Radiation therapy with or without primary limited surgery for operable breast cancer: a 20 year experience at the Marseilles Cancer Institute. *Cancer* **49:** 30–34.

50. Osborne, M. P., N. Ormiston, C. L. Harmer, J. A. McKinna, J. Baker, and W. P. Greening. 1984. Breast conservation in the treatment of early breast cancer. A 20-year follow-up. *Cancer* **53:** 349–355.

51. Harris, J. R. and S. Hellman. 1983. Primary radiation therapy for early breast cancer. *Cancer* **51:** 2547–2552.

52. Montague, E. D. and G. H. Fletcher. 1985. Local regional effectiveness of surgery and radiation therapy in the treatment of breast cancer. *Cancer* **55:** 2266–2272.

53. Prosnitz, L. R., I. S. Goldenberg, R. A. Packard, M. B. Levene, J. Harris, S. Hellman, et al. 1977. Radiation therapy as initial treatment for early stage cancer of the breast without mastectomy. *Cancer* **39:** 917–923.

54. Fisher, B. 1980. Laboratory and clinical research in breast cancer—a personal adventure: the David A. Karnofsky memorial lecture. *Cancer Res.* **40:** 3863–3874.

55. Fisher, B., C. Redmond, E. R. Fisher, M. Bauer, N. Wolmark, L. Wickerham, et al. 1985. Ten-year results of a randomized clinical trial comparing radical mastectomy and total mastectomy with or without radiation. *N. Engl. J. Med.* **312**: 674–681.

56. Fisher, B., N. Wolmark, C. Redmond, M. Deutsch, and E. R. Fisher. 1981. Findings from NSABP Protocol No. B–04: comparison of radical mastectomy with alternative treatments. II. The clinical and biological significance of medial-central breast cancers. *Cancer* **48**: 1863–1872.

57. Veronesi, U. 1987. Rationale and indications for limited surgery in breast cancer: current data. *World J. Surg.* **11**: 493–498.

58. Veronesi, U., R. Saccozzi, M. Del Vecchio, A. Banfi, C. Clemente, M. De Lena, et al. 1981. Comparing radical mastectomy with quadrantectomy, axillary dissection, and radiotherapy in patients with small cancers of the breast. *N. Engl. J. Med.* **305**: 6–11.

59. Veronesi, U., B. Salvadori, A. Luini, A. Banfi, R. Zucali, M. Del Vecchio, et al. 1990. Conservative treatment of early breast cancer. Long-term results of 1232 cases treated with quadrantectomy, axillary dissection, and radiotherapy. *Ann. Surg.* **211**: 250–259.

60. Fisher, B., M. Bauer, R. Margolese, R. Poisson, Y. Pilch, C. Redmond, et al. 1985. Five-year results of a randomized clinical trial comparing total mastectomy and segmental mastectomy with or without radiation in the treatment of breast cancer. *N. Engl. J. Med.* **312**: 665–673.

61. Fisher, B. and S. Anderson. 1994. Conservative surgery for the management of invasive and noninvasive carcinoma of the breast: NSABP trials. National Surgical Adjuvant Breast and Bowel Project. *World J. Surg.* **18**: 63–69.

62. Fisher, B., C. Redmond, R. Poisson, R. Margolese, N. Wolmark, L. Wickerham, et al. 1989. Eight-year results of a randomized clinical trial comparing total mastectomy and lumpectomy with or without irradiation in the treatment of breast cancer. *N. Engl. J. Med.* **320**: 822–828.

63. Fisher, B., S. Anderson, C. K. Redmond, N. Wolmark, D. L. Wickerham, and W. M. Cronin. 1995. Reanalysis and results after 12 years follow-up in a randomized clinical trial comparing total mastectomy with lumpectomy with or without irradiation in the treatment of breast cancer. *N. Engl. J. Med.* **333**: 1456–1461.

64. Stablein, D. M., and the staff of the EMMES Corporation. March 30, 1994. A reanalysis of NSABP Protocol B–06: final report.

65. Clark, R. M., P. B. McCulloch, M. N. Levine, M. Lipa, R. H. Wilkinson, L. J. Mahoney, et al. 1992. Randomized clinical trail to assess the effectiveness of breast irradiation following lumpectomy and axillary dissection for node-negative breast cancer. *J. Natl. Cancer Inst.* **84**: 683–689.

66. Haffty, B. G., N. B. Goldberg, M. Rose, B. Heil, D. Fischer, M. Beinfield, C. McKhann, and J. B. Weissberg. 1989. Conservative surgery with radiation therapy in clinical stage I and II breast cancer. Results of a 20-year experience. *Arch. Surg.* **124**: 1266–1270.

67. Jacobson, J. A., D. N. Danforth, K. H. Cowan, T. d'Angelo, S. M. Steinberg, L. Pierce, et al. 1995. Ten-year results of a comparison of conservation with mastectomy in the treatment of stage I and II breast cancer. *N. Engl. J. Med.* **332**: 907–911.

68. Mansfield, C. M., L. T. Komarnicky, G. F. Schwartz, A. L. Rosenberg, L. Krishnan, W. R. Jewell, et al. 1995. Ten-year results in 1070 patients with stages I and II breast cancer treated by conservative surgery and radiation therapy. *Cancer* **75**: 2328–2336.

69. Sarrazin, D., M. Le, J. Rouesse, G. Contesso, J. Y. Petit, J. Lacour, J. Viguier, and C. Hill. 1984. Conservative treatment versus mastectomy in breast cancer tumors with macroscopic diameter of 20 millimeters or less. The experience of the Institut Gustave-Roussy. *Cancer* **53**: 1209–1213.

70. Stehlin, J. S., Jr., P. D. de Ipolyi, P. J. Greeff, A. E. Gutierrez, R. J. Hardy, and S. L. Dahiya. 1987. A ten-year study of partial mastectomy for carcinoma of the breast. *Surg. Gynecol. Obstet.* **165:** 191–198.

71. Recht, A. 1996. Selection of patients with early stage invasive breast cancer for treatment with conservation surgery and radiation therapy. *Semin. Oncol.* **23:** 19–30.

72. Winchester, D. P. and J. D. Cox. 1992. Standards for breast-conservation treatment. *CA Cancer J. Clin.* **42:** 134–162.

73. Fisher, B., N. Wolmark, E. R. Fisher, and M. Deutsch. 1985. Lumpectomy and axillary dissection for breast cancer: surgical, pathological, and radiation considerations. *World J. Surg.* **9:** 692–698.

74. Margolese, R., R. Poisson, H. Shibata, Y. Pilch, H. Lerner, and B. Fisher. 1987. The technique of segmental mastectomy (lumpectomy) and axillary dissection: a syllabus from the National Surgical Adjuvant Breast Project workshops. *Surgery* **102:** 828–834.

75. Fisher, B., N. Wolmark, M. Bauer, C. Redmond, and M. Gebhardt. 1981. The accuracy of clinical nodal staging and of limited axillary dissection as a determinant of histologic nodal status in carcinoma of the breast. *Surg. Gynecol. Obstet.* **152:** 765–772.

76. Pigott, J., R. Nichols, W. A. Maddox, and C. M. Balch. 1984. Metastases to the upper levels of the axillary nodes in carcinoma of the breast and its implications for nodal sampling procedures. *Surg. Gynecol. Obstet.* **158:** 255–259.

77. Rosen, P. P., M. L. Lesser, D. W. Kinne, and E. J. Beattie. 1983. Discontinuous or "skip" metastases in breast carcinoma. Analysis of 1228 axillary dissections. *Ann. Surg.* **197:** 276–283.

78. Schwartz, G. F., D. M. D'Ugo, and A. L. Rosenberg. 1986. Extent of axillary dissection preceding irradiation for carcinoma of the breast. *Arch. Surg.* **121:** 1395–1398.

79. Kinne, D. W. 1991. The surgical management of primary breast cancer. *CA Cancer J. Clin.* **41:** 71–84.

80. Recht, A. and M. J. Houlihan. 1995. Axillary lymph nodes and breast cancer: a review. *Cancer* **76:** 1491–1512.

81. Ruffin, W. K., A. Stacey-Clear, J. Younger, and H. C. Hoover, Jr. 1995. Rationale for routine axillary dissection in carcinoma of the breast. *J. Am. Coll. Surg.* **180:** 245–251.

82. Baxter, N., D. McCready, J. A. Chapman, E. Fish, H. Kahn, W. Hanna, M. Trudeau, and H. L. Lickley. 1996. Clinical behavior of untreated axillary nodes after local treatment for primary breast cancer. *Ann. Surg. Oncol.* **3:** 235–240.

83. Cady, B., M. D. Stone, and J. Wayne. 1993. New therapeutic possibilities in primary invasive breast cancer. *Ann. Surg.* **218:** 338–347.

84. Silverstein, M. J., E. D. Gierson, J. R. Waisman, W. J. Colburn, and P. Gamagami. 1995. Predicting axillary node positivity in patients with invasive carcinoma of the breast by using a combination of T category and palpability. *J. Am. Coll. Surg.* **180:** 700–704.

85. Rosner, D., W. W. Lane, and R. Penetrante. 1991. Ductal carcinoma *in situ* with microinvasion. A curable entity using surgery alone without need for adjuvant therapy. *Cancer* **67:** 1498–1503.

86. Wong, J. H., K. H. Kopald, and D. L. Morton. 1990. The impact of microinvasion on axillary node metastases and survival in patients with intraductal breast cancer. *Arch. Surg.* **125:** 1298–1301.

87. Chontos, A. J., D. P. Maher, E. R. Ratzer, and M. E. Fenoglio. 1997. Axillary lymph node dissection: is it required in T1a breast cancer? *J. Am. Coll. Surg.* **184:** 493–498.

88. Mustafa, I. A., B. Cole, H. J. Wanebo, K. I. Bland, and H. R. Chang. 1997. The impact of histopathology on nodal metastases in minimal breast cancer. *Arch. Surg.* **132:** 384–390.

89. White, R. E., M. P. Vezeridis, M. Konstadoulakis, B. F. Cole, H. J. Wanebo, and K. I. Bland. 1996. Therapeutic options and results for the management of minimally invasive carcinoma of the breast: influence of axillary dissection for treatment of T1α and T1β lesions. *J. Am. Coll. Surg.* **183:** 575–582.

90. Albertini, J. J., G. H. Lyman, C. Cox, T. Yeatman, L. Balducci, N. Ku, et al. 1996. Lymphatic mapping and sentinel node biopsy in the patient with breast cancer. *JAMA* **276:** 1818–1822.

91. Giuliano, A. E., A. M. Barth, B. Spivack, P. D. Beitsch, and S. W. Evans. 1996. Incidence and predictors of axillary metastasis in T1 carcinoma of the breast. *J. Am. Coll. Surg.* **183:** 185–189.

92. Giuliano, A. E., D. M. Kirgan, J. M. Guenther, and D. L. Morton. 1994. Lymphatic mapping and sentinel lymphadenectomy for breast cancer. *Ann. Surg.* **220:** 391–398.

93. National Institutes of Health Consensus Conference. 1991. Treatment of early-stage breast cancer. *JAMA* **265:** 391–395.

94. Osteen, R. T., B. Cady, J. S. Chmiel, R. E. Clive, R. L. Doggett, M. A. Friedman, et al. 1994. 1991 national survey of carcinoma of the breast by the Commission on Cancer. *J. Am. Coll. Surg.* **178:** 213–219.

95. National Cancer Data Base. 1995. American Cancer Society, update 1996. **2:** 6.

96. Tarbox, B. B., J. K. Rockwood, and C. M. Abernathy. 1992. Are modified radical mastectomies done for T1 breast cancers because of surgeon's advice or patient's choice? *Am. J. Surg.* **164:** 417–420.

97. Albain, K. S., S. R. Green, A. S. Lichter, L. F. Hutchins, W. C. Wood, I. C. Henderson, et al. 1996. Influence of patient characteristics, socioeconomic factors, geography, and systemic risk on the use of breast-sparing treatment in women enrolled in adjuvant breast cancer studies: an analysis of two intergroup trials. *J. Clin. Oncol.* **14:** 3009–3017.

98. Kotwall, C. A., D. L. Covington, R. Rutledge, M. P. Churchill, and A. A. Meyer. 1996. Patient, hospital, and surgeon factors associated with breast conservation surgery. A statewide analysis in North Carolina. *Ann. Surg.* **224:** 419–426.

99. Polednak, A. P. 1997. Predictors of breast-conserving surgery in Connecticut, 1990–1992. *Ann. Surg. Oncol.* **4:** 259–263.

100. Dowlatshahi, K., M. L. Yaremko, L. F. Kluskens, and P. M. Jokich. 1991. Nonpalpable breast lesions: findings of stereotaxic needle-core biopsy and fine-needle aspiration cytology. *Radiology* **181:** 745–750.

101. Israel, P. Z. and R. E. Fine. 1995. Stereotactic needle biopsy for occult breast lesions: a minimally invasive alternative. *Am. Surg.* **61:** 87–91.

102. Mitnick, J. S., M. F. Vazquez, P. I. Pressman, M. N. Harris, and D. F. Roses. 1996. Stereotactic fine-needle aspiration biopsy for the evaluation of nonpalpable breast lesions: report of an experience based on 2,988 cases. *Ann. Surg. Oncol.* **3:** 185–191.

103. Julian, T. Personal communication.

104. Dowlatshahi, K. Personal communication.

105. Muntaz, H., M. A. Hall-Craggs, A. Wotherspoon, M. Paley, G. Buonaccorsi, Z. Amin, et al. 1996. Laser therapy for breast cancer: MR imaging and histopathologic correlation. *Radiology* **200:** 651–658.

106. Staren, E. D., M. S. Sabel, L. M. Gianakakis, G. A. Wiener, V. M. Hart, M. Gorski, et al. 1997. Cryosurgery of breast cancer. *Arch. Surg.* **132:** 28–33.

107. Rand, R. W., R. P. Rand, F. Eggerding, L. Den Besten, and W. King. 1987. Cryolumpectomy for carcinoma of the breast. *Surg. Gynecol. Obstet.* **165:** 392–396.

108. Fisher, B., R. G. Ravdin, R. K. Ausman, N. H. Slack, G. E. Moore, and R. J. Noer. 1968. Surgical adjuvant chemotherapy in cancer of the breast: results of a decade of cooperative investigation. *Ann. Surg.* **168:** 337–356.

109. Bonadonna, G., E. Brusamolino, P. Valagussa, A. Rossi, L. Brugnatelli, C. Brambilla, et al. 1976. Combination chemotherapy as an adjuvant treatment in operable breast cancer. *N. Engl. J. Med.* **294:** 405–410.

110. Bonadonna, G., P. Valagussa, A. Moliterni, M. Zambetti, and C. Brambilla. 1995. Adjuvant cyclophosphamide, methotrexate, and fluorouracil in node-positive breast cancer: the results of 20 years of follow-up. *N. Engl. J. Med.* **332:** 901–906.

111. Jones, S. E., T. E. Moon, G. Bonadonna, P. Valagussa, S. Rivkin, A. Buzdar, E. Montague, and T. Powles. 1987. Comparison of different trials of adjuvant chemotherapy in stage II breast cancer using a natural history data base. *Am. J. Clin. Oncol.* **10:** 387–395.

112. Smalley, R. V., J. Carpenter, A. Bartolucci, C. Vogel, and S. Krauss. 1977. A comparison of cyclophosphamide, adriamycin, 5-fluorouracil (CAF) and cyclophosphamide, methotrexate, 5-fluorouracil, vincristine, prednisone (CMFVP) in patients with metastatic breast cancer: a Southeastern Cancer Study Group project. *Cancer* **40:** 625–632.

113. Sledge, G. W., Jr. 1996. Adjuvant therapy for early stage breast cancer. *Semin. Oncol.* **23:** 51–54.

114. Early Breast Cancer Trialists' Collaborative Group. 1992. Systemic treatment of early breast cancer by hormonal, cytotoxic, or immune therapy. 133 randomized trials involving 31,000 recurrences and 24,000 deaths among 75,000 women. *Lancet* **339:** 1–5, 71–85.

115. Glick, J. H., R. D. Gelber, A. Goldhirsch, and H. J. Senn. 1992. Meeting highlights: adjuvant therapy for primary breast cancer. *J. Natl. Cancer Inst.* **19:** 1479–1485.

116. National Cancer Institute. 1995. Clinical announcement: adjuvant therapy of breast cancer—tamoxifen update.

117. Fisher, B., J. Dignam, J. Bryant, A. DeCillis, D. L. Wickerham, N. Wolmark, et al. 1996. Five versus more than five years of tamoxifen therapy for breast cancer patients with negative lymph nodes and estrogen receptor-positive tumors. *J. Natl. Cancer Inst.* **88:** 1529–1542.

118. Cuenca, R. E., J. Giachino, M. A. Arredondo, R. Hempling, and S. B. Edge. 1996. Endometrial carcinoma associated with breast carcinoma: low incidence with tamoxifen use. *Cancer* **77:** 2058–2063.

119. McGuire, W. L., A. K. Tandon, D. C. Allred, G. C. Chamness, P. M. Ravdin, and G. M. Clark. 1992. Prognosis and treatment decisions in patients with breast cancer without axillary node involvement. *Cancer* **70:** 1775–1781.

120. Goldhirsch, A., W. C. Wood, H. J. Senn, J. H. Glick, and R. D. Gelber. 1995. Meeting highlights: international consensus panel on the treatment of primary breast cancer. *J. Natl. Cancer Inst.* **87:** 1441–1445.

121. Consensus conference. 1985. Adjuvant chemotherapy for breast cancer. *JAMA* **254:** 3461–3463.

122. Bauer, R. L., E. Busch, E. Leven, and S. B. Edge. 1995. Therapy for inflammatory breast cancer: impact of doxorubicin-based therapy. *Ann. Surg. Oncol.* **2:** 288–294.

123. Fisher, B., A. B. Brown, E. Mamounas, S. Wieand, A. Robidoux, R. G. Margolese, et al. 1997. Effect of preoperative chemotherapy on local-regional disease in women with operable breast cancer: findings from National Surgical Adjuvant Breast and Bowel Project B-18. *J. Clin. Oncol.* **15:** 2483–2493.

124. Singletary, S. E., M. D. McNeese, and G. N. Hortobagyi. 1992. Feasibility of breast-conservation surgery after induction chemotherapy for locally advanced breast carcinoma. *Cancer* **69:** 2849–2852.

125. Veronesi, U., G. Bonadonna, S. Zurrida, V. Galimberti, M. Greco, C. Brambilla, et al. 1995. Conservation surgery after primary chemotherapy in large carcinomas of the breast. *Ann. Surg.* **222:** 612–618.

126. Peters, W. P., M. Ross, J. J. Vredenburgh, B. Meisenberg, L. B. Marks, E. Winer, et al. 1993. High-dose chemotherapy and autologous bone marrow support as consolidation after standard-dose adjuvant therapy for high-risk primary breast cancer. *J. Clin. Oncol.* **11:** 1132–1143.

127. Seidman, A. D. 1996. Chemotherapy for advanced breast cancer: a current perspective. *Semin. Oncol.* **23:** 55–59.

19

Breast Cancer Therapy
Using Monoclonal Antibodies Against
Epidermal Growth Factor Receptor and HER-2

Zhen Fan and John Mendelsohn

1. INTRODUCTION

The importance of growth factors for tumor cell growth is inferred from many experimental observations *(1–3)*. A large number of oncogenes code for molecules that are growth factors, their receptors, or signal-transducing molecules that are activated by the receptors *(4,5)*. These oncogenes have been shown to play causal roles in cell transformation and tumorigenesis *(6–8)*. Clinical studies also indicate that overexpression of growth factor receptors, such as epidermal growth factor receptor (EGFR) and HER-2 (reviewed in Chapter 2), which occurs commonly in human cancers, including breast cancers, often correlates with poorer prognosis *(9–12)*. Inhibitors that block the activities of growth factor receptors or the transduction pathways of receptor downstream signaling can inhibit the proliferation of cultured, and, in some studies, xenografted cancer cell lines. Thus, these inhibitors may be potential new drugs for the treatment of human cancer *(13)*.

The potential therapeutic uses of monoclonal antibodies (MAbs) in the treatment of human cancer have attracted considerable interest in the past two decades. Related research has focused primarily upon MAbs as activators of host immune molecules and immune cells, or MAbs as carriers to deliver cytotoxic agents or radioactive isotopes to specific targets. Alternatively, antibodies with the capacity to bind and block ligand-induced activation of growth factor receptors can also serve as pharmacological agents to interfere with the physiological function of cell membrane receptors. There are "experiments of nature" in which stable physiological changes resulting in disease are observed when patients develop antibodies against certain receptors. These include antibodies against receptors for acetylcholine (in patients with myasthenia gravis), receptors for thyroid-stimulating hormone (in some patients with hypothyroidism or hyperthyroidism), and receptors for insulin (in patients with a rare form of diabetes mellitus).

How might selectivity be obtained with such MAbs directed against growth factor receptors? Advantage may be taken of quantitative differences in the expression of specific growth receptors, such as the EGFR, in tumor cells compared with normal

From: Breast Cancer: *Molecular Genetics, Pathogenesis, and Therapeutics*
Edited by: A. M. Bowcock © Humana Press Inc., Totowa, NJ

cells. MAbs that block receptor activation also can exploit the fact that cancer cells are deficient in growth control, and display a degree of miscoordination that is not found in normal cells. If normal cells are deprived of serum (growth factors), biochemical processes are coordinated, so that the cells typically enter into a quiescent Go phase, from which they can be rescued when serum or growth factors are replenished *(14,15)*. If cultured transformed cells are deprived of serum or growth factors, although proliferation ceases, DNA synthesis may continue at an appreciable level, in many cases accompanied by imbalanced cell proliferation and cell death *(14)*. This may be because the checkpoints, which interrupt cell cycle traversal in normal cells if there is a problem with DNA replication or other essential cellular functions, are malfunctioning in malignant cells *(16,17)*. Another approach with antireceptor MAbs is to take advantage of the need for a cocktail of growth factors to support the proliferation of cultured cell lines *(2)*. Thus, combinations of MAbs against two or more receptors may provide even more selectivity for particular types of targeted cells.

In human breast cancer, the EGFR and HER-2 appear to be two of the most important growth factors controlling growth. This review presents current progress and strategies using MAbs directed against the EGFR and HER-2 in inhibiting the proliferation of human breast cancer cells. This could lead to novel clinical approaches to the treatment of breast cancer patients.

2. EGFR AND BREAST CANCER THERAPY

2.1. EGFR and Breast Cancer

The EGFR and its ligands have an important role in the regulation of growth of human breast cancer *(18)*. The EGFR is a 170 kDa glycoprotein in the plasma membrane, composed of an extracellular binding domain, a transmembrane lipophilic segment, and an intracellular protein tyrosine kinase domain with a regulatory carboxyl terminal segment *(19,20)*. The most widely expressed ligands for EGFRs are EGF and transforming growth factor-alpha (TGF-α). Following binding of ligand, EGFRs form homodimers, which results in the activation of the intrinsic tyrosine kinase *(19,20)*. Activation of the tyrosine kinase triggers a series of signal-transduction pathways that ultimately lead to cell growth and proliferation.

The role of EGFRs in breast cancer has been under study for nearly two decades *(21)*. EGFR expression is found in established breast carcinoma cell lines, as well as in primary breast carcinoma cells. Following up a report that EGF stimulated proliferation of MCF-7 breast cancer cells in chemically defined growing medium *(21)*, Fitzpatrick et al. showed that each of 13 breast cancer cell lines, which grow attached to the surface of culture dishes, express high-affinity EGFRs in varying amounts, and that some (but not all) of these lines were stimulated by addition of EGF to serum-free medium *(22)*. The same authors noted that EGF binding to specimens of primary human breast tumors was independent of estrogen binding, and, in fact, 20% of tumors were positive for EGFRs and negative for estrogen receptor (ER) *(23)*. Subsequent reports have found a significant inverse correlation between the expression of EGFRs and ERs in primary breast tumors *(24–26)*, and a significantly more frequent expression of EGFRs on metastases than that on primary tumors *(10)*. Davidson et al. examined breast cancer cell lines and found that high levels of EGFR expression are associated with absent ERs *(27)*. Aside from one cell line, MDA-MB-468 *(28)*, the gene for EGFR is not amplified, and increased transcription is felt to explain the high levels of receptor observed in mammary cell lines *(27)*.

Increased expression of EGFR ligand was also observed. Messenger RNA for TGF-α was expressed in more than half of primary breast adenocarcinoma specimens examined *(28,29)*, and immunoreactive and biologically active TGF-α was significantly higher in malignant effusions from breast cancer patients than in effusions from noncancer patients *(30)*. Studies with established breast cancer cell lines also have demonstrated TGF-α production *(31)*. The level of TGF-α may be regulated by estrogen, which can induce increased TGF-α production in a number of breast cancer lines *(29,32)*.

TGF-α stimulates the growth and development of mammary epithelial cells, and is implicated in the tumorigenesis of human breast cancer. One study with mouse mammary tumor virus (MMTV)-TGF-α transgenic mice exhibited terminal duct and alveolar hyperplasia in both virgin and pregnant mice in 3 of 10 founder lines *(33)*. With longer observation, lobular hyperplasia, cystic hyperplasia, adenoma, and adenocarcinoma were also observed. Two other studies with TGF-α transgene driven by mouse metallothioneine promoter also revealed adenomas and adenocarcinomas after 6–14 mo of latency *(34,35)*. TGF-α may promote mammary tumorigenesis by selectively stimulating secretory epithelial cell proliferation during lactation, and prolonging cell survival during involution *(36)*. The c-*myc* oncogene, which is commonly amplified in breast cancer, can interact synergistically with TGF-α to promote phenotypic transformation of mammary epithelial cells. Bitransgenic mice carrying the TGF-α and c-*myc* transgenes showed markedly decreased tumor latency, increased tumor growth, and even induction of mammary tumors in virgin female and male mice *(37,38)*.

Clinical studies of primary breast cancer specimens by Harris et al. have revealed important correlation between the levels of EGFRs and both prognosis and response to therapy. Both relapse-free survival and total survival were significantly shorter for EGFR-positive as compared with EGFR-negative tumors *(9,10)*. There also was evidence for lack of response to endocrine therapy in patients with EGFR-positive tumors *(39)*. In fact, EGFR status was as good as ER status for predicting an objective response to estrogen therapy *(39)*.

2.2. Anti-EGFR MAbs

MAbs 225 IgG1 and 528 IgG2a are among the best-studied anti-EGFR MAbs for their capabilities to inhibit tumor-cell proliferation *(40–43)*. They bind to the receptor with affinity comparable to the natural ligand (Kd = 1–2 n*M*), and compete with ligand for receptor binding. Unlike the natural ligands, the binding of MAb 225 or 528 to receptors does not activate the receptor tyrosine kinase, but prevents ligand-induced receptor activation *(44)*. The MAbs can induce EGFR dimerization through simultaneous bivalent binding to two EGFRs, and can induce MAb–receptor complex internalization *(45)*. The initial rates of internalization of EGFRs are the same in the presence of EGF or antireceptor MAb *(46)*. However, subsequent receptor processing and catabolism appear to occur through a slower pathway when the receptor is bound to antibody *(47)*, possibly because of the differences in receptor tyrosine phosphorylation *(46,47)*.

The MAbs can block EGF- and TGF-α-induced stimulation of growth in a variety of cultured cell lines, including breast cell lines *(43)*. The inhibitory effects of MAbs 225 and 528 on malignant cells were first demonstrated with A431 vulvar squamous carcinoma cells, which express both EGFRs and TGF-α in large quantities *(40–42)*. Later, similar observations have been found in a variety of other cultured malignant and non-malignant cell lines, and in some xenografted malignant cell lines *(48)*. The capability of MAbs to inhibit cell proliferation does not necessarily require the presence of Fc fragment of the MAb, since the F(ab')2 fragment of MAb 225 can produce effects comparable to the intact MAb 225 in preventing the growth of A431 xenografts in nude mice *(49)*.

Other murine anti-EGFR MAbs that have antiproliferative effects similar to MAbs 225 and 528 include MAb 108 *(50)* and MAb 425 *(51)*. MAb 455 *(40)* and R1, which was the first MAb against the EGFR *(52)*, do not block binding of ligand to EGFRs, and do not inhibit cell proliferation. Recently, a rat MAb ICR62 with similar antiproliferative effects also has been reported *(53,54)*.

2.3. Biochemical Mechanism of Growth Inhibition by Anti-EGFR MAbs

It is postulated that growth inhibition induced by anti-EGFR MAbs results from mAb-mediated interruption of the EGFR autocrine loop *(43)*. However, the intracellular mechanisms explaining how blockade of EGFR-mediated signal transduction leads to arrest of the cell cycle in G1 phase *(55–59)*, or induction of apoptosis, in rare cases *(60)*, are still not fully understood.

The cell cycle engine, driving cells to traverse sequential phases of the cell cycle, is composed of a series of serine/threonine kinases known as cyclin-dependent kinases (CDKs) *(61,62)*. The order and timing of cell-cycle events are tightly associated with the temporal activation and inactivation of CDKs during cell-cycle traversal. The activities of CDKs are regulated by cyclins, the activating partners of CDK, and the opposing partners, called CDK inhibitors. In addition, the activities of CDKs can also be regulated at the levels of synthesis/degradation and phosphorylation/dephosphorylation of the CDK molecules *(61,62)*. The retinoblastoma protein (RB) or the RB-related proteins (p107 and p130) are putative substrates of CDKs. RB family proteins are dephosphorylated as cells exit mitosis, and remain hypophosphorylated during early G1 phase, serving as molecular guardians that prevent cell-cycle progression through G1 phase. When cell-cycle traversal reaches the restriction point in G1 phase, RB or RB-related proteins are hyperphosphorylated by CDK/cyclin complexes, which results in concomitant liberation and activation of members of the E2F family of transcription factors necessary for S-phase entry *(61,62)*.

The authors examined the cell cycle effects of EGFR blockade on cultured MCF-10A nonmalignant human mammary epithelial cells, which were originally derived from human fibrocystic mammary tissue *(63)*. These cells are immortalized, but still depend on exogenously supplied EGF for optimal growth. Complete G1 arrest was rapidly induced after withdrawal of EGF from the culture medium. These cells remained arrested in G1 phase for a long time (80 d) without dying, and they could re-enter the cell cycle when EGF was replenished *(55)*. The rate of G1 arrest upon EGF withdrawal could be accelerated by addition of anti-EGFR MAb 225 to the culture medium. The cell cycle arrest was temporally associated with an increase in the levels of p27^{Kip1}, a CDK inhibitor, and a decrease in the levels of cyclin D1. Changes in the levels of other known CDK inhibitors were not observed. The increased p27^{Kip1} was associated with CDK2, and CDK2 kinase activity was markedly inhibited. A reduction of cyclin D1-associated kinase activity was also observed *(55)*.

The involvement of p27^{Kip1} in the induction of G1 arrest, mediated by EGFR blockade with anti-EGF MAb 225, was also observed in several other types of human cancer cell lines, including A431 vulvar squamous carcinoma cells *(56)*, DiFi colon adenocarcinoma cells *(57)*, and DU145 prostate adenocarcinoma cells *(58)*.

2.4. Growth Inhibition of Breast Cancer Cells by Anti-EGFR MAbs

A series of observations suggested that blockade of EGFR and TGF-α autocrine pathways by MAbs can inhibit proleration of breast cancer cells. Collaborative studies were undertaken between the authors' laboratory and the laboratories of Bates, Stampfer, Dickson, Lippman, Salomon, Arteaga, and Osborne, using anti-EGFR MAbs 225 or 528 to characterize the prevalence of the EGFR-mediated autocrine pathway in cultured nonmalignant and malignant human breast cells *(49,55,59,64–67)*.

MCF-10A cells grow in culture medium supplemented with exogenous TGF-α or EGF. They also produce the ligand, but in quantities inadequate to stimulate optimal proliferation *(49,55)*. The introduction of either c-Ha-*ras* or TGF-α into MCF-10A cells led to in vitro transformation *(64)*. These MCF-10A c-Ha-*ras* or TGF-α transfectants exhibited enhanced growth rate in serum-free medium, and could grow as clones in soft agar. Treatment of cultures with either EGFR-blocking MAb or TGF-α-neutralized MAb could inhibit proliferation, and eliminate the capacity for anchorage-independent growth *(64)*.

Nonmalignant human breast epithelial cell line 184 is derived from a reduction mammoplasty. The cells make large quantities of TGF-α in culture. Growth of these cells was also completely inhibited in the presence of MAb 225 *(59)*.

MDA-MB-468 breast adenocarcinoma cells have an amplified, but not rearranged, EGFR gene, and express approx 1×10^6 EGFRs/cell *(65,68,69)*. Studies in vitro have shown that the proliferation of MDA-MB-468 cells is inhibited in the presence to MAbs 225 or 528 *(65)*.

Inhibition of anchorage-dependent growth of MCF-10A, 184, and MDA-MB-468 cells by anti-EGFR MAb, in the absence of exogenous EGF, suggests that the antibodies were acting to block access of an endogenously produced ligand to the EGFR. Therefore, these cells appear to have an active and obligatory autocrine pathway.

MCF-7 breast adenocarcinoma cells do not ordinarily require EGF or TGF-α for growth in culture *(21)*. However, studies with MCF-7 cells, cultured under estrogen-deprived conditions, demonstrated that MCF-7 cell proliferation required addition of exogenous TGF-α, and that addition of anti-EGFR MAb 528 could block this growth response *(67)*. There are other breast cancer cell lines that do not appear to be stimulated by TGF-α or EGF under any conditions, and they ignore the presence of anti-EGFR MAb. These include MDA-MB-231 cells, which express both EGFRs and TGF-α, and HS578T cells, which express EGFRs, but not TGF-α *(43)*. The data suggest that the presence of a potential autocrine EGFR pathway does not always indicate dependence on this pathway for proliferation at usual conditions in cell culture.

2.5. Preclinical Studies with Anti-EGFR MAbs on Breast Cancer Cell Xenografts

In vivo effects of treatment with anti-EGFR MAbs were assayed immediately after implantation of xenografts of human breast adenocarcinoma MDA-MB-468 cells. A treatment schedule of intraperitoneal injections twice weekly was selected, based on a measured MAb half-life in serum of 3 d *(49)*. The administration of 2 mg of MAb 528 intraperitoneally twice a week resulted in a marked inhibition of tumor growth *(70)*. Another set of experiments with rat MAb ICR62 against the EGFR used a dose schedule of 200 μg/d for five consecutive days, and three times weekly thereafter. This also abolished growth of MDA-MB-468 xenografts *(54)*. These observations demonstrated that treatment with anti-EGFR MAb results in marked inhibition of tumor growth in mice bearing subcutaneous xenografts of cancer cell lines that express high levels of EGFRs. However, this treatment could not consistently eliminate xenografts that were well established *(71)*. Since the majority of patients with advanced breast carcinoma have well-established tumor masses, anti-EGFR MAbs alone will probably not be curative in this setting.

One approach to meet this challenge is the application of combination treatment with a chemotherapeutic agent and an anti-EGFR MAb *(50,71,72)*. This may be a promising strategy for a number of reasons. First, tissue culture data with cells that depend on EGFR activation by endogenous TGF-α for growth demonstrate that, when these cells are cultured at low density, the addition of exogenous growth factor is required for optimal proliferation *(72)*. Growth of these cells is inhibited by anti-EGFR MAbs *(72)*. By reducing the number of viable tumor cells, chemotherapy decreases the bulk of tumor burden, and, as a consequence, may result in a reduced concentration of endogenous growth factors in the immediate environment of the remaining tumor cells, and, therefore, may induce an increased susceptibility to the antitumor effects of anti-EGFR MAbs. Second, it has been shown in recent years that the death of cells exposed to chemotherapy and the death of cells deprived of essential growth factors both involve programmed cell death (apoptosis) *(73–76)*. Because of mutations in p53 and other key regulatory molecules, malignant cells often disobey checkpoint signals that control cell proliferation. The authors hypothesize that this situation could render cancer cells more susceptible to irreparable damage, if they simultaneously ignore two separate checkpoints activated both by blockade of mitogenic growth signals (G1 checkpoint) and by DNA damage induced by concurrent chemotherapy (G2 checkpoint) *(76)*. Finally, growth factors in serum can become survival factors for some experimentally derived cell lines *(77)*. It is possible that cellular damage from chemotherapy can convert ligands for the EGFR from growth factors into survival factors.

The authors' laboratory first studied the chemotherapeutic agent doxorubicin, an anthracycline that is one of the most active drugs for breast cancer treatment *(72)*. Experiments with MDA-MB-468 cell cultures and xenografts explored the antitumor effects of combined therapy. Culture of MDA-MB-468 cells with doxorubicin at various concentrations (0–10 n*M*) for 2 d, in combination with MAb 528 or MAb 225, produced an additive inhibition of growth, increasing the inhibitory effects of doxorubicin by 37%. The increased antitumor activity was not observed when cells were treated with doxorubicin in combination with the nonblocking anti-EGFR MAb 455 *(72)*. We next explored the effects of combination therapy on well-established MDA-

MB-468 breast adenocarcinoma cell xenografts more than 0.2 cm^3 in size. In untreated animals, tumors grew rapidly. Doxorubicin alone, at the maximally tolerated dose of 100 µg/20 g body wt on two successive days, did not have a noticeable antitumor activity, and treatment with intraperitoneal injections with MAb 528 or 225 (2 mg twice a week for 10 doses) only slowed tumor xenograft growth. However, the combination therapy with doxorubicin and MAb resulted in marked antitumor activity, with complete eradication of the xenografts (72). Another series of experiments was carried out with combination treatment of MAb 225 with paclitaxel, a promising chemotherapeutic agent acting on tubulin, on MDA-MB-468 breast adenocarcinoma cells. In this case, the tumors were quite sensitive to paclitaxel therapy, and suboptimal drug doses were used to assess the effect of concurrent treatment with MAb 225. The results again demonstrated elimination of well-established xenografts by combined therapy (78). Similar results were also obtained with other types of cancer cell xenografts, including A431 human vulvar squamous carcinoma cells (71) and DU-145 human prostate adenocarcinoma cells (79).

2.6. Clinical Trials with Anti-EGFR MAbs

A phase-I trial of anti-EGFR MAb therapy was carried out with escalating single doses of murine MAb 225 IgG1 in patients with advanced squamous cell carcinoma of the lung (80). The goals of this phase-I trial were to define the toxicity and pharmacokinetics of ^{111}In-MAb 225 in patients, and to determine if ^{111}In-MAb 225 localized to sites of squamous carcinoma of the lung. These tumors express high levels of EGFRs. Patients, in groups of three, received a single 1-h infusion of labeled MAb 225 in gradually increasing doses. Imaging studies revealed visualization of each primary tumor in patients who received 40 mg MAb or more, and could detect all presumed sites of metastatic disease with diameter more than 1 cm (determined by CT scan or X-ray). Percent injected dose in the tumor at 72 h, determined by area of interest scanning with a gamma camera, was 3.4% in patients who received 120 mg MAb. There was substantial liver uptake of labeled MAb, presumably because of the well-described clearing capacity of parenchymal and phagocytic cells in the liver, as well as the presence of EGFRs on the hepatocytes. Most importantly, no toxicity was observed in patients treated with up to 300 mg of anti-EGFR MAb. The serum concentration of ^{111}In-225 MAb was more than 20 nM for more than 3 d, when the administered dose was escalated to 120 mg and above. The authors' experimental research on cell culture has indicated that this concentration of MAb could completely saturate EGFRs, if it was achieved in tissues. As expected, all patients produced human antimouse IgG antibodies. The authors concluded that patients can tolerate the presence of saturating concentrations of an EGFR-blocking MAb in their blood for a period of more than 3 d without side effects.

Other laboratories have also produced MAbs against the EGFR that have been studied in clinical trials. MAb 425 IgG2a, which has many properties similar to MAb 528 IgG2a, has been used to image recurrent malignant gliomas (81). Therapy was attempted with ^{125}I-labeled MAb in this trial. No significant toxicities were observed. Phase-I trials have also been performed with MAb RG83852 (MAb 108) (82), which has been shown to selectively bind to the high-affinity EGFR, and to inhibit the proliferation of tumor cells overexpressing EGFR in culture and in xenografts (50). At doses greater than 200 mg/m^2, high levels of EGFR saturation with MAb were observed in biopsied specimens, and no toxicity was observed *(82)*. MAb Rl does not block EGF binding, and has not been shown to inhibit cell proliferation. In a clinical trial, radioactive labeled MAb Rl demonstrated imaging of glioblastomas with greater specificity than an isotype-matched control MAb *(83)*.

Murine MAbs are immunogenic, and all patients in the authors' clinical phase-I trial with MAb 225 produced human antimouse IgG antibodies *(80)*. This would have precluded the administration of repeated doses of the murine MAb at levels required to maintain a receptor-saturating level of MAb 225 in serum. Therefore, a human/murine chimeric version of MAb 225 was produced with the human IgG1 isotype. The chimeric MAb 225 (C225) fully retains the activity of murine MAb 225 in competing with EGF for receptor binding, and produces a similar spectrum of antitumor activity on a variety of cultured and xenografted human cancer cell lines *(84)*.

A phase-I study with MAb C225 was carried out in patients with EGFR-overexpressing tumors from head and neck, kidney, ovary, breast, prostate, and pancreas *(85)*. Escalating doses were administered to different subjects, first as single intravenous infusions, and then as repeated weekly infusions for up to 12 doses. Saturating levels in the blood were again achieved and maintained with the weekly doses of 100 mg/m^2, without evidence of toxicity. Clinical-phase Ib/IIa studies are currently examining repeated administration of MAb C225, in combination with appropriate chemotherapy, in patients with breast cancer (MAb C225 with paclitaxel), as well as in patients with other types of cancer, such as prostate cancer (MAb C225 with doxorubicin) and head and neck cancer (MAb C225 with cisplatinum).

3. HER-2 RECEPTOR AND BREAST CANCER THERAPY

3.1. Overexpression of HER-2 in Breast Cancer

The c-*erb*B-2 protooncogene (also known as *neu* in rat) codes for a 185 kDa transmembrane glycoprotein, HER-2, with intrinsic tyrosine kinase activity that resembles the receptor for EGF *(86–88)*. Despite extensive sequence homology between HER-2 and the EGFR, EGF and TGF-α do not bind to HER-2 *(89)*. No direct ligand for the HER-2 receptor has been identified yet. However, HER-2 can be transactivated by EGF through heterodimerization with the EGFR *(90)*. It also can be transactivated by *neu* differentiation factor (NDF)/heregulin (HRG) through heterodimerization with HER-3 or HER-4 receptors, the other two members of the EGFR family *(91,92)*.

HER-2 is normally expressed at low levels in a variety of human secretory epithelial tissues *(93)*. Amplification of HER-2 has been implicated as an important event in the genesis of human breast cancer. Transgenic mice bearing either an activated form of HER-2 or the wild-type proto-oncogene, under the transcriptional control of the mouse mammary tumor virus (MMTV) promotor-enhancer, frequently develop mammary carcinomas *(94,95)*. Induction of mammary tumors in transgenic mice expressing HER-2 is associated with activation of the receptor's intrinsic tyrosine kinase *(96)*.

Approximately 30% of human breast cancers have amplification of HER-2 *(11)*, often in conjunction with mutation in p53. Bitransgenic mice carrying MMTV-*neu* and mutant p53 (172Arg to His) genes reduced tumor latency from 234 d in MMTV-*neu* transgenic mice to 154 d in the bitransgenic mice, indicating strong cooperativity of HER-2 with p53 mutation *(97)*.

Slamon et al. have published extensive studies examining HER-2 mRNA and protein levels in primary human breast tumor specimens, which demonstrate a poorer clinical outcome for breast cancers from node-positive patients, and for ovarian cancers, when HER-2 is expressed at high levels (>5-fold increase) *(11)*. A review of results from many publications has been provided by Gullick, who concludes that the larger studies demonstrate a significant association between elevated levels of EGFR and/or HER-2, and poor clinical prognosis of breast cancer *(98)*.

3.2. Anti-HER-2 MAbs and Growth Inhibition by Anti-HER-2 MAbs

MAb 7.16.4 IgG2a, directed against murine HER-2, exerts a cytostatic effect on the growth of HER-2-transformed NIH3T3 fibroblasts *(99)*, and inhibits anchorage-independent growth of the ethylnitrosourea-induced rat neuroblastoma cell line *(100)*, from which HER-2 was originally isolated and characterized. This antibody can revert HER-2-transformed cells to the nontransformed phenotype, determined by capacity for anchorage-independent growth in soft agar *(99)*. In combination with an anti-EGFR MAb 425, MAb 7.16.4 can also reverse the phenotype of cells transformed by co-expression of EGFR and HER-2 *(101)*.

Several groups have produced MAbs against human HER-2, and demonstrated that the proliferation of human cancer cell lines that overexpress HER-2 can be inhibited by these MAbs *(102–106)*. Among them, MAb 4D5 has been most thoroughly studied for its potential to inhibit tumor-cell proliferation *(107)*, especially in breast and ovarian cancer *(108)*, and has been humanized for clinical trial *(109)*.

There was a correlation between the levels of HER-2 expression and sensitivity to the growth inhibitory effect of anti-HER-2 MAbs against a panel of human breast cancer cell lines. Cell lines with minimal expression of HER-2 (MCF-7, MDA-MB-231, ZR-75-1, MDA-MB-436, and so on) were not inhibited in the presence of anti-HER-2 MAbs in culture. Cell lines with higher levels of HER-2 expression (MDA-MB-175, MDA-MB-453, MDA-MB-361, and so on) were increasingly more sensitive to antibody-mediated growth inhibition. SKBR-3 and BT-474 are two breast cancer cell lines expressing very high levels of HER-2, and they were the most sensitive to anti-HER-2 antibody-mediated growth inhibition. However, experimental elevation of functional HER-2 expression to high levels in human breast cancer cell line MCF-7 did not result in growth inhibition by MAb 4D5, compared with the corresponding control-vector transfected MCF-7 cells *(110)*. In addition, different tissues may display differential responses to anti-HER-2 MAb. MAb 4D5 inhibited the growth of several cell lines derived from breast, ovarian, and lung cancers, but did not inhibit the growth of cell lines from colon or gastric adenocarcinomas with increased expression of this receptor *(111)*.

Similar to the inhibitory effects of anti-EGFR MAbs on most cell lines studied, the effects of anti-HER-2 MAbs are merely cytostatic on the proliferation of HER-2-overexpressing cell lines. MAbs reactive with distinct domains of the HER-2 may exert synergistic antitumor effects in vivo *(112)*. In order to enhance the antitumor activity of anti-HER-2 MAb, several groups have reported the combination of conventional chemotherapy with anti-HER-2 MAb. In an early study, Hancock et al. reported that anti-HER-2 MAb Tab250 markedly enhanced the antitumor effects of cisplatinum, both in culture and on human SKOV-3 ovarian tumor xenografts *(113)*. Using the same antibody, Arteaga et al. have shown enhanced etoposide or cisplatinum-induced cytotoxicity against human breast carcinoma cells, and proposed a possible direct association between HER-2 receptor signal transduction and inhibition of drug-induced DNA repair *(114)*. Studies by Slamon et al. showed that MAb 4D5 potentiates the cytotoxicity of chemotherapeutic drugs, including doxorubicin, carboplatinum, and cisplatinum, on human breast adenocarcinoma cells *(115,116)*. In the case of cisplatinum, they have further demonstrated that MAb 4D5 promotes sensitivity to chemotherapy by interfering with the repair of cisplatinum-induced DNA damage in breast and ovarian carcinoma cells *(116)*. The authors' laboratory has explored the combination of MAb 4D5 with paclitaxel in BT-474 breast cancer cells, and also observed an additive effect on anchorage-dependent growth of these cells *(117)*.

3.3. Preclinical Studies and Clinical Trials with Anti-HER-2 MAbs

Anti-HER-2 MAbs have been shown to inhibit the proliferation of xenografted human cancer cell lines *(112,117–119)*. In the studies with xenografts of BT-474 human breast cancer cells, the authors' laboratory observed that treatment with intraperitoneal injections of MAb 4D5 (1 mg/kg) eradicated well-established tumors *(117)*. This laboratory has also demonstrated that treatment of BT-474 breast cancer cell xenografts with lower doses of MAb 4D5 (0.3 mg/kg), in combination with paclitaxel or doxorubicin, produced striking antitumor effects, resulting in the suppression or cure of well-established xenografts *(117)*.

Clinical phase-I study with humanized MAb 4D5 (known as Herceptin™) showed no toxicities after weekly administration of Herceptin™, for periods of more than 1 yr. Two clinical phase-II studies in patients with refractory breast cancer overexpressing of HER-2 have been reported. Treatment of breast cancer patients with weekly injections of Herceptin™ alone induced objective partial responses in 10% of patients, as well as one complete response *(120)*. The importance of this observation is that it provides evidence that antireceptor MAb therapy can produce remission in human cancer. Another phase-II trial utilized Herceptin™, in combination with cisplatinum chemotherapy, for advanced breast cancer. The combination of Herceptin™ and cisplatinum resulted in a 25% partial response rate, which was higher than that expected with cisplatinum alone *(121)*. Results of a recent phase-III study on 469 breast cancer patients who had tumors that overexpressed HER-2 were recently presented at the annual meeting of the American Association of Clinical Oncology in May, 1998 *(122)*. Patients were treated with Herceptin™ in combination with paclitaxel or with Herceptin™ in combination with anthracycline plus cyclophosphamide *(123)*. Adding Herceptin™ to chemotherapy increased the number of breast cancer patients who had a complete or partial response from 32% (74 out of 234 patients) to 49% (114 out of 235), a 53% increase. The median time to disease progression was increased by 65% (from 4.6 to 7.6 mo) for patients treated with chemotherapy and Herceptin™. In addition, approximately 28% of breast cancer patients treated with Herceptin™ plus chemotherapy did not show evidence of tumor progression at 1 yr, compared to 14% of the patients treated with chemotherapy alone. Cardiac toxicity was significantly increased in the group receiving Herceptin™ plus anthracycline. A second clinical trial evaluated the overall response rate and safety as primary endpoints when using Herceptin™ as a single agent (without chemotherapy) *(124)*. The study included 222 patients. The independent Response Evaluation Committee (REC)-determined overall response rate was 16% (34 out of 213 patients), with 8 patients (4%) experiencing a complete response and 26 patients experiencing a partial response. The median duration of response was 9 mo *(123)*.

Based on these positive results, Herceptin™ was approved by U.S. Food and Drug Administration (FDA) for use in patients with metastatic breast cancer who have tumors that overexpress HER2 *(125)*. A panel of FDA advisors voted unanimously on September 1998 that Herceptin™ offered benefit to breast cancer patients who had failed conventional chemotherapy, and it could be used as first-line therapy together with paclitaxel. However, they recommended that Herceptin™ should not be used with anthracyclines as the increased risk of cardiac dysfunction outweighed the benefits *(126)*.

4. CONCLUDING REMARKS

In summary, there are ample and sound experimental data supporting the hypothesis that the EGFR and HER-2 are suitable targets for the therapy of human breast cancer. Laboratory studies with antibodies against the EGFR or HER-2, either alone or in combination with chemotherapy, were promising, and have led to the current ongoing clinical trials with human/murine chimeric anti-EGFR MAb C225 and humanized anti-HER-2 MAb 4D5 (Herceptin™) on human cancers, including breast cancer. These trials will eventually determine the feasibility of this novel approach in the treatment of human cancer.

REFERENCES

1. Barnes, D. and G. Sato. 1980. Serum-free cell culture: a unifying approach. *Cell* **22:** 649–655.
2. Sporn, M. B. and A. B. Roberts. 1985. Autocrine growth factors and cancer. *Nature* **313:** 745–747.
3. Aaronson, S. A. 1991. Growth factors and cancer. *Science* **254:** 1146–1153.
4. Weinberg, R. A. 1989. *Oncogenes and the Molecular Origin of Cancer*, Cold Spring Harbor Laboratories, Cold Spring Harbor, NY.
5. DeVita, V. T., Jr., S. Hellman, and S. A. Rosenberg. 1997. *Cancer: Principal of Oncology,* 5th ed. Lippincott-Raven, Philadelphia, PA.
6. Rosenthal, A., P. B. Lindquist, T. S. Bringman, D. V. Goeddel. and R. Derynck. 1986. Expression in rat fibroblasts of a human transforming growth factor-alpha cDNA results in transformation. *Cell* **46:** 301–309.
7. DiFiore, P. P., J. H. Pierce, T. P. Fleming, R. Hazan, A. Ullrich, C. R. King, J. Schlessinger, and S. A. Aaronson. 1987. Overexpression of the human EGF receptor confers an EGF-dependent transformed phenotype to NIH3T3 cells. *Cell* **51:** 1063–1070.
8. Velu, T. J., L. Beguinot, W. C. Vass, K. Zhang, I. Pastan, and D. R. Lowy. 1987. Epidermal growth factor-dependent transformation by a human EGF receptor proto-oncogene. *Science* **238:** 1408–1410.
9. Sainsbury, J. R. C., A. J. Malcolm, D. R. Appleton, J. R. Farndon, A. L. Harris. 1985. Presence of epidermal growth factor receptor as an indicator of poor prognosis in patients with breast cancer. *J. Clin. Pathol.* **38:** 1225–1228.
10. Harris, A. L., S. Nicholson, J. R. C. Sainsbury, J. R. Farndon, and C. Wright. 1989. Epidermal growth factor receptors in breast cancer: association with early relapse and

death, poor response to hormones and interactions with neu. *J. Steroid Biochem.* **34:** 123–131.

11. Slamon, D. J., G. M. Clark, S. G. Wong, W. J. Levin, A. Ullrich, and W. L. McGuire. 1987. Human breast cancer: correlation of relapse and survival with amplification of the HER-2/neu oncogene. *Science* **235:** 177–182.

12. Wright, C., B. Angus, S. Nicholson, J. R. C. Sainsbury, J. Cairns, W. J. Gullick, et al. 1989. Expression of c-erbB-2 oncoprotein: a prognostic indicator in human breast cancer. *Cancer Res.* **49:** 2087–2090.

13. Levitzki, A. and A. Gazit. 1995. Tyrosine kinase inhibition, an approach to drug development. *Science* **267:** 1782–1788.

14. Holley, R. W. 1975. Control of growth of mammalian cells in cell culture. *Nature* **258:** 487–490.

15. Pardee, A. B., R. Dubrow, J. L. Hamlin, and R. F. Kletzien. 1978. Animal cell cycle. *Annu. Rev. Biochem.* **47:** 715–750.

16. Hartwell, L. and T. Weinert. 1991. Genetic control of mitotic fidelity in yeast and its relations to cancer, in *Origins of Human Cancer* (Brugge, J., T. Curran, E. Harlow, F. McCormick, eds.), Cold Spring Harbor Laboratories, Cold Spring Harbor, NY, pp. 45–49.

17. Van de Woude, G. F., N. Schulz, R. Zhou, R. S. Paules, I. Daar, N. Yew, and M. Oskarsson. 1990. Cell cycle regulation, oncogenes, and antineoplastic drugs, in *Accomplishments in Cancer Research* of the General Motors Cancer Research Foundation (Fortner, J. G. and J. E. Rhoads, eds.), Lippincott, Philadelphia, PA, pp. 128–143.

18. Harris, A. L. 1989. Epidermal growth factor in human breast cancer. *Recent Results Cancer Res.* **113:** 70–77.

19. Carpenter, G. 1987. Receptors for epidermal growth factor and other polypeptide mitogens. *Ann. Rev. Biochem.* **56:** 881–914.

20. Lichtner, R. B. and R. N. Harkins. 1997. Signal transduction by EGF receptor tyrosine kinase, in *EGF Receptor in Tumor Growth and Progression* (Lichtner, R. B. and R. N. Harkins, eds.), Ernst Schering Research Foundation Workshop 19, Springer-Verlag, Heidelberg, 1–17.

21. Osborne, C., B. Hamilton, G. Titus, and R. Livingston. 1980. Epidermal growth factor stimulation of human breast cancer cells in culture. *Cancer Res.* **40:** 2361–2366.

22. Fitzpatrick, S. L., M. P. LaChance, and G. S. Schultz. 1984. Characterization of epidermal growth factor receptor and action on human breast cancer cells in culture. *Cancer Res.* **44:** 3442–3447.

23. Fitzpatrick, S. L., J. B. Brightwell, J. L. Wittliff, G. H. Barrows, and G. S. Schultz. 1984. Epidermal growth factor binding by breast tumor biopsies and relationship to estrogen receptor and progestin receptor levels. *Cancer Res.* **44:** 3448–3453.

24. Perez, R., M. Pascual, A. Macias, and A. Lage. 1984. Epidermal growth factor receptors in human breast cancer. *Breast Cancer Res. Treatment* **4:** 189–193.

25. Sainsbury, J. R. C., G. V. Sherbet, J. R. Farndon, and A. L. Harris. 1985. Epidermal growth factor receptors and oestrogen receptors in human breast cancer. *Lancet* **1:** 364–366.

26. Koenders, P. G., L. K. V. A. M. Beex, A. Geutz-Moespot, J. J. T. M. Heuvel, C. B. M. Kienhuis, and T. J. Benraad. 1991. Epidermal growth factor receptor-negative tumors are predominantly confined to the subgroup of estradiol receptor-positive human primary breast cancers. *Cancer Res.* **51:** 4544–4548.

27. Davidson, N. E., E. P. Gelmann, M. E. Lippman, and R. B. Dickson. 1987. Epidermal growth factor receptor gene expression in estrogen receptor-positive and negative human breast cancer cell lines. *Mol. Endocrinol.* **1:** 216–223.

28. Filmus, J., J. M. Trent, M. N. Pollak, and R. N. Buick. 1987. Epidermal growth factor receptor gene-amplified MDA-MB-468 breast cancer cell line and its nonamplified variant. *Mol. Cell. Biol.* **7:** 251–257.

29. Bates, S. E., N. E. Davidson, E. M. Valverius, C. E. Freter, R. B. Dickson, J. P. Tam, et al. 1988. Expression of transforming growth factor-α and its messenger ribonucleic acid in human breast cancer: its regulation by estrogen and its possible functional significance. *Mol. Endocrinol.* **2:** 543–555.

30. Ciardiello, F., N. Kim, D. S. Liscia, C. Bianco, R. Lidereau, G. Merlo, et al. 1989. mRNA expression of transforming growth factor alpha in human breast carcinomas and its activity in effusions of breast cancer patients. *J. Natl. Cancer Inst.* **81:** 1165–1171.

31. Dickson, R. B., S. E. Bates, M. E. McManaway, and M. E. Lippman. 1986. Characterization of estrogen responsive transforming activity in human breast cancer cell lines. *Cancer Res.* **46:** 1707–1713.

32. Dickson, R. B., K. K. Huff, E. M. Spencer, and M. E. Lippman. 1985. Induction of epidermal growth factor-related polypeptides by 17β-estradiol in MCF-7 human breast cancer cells. *Endrocrinology* **118:** 138–142.

33. Matsui, Y., S. A. Halter, J.T. Holt, B.L. Hogan, R. J. Coffey. 1990. Development of mammary hyperplasia and neoplasia in MMTV-TGF alpha transgenic mice. *Cell* **61:** 1147–1155.

34. Jhappan, C., C. Stahle, R. N. Harkins, N. Fausto, G.H. Smith, G. T. Merlino. 1990. TGF-αlpha overexpression in transgenic mice induces liver neoplasia and abnormal development of the mammary gland and pancreases. *Cell* **61:** 1137–1146.

35. Sandgren, E. P., N.C. Luetteke, R. D. Plamiter, R.L. Brisnster, D.C. Lee. 1990. Overexpression of TGF alpha in transgenic mice: induction of epithelial hyperplasia pancreatic metaplasia, and carcinoma of the breast. *Cell* **61:** 1121–1135.

36. Smith, G.H., R. Sharp, E. C. Kordon, C. Jhappan, G. Merlino. 1995. Transforming growth factor-alpha promotes mammary tumorigenesis through selective survival and growth of secretory epithelial cells. *Am. J. Pathol.* **147:** 1081–1096.

37. Amundadottir, L. T., M.D. Johnson, G. Merlino, G. H. Smith, R.B. Dickson. 1995. Synergistic interaction of transforming growth factor alpha and c-*myc* in mouse mammary and salivary gland tumorigenesis. *Cell Growth Differ.* **6:** 737–748.

38. Sandgren, E. P., J. A. Schroeder, T. H. Qui, R. D. Palmiter, R. L. Brinster, D. C. Lee. 1995. Inhibition of mammary gland involution is associated with transforming growth factor alpha but not c-*myc*-induced tumorigenesis in transgenic mice. *Cancer Res.* **55:** 3915–3927.

39. Nicholson, S., P. Halcrow, J. R. Farndon, J. R. C. Sainsbury, P. Chambers, and A. L. Harris. 1989. Expression of epidermal growth factor receptors associated with lack of response to endocrine therapy in recurrent breast cancer. *Lancet* **1:** 182–185.

40. Sato, J. D., T. Kawamoto, A. D. Le, J. Mendelsohn, J. Polikoff, and G. H. Sato. 1983. Biological effect in vitro of monoclonal antibodies to human EGF receptors. *Mol. Biol. Med.* **1:** 511–529.

41. Kawamoto, T., J. D. Sato, A. D. Le, J. Polikoff, G. H. Sato, and J. Mendelsohn. 1983. Growth stimulation of A431 calls by EGF: identification of high affinity receptors for epidermal growth factor by an anti-receptor monoclonal antibody. *Proc. Natl. Acad. Sci. USA* **80:** 1337–1341.

42. Gill, G. N., T. Kawamoto, C. Cochet, A. Le, J. D. Sato, H. Masui, C. L. MacLeod, and J. Mendelsohn. 1984. Monoclonal anti-epidermal growth factor receptor antibodies which are inhibitors of epidermal growth factor binding and antagonists of epidermal growth factor-stimulated tyrosine protein kinase activity. *J. Biol. Chem.* **259:** 7755–7760.

43. Mendelsohn, J. 1990. The epidermal growth factor receptor as a target for therapy with antireceptor monoclonal antibodies. *Semin. Cancer Biol.* **1:** 339–344.

44. Fan, Z., J. Mendelsohn, H. Masui, and R. Kumar. 1993. Regulation of epidermal growth factor receptor in NIH3T3/HER14 cells by antireceptor monoclonal antibodies. *J. Biol. Chem.* **268:** 21,073–21,079.

45. Fan, Z., Y. Lu, X. Wu, and J. Mendelsohn. 1994. Antibody-induced epidermal growth factor receptor dimerization mediates inhibition of autocrine proliferation of A431 squamous carcinoma cells. *J. Biol. Chem.* **269:** 27,595–27,602.

46. Sunada, H., B. Magun, J. Mendelsohn, and C. L. MacLeod. 1986. Monoclonal antibody against EGF receptor is internalized without stimulating receptor phosphorylation. *Proc. Natl. Acad. Sci. USA* **83:** 3825–3829.

47. Sunada, H., P. Yu, J. S. Peacock, and J. Mendelsohn. 1990. Modulation of tyrosine serine and threonine phosphorylation and intracellular processing of the epidermal growth factor receptor by anti-receptor monoclonal antibody. *J. Cell. Physiol.* **142:** 284–292.

48. Mendelsohn, J., J. Baselga, X. Wu, D. Peng, C. Brown, J. L. Chou, H. Masui, and Z. Fan. 1997. EGF receptor inhibition by antibody as anticancer therapy, in *EGF Receptor in Tumor Growth and Progression* (Lichtner, R. B. and R. N. Harkins, eds.), Ernst Schering Research Foundation Workshop 19, Springer-Verlag, Heidelberg, pp. 234–251.

49. Fan, Z., H. Masui, I. Atlas, and J. Mendelsohn. 1993. Blockade of epidermal growth factor receptor function by bivalent and monovalent fragments of 225 anti-epidermal growth factor receptor monoclonal antibodies. *Cancer Res.* **53:** 4322–4328.

50. Aboud-Pirak, E., E. Hurwitz, M. E. Pirak, F. Bellot, J. Schlessinger, and M. Sela. 1988. Efficacy of antibodies to epidermal growth factor receptor against KB carcinoma in vitro and in nude mice. *J. Natl. Cancer Inst.* **21:** 1605–1611.

51. Rodeck, U., M. Herlyn, D. Herlyn, C. Molthoff, B. Atkinson, M. Varello, Z. Steplewski, and H. Koprowski. 1987. Tumor growth modulation by a monoclonal antibody to the epidermal growth factor receptor: immunologically mediated and effector cell-independent effects. *Cancer Res.* **47:** 3692–3696.

52. Waterfield, M. D., E. L. V. Mayes, P. Stroobant, P. L. P. Bennett, S. Young, P. N. Goodfellow, G. S. Banting, and B. Ozanne. 1982. A monoclonal antibody to the human epidermal growth factor receptor. *J. Cell. Biochem.* **20:** 149–161.

53. Modjtahedi, H., J. Styles, and C. Dean. 1993. The human EGF receptor as a target for cancer therapy: six new rat mAbs against the receptor on the breast carcinoma MDA-MB-468. *Br. J. Cancer* **67:** 247–253.

54. Modjtahedi, H., S. Eccles, G. Box, J. Styles, and C. Dean. 1993. Immunotherapy of human tumour xenografts over-expressing the EGF receptor with rat antibodies that block growth factor-receptor interaction. *Br. J. Cancer* **67:** 254–261.

55. Chou, J.-L., Z. Fan, A. Koff, and J. Mendelsohn. 1996. EGF receptor blockage induces reversible growth arrest and changes in proteins that regulate the cell cycle in human mammary epithelial cells. *Proc. Am. Assoc. Cancer Res.* **37:** 10 (Abstract #68).

56. Fan, Z., B.Y. Shang, Y. Lu, J.-L. Chou, and J. Mendelsohn. 1997. Reciprocal changes in p27[Kip1] and p21[Cip1] in growth inhibition mediated by blockade or overstimulation of epidermal growth factor receptors. *Clin. Cancer Res.* **3:** 1943–1948.

57. Wu, X., M. Rubin, Z. Fan, T. DeBlasio, T. Soos, A. Koff, and J. Mendelsohn. 1996. Involvement of p27[Kip1] in G1 arrest mediated by an anti-epidermal growth factor receptor monoclonal antibody. *Oncogene* **12:** 1397–1403.

58. Peng, D., Z. Fan, Y. Lu, T. DeBlasio, H. Scher, and J. Mendelsohn. 1996. Anti-epidermal growth factor receptor monoclonal antibody 225 upregulates p27[Kip1] and induces G1 arrest in prostatic cancer cell line DU145. *Cancer Res.* **56:** 3666–3669.

59. Stampfer, M. R., C. H. Pan, J. Hosoda, J. Bartholomew, J. Mendelsohn, and P. Yaswen. 1993. Blockage of EGF receptor signal transduction causes reversible arrest of normal and immortal human mammary epithelial cells with synchronous re-entry into the cell cycle. *Exp. Cell Res.* **208:** 175–188.

60. Wu, X., Z. Fan, H. Masui, N. Rosen, and J. Mendelsohn. 1995. Apoptosis induced by an anti-EGF receptor monoclonal antibody in a human colorectal carcinoma cell line and its delay by insulin. *J. Clin. Invest.* **95:** 1897–1905.

61. Weinberg, R. A. 1995. The Retinoblastoma protein and cell cycle control. *Cell* **81:** 323–330.
62. Morgan, D. O. 1995. Principles of CDK regulation. *Nature* **374:** 131–134.
63. Soule, H. D., T. M. Malony, S. R. Wolman, W. D. Peterson, Jr., R. Brenz, C. M. McGrath, et al. 1990. Isolation and characterization of a spontaneously immortalized human breast epithelial cell line, MCF-10. *Cancer Res.* **50:** 6075–6086.
64. Ciardiello, F., M. McGeady, L., N. Kim, F. Basolo, N. Hynes, B. C. Langton, et al. 1990. TGF-α expression in enhanced human mammary epithelial cells transformed by an activated c-Ha-ras protooncogene but not by the c-neu protooncogene and overexpression of the TGF-α cDNA leads to transformation. *Cell Growth Differ.* **1:** 407–420.
65. Ennis, B. W., E. M. Valverius, M. E. Lippman, F. Bellot, R. Kris, J. Schlessinger, et al. 1989. Monoclonal anti-EGF receptor antibodies inhibit the growth of malignant and non-malignant human mammary epithelial cells. *Mol. Endocrinol.* **3:** 1830–1838.
66. Arteaga, C. L., E. Coronado, and C. K. Osborne. 1988. Blockade of the epidermal growth factor receptor inhibits transforming growth factor a-induced but not estrogen-induced growth of hormone-dependent human breast cancer. *Mol. Endocrinol.* **2:** 1064–1069.
67. Bates, S. E., E. M. Valverius, B. W. Ennis, D. A. Bronzert, J. P. Sheridan, M. R. Stampfer, et al. 1990. Expression of the TGF-α/EGF receptor pathway in normal human breast epithelial cells. *Endocrinology* **126:** 596–607.
68. Filmus, J., M. N. Pollak, R. Cailleau, and R. N. Buick. 1985. MDA-MB-468, a human breast cancer cell line with a high number of epidermal growth factor (EGF) receptors, has an amplified EGF receptor gene and is growth inhibited by EGF. *Biochem. Biophys. Res. Commun.* **128:** 898–905.
69. Prasad, K. A. N. and J. G. Church. 1991. EGF-dependent growth inhibition in MDA-MB-468 cells human breast cancer cells is characterized by late G1 arrest and altered gene expression. *Exp. Cell Res.* **195:** 20–26.
70. Mendelsohn, J. 1989. Potential clinical applications of anti-EGF receptor monoclonal antibodies, in *The Molecular Diagnostics of Human Cancer: Cancer Cells*, vol. 7 (Furth, M. and M. Greaves, eds.), Cold Spring Harbor Laboratory, Cold Spring Harbor, NY, pp. 359–362.
71. Fan, Z., J. Baselga, H. Masui, and J. Mendelsohn. 1993. Antitumor effect of anti-epidermal growth factor receptor monoclonal antibodies plus cis-diamminedichloroplatinum on well established A431 cell xenografts. *Cancer Res.* **53:** 4637–4642.
72. Baselga, J., L. Norton, H. Masui, A. Pandiella, K. Coplan, W. H. Miller, and J. Mendelsohn. 1993. Anti-tumor effects of doxorubicin in combination with anti-epidermal growth factor receptor monoclonal antibodies. *J. Natl. Cancer Inst.* **85:** 1327–1333.
73. Rowan, S. and D. E. Fisher. 1997. Mechanism of apoptotic cell death. *Leukemia* **11:** 457–465.
74. Vaux, D. L. and A. Strasser. 1996. The molecular biology of apoptosis. *Proc. Natl. Acad. Sci. USA* **93:** 2239–2244.
75. Lowe, S. W. 1995. Cancer therapy and p53. *Curr. Opin. Oncol.* **7:** 547–553.
76. Mendelsohn, J. and Z. Fan. 1997. Epidermal growth factor receptor family and chemosensitization. *J. Natl. Cancer Inst.* **89:** 341–343(Editorial).
77. Evan, G. I., A. H. Wyllie, C. S. Gilbert, T. D. Littlewood, H. Land, M. Brooks, C. M. Waters, L. Z. Penn, and D. C. Hancock. 1992. Induction of apoptosis in fibroblasts by c-*myc* protein. *Cell* **69:** 119–128.
78. Baselga, J., L. Norton, K. Coplan, R. Shalaby, and J. Mendelsohn. 1994. Antitumor activity of paclitaxel in combination with anti-growth factor receptor monoclonal antibodies in breast cancer xenografts. *Proc. Am. Assoc. Cancer Res.* **35:** 380(Abstract).
79. Prewett, M., P. Rockwell, R. F. Rockwell, N. A. Giorgio, J. Mendelsohn, H. I. Scher, and N. I. Goldstein. 1996. The biological effects of C225, a chimeric monoclonal antibody to

the EGFR, on human prostate carcinoma. *J. Immunother. Emphasis Tumor Immunol.* **19:** 416–427.

80. Divgi, C. R., C. Welt, M. Kris, F. X. Real, S. D. J. Yeh, R. Gralla, et al. 1991. Phase I and imaging trial of indium-111 labeled anti-EGF receptor monoclonal antibody 225 in patients with squamous cell lung carcinoma. *J. Natl. Cancer Inst.* **83:** 97–104.
81. Brady, L. W., D. V. Woo, A. Marko, S. Dadparvar, U. Karlsson, M. Rackover, et al. 1990. Treatment of malignant gliomas with 125I-labeled monoclonal antibody against epidermal growth factor receptor. *Antibody Immunoconjugate Radiopharm.* **3:** 169–179.
82. Perez-Soler, R., N. J. Donato, D. M. Shin, M.G. Rosenblum, H.-Z. Zhang, C. Tornos, et al. 1994. Tumor epidermal growth factor receptor studies in patients with non-small-cell lung cancer or head and neck cancer treated with monoclonal antibody RG83852. *J. Clin. Oncol.* **12:** 730–739.
83. Kalofonos, H. P., T. R. Pawlikowska, A. Hemingway, N. Courtenay-Luck, B. Dhokia, D. Snook, et al. 1989. Antibody guided diagnosis and therapy of brain gliomas using radio-labeled monoclonal antibodies against epidermal growth factor receptor and placental alkaline phosphatase. *J. Nucl. Med.* **30:** 1636–1645.
84. Goldstein, N. I., M. Prewett, K. Zuklys, P. Rockwell, and J. Mendelsohn. 1995. Biological efficacy of a chimeric antibody to the epidermal growth factor receptor in a human tumor xenograft model. *Clin. Cancer Res.* **1:** 1311–1318.
85. Bos, M., J. Mendelsohn, C. Bowden, D. Pfister, M. R. Cooper, R. Cohen, et al. 1996. Phase I studies of anti-epidermal growth factor receptor chimeric monoclonal antibody C225 in patients with EGFR overexpressing tumors. *Proc. Am. Soc. Clin. Oncol.* **15:** 443(Abstract).
86. Coussens, L., T. L. Yang-Feng, Y. C. Liao, E. Chen, A. Gary, J. McGrath, et al. 1985. Tyrosine kinase receptor with extensive homology to EGF receptor shares chromosomal location with *neu* oncogene. *Science* **230:** 1132–1139.
87. Akiyama, T., C. Sudo, H. Ogawara, K. Toyoshima, and T. Yamamoto. 1986. The product of the human c-erbB2 gene: a 185,000 dalton glycoprotein with tyrosine kinase activity. *Science* **232:** 2644–1646.
88. Stern, D. F., P. A. Hefferman, and R. A. Weinberg. 1986. p185, a product of the *neu* proto-oncogene, is a receptor-like protein associated with tyrosine kinase activity. *Mol. Cell. Biol.* **6:** 1729–1740.
89. Schechter, A. L., M.-C. Hung, L. Vaidyanathan, R. A. Weinberg, T. L. Yang-Feng, U. Francke, A. Ullrich, and L. Coussens. 1985. The *neu* gene: an erb-B-homologous gene distinct from and unlinked to the gene encoding the EGF receptor. *Science* **229:** 976–978.
90. Lupu, R., R. Colomer, G. Zugmaier, J. Sarup, M. Shepard, D. Slamon, and M. E. Lippman. 1990. Direct interaction of a ligand for the erbB2 oncogene product with the EGF receptor and p185erbB2. *Science* **249:** 1552–1555.
91. Lewis, G. D., J. A. Lofgren, A. E. McMurtrey, A. Nuijens, B. M. Fendly, K. D. Bauer, and M. X. Sliwkowski. 1995. Growth regulation of human breast and ovarian tumor cells by heregulin: evidence for the requirement of ErbB2 as a critical component in mediating heregulin responsiveness. *Cancer Res.* **56:** 1457–1465.
92. Earp, H. S., T. L. Dawson, X. Li, and H. Yu. 1995. Heterodimerization and functional interaction between EGF receptor family members: a new signaling paradigm with implications for breast cancer research. *Breast Cancer Res. Treatment* **35:** 115–132.
93. Press, M. F., C. Cordon-Cardo, and D. J. Slamon. 1990. Expression of the HER-2/neu proto-oncogene in normal human adult and fetal tissues. *Oncogene* **5:** 953–962.
94. Muller, W. J., E. Sinn, P. K. Pattengale, R. Wallace, and P. Leder. 1988. Single-step induction of mammary adenocarcinoma in transgenic mice bearing the activated c-neu oncogene. *Cell* **54:** 105–115.

95. Bouchard, L., L. Lamarre, P. J. Tremblay, and P. Jolicoeur. 1989. Stochastic appearance of mammary tumors in transgenic mice carrying the MMTV/c-neu oncogene. *Cell* **57:** 931–936.

96. Guy, C. T., M. A. Webster, M. Schaller, T. J. Parsons, R. D. Cardiff, and W. J. Muller. 1992. Expression of the *neu* protooncogene in the mammary epithelium of transgenic mice induces metastatic disease. *Proc. Natl. Acad. Sci. USA* **89:** 10,578–10,582.

97. Li, B., J. M. Rosen, J. McMenamin-Balano, W. J. Muller, and A. S. Perkins. 1997. Neu/ERBB2 cooperates with p53-172H during mammary tumorigenesis in trangenic mice. *Mol. Cell. Biol.* **17:** 3155–3163.

98. Gullick, W. J. 1990. The role of the epidermal growth factor receptor and the c-erbB-2 protein in breast cancer. *Int. J. Cancer* **5(Suppl.):** 55–61.

99. Drebin, J. A., V. C. Link, D. F. Stern, R. A. Weinberg, and M. I. Greene. 1985. Down-regulation of an oncogene protein product and reversion of the transformed phenotype by monoclonal antibodies. *Cell* **41:** 695–706.

100. Drebin, J. A., V. C. Link, R. A. Weinberg, and M. I. Greene. 1986. Inhibition of tumor growth by a monoclonal antibody reactive with an oncogene-encoded tumor antigen. *Proc. Natl. Acad. Sci. USA* **83:** 9129–9133.

101. Wada, T., J. N. Meyers, Y. Kokai, V. I. Brown, J. Hamuro, C. M. LeVea and M. I. Greene. 1990. Anti-receptor antibodies reverse the phenotype of cells transformed by two inter-acting proto-oncogene encoded receptor proteins. *Oncogene* **5:** 489–495.

102. Dougall, W. C. and M. I. Greene. 1994. Biological studies and potential therapeutic applications of monoclonal antibodies and small molecules reactive with the neu/c-erbB-2 protein. *Cell Biophys.* **24/25:** 209–218.

103. Stancovski, I., E. Hurwitz, O. Leitner, A. Ullrich, Y. Yarden, and M. Sela. 1991. Mechanistic aspects of the opposing effects of monoclonal antibodies to the ERBB2 receptor on tumor growth. *Proc. Natl. Acad. Sci. USA* **88:** 8691–8695.

104. Hurwitz, E., I. Stancovski, M. Sela, and Y. Yarden. 1995. Suppression and promotion of tumor growth by monoclonal antibodies to ErbB-2 differentially correlate with cellular uptake. *Proc. Natl. Acad. Sci. USA* **92:** 3353–3357.

105. McKenzie, S. J., P. J. Marks, T. Lam, J. Morgan, D. L. Panicali, K. L. Trimpe, and W. P. Carney. 1989. Generation and characterization of monoclonal antibodies specific for the human *neu* oncogene product, p185. *Oncogene* **4:** 543–548.

106. Kasprzyk, P. G., S. U. Song, P. P. DiFiore, and C. R. King. 1992. Therapy of an animal model of human gastric cancer using a combination of anti-erbB-2 monoclonal antibodies. *Cancer Res.* **52:** 2771–2776.

107. Fendly, B. M., M. Winget, R. M. Hudziak, M. T. Lipari, M. A. Napier, and A. Ullrich. 1990. Characterization of murine monoclonal antibodies reactive to either the human epidermal growth factor receptor or HER-2/neu gene product. *Cancer Res.* **50:** 1550–1558.

108. Slamon, D. J., W. Godolphin, L. A. Jones, J. A. Hólt, S. G. Wong, D. E. Keth, et al. 1989. Studies of the HER-2/neu proto-oncogene in human breast and ovarian cancer. *Science* **244:** 707–712.

109. Carter, P., L. Presta, C. M. Gorman, J. B. Rideway, D. Henner, W. L. Wong, et al. 1992. Humanization of an anti-p185HER2 antibody for human cancer therapy. *Proc. Natl. Acad. Sci. USA* **89:** 4285–4289.

110. Benz, C. C., G. K. Scott, J. C. Sarup, R. M. Johnson, D. Tripathy, E. Coronado, H. M. Shepard, and C. K. Osborne. 1993. Estrogen-dependent, tamoxifen-resistant tumorigenic growth of MCF-7 cells transfected with HER2/neu. *Breast Cancer Res. Treatment* **24:** 85–95.

111. Lewis, G. D., I. Figari, B. Fendly, W. L. Wong, P. Carter, C. Gorman, and H. M. Shepard. 1993. Differential response of human tumor cell lines to anti-p185HER2 monoclonal antibodies. *Cancer Immunol. Immunother.* **37:** 255–263.

112. Drebin, J. A., V. C. Link, and M. I. Greene. 1988. Monoclonal antibodies reactive with distinct domains of the *neu* oncogene-encoded p185 molecule exert synergistic anti-tumor effects in vivo. *Oncogene* **2**: 273–277.

113. Hancock, M. C., B. C. Langton, T. Chan, P. Toy, J. J. Monahan, R. P. Mischak, and L. K. Shawver. 1991. A monoclonal antibody against the c-erbB-2 protein enhances the cytotoxicity of cis-diamminedichloroplatinum against human breast and ovarian tumor cell lines. *Cancer Res.* **51**: 4575–4580.

114. Arteaga, C. L., A. R. Winnier, M. C. Poirier, D. M. Lopez-Larraza, L. K. Shawver, S. D. Hurd, and S. J. Stewart. 1994. p185 c-erbB-2 signaling enhances cisplatin-induced cytotoxicity in human breast carcinoma cells: association between an oncogenic receptor tyrosine kinase and drug-induced DNA repair. *Cancer Res.* **54**: 3758–3765.

115. Pegram, M. D., R. J. Pietras, and D. J. Slamon. 1992. Monoclonal antibody to HER-2/neu gene product potentiates cytotoxicity of carboplatin and doxorubicin in human breast tumor cells. *Proc. Am. Assoc. Cancer Res.* **33**: 442(Abstract).

116. Pietras, R. J., B. M. Fendly, V. R. Chazin, M. D. Pegram, S. B. Howell and D. J. Slamon. 1994. Antibody to HER-2/neu receptor blocks DNA repair after cisplatin in human breast and ovarian cancer cells. *Oncogene* **9**:1829–1838.

117. Baselga, J., L. Norton, R. Shalaby, and J. Mendelsohn. 1994. Anti-HER-2 humanized monoclonal antibody (mAb) alone and in combination with chemotherapy against human breast carcinoma xenografts. *Proc. Am. Assoc. Clin. Oncol.* **13**: 63(Abstract).

118. Tokuda, Y., Y. Ohnishi, K. Shimamura, M. Iwasawa, M. Yoshimura, Y. Ueyama, et al. 1996. In vitro and in vivo anti-tumor effects of a humanized monoclonal antibody against c-erbB-2 product. *Br. J. Cancer* **73**: 1362–1365.

119. Ohnishi, Y., H. Nakamura, M. Yoshimura, Y. Tokuda, M. Iwasawa, Y. Ueyama, N. Tamaoki, and K. Shimamura. 1995. Prolonged survival of mice with human gastric cancer treated with an anti-c-erbB-2 monoclonal antibody. *Br. J. Cancer* **71**: 969–973.

120. Baselga, J., D. Tripathy, J. Mendelsohn, S. Baughman, C. C. Benz, L. Dantis, et al. 1996. Phase II study of weekly intravenous recombinant humanized anti-p185HER2 monoclonal antibody in patients with HER2/neu-overexpressing metastatic breast cancer. *J. Clin. Oncol.* **14**: 737–744.

121. Pegram, M, A. Lipton, R. Pietras, D. Hayes, B. Weber, J. Baselga, et al. 1995. Phase II study of intravenous recombinant humanized anti-p185 HER-2 monoclonal antibody (rhuMAb HER-2) plus cisplatinum in patients with HER-2/neu overexpressing metastatic breast cancer. *Proc. Am. Soc. Clin. Oncol.* **14**: 106(Abstract).

122. Slamon, D., B. Leyland-Jones, S. Shak, V. Paton, A. Bajamonde, T. Fleming, W. Eiermann, J. Wolter, J. Baselga, and L. Norton. 1988. Addition of Herceptin™ (humanized anti-HER2 antibody) to first line chemotherapy for HER2 overexpressing metastatic breast cancer (HER2+/MBC) markedly increases anticancer activity: a randomized multinational controlled phase III trial. *Proc. Am. Soc. Clin. Oncol.* **17**: 98a.

123. Source from Genentech, Inc. http://www.gene.com/pressrelease/1998/05_18_98_herceptin.html.

124. Cobleigh, M. A., C. L. Vogel, D. Tripathy, N. J. Roberts, S. Scholl, S. L. Fehren-bacher, V. Paton, S. Shak, G. Lieberman, and D. Slamon. 1998. Efficacy and safety of Herceptin™ (humanized anti-HER2 antibody) as a single agent in 222 women with HER2 overexpressing who relapsed following chemotherapy for metastatic breast cancer. *Proc. Am. Soc. Clin. Oncol.* **17**: 97a.

125. Source from Genentech, Inc. http://www.gene.com/pressrelease/1998/09_25_98.html.

126. Source from Genentech, Inc. http://www.gene.com/pressrelease/1998/09_02_98.html.

20

Towards the Therapeutic Targeting
of Matrix Metalloproteinases in Breast Cancer

Erik W. Thompson and George W. Sledge, Jr.

1. OVERVIEW

Matrix metalloproteinases are involved in extracellular matrix remodeling around breast carcinomas, and may also be employed by endothelial cells for angiogenesis and invading carcinoma cells for metastasis. The relative contributions of different MMPs to breast cancer progression is summarized, and the findings with matrix metallo-proteinase inhibitors in vitro and in vivo is discussed. Recent experiences from clinical trials of MMP inhibitors are described, and the limitations of the testing model, as well as problems in interpretation are highlighted.

2. WHY MMPS

Breast cancer is the leading cause of cancer in women in the United States, and the second leading cause of cancer deaths. In virtually all cases, death results from invasion and metastasis. Invasion and metastasis are now thought to occur as the result of complex, multistep processes, which have been studied extensively in recent years. Because cancers are capable of dissolving basement membranes surrounding breast ducts, dissolving the surrounding stroma, dissolving the basement membrane surrounding blood vessels (in both intravasation and extravasation), and inducing neovascularization, evidence has pointed to dysregulation of normal tissue remodeling as playing a central role for both invasion and metastasis *(1–3)*. Matrix metalloproteinases (MMPs) represent a major class of effector molecules for such remodeling of extracellular matrix *(4,5)*, and thus represent a potential therapeutic target for limiting the growth and spread of breast carcinoma. The MMPs are evolutionarily highly conserved proteins, being found not only in mammals but also, for instance, as the hemorrhagic component of rattlesnake venom *(6)*. In humans, the MMP family comprises a growing number (currently 16) of independent gene products with significant domain homologies *(4,5)*. It is interesting to note that many of the MMP's discovered in the last 5 years were discovered or codiscovered in breast cancer : MMP-11 *(7)*, MMP-13 *(8)*, MMP-14 *(9)*, MMP-17 *(10)* and MMP-19 *(11)*. Many of the MMP's have been localized in breast cancer, particularly MMP-2 (gelatinase A), collagenase 3 or MMP-13, stromelysin-3, and MMP-9, where they are predominantly produced by the

From: Breast Cancer: *Molecular Genetics, Pathogenesis, and Therapeutics*
Edited by: *A. M. Bowcock* © *Humana Press Inc., Totowa, NJ*

host stroma cells, as recently reviewed *(12–14)*, (*see* also Chapter 14). In this article, we will summarize recent developments in the use of specific MMP inhibitors in a variety of cancer model systems, and in particular focus on our own studies with human breast carcinoma cell lines.

3. MMP PRODUCTION/UTILIZATION BY HBC CELL LINES

Although the bulk of evidence suggests that MMP production occurs primarily in the stromal cells surrounding the tumor *(12–14)*, analysis of breast cancer cell lines has revealed the expression of certain MMP's by those cell lines which have adopted or retained an invasive, metastatic phenotype in nude mice (reviewed in ref. *15*). The elaboration of otherwise stromally expressed enzymes is consistent with a number of other mesenchymal-like traits in these cells, including a stellate morphology in culture, lack of E-cadherin expression, vimentin rather than keratin expression, and the expression of the c-ets-1 transcription factor *(16–19)*. This phenotype, typified by vimentin expression, is thought to arise by a process resembling the epithelial to mesenchymal transition (EMT) which epithelial cells undergo prior to embryologic migration (reviewed in refs. *13* and *20*). Vimentin expression has been studied in breast carcinoma, where it associates with high growth fraction, poor nuclear grade and lack of estrogen receptor and in some studies with poor survival (reviewed in ref. *21*). Although some of these invasive cell lines express MMP-9 or MMP-2, all are capable of elaborating a cell surface mechanism for activation of MMP-2 *(22–24)*. Such activation, at least in vitro, is not automatic, and requires that the cells be cultured on a fibrillar collagen gel substratum or stimulated with the lectin Concanavalin A *(22–27)*. Accumulated data in our laboratory have implicated the first of the membrane type MMP's, MT-MMP1, in this process, and MT1-MMP is also abundantly expressed in breast tumors *(9,12,13,28)*. Thus, although stromal MMP production may support the growth and invasion of breast cancers through local spacial expansion and facilitation of angiogenesis, invasive breast cancer cells may also directly employ their own membrane-associated MMP's for tissue invasion.

4. NATURAL MMP INHIBITORS

Because MMPs appear to be important in invasion and metastasis, efforts to inhibit their activity represent a promising therapeutic approach. Under physiologic conditions enzymatic degradation by activated MMPs is balanced by tissue inhibitors of metalloproteinases (TIMPs) *(29,30)*. Four TIMPs have been reported to date, TIMP-3 *(31,32)* being ECM-associated in contrast to TIMP-1 and TIMP-2, which are predominantly secreted *(4)*. TIMP-4 was very recently discovered through EST library screening, and found to be specifically down-regulated in the stroma adjacent to breast tumors *(33)*. All TIMP's block the active sites of all active MMP species *(4)*, and gelatinase A/MMP-2, and its 92-kDa counterpart gelatinase B/MMP-9, also interact with the TIMP's while in the latent form (i.e. before activation), forming stable stoichiometric complexes with TIMP-2 *(34,35)* and TIMP-1 *(36)* respectively. TIMP-1 and TIMP-2 are both expressed in human breast cancers *(37–41)* and breast cancer cell lines (Table 1 and ref. *42*). TIMPs are effective inhibitors of both amnion (43,44) and Boyden chamber *(45–47)* assays for basement membrane invasiveness. In experimental model sys-

Table 1
Matrix-Metalloproteinase Family Status of HBC Cell Lines[a]

Cell Line	MCF-7	T47-D	MDA-MB-468	Sk-Br-3	MCF-7-ADR	BT549	MDA-MB-436	MDA-MB-435	MDA-MB-231	Hs578T
ER	+	+	–	–	–	–	–	–	–	–
UVO	+	+	+	–	–	–	–	–	–	–
VIM	–	–	–	–	+	+	+	+	+	+
INV	Low	Low	Low	Low	High	High	High	High	High	High
MG	Spheroid	Spheroid	Spheroid	Cluster	Stellate	Stellate	Stellate	Stellate	Stellate	Stellate
In vivo	P	P	P	N	P	N	LI	LI	LI	HM
MMP-2	–	+/–	–	–	–	+/–	++++	–	+/–	++++
TIMP-2	++	++++	++	++++	+++++	+++	+++++	+++++	+++++	+++
MMP-9	+++	+/–	–	+++	+++	+++	–	–	–	–
TIMP-1	+++	+++	+++	+	+++	++	+++++	+++++	+++	+++
MMP-2 ACT'N	–	–	nd	–	+	++++	++	++	+++++	++++

[a]Prognostic factor expression, invasiveness in vitro and in nude mice, and MMP family expression. The prognostic factors estrogen receptor (ER), uvomorulin (UVO), and vimentin (VIM) are indicated as either positive (+) or negative (–). Invasiveness in the Boyden chamber assay (INV) is scored as low or high, and matrigel outgrowth morphology is listed as either spherical, clusters of rounded cells (cluster), or invasive, stellate outgrowths (stellate). Nude mouse activity is listed as nontumorigenic (N), primary tumor only (P), peritoneal extension through local invasion (LI), or hematogenous metastasis (HM). Relative levels of secretion of MMP-2, MMP-9, TIMP-1, and TIMP-2 as determined by ELISA analysis (in collaboration with Stanley Zuker) of cell-number standardized, 20-fold concentrated aliquots of conditioned media from the various HBC cell lines. In addition, capacity to activate endogenous or exogenous MMP-2 when cultured on collagen gels (MMP-2 ACT'N) is listed. The values are expressed in terms of relative expression compared to the maximum. + is 0–20%; ++, 20–40%; +++, 40–60%; ++++, 60–80%; +++++, 80–100%.

439

tems, transfection of highly metastatic cell lines with TIMPs results in suppression of metastatic ability, suggesting that it is possible to redress the imbalance seen in cancers *(48–50)*. Although this approach has proven useful in delineating the role of MMP's, it is not currently clinically practical, owing to limitations in gene therapy of human tumors.

Specific increases in proteolytic activity could result from either overexpression of MMP or underexpression of TIMP *(2)*. An increasing number of studies are demonstrating significant correlations between levels of one or another TIMP expression and prognosis in various cancers. This is perhaps because inhibitors are often upregulated in concordance with their respective enzymes, and the elevated levels of TIMP may represent the host tissues efforts to protect itself from the tumor induced MMP's. Notably, TIMP-2 in breast cancer correlated better with disease recurrence than MMP-2 in a recent breast cancer study *(37)*, as also seen with TIMP-1 expression in colorectal tumors *(51)*. A comprehensive analysis of human cell lines and tumor tissues associated a general upregulation of TIMP-1 with metastatic potential *(29)*, although downregulated TIMP-1 mRNA has also been associated with metastatic potential of SP1 murine mammary adenocarcinoma cells *(52)*. We have also seen that TIMP levels tend to be higher in the invasive HBC cell lines, especially when examined at the RNA level (not shown and Table 1). The basis for these unexpected correlations is not clear. They may simply be more easily measured surrogate markers indicating overall upregulation of MMP's, or it is possible that secondary activities of TIMPs may aid the tumor progression. TIMP-2 has been implicated in MMP-2 activation, and it is worth noting that TIMP-2 has direct cell growth effects *(53–57)*.

5. SYNTHETIC MMP INHIBITORS

Numerous MMP inhibitors have been described in recent years; a partial listing of published compounds and their activities are shown in Table 2. A summary of their activities in vitro, in vivo cancer models is shown in Tables 3–5.

Crystallographic studies of MMPs and their inhibitors have revealed several important facts:

1. The active sites of collagenolytic enzymes characterized by the Zn-binding sequence HExGHxxGxxH are virtually superimposable *(58)*. This is true not only for the mammalian metalloproteinases, but also for structurally related snake venom enzymes *(58,59)*.
2. An exceptionally deep primary specificity site provides the primary target for most of the studied MMP inhibitors, and all of the highly specific inhibitors studied to date ligate the active site Zn atom in the apical position *(60–62)*.
3. Side chain differences along the extended binding site of different MMPIs are probably responsible for inhibitors' different specificity's.

Perhaps the best described of the MMP inhibitors is batimastat. Batimastat (BB-94) ([4-*N*-hydroxyamino)-2R-isobutyl-3S-(thienyl-thiomethyl)succinyl]-L-phenylalanine-*N*-methylamide) is the first of a new class of agents specifically developed to inhibit MMP activity. Crystallographic analysis of BB-94 bound to the rattlesnake venom metalloproteinase Ht-d demonstrates its striking ability to penetrate and almost completely occupy the S1' site *(60)*. Batimastat inhibits MMPs in vitro with the follow-

Table 2
Synthetic MMP Inhibitors

Compound	Activity	Reference
Batimastat (BB-94)	3–20 nM	(63)
Marimastat (BB-2516)		
Glaxo RO31-4724	9 nM	(94)
SCH 47890	0.12 μM*	
Rattlesnake venom inhibitor	3.5 μM^	(6)
GM6001		(95)
SC44463		(96)
Tetracyclines	15–350 μM	(107,108)
(minocycline		
doxycycline		
chemically modified		
tetracyclines)		
AG3340	38–270 pM^	(104)
APB-3206	0.7–5 μM	(105)
CT17346	200 nM	(106)

Activity refers to IC 50 except where otherwise stated; *, D_d; ^, K_i.

Table 3
MMP-Targeted Tumor Studies In Vivo

Inhibitor	Results	Reference
TIMP-1	B16F10 cells i/v, rTIMP-1 i/p decreased # but not size of lung mets. No inhibition sc growth	(44)
	4R cells: rTIMP1 i/p decreased # but not size of lung mets	(97)
	Gastric ca/chick embryo: TIMP1 transfection reduces liver metastasis	(48)
	B16-F10 melanoma i/v: TIMP1 transfection reduces # and size of i/v mets, and reduces s/c tumor growth	(50) (109)
TIMP-2	4R cells, local invasion, i/v injection, growth	(49)
SC44463	Melanoma, fibrosarcoma experimental metastasis (i/v)	(96)
be16627b	Colon carcinoma s/c growth	(87)
Cell Tech	Various tumor models	(90)
(CT 1746)	Lewis lung carcinoma	(106)
BB-94	Ovarian ascites, tumor burden, survival	(63)
batimastat	B16-BL6, growth, spread	(64)
	Colon carcinoma, caecal growth and liver spread	(65)
	Colon carcinoma:	
	i/v lung met model: wt. not #	
	i/p hepatic met model: size and #	
	Hemangioma growth	(68)
	MDA-MB–135 recurrence	(69)
	MDA-MB–135 ascites	(70)

Table 4
MMP-Targeted Tumor Studies In Vitro

Inhibitor	Results	Reference
TIMP-1	Purified TIMP-1 inhibits amnion assay	*(100)*
	rTIMP1 inhibits invasion of B16F10 cells in amnion assay	*(44)*
	4R cells: rTIMP1 blocks collagen degradation	*(97)*
	TIMP-1 knockout stimulates invasiveness of ES cells	*(101)*
TIMP-2	4R cells transfection, smooth muscle ECM invasion	*(49)*
	HT-1080 tibrosarcoma cells matrigel invasion	*(47)*
SC44463	Melanoma, fibrosarcoma	*(96)*
anti-MMP's	Amnion invasion assay	*(100)*
	Monoclonals/reconst. BM	*(102)*
	Anti-MMP-2/matrigel	*(103)*
	MMP-autoinhibitor domain	*(103)*

Table 5
MMP and Angiogenesis Studies In Vitro and In Vivo

Inhibitor	Results	Reference
MMP antibodies	Amnion Assay	*(100)*
TIMP-1	Amnion assay	*(100)*
	In vitro matrigel assay	
TIMP-2	In vitro matrigel assay	
GM6001 galardin	Corneal angiogenesis in vivo	*(95)*
BB-94 batimastat	Angiogenesis in vitro and hemangioma growth	*(110)*
	Angiogenesis in vitro	*(67)*

ing IC_{50}'s: interstitial collagenase, 3 nM; stromelysin, 20 nM; Mr 72,000 type IV colla-genase, 4 nM; Mr 92,000 type IV collagenase, 4 nM; and matrilysin, 6 nM *(63)*. Batimastat has been shown to inhibit human ovarian cancer cells growth in an in vivo model, to prevent the metastasis of B16-BL6 murine melanoma cells in an experimen-tal metastasis model system, and to inhibit growth and prevent metastasis of human colon cancer cells in nude mice *(63–66)*. In addition, batimastat inhibits angiogenesis in vitro and in vivo *(67,68)*.

There is little data available regarding batimastat or other inhibitors in breast cancer. Early studies in vitro with SC44463 *(see* Table 2) showed inhibition of the MDA-MB-231 HBC cell line in two different in vitro invasion assays employing Matrigel *(16)*; The Boyden chamber chemoinvasion assay and the Matrigel outgrowth assay. Further-more, one of our laboratories, working with the MDA-MB-435 nude mouse xenograft model of breast cancer metastasis, has demonstrated that readily achievable levels of batimastat decrease the number and volume of lung metastases, as well as local-regional tumor regrowth *(69)*. These data also demonstrate in vitro inhibition of MMPs (by gelatin zymography) without inhibition (in vivo) of MMP mRNA expression, con-sistent with the known mechanism of batimastat. Low et al. *(70)* also showed that batimastat-mediated inhibition does not occur while MDA-MB-435 cells are growing as ascites. Eccles et al., using a rat breast carcinoma metastasis model, have generated data similar to that seen in the MDA-MB-435 xenograft model of metastasis *(71)*, and such exciting synergism was also reported recently against colon cancer orthotopic zenografts *(66)*. Recent data from the nude mouse xenograft model of breast cancer metastasis suggests synergistic anti-metastatic activity of batimastat when combined with the tetracycline analog doxycycline *(72)*.

Tetracyclines, long valued as antimicrobial agents, have multiple effects on eukaryotic cells. These include MMP inhibition *(73,74)*, inhibition of growth *(75–77)*, and inhibition of angiogenesis *(72,76,77)*. It is uncertain to whether these effects are interrelated, though endothelial cell growth inhibition and MMP inhibition are separable in vitro, as are antimicrobial and MMP effects *(73,76)*. Similarly, it is uncertain how these cellular and tissue effects are mediated at a subcellular level. Inhibition of proliferation is thought to be due to inhibition of mitochondrial protein synthesis *(78)*. Other suggested mechanisms include chelation of calcium and zinc (for MMP inhibition) and inhibition of MMP gene expression (for MMP inhibition). Tetracyclines inhibit tumor growth and metastasis in several model systems. Van den Bogert and colleagues demonstrated the effectiveness of tetracyclines as cytotoxic agents in rat leukemias *(79)* and renal and prostate cancers in vitro *(77)*; Teicher et al. have demonstrated the effectiveness of minocycline as a modulator of chemotherapy, radiation therapy, and hyperthermia in rat fibrosarcomas *(80)*, and both minocycline and doxycycline have been shown to inhibit ascitic fluid production in a similar system *(81)*; minocycline inhibits metastasis in a rat adenocarcinoma experimental metastasis system *(82)*.

Tetracyclines are less well examined in breast cancer. Sotomayor et al. were unable to demonstrate significant anti-tumor effect in murine EMT-6 breast cancer in vitro, though this may have been related to the brief (24 h) exposure time employed *(83)*, as others have demonstrated growth inhibition in vivo in a murine mammary cancer model with prolonged drug exposure *(78)*. The tetracycline derivative doxycycline has several effects on human breast cancer cells, including:

1. In vitro inhibition of MMP activity (demonstrated by gelatin zymography);
2. In vitro inhibition of invasion;
3. In vitro inhibition of proliferation;
4. In vivo inhibition of breast cancer growth;
5. In vivo inhibition of MMP mRNA expression *(75)*. It is unknown whether tetracyclines have anti-angiogenic effects in breast cancer.

These data suggest that tetracyclines might represent a novel and exciting therapeutic approach for breast cancer. This potential clinical application is bolstered by the widespread, long-standing and safe use of tetracyclines for infectious disease, and (more to the point) by their recent and effective use in the settings of gingivitis and rheumatoid arthritis, two disorders characterized by MMP-related dysregulation of tissue remodeling *(84,85)*. Because the antibiotic effects of the tetracycline are separable from their MMP inhibitory effects, tetracycline analogs (so-called chemically modified tetracyclines, or CMTs) with specific MMP inhibitory activity have recently been developed *(73)*. These analogs have increased potency in vitro compared to classic antibiotic tetracyclines, and might therefore result in a preferable toxicity profile in vivo.

6. CLINICAL DEVELOPMENT OF MMP INHIBITORS

MMP inhibitors offer both significant promise and real challenges to the clinician. The promise is obvious: given the integral involvement of the MMPs in invasion, metastasis, and angiogenesis, inhibition of these processes could add an important new weapon to our therapeutic armamentarium. Our observations of growth inhibition join a growing body of evidence supporting a role for MMP's in tumor growth. Primary tumor growth inhibition has been a constant finding after treatment with BB-94. Batimastat treatment caused ovarian carcinoma growing as a loose ascites deposit to become compacted inside a stromal sheath, with significantly reduced tumor biomass and prolonged mouse survival *(63)*. Growth effects were also seen after transfection of activated matrilysin into colon carcinoma cells *(86)*, and we have seen the same after either MMP-2 or MT1-MMP transfection into MCF-7 HBC cells (unpublished). Inhibition of the HT1080 growth in vivo with a novel microbial-derived MMP inhibitor was reported by Naito et al. *(87)*, and increased primary tumor growth was seen after transfection of activated matrilysin into colon carcinoma cells *(88)*. Transfection of MMP-11 (stromelysin-3) into MCF-7 cells reduced the latency period and thus stimulated tumorigenicity *(89)*. Recently, Conway et al. *(90)*, using a panel of synthetic MMP inhibitors with differential inhibitory profiles, selectively inhibited primary tumor growth rather than metastasis of a number of cell lines, and showed that the growth was more likely due to gelatinases (MMP-2, MMP-9) than either interstitial collagenase or stromelysins 1 or 2. Thus, primary tumor growth appears somewhat dependent on MMP activity, either directly through local proliferative effects and space expansion or indirectly through enhanced vascularization. Because synthetic MMP inhibitors offer the promise of great specificity, in theory they might offer a considerably less toxic alternative to more standard chemotherapeutic agents.

MMP inhibitors offer equally real challenges. MMP inhibition could be expected to play a useful role in the setting of micrometastatic breast cancer, preventing its transition to overt metastatic disease. But because this therapy might be expected to have tumoristatic rather than tumoricidal effects, it could well be ineffective (as measured by classic objective response measures). The patient with a kilogram of disseminated tumor, with extant and extensive vasculature and a fully developed tumor microenvironment, is unlikely to have her fate altered by an MMP inhibitor administered alone. Similarly, a bulky tumor may well harbor inhibitor-resistant clones not found in a smaller tumor, although the indications that MMP's are produced largely by the normal stromal cells may lead to less resistance . Alternatively, the occurrence of multiple redundant systems mediating growth, invasion, and metastasis may be expected to come in to play in larger as opposed to smaller tumors. And because patients with extensive disease are exactly the group utilized in Phase I and II clinical trials, MMP inhibitors stand a significant *a priori* likelihood of apparent failure.

A potential solution to this dilemma would be to proceed to Phase III (randomized) trials in an adjuvant (micrometastatic) setting immediately following the completion of Phase I trials adequate to demonstrate the safety of acutely and chronically administered MMP inhibitors. Although Phase II trials could well be performed (perhaps following treatment with systemic combination chemotherapy for metastatic breast cancer), their (anticipated) failure should not represent a valid barrier to more extensive trials in more limited disease states.

The first MMP inhibitor to enter clinical trials was batimastat *(91)* which has been recently superseded by marimastat, an orally active analog of batimastat *(92)*. In Phase I trials of marimastat, the (unexpected) dose limiting toxicity has been musculoskeletal toxicity, particularly tendonitis/bursitis *(92)*. This side effect is dose-related and reversible with cessation of therapy. Whether this side effect is specific to marimastat, or generic to MMP inhibitors, will await clinical trials with other agents in this class. It is possible that MMP inhibitors with different structures may have a different spectrum of side effects, though this is currently unknown. This is a potentially important issue for a drug where chronic administration may be required. Similarly, it is unknown whether broad-spectrum MMP inhibition will be required to prevent disease progression, or whether agents targeting one or only a few of the MMPs will suffice. Given the propensity of new agents to develop unexpected toxicities, a highly specific MMP inhibitor might induce fewer long-term side effects; but would it suffice to halt the cancer?

Two recently initiated trials demonstrate how these agents might be developed. The Eastern Cooperative Oncology Group (ECOG) has initiated a prospective, randomized Phase III trial in metastatic breast cancer. In this trial (E2196), patients receive systemic chemotherapy for 6–8 cycles, following which they are randomized to receive marimastat or a control arm. The primary clinical endpoint in this trial is time to progression (TTP), testing the hypothesis that matrix metalloproteinase inhibition will prevent tumor regrowth or progression.

A second trial is being conducted in a limited institution setting by participating ECOG institutions. In this phase I/pilot trial, patients with early stage breast cancer receive marimastat in an adjuvant setting either following completion of adjuvant adriamycin-based chemotherapy, or concomitantly with adjuvant hormonal therapy with tamoxifen. The major endpoints in this trial revolve around pharmacokinetic and safety questions for chronically administered MMP inhibition therapy, a necessary prelude to a large adjuvant Phase III trial.

The use of agents like the MMP inhibitors will require new patterns of thought for practicing clinicians. Care of breast cancer (and other malignancies) has often been conceived of as requiring the elimination of the last cancer cell, or at least reduction of tumor mass to a point where the body's immune surveillance system can "mop up" the last tumor cells. The MMP inhibitors require us to think of micrometastatic disease much as the endocrinologist conceives of insulin-dependent diabetes mellitus: a chronic disease whose ravages might be controlled through the chronic administration of a highly selective drug. This chronic drug might not (like the administration of insulin itself) be without toxicity, and it might not (again like insulin) represent either a cure for the underlying disease or a perfect and final solution to every complication of that disease. But it might offer many patients years of useful, high-quality life. If so, the MMP inhibitors will have fulfilled their promise.

REFERENCES

1. Liotta, L. A. 1986. Tumor invasion and metastases-role of the extracellular matrix: rhoads memorial award lecture. *Cancer Res.* **46:** 1–7.
2. Liotta, L. A., P. S. Steeg, and W. G. Stetler-Stevenson. 1991. Cancer metastasis and angiogenesis: An imbalance of positive and negative regulation. *Cell* **64:** 327–336.

3. Liotta, L. A., W. G. Stetler-Stevenson, and P. S. Steeg. 1991. Cancer invasion and metastasis: positive and negative regulatory elements. *Cancer Invest.* **9**: 543–551.

4. Woessner, J. F., Jr. 1991. Matrix metalloproteinases and their inhibitors in connective tissue remodeling. *FASEB J.* **5**: 2145–2154.

5. Birkedal-Hansen, H., W. G. Moore, M. K. Bodden, L. F. Windsor, B. Birkedal-Hansen, A. De Carlo, and J. A. Engler. 1993. Matrix metalloproteinases: A review. *Crit. Rev. Oral Biol. Med.* **4**: 197–250.

6. Zhang, D., I. Botos, F. X. Gomis-Ruth, R. Doll, C. Blood, F. G. Njoroge, J. W. Fox, W. Bode, and E. F. Meyer. 1994. Structural interaction of natural and synthetic inhibitors with the venom metalloproteinase, atrolysin c (form d). *Proc. Natl. Acad. Sci. USA* **91**: 8447–8451.

7. Basset, P., J. P. Bellocq, C. Wolf, I. Stoll, P. Hutin, J. M. Limacher, O. L. Podhajcer, M. P. Chenard, M. C. Rio, and P. Chambon. 1990. A novel metalloproteinase gene specifically expressed in stromal cells of breast carcinomas. *Nature* **348**: 699–704.

8. Freije, J. M., I. Diez-Itza, M. Balbin, L. M. Sanchez, R. Blasco, J. Tolivia, and C. Lopez-Otin. 1994. Molecular cloning and expression of collagenase-3, a novel human matrix metalloproteinase produced by breast carcinomas. *J. Biol. Chem.* **269**: 16,766–16,773.

9. Okada, A., J. P. Bellocq, N. Rouyer, M. P. Chenard, M. C. Rio, P. Chambon, and P. Basset. 1994. Membrane-type matrix metalloproteinase (MT-MMP) gene is expressed in stromal cells of human colon, breast, and head and neck carcinomas. *Proc. Natl. Acad. Sci. USA* **92**: 2730–2734.

10. Puente, X. S., A. M. Pendas, E. Llano, G. Velasco, and C. Lopez-Otin. 1996. Molecular cloning of a novel membrane-type matrix metalloproteinase from a human breast carcinoma. *Cancer Res.* **56**: 944–949.

11. Pendas, A. M., V. Knauper, X. S. Puente, E. Llano, M. G. Mattei, S. Apte, G. Murphy, and C. Lopez-Otin. 1997. Identification and characterization of a novel human matrix metalloproteinase with unique structural characteristics, chromosomal location, and tissue distribution. *J. Biol. Chem.* **272**: 4281–4286.

12. Heppner, K. J., L. M. Matrisian, R. A. Jensen, and W. H. Rodgers. 1996. Expression of most matrix metalloproteinase family members in breast cancer represents a tumor-induced host response. *Am. J. Pathol.* **149**: 273–282.

13. Polette, M. and P. Birembaut. 1996. Matrix metalloproteinases in breast cancer. *Breast J.* **2**: 209–220.

14. MacDougall, J. R. and L. M. Matrisian. 1995. Contributions of tumor and stromal matrix metalloprteinases to tumor progression, invasion and metastasis. *Cancer Metastasis Rev.* **14**: 351–362.

15. Thompson, E. W., M. Yu, J. Bueno, L. Jin, S. N. Maiti, F. L. Palao-Marco, H. Pulyaeva, J. W. Tamborlane, R. Tirgari, I. Wapnir, and H. S. Azzam. 1994. Collagen induced MMP–2 activation in human breast cancer. *Breast Cancer Res. Treat.* **31**: 357–370.

16. Bae, S. N., G. Arand, H. Azzam, P. Pavasant, J. Torri, T. L. Frandsen, and E. W. Thompson. 1993. Molecular and cellular analysis of basement membrane invasion by human breast cancer cells in matrigel-based in vitro assays. *Breast Cancer Res. Treat.* **24**: 241–255.

17. Thompson, E. W., S. Paik, N. Brunner, C. L. Sommers, G. Zugmaier, R. Clarke, T. B. Shima, J. Torri, S. Donahue, M. E. Lippman, G. R. Martin, and R. B. Dickson.1992. Association of increased basement membrane invasiveness with absence of estrogen receptor and expression of vimentin in human breast cancer cell lines. *J. Cell Physiol.* **150**: 534–544.

18. Sommers, C. L., S. W. Byers, E. W. Thompson, J. A. Torri, and E. P. Gelmann. 1994. Differentiation state and invasiveness of human breast cancer cell lines. *Breast Cancer Res. Treat.* **31**: 325–335.

19. Gilles, C., M. Polette, P. Birembaut, N. Brunner, and E. W. Thompson. 1997. Expression of c-ets-1 mRNA is associated with an invasive, EMT-derived phenotype in breast carcinoma cell lines. *Clin. Exp. Metastasis*, in press.

20. Savagner, P., B. Boyer, A. M. Valles, J. Jouanneau, and J. P. Thiery. 1994. 52 Modulations of the epithelial phenotype during embryogenesis and cancer progression. *Cancer Treat. Res.* **71**: 229–249.

21. Gilles, C. and E. W. Thompson. 1996. The epithelial to mesenchymal transition and metastatic progression in carcinoma. *Breast J.* **2**: 83–96.

22. Azzam, H. S., G. Arand, M. E. Lippman, M. E., and W. Thompson. 1993. Association of MMP-2 activation potential with metastatic progression in human breast cancer cell lines independent of MMP- 2 production. *J. Natl. Cancer Inst.* **85**: 1758–1764.

23. Pulyaeva, H., D. Washington, J. Bueno, H. Sato, M. Seiki, N. Azumi, and E. W. Thompson. 1997. MT1-MMP correlates with MMP-2 activation potential seen after epithelial to mesenchymal transition in human breast carcinoma cells. *Clin. Exp. Metastasis* **15**: 111–120.

24. Gilles, C., M. Polette, M. Seiki, P. Birembaut, and E. W. Thompson. 1997. Collagen type I-induced MT1-MMP expression and MMP–2 activation: Implication in the metastatic progression of breast carcinoma. *Lab. Invest.* **76**: 651–660.

25. Azzam, H. S. E. W. and Thompson. 1992. Collagen-induced activation of the Mr 72,000 type IV collagenase in normal and malignant human fibroblastoid cells. *Cancer Res.* **52**: 4540–4544.

26. Yu, M., H. Sato, M. Seiki, and E. W. Thompson. 1995. Complex regulation of membrane-type matrix metalloproteinase expression and matrix metalloproteinase-2 activation by concanavalin A in MDA-MB-231 human breast cancer cells. *Cancer Res.* **55**: 3272–3277.

27. Maiti, S. N., M. Yu, J. Bueno, R. H. Tirgari, F. L. Palao-Marco, H. Pulyaeva, and E. W. Thompson. 1994. 66 Differential regulation of matrix metalloproteinase-2 activation in human breast cancer cell lines. *Ann. NY Acad. Sci.* **732**: 456–458.

28. Polette, M., B. Nawrocki, C. Gilles, H. Sato, H., Seiki, M. Tournier, and P. Birembaut. 1996. MT-MMP expression and localization in human breast and lung cancer. *Virchows Arch.* **428**: 29–35.

29. Stetler-Stevenson, W. G., P. D. Brown, M. Onisto, A. T. Levy, and L. A. Liotta. 1990. Tissue inhibitor of metalloproteinases-2 (timp-2) mrna expression in tumor cell lines and human tumor tissues. *J. Biol. Chem.* **265**: 13,933–13,938.

30. Matrisian, L. M. 1992. The matrix-degrading metalloproteinases. *Bioessays* **14**: 455–463.

31. Leco, K. J., R. Khokha, N. Pavloff, S. P. Hawkes, and D. R. Edwards. 1994. Tissue inhibitor of metalloproteinases-3 (timp-3) is an extracellular matrix-associated protein with a distinctive pattern of expression in mouse cells and tissues. *J. Biol. Chem.* **269**: 9352–9360.

32. Uria, J. A., A. A. Ferrando, G. Velasco, G., Freije, and C. Lopez-Otin. 1994. Structure and expression in breast tumors of human timp–3, a new member of the metalloproteinase inhibitor family. *Cancer Res.* **54**: 2091–2094.

33. Greene, J., M. Wang, Y. E. Liu, L. A. Raymond, C. Rosen, and Y. E. Shi. 1996. Molecular cloning and characterization of human tissue inhibitor of metalloproteinase 4. *J. Biol. Chem.* **271**: 30,375–30,380.

34. Stetler-Stevenson, W. G., H. C. Krutzsch, H. C., and L. A. Liotta. 1989. Tissue inhibitor of metalloproteinase (timp-2). a new member of the metalloproteinase inhibitor family. *J. Biol. Chem.* **264**: 17,374–17,378.

35. Goldberg, G. I., B. L. Marmer, G. A. Grant, A. Z. Eisen, S. Wilhelm, and C. S. He. 1989. Human 72-kilodalton type iv collagenase forms a complex with a tissue inhibitor of metalloproteases designated timp-2. *Proc. Natl. Acad. Sci. USA* **86**: 8207–8211.

36. Wilhelm, S. M., I. E. Collier, B. L. Marmer, A. Z. Eisen, G. A. Grant, and G. I. Goldberg. 1989. Sv40-transformed human lung fibroblasts secrete a 92-kda type iv collagenase which is identical to that secreted by normal human macrophages [published erratum. 1990. *J. Biol. Chem.* **265(36):** 22,570]. *J. Biol. Chem.* **264:** 17,213–17,221.

37. Visscher, D. W., M. Hoyhtya, S. K. Ottosen, C. M.Liang, F. H. Sarkar, J. D. Crissman, and R. Fridman. 1994. Enhanced expression of tissue inhibitor of metalloproteinase-2 (timp-2) in the stroma of breast carcinomas correlates with tumor recurrence. *Int. J. Cancer* **59:** 339–344.

38. Alessandro, R., S. Minafra, I. Pucci-Minafra, M. Onisto, S. Garbisa, A. Melchiori, L. Tetlow, and D. E. Woolley. 1993. Metalloproteinase and timp expression by the human breast carcinoma cell line 8701-bc. *Int. J. Cancer* **55:** 250–255.

39. Clavel, C., M. Polette, M. Doco, I. Binninger, and P. Birembaut. 1992. Immuno-localization of matrix metallo-proteinases and their tissue inhibitor in human mammary pathology. *Bull. Cancer* (Paris) **79:** 261–270.

40. Polette, M., C. Clavel, M. Cockett, S. Girod de Bentzmann, G. Murphy, and P. Birembaut. 1993. Detection and localization of mRNAs encoding matrix metalloproteinases and their tissue inhibitor in human breast pathology. *Invasion Metastasis* **13:** 31–37.

41. Poulsom, R., A. M. Hanby, M. Pignatelli, R. E. Jeffery, J. M. Longcroft, L. Rogers, and G. W. Stamp. 1993. Expression of gelatinase a and timp-2 mrnas in desmoplastic fibro-blasts in both mammary carcinomas and basal cell carcinomas of the skin. *J. Clin. Pathol.* **46:** 429–436.

42. Thompson, E. W., J. Yoon, M. B. Burgess, R. B. Dickson, G. I. Goldberg, M. E. Lippman, and F. G. Kern. Matrix metalloproteinase family analysis in human breast cancer cell lines of differential in vivo and in vitro invasiveness. *Proc. Am. Assoc. Cancer Res.* **32:** 711,991 (Abstract).

43. Thorgeirsson, U. P., L. A. Liotta, T. Kalebic, I. M. Margulies, K. Thomas, M. Rios-Candelore, and R. G. Russo. 1982. Effect of natural protease inhibitors and a chemoattractant on tumor cell invasion in vitro. *J. Natl. Cancer Inst.* **69:** 1049–1054.

44. Schultz, R. M., S. Silberman, B. Persky, A. S. Bajkowski, D. F. Carmichael. 1988. Inhi-bition by human recombinant tissue inhibitor of metalloproteinases of human amnion invasion and lung colonization by murine B16-F10 melanoma cells.

45. Reich, R., S. H. Alder, G. R. Martin, and L. S. Royce. 1989. Use of in vitro assays to define the malignant activities of tumor cells to screen for antimetastatic drugs. *Alterna-tive Methods Toxocol.* **7:** 11–22.

46. Lee, K., S. Rha, S. Kim, J. Kim, J. Roh, B. Kim, and H. Chung. 1996. Sequential activa-tion and production of matrix metalloproteinase-2 during breast cancer progression. *Clin. Exp. Metastasis* **14:** 512–519.

47. Albini, A., A. Melchiori, L. Santi, L. A. Liotta, P. D. Brown, and W. G. Stetler-Stevenson. 1991. Tumor cell invasion inhibited by timp-2 [see comments]. *J. Natl. Cancer Inst.* **83:** 775–779.

48. Tsuchiya, Y., H. Sato, Y. Endo, Y. Okada, M. Mai, T. Sasaki, and M. Seiki. 1993. Tissue inhibitor of metalloproteinase 1 is a negative regulator of the metastatic ability of a human gastric cancer cell line, KK1S, in the chick embryo.

49. De Clerck, Y. A., N. Perez, H. Shimada, T. C. Boone, K. E. Langley, and S. M. Taylor. 1992. Inhibition of invasion and metastasis in cells transfected with an inhibitor of metalloproteinases. *Cancer Res.* **52:** 701–708.

50. Khokha, R. 1994. Suppression of the tumorigenic and metastatic abilities of murine b16-f10 melanoma cells in vivo by the overexpression of the tissue inhibitor of the metalloproteinases-1. *J. Natl. Cancer Inst.* **86:** 299–304.

51. Zeng, Z., A. Cohen, Z. Zhang, W. G. Stetler-Stevenson, and J. Guillem. 1995. Elevated tissue inhibitor of metalloproteinase 1 RNA in colorectal carcinoma stroma correlates with lymph node and distant metastases. *Clin. Cancer Res.* **1:** 899–906.

52. Ponton, A., B. Coulombe, and D. Skup, D. 1991. Decreased expression of tissue inhibitor of metalloproteinases in metastatic tumor cells leading to increased levels of collagenase activity. *Cancer Res.* **51:** 2138–2143.

53. Nemeth, J. A. and C. L. Goolsby. 1993. Timp-2, a growth-stimulatory protein from sv40-transformed human fibroblasts. *Exp. Cell Res.* **207:** 376–382, 1993.

54. Hayakawa, T., K. Yamashita, E. Ohuchi, and A. Shinagawa. 1994. Cell growth-promoting activity of tissue inhibitor of metalloproteinases-2 (timp-2). *J. Cell Sci.* **107:** 2373–2379.

55. Nemeth, J. A., A. Rafe, M. Steiner, and C. L. Goolsby. 1996. Timp-2 growth-stimulatory activity: a concentration- and cell type-specific response in the presence of insulin. *Exp. Cell Res.* **224:** 110–115.

56. Yamashita, K., M. Suzuki, H. Iwata, T. Koike, M. Hamaguchi, A. Shinagawa, T. Noguchi, and T. Hayakawa. 1996. Tyrosine phosphorylation is crucial for growth signaling by tissue inhibitors of metalloproteinases (timp-1 and timp-2). *FEBS Lett.* **396:** 103–107.

57. Corcoran, M. L., M. R. Emmert-Buck, J. L. McClanahan, M. Pelina-Parker, and W. Stetler-Stevenson. 1996. G. Timp-2 mediates cell surface binding of mmp-2. *Adv. Exp. Med. Biol.* **389:** 295–304.

58. Bode, W., F. X. Gomis-Ruth, and W. Stockler. 1993. Astacins, serralysins, snake venom and matrix metalloproteinases exhibit identical zinc-binding environments (hexxhxxgxxh and met-turn) and topologies and should be grouped into a common family, the 'metzincins'. *FEBS Lett.* **331:** 134–140.

59. Bode, W., L. F. Kress, E. F. Meyer, E. F.,and F. X. Gomis-Ruth. 1994. The crystal structure of adamalysin ii, a zinc-endopeptidase from the snake venom of the eastern diamondback rattlesnake crotalus adamanteus. *Braz. J. Med. Biol. Res.* **27:** 2049–2068.

60. Botos, I., L. Scapozza, D. Zhang, L. A. Liotta, and E. F. Meyer. 1996. Batimastat, a potent matrix mealloproteinase inhibitor, exhibits an unexpected mode of binding. *Proc. Natl. Acad. Sci. USA* **93:** 2749–2754.

61. Gooley, P. R., J. F. O'Connell, A. I. Marcy, G. C. Cuca, S. P. Salowe, B. L. Bush, J. D. Hermes, C. K. Esser, W. K. Hagmann, J. P. Springer, et al. 1994. The nmr structure of the inhibited catalytic domain of human stromelysin-1. *Nat. Struct. Biol.* **1:** 111–118.

62. Stams, T., J. C. Spurlino, D. L. Smith, R. C. Wahl, T. F. Ho, M. W. Qoronfleh, T. M. Banks, and B. Rubin. 1994. Structure of human neutrophil collagenase reveals large s1' specificity pocket. *Nat. Struct. Biol.* **1:** 119–123.

63. Davies, B., P. D. Brown, N. East, M. J. Crimmin, and F. R. Balkwill. 1993. A synthetic matrix metalloproteinase inhibitor decreases tumor burden and prolongs survival of mice bearing human ovarian carcinoma xenografts. *Cancer Res.* **53:** 2087–2091.

64. Chirivi, R. G., A. Garofalo, M. J. Crimmin, L. J. Bawden, A. Stoppacciaro, P. D. Brown, and R. Giavazzi, R. 1994. Inhibition of the metastatic spread and growth of b16-bl6 murine melanoma by a synthetic matrix metalloproteinase inhibitor. *Int. J. Cancer* **58:** 460–464.

65. Wang, X., X. Fu, P. D. Brown, M. J. Crimmin, and R. M. Hoffman. 1994. Matrix metalloproteinase inhibitor bb–94 (batimastat) inhibits human colon tumor growth and spread in a patient-like orthotopic model in nude mice. *Cancer Res.* **54:** 4726–4728.

66. An, Z., X. Wang, N. Willmott, S. K. Chander, S. Tickle, A. J. Docherty, A. Mountain, A. T. Millican, J. R. Morphy, J. P. Porter, O. Epemolu, T. Kubota, A. R. Moossa, and R. M. Hoffman. 1997. Conversion of highly malignant colon cancer from an aggresive to a controlled disease by oral administration of a metalloproteinase inhibitor. *Clin. Exp. Metastasis* **15:** 184–195.

67. Fisher, C., S. Gilbertson-Beadling, E. A. Powers, G. Petzold, R. Poorman, and M. A. Mitchell, M. A. Interstitial collagenase is required for angiogenesis in vitro. *Dev. Biol.* **162:** 499–510.

68. Taraboletti, G., A. Garofalo, D. Belotti, et al. 1995. Inhibition of angiogenesis and murine hemangioma growth by Batimastat, a synthetic inhibitor of matrix metalloproteinases. *J. Natl. Cancer Inst.* **87:** 293–298.

69. Sledge, G. W., Jr., M. Qulali, R. Goulet, E. A. Bone, R. S. Fife. 1995. Effect of matrix metalloproteinase inhibitor batimastat on breast cancer regrowth and metastasis in athymic mice. *J. Natl. Cancer Inst.* **87:** 1546–1550.

70. Low, J. A., M. D. Johnson, E. A. Bone, and R. B. Dickson. 1996. The matrix metalloproteinase inhibitor batimasat (BB-94) retards human breast cancer solid tumor growth but not ascites formation in nude mice. *Clin. Cancer Res.* **2:** 1207–1214.

71. Eccles, S., G. Box, W. Court, E. Bone, and P. Brown. 1996. Control of lymphatic and blood borne metastasis of a rat breast carcinoma xenograft model of human breast carcinoma by the matrix metalloproteinase inhibitor, batimastat. *Proc. Am. Assoc. Cancer Res.* **37:** (Abstract).

72. Tamargo, R. J., R. A. Bok, and H. Brem. 1991. Angiogenesis inhibition by minocycline. *Cancer Res.* **51:** 672–675.

73. Golub, L. M., T. F. McNamara, G. D'Angelo, R. A. Greenwald, and N. S. Ramamurthy. 1987. A non-antibacterial chemically-modified tetracycline inhibits mammalian collagenase activity. *J. Dent. Res.* **66:** 1310–1314.

74. Golub, L. M., Lee, H. M., Lehrer, G., Nemiroff, A., McNamara, T. F., Kaplan, R., and Ramamurthy, N. S. Minocycline reduces gingival collagenolytic activity during diabetes. preliminary observations and a proposed new mechanism of action. *J. Periodont. Res.* **18:** 516–526, 1983.

75. Fife, R. S. and G. W. Sledge. 1995. Effects of doxycycline on in vitro growth, migration, and gelatinase activity of breast carcinoma cells. *J. Lab. Clin. Med.* **125:** 407–411.

76. Guerin, C., J. Laterra, T. Masnyk, L. M. Golub, and H. Brem. 1992. Selective endothelial growth inhibition by tetracyclines that inhibit collagenase. Biochem. Biophys. Res. Commun. **188:** 740–745.

77. van den Bogert, C., B. H. Dontje, M. Holtrop, T. E. Melis, J. C. Romijn, J. W. van Dongen, and A. M. Kroon. 1986. Arrest of the proliferation of renal and prostate carcinomas of human origin by inhibition of mitochondrial protein synthesis. *Cancer Res.* **46:** 3283–3289.

78. Kroon, A. M., B. H. Dontje, M. Holtrop, and C. van den Bogert. 1984. The mitochondrial genetic system as a target for chemotherapy: tetracyclines as cytostatics. *Cancer Lett.* **25:** 33–40.

79. van den Bogert, C., Dontje, B. H., and Kroon, A. M. The antitumour effect of doxycycline on a t-cell leukaemia in the rat. Leuk. Res. **9:** 617–623, 1985.

80. Teicher, B. A., S. A. Holden, C. J. Liu, G. Ara, and T. S. Herman. 1994. Minocycline as a modulator of chemotherapy and hyperthermia in vitro and in vivo. *Cancer Lett.* **82:** 17–25.

81. Wakai, K., E. Ohmura, T. Satoh, H. Murakami, O. Isozaki, N. Emoto, H. Demura, K. Shizume, and T. Tsushima. 1994. Mechanism of inhibitory actions of minocycline and doxycycline on ascitic fluid production induced by mouse fibrosarcoma cells. *Life Sci.* **54:** 703–709.

82. Masumori, N., T. Tsukamoto, N. Miyao, Y. Kumamoto, I. Saiki, and J. Yoneda. 1994. Inhibitory effect of minocycline on in vitro invasion and experimental metastasis of mouse renal adenocarcinoma. *J. Urol.* **151:** 1400–1404.

83. Sotomayor, E. A., B. A. Teicher, G. N. Schwartz, S. A. Holden, K. Menon, T. S. Herman, and E. Frei, 3rd. 1992. Minocycline in combination with chemotherapy or radiation therapy in vitro and in vivo. *Cancer Chemother. Pharmacol.* **30:** 377–384.

84. Lee, W., S. Aitken, G. Kulkarni, P. Birek, C. M. Overall, J. Sodek, and C. A. McCulloch. 1991. Collagenase activity in recurrent periodontitis: relationship to disease progression and doxycycline therapy. *J. Periodont. Res.* **26:** 479–485.

85. Tilley, B. C., G. S. Alarcon, S. P. Heyse, D. E. Trentham, R. Neuner, D. A. Kaplan, D. O. Clegg, J. C. Leisen, L. Buckley, S. M. Cooper, et al. 1995. Minocycline in rheumatoid

arthritis. a 48-week, double-blind, placebo-controlled trial. mira trial group [see comments]. *Ann. Intern. Med.* **122:** 81–89.

86. Witty, J. P., S. McDonnell, K. J. Newell, P. Cannon, M. Navre, R.f J. Tressler, and L. M. Matrisian. 1994. Modulation of matrilysin levels in colon carcinoma cell lines affects tumorigenicity in vivo. *Cancer Res.* **54:** 4805–4812.

87. Naito, K., N. Kanbayashi, S. Nakajima, T. Murai, K. Arakawa, S. Nishimura, and A. Okuyama. 1994. Inhibition of growth of human tumor cells in nude mice by a metalloproteinase inhibitor. *Int. J. Cancer* **58:** 730–735.

88. Powell, W. C., J. D. Knox, M. Navre, T. M. Grogan, J. Kittelson, R. B. Nagle, and G. T. Bowden. 1993. Expression of the metalloproteinase matrilysin in DU-145 cells increases their invasive potential in severe combined immunodeficient mice. *Cancer Res.* **53:** 417–422.

89. Noel, A. C., O. Lefebvre, E. Maquoi, L. Van Hoorde, M. P. Chenard, M. Mareel, J. M. Foidart, P. Basset, and M. C. Rio. 1996. Stromelysin-3 expression promotes tumor take in nude mice. *J. Clin. Invest.* **97:** 1924–1930.

90. Conway, J. G., S. J. Trexler, J. A. Wakefield, B. E. Marron, D. L. Emerson, D. M. Bickett, D. N. Deaton, D. Garrison, M. Elder, A. McElroy, N. Willmott, A. J. Dockerty, and G. M. McGeehan. 1996. Effect of matrix metalloproteinase inhibitors on tumor growth and spontaneous metastasis. *Clin. Exp. Metastasis* **14:** 115–124.

91. Wojtowicz-Praga, S., J. Low, J. Marshall, E. Ness, R. B. Dickson, J. Barter, M. Sale, P. McCann, J. Moore, A. Cole, and M. J. Hawkins. 1996. Phase I trial of a novel matrix metalloproteinase inhibitor batimastat (BB-94) in patients with advanced cancer. Invest. New Drugs, **14:** 193–202.

92. Wojtowicz-Praga, S., J. Low, R. Dickson, et al. 1996. Pharmacokinetics (PK) of marimastat (BB 2516), a novel matrix metalloproteinase inhibitor administered orally to patients with matastatic lung cancer. *Proc. Am. Assoc. Cancer Res.* **15:** (Abstract).

93. Fransden, T. L., B. E. Boysen, S. Jirus, M. Spang-Thomsen, K. Dano, E. W. Thompson, and N. Brunner. 1992. Experimental models for the study of human cancer cell invasion and metastasis. *Fibrinolysis* **6:** 71–76.

94. Borkakoti, N., F. K. Winkler, D. H. Williams, A. D'Arcy, M. J. Broadhurst, P. A. Brown, W. H. Johnson, and E. J. Murray. 1994. Structure of the catalytic domain of human fibroblast collagenase complexed with an inhibitor. *Nat. Struct. Biol.* **1:** 106–110.

95. Galardy, R. E., D. Grobelny, H. G. Foellmer, and L. A. Fernandez. 1994. Inhibition of angiogenesis by the matrix metalloprotease inhibitor n-[2r-2-(hydroxamidocarbonymethyl)-4-methylpentanoyl)]-l-tryptophan methylamide. *Cancer Res.* **54:** 4715–4718.

96. Reich, R., E. W. Thompson, Y. Iwamoto, G. R. Martin, J. R. Deason, G. C. Fuller, and R. Miskin. 1988. Effects of inhibitors of plasminogen activator, serine proteinases, and collagenase IV on the invasion of basement membranes by metastatic cells.

97. Alvarez, O. A., D. F. Carmichael, and Y. A. De Clerck. 1990. Inhibition of collagenolytic activity and metastasis of tumor cells by a recombinant human tissue inhibitor of metalloproteinases. *J. Natl. Cancer Inst.* **82:** 589–595.

98. Watson, S. A., T. M. Morris, G. Robinson, M. J. Crimmin, P. D. Brown, and J. D. Hardcastle. 1995. Inhibition of organ invasion by the matrix metalloproteinase inhibitor batimastat (bb-94) in two human colon carcinoma metastasis models. *Cancer Res.* **55:** 3629–3633.

99. Schnaper, H. W, D. S. Grant, W. G. Stetler-Stevenson, et al. 1993. Type IV collageneases and TIMPs modulate endothelial cell morphogenesis in vitro. *J. Cell Physiol.* **156:** 235–246.

100. Mignatti, P., Tsuboi, R., Robbins, E., and Rifkin, D. B. 1989. In vitro angiogenesis on the human amniotic membrane: requirement for basic fibroblast growth factor-induced proteinases. *J. Cell Biol.* **108:** 671–682.

101. Alexander, C. M. and Z. Werb. 1992. Targeted disruption of the tissue inhibitor of metalloproteinases gene increases the invasive behavior of primitive mesenchymal cells derived from embryonic stem cells in vitro. *J. Cell Biol.* **118**: 727–739.

102. Hoyhtya, M., E. Hujanen, T. Turpeenniemi-Hujanen U. Thorgeirsson, L. A. Liotta, and K. Tryggvason. 1990. Modulation of type-IV collagenase activity and invasive behavior of metastatic human melanoma (A2058) cells in vitro by monoclonal antibodies to type-IV collagenase. *Int. J. Cancer* **46(2)**: 282–286.

103. Melchiori, A., A. Albini, J. M. Ray, and W. G. Stetler-Stevenson. 1992. Inhibition of tumor cell invasion by a highly conserved peptide sequence from the matrix metalloproteinase enzyme prosegment. *Cancer Res.* **52**: 2353–2356.

104. Collier, M. A., G. J. Yuen, S. K. Bansai, et al. 1997. A Phase I study of the matrix metalloproteinase (MMP) inhibitor AG3340 given in single doses to healthy volunteers. Proc. Am. Assoc. *Cancer Res.* **38**: 221 (Abstract 1491).

105. Shono, T., M. Ono, S. Jimi, et al. 1997. A novel synthetic matrix metalloproteinase inhibitor OPB–3206: Inhibition of tumor growth, metastasis, and angiogenesis. *Proc. Am. Assoc. Cancer Res.* **38**: 525 (Abstract 3523).

106. Anderson, I. C., M. A. Shipp, A. J. P. Docherty, B. and A. Teicher. 1996. Combination therapy including a gelatinase inhibitor and cytotoxic agent reduces local invasion and metastasis in murine Lewis lung carcinoma. *Cancer Res.* **56**: 715–718.

107. Burns, F. R., M. S. Stack, R. D. Gray, and C. A. Paterson. 1989. Inhibition of purified collagenase from alkali-burned rabbit corneas. *Invest. Opthalmol. Vis. Sci.* **30**: 1569–1575.

108. Gilbertson-Beadling, S., E. A. Powers, M. Stamp-Cole, et al. 1995. The tetracycline analogs minocycline and doxycycline inhibit angiogenesis in vitro by a non-metalloproteinase-dependent mechanism. *Cancer Chemother. Pharmacol.* **36**: 418–424.

109. Khoka, R. 1994. Suppression of the tumorigenic and metastatic abilities of murine B16-F10 melanoma cells in vivo by the overexpression of the tissue inhibitor of the metalloproteinases-1. *J. Natl. Cancer Inst.* **86**: 299–304.

110. Taraboletti, G., A. Garofalo, D. Belotti, et al. 1995. Inhibition of angiogenesis and murine hemangioma growth by Batimastat, a synthetic inhibitor of matrix metalloproteinases. *J. Natl. Cancer Inst.* **87**: 293–298.

21

MUC1 Mucin as a Tumor Antigen in Breast Cancer

Pawel Ciborowski, Elisabeth M. Hiltbold,
Simon M. Barratt-Boyes, and Olivera J. Finn

1. INTRODUCTION

Diagnosis and treatment of breast cancer is greatly facilitated by detailed knowledge of the important molecules and functions that distinguish the transformed cell from its normal counterpart. The last decade of research has witnessed a remarkable progress in this endeavor, starting from characterizing products of mutated genes responsible for causing or maintaining the transformed state, to characterizing products of nonmutated genes whose posttranslational modifications mark them as tumor-specific. MUC1 mucin belongs to the latter category. It has been intensely studied in relationship to breast cancer by scientists in different disciplines for several compelling reasons. Unlike many other breast-cancer related molecules that are each expressed only in a small subset of breast tumors, MUC1 is expressed by most breast cancers, the primary tumor as well as its metastases. In fact, those interested in tumor metastases have postulated an important role for MUC1 in promoting metastases. Molecular biologists have been fascinated by the effect that malignant transformation has on the increased activity of the MUC1 gene promoter, cell biologists have tried to understand why MUC1 is strictly polarized in its expression to the apical surface of normal ductal epithelia and why is that polarization lost in malignant cells, and biochemists have tried to understand drastic differences in glycosylation of MUC1 on normal vs malignant cells. Tumor immunologists have assumed that every one of the aforementioned changes could make this molecule appear foreign to the immune system and have defined biological and biochemical characteristics of this molecule that make it an especially attractive candidate for a tumor-specific target and a tumor-specific vaccine.

2. STRUCTURE AND FUNCTION OF MUC1 MUCIN

Mucins are a family of high molecular-weight glycoproteins produced by epithelial cells. Highly branched O-linked oligosaccharides and N-linked glycans account for more than 50% of dry weight of these proteins. MUC1 is the only transmembrane mucin of the nine identified so far *(1,2)*. Over the last decade of extensive studies, various other names have been assigned to this molecule such as: polymorphic epithelial mucin (PEM), episialin, human milk fat globule (HMFG) antigen, DF3 antigen, epitectin, and so on. In order to follow Human Genome Mapping conventions and to be

From: Breast Cancer: *Molecular Genetics, Pathogenesis, and Therapeutics*
Edited by: A. M. Bowcock © Humana Press Inc., Totowa, NJ

consistent with all other publications from our group we will use MUC1 to describe transmembrane mucin that is a product of the *MUC1* gene.

MUC1 can be found in breast, lung, pancreatic, ovarian, uterine, colonic, gastric, and gallbladder epithelia. In normal ductal epithelia of these tissues, mucin expression is highly polarized to the apical surface facing the lumen of the duct. It has been well-accepted that some of the functions shared by all mucins, including MUC1, are to lubricate the surfaces of ducts, protect the epithelial cells from pathogens and digestive enzymes, and to modulate the often harsh environment inside the ducts. More recently, formal studies have been initiated by several groups to examine other potential functions of MUC1, such as its role in tumor progression and metastasis, in cell-cell and/or cell-matrix proteins interactions, in signal transduction , and as a ligand for P- and E-selectins by being a carrier of Lewis[x] and sialyl-Lewis[a] carbohydrates.

MUC1 mucin is abundantly expressed on the surface of malignant cells originating from ductal epithelia. In tumors, such as breast cancer, there is a loss of polarized expression of MUC1. This and an overall increase in MUC1 production causes MUC1 mucin to be aberrantly glycosylated, leading to the expression of tumor-specific forms.

2.1. The Protein Backbone

The complete structure of the gene encoding MUC1 and its product has been elucidated *(3)*. The protein backbone of the MUC1 mucin consists of a number of distinct domains (Fig. 1). The major portion of the protein is the central region consisting of a variable number of tandem repeats, perfectly conserved stretches of 20 amino acids (a.a.) rich in proline (25%), threonine (15%), and serine (10%). Both serine and threonine residues are potential sites of O-glycosylation. The variability of the number of tandem repeats (from 20–120 per molecule) is owing to allelic polymorphism exhibited by genes encoding mucins, leading to large differences in molecular weight of the protein. The region from the N-terminus to the first tandem repeat is 127 a.a. long consisting of the signal peptide followed by 104 a.a. corresponding to degenerate repeats. This part of the molecule is rich in threonine (16%) and serine (18%) residues that are not O-glycosylated. C-terminal to the tandem-repeat region is another region (227 a.a.) consisting of degenerate repeats rich in threonine (11%) and serine (18%) residues that are not O-glycosylated and five N-glycosylation sites that are glycosylated. A 31 a.a. long hydrophobic membrane-spanning domain, and a 69 a.a. long cytoplasmic domain complete the molecule. In MUC1, unlike in other mucins, the cysteine residues in the C-terminal region do not form functional disulfide bonds. The fact that MUC1 is a transmembrane molecule is very important for its role as a tumor-specific antigen. Cell-surface molecules are much better targets of anti-tumor therapies, especially those based on specific antibodies, than are secreted molecules.

The MUC1-protein precursor undergoes proteolytic modification immediately after translation is completed. The two resulting parts of the molecule remain associated through noncovalent sodium dodecyl sulfate (SDS)-sensitive forces. It has been reported that in addition to the major transmembrane form characterized by numerous tandem repeats, other minor forms of MUC1 can be found such as a secreted form and a form devoid of tandem repeats. These are considered to be a result of differential

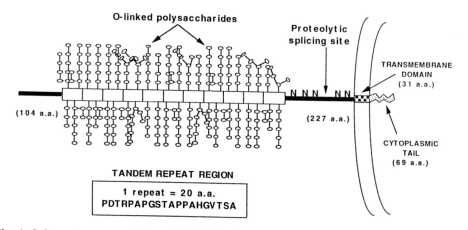

Fig. 1. Schematic representation of MUC1, a heavily glycosylated transmembrane protein.

splicing events. The existence of these minor forms is a relatively recent observation and their functional significance, especially as related to breast cancer, is currently being explored *(4)*. The most intensely studied form has been MUC1 consisting primarily of tandem repeats. The highly conserved, proline rich repetitive sequence PDTRPAPGSTAPPAHGVTSA is folded into an interesting three-dimensional structure elucidated by nuclear magnetic resonance (NMR) correlation spectroscopy, circular-dichroism (CD) spectroscopy, and intrinsic-viscosity (η) measurements of synthetic peptides *(5)*. It forms a stable type II β-turn with evenly spaced (every 20 amino acids) protruding "knobs" with the PDTRP sequence on the tip of each "knob". The stability of the "knobs" and the overall conformation of the molecule is enhanced and maintained in solutions by the multiplicity of the repeats *(6)*. We will discuss later in this chapter the consequences that this particular structure has on the recognition of MUC1 by the immune system.

2.2. Post-Translational Modifications of MUC1 in Tumor Cells and Normal Cells

MUC1 molecule undergoes a complex process of post-translational modifications before it is transported to the cell surface as a fully mature glycoprotein. Two early precursors have been identified after initiation of biosynthesis. Both are N-glycosylated and are different in molecular weight owing to a proteolytic cleavage of a 20 kDa fragment within 53–71 amino acids N-terminal to its transmembrane domain *(7)*. This is an early event that occurs approximately 1–2 min. after initiation of biosynthesis and therefore thought to take place in the endoplasmic retirculum (ER) *(8)*. Both fragments are then joined together noncovalently, but with a sufficiently strong association to keep the integrity of the molecule. It has been speculated that this proteolysis plays a role in intracellular transport and/or glycosylation. However, MUC1 devoid of tandem repeats does not undergo this proteolytic alteration and is still transported to the cell surface, as is the secreated form of MUC1 in which the proposed alternative splicing excludes the site of the cleavage. Clearly, further study is required to determine the exact role of post-translational proteolytic modification of the transmembrane form of

MUC1. The late precursor of the transmembrane form can be identified around 20–25 min after the initiation of biosynthesis; the time required for transit of the newly synthesized molecule from ER to Golgi. This form is O-glycosylated but not yet fully sialylated. It is transported to the plasma membrane and can be detected on the cell surface around 20–25 min later *(9)*. To be further glycosylated/sialylated all forms of MUC1 are repeatedly internalized and recycled through the trans-Golgi network until they are released into the outside environment or degraded when directed into the lysosomal pathway *(10)*. Each cycle is completed within 143 min, and an average MUC1 molecule undergoes 10 cycles before it is released into the environment within 24 h of its half-life *(10)*. The intracellular transit time of MUC1 may be affected by aberrant glycosylation *(11)*, making this process in tumor cells different than in normal cells. Our own observations indicate that underglycosylated tumor forms of MUC1 are preferentially retained on the surface of cancer cells, whereas the fully glycosylated forms are abundantly present in body fluids of cancer patients (unpublished data). Any change in the time it takes a molecule to be pocessed in any particular compartment of the cell, or any change in processing that this entails, affects the presentation of this molecule by the tumor cell or by surrounding antigen presenting cells to the immune system.

2.3. Normal and Aberrant O-Glycosylation

In vitro O-glycosylation of the tandem repeat region of MUC1 is a sequentially ordered process depending on the primary amino-acid sequence, length of the peptide, and relative position of the residues to be glycosylated *(12,13)*. Using the PDTRP sequence in the tandem repeat as an orientation marker, the threonine residue that is located N-terminally to this region is glycosylated first. Second is the threonine residue that is C-terminal to the immunodominant region, followed by glycosylation of the adjacent serine residue. There is no evidence that the threonine within the PDTRP sequence is glycosylated and glycosylation of the second serine residue within the tandem repeat remains undetermined. In normal breast epithelial cells, the GalNAc-T/S precursors are further glycosylated leading to the formation of long and branched polysaccharides with low relative contents of sialic acid *(1)*. In contrast, in breast-cancer cells, as well as in other cancer cells originating from ductal epithelial tissue, further glycosylation is prematurely terminated, leading to the accumulation of precursors such as 3GalNAcα1(O-Ser/Thr, known as a tumor-specific carbohydrate antigen Tn, Galβ1(3GalNAcα1)-O-Ser/Thr, known as T or TF antigen, and their sialylated forms: sTn and sT (sTF). These alterations in glycosylation have been found to be owing to both changes in the glycosylation machinery of the tumor cells *(1)* , as well as the increased level of production of MUC1.

3. MUC1 MUCIN AS A TUMOR ANTIGEN

All the aforementioned changes that during tumorigenesis affect breast epithelium, and MUC1 in particular, do not go unnoticed by the immune system. The premature truncation of oligosaccharide sidechains on tumor mucin has the effect of uncovering the polypeptide backbone of the molecule, and this in turn leads to exposure of antigenic epitopes that are recognized by the immune system. In addition, the MUC1 protein is no longer sequestered on the apical surface of an ordered ductal epithelium, as in the normal breast, but instead is abundantly expressed over the entire tumor cell surface, increasing the likelihood that cells of the immune system will encounter the antigen. Most importantly, B- and T-lymphocytes, which engage the tumor-associated MUC1 epitopes do so specifically; they do not recognize the glycosylated mucin protein expressed on normal breast epithelium. This, by definition, makes MUC1 a tumor-specific antigen.

The first indication that MUC1 mucin expressed by human adenocarcinomas was a tumor-specific antigen came from the characterization of murine monoclonal antibodies (MAbs) raised against whole tumor cells or human milk fat globule membranes. It was already appreciated at the time that MUC1 mucin was underglycosylated on breast-cancer cells as compared to normal tissue (14), and as a result it was possible to generate MAbs that recognized this difference. One antibody in particular, SM-3, was found to react with a core-protein epitope on breast-tumor cells and not on normal breast tissue (15). Using overlapping peptides of 8 amino acids in length, the target epitope of SM-3 was identified as the PDTRP sequence (16), which was later found on the tip of the immunodominant "knob" present within each tandem repeat (6). In fact, the majority of MUC1-specific MAbs appear to recognize this peptide sequence (17), probably because it extends out from the polypeptide backbone and hence is accessible to antibody binding. Surprisingly, however, a proportion of these antibodies are able to bind to normal, fully-glycosylated mucin, in contrast to the tumor-specific SM-3 antibody. This indicates that the peptide region is accessible to some antibodies despite the long oligosaccharide side-chains present on normal breast epithelial mucin. As we shall see, tumor-specific T-cells also recognize this peptide sequence, in perhaps the same manner as SM-3.

In breast cancer patients, tumor-reactive T-cells can be isolated from peritumoral lymph nodes resected at surgery, and these cells can be maintained and expanded by repeated stimulation in culture with allogeneic tumor cell lines (18). The original studies were done using a cytotoxic T-cell line derived from a patient with pancreatic cancer, another tumor type that expresses MUC1. This T-cell line was shown to kill 80% of pancreatic-tumor cell lines and all breast-tumor cell lines tested, but was shown not to react with melanoma, colon carcinoma, and a number of other tumor cell lines (18). The common feature between the tumor cells targeted by this T-cell line was expression of the MUC1 mucin antigen. To confirm that mucin was indeed the target antigen, inhibition studies were done that demonstrated that purified mucin protein and the MAb SM-3 both prevented T-cell-mediated cytolysis of tumor. Hence it appeared that the T-cells were recognizing the same epitope on the tandem-repeat region of mucin recognized by antibody SM-3. This was later defined as the immunodominant epitope on the tip of the "knob."

These in vitro studies identified MUC1 mucin as the target antigen for the tumor-specific cytotoxic T-cells (CTL), and also uncovered a highly unconventional mode of killing. Numerous tumor cell lines were killed despite having disparate major histocompatability complex (MHC) antigens, suggesting that the T-cells could target tumor-associated mucin independently of the MHC. In general, T-cells that express the αβ T-cell receptor recognize antigens that have been processed and presented as small peptide fragments associated with MHC molecules, and this recognition is restricted to target cells that bear the same MHC molecules as the T-cell. In these studies, however, the tumor cell killing was independent of MHC and was directed towards MUC1 mucin expressed as a native molecule at the tumor-cell surface. The results were soon repeated using T-cells isolated from a breast cancer patient and again using CTL from ovarian malignant tumors *(19,20)*. All these tumor types express the same underglycosylated MUC1 mucin molecule.

The hypothesis that was developed to explain the mechanism of antigen-specific but MHC-unrestricted recognition of MUC1 mucin was that a single T-cell was able to interact with multiple epitopes present in the extracellular domain of a single mucin molecule, and that this interaction could take place simultaneously, resulting in cross-linking of the T-cell receptor and subsequent T-cell activation. This model would explain the observation that T-cells from one patient could kill tumor cells from MHC-disparate individuals, as there would be no direct involvement in the MHC in antigen presentation to the T-cell. The hypothesis was supported by studies of mucin-specific T-cell lines from breast- and pancreatic-cancer patients, which were established using autologous or allogeneic mucin-transfected B cells as a source of antigen *(21)*. CTL stimulated with allogeneic transfectants killed mucin-transfected cells from the host, demonstrating that the T-cell lines were specific for mucin and not allogeneic antigens. Furthermore, the mucin-transfected targets required treatment with a competitive inhibitor of O-linked glycosylation, phenyl-GalNAc, to be recognized. This treatment presumably mimicked the state of underglycosylation present on tumor cells.

As previously stated, the epitope recognized by the MHC-unrestricted T-cells as well as tumor-specific antibodies resides on the polyproline-rich knob-like structure tandemly repeated along the polypeptide core of the tumor MUC1. It is an immunodominant epitope recognized by all breast cancer patients. Reactivity to other epitopes has been detected in T-cells from some patients *(22)*. The additional epitopes identified to date also reside in the tandem-repeat region of mucin, but are recognized in an MHC-restricted fashion. However, these antigens are not tumor specific; the epitope is not mutated on tumor cells and so potentially the same epitope could be presented by normal epithelium as well as breast-tumor epithelium. Their utility in the anti-tumor responses is, for the time being, considered limited. The major focus of mucin-based vaccine approaches against breast cancer, discussed in the following section, has been the tandem-repeat region of the molecule. This provides an opportunity to target the tumor-specific "knob" through stimulation of the MHC-unrestricted CTL, and also to test if MHC-restricted responses to other epitopes can be generated and be tumor-specific. In addition to peptide epitopes, the oligosaccharide side-chains on tumor-associated mucin may elicit a tumor-specific immune response. Attempts have been made to elicit protective immunity to Tn and T antigens and the sialylated counterparts sTn and sT *(23)*. It is also of great interest to determine if the tandem-repeat region contains epitopes that could bind to MHC class II molecules for stimulation of helper T-cells. T helper cell responses to mucin are required for generation of long-term immunologic memory for the tumor. Tumor-specific immune response is likely to be fundamental not only in the elimination of tumor but in prevention of the establishment of any future micrometastases which, if allowed to develop, can have disastrous consequences.

4. MUC1 MUCIN AS A CANCER VACCINE

In order to target effective immune responses to the unique, aberrant expression of MUC1 by tumor cells, there have been numerous attempts to incorporate this tumor antigen into various vaccine formulations. The goals of these studies have been to elicit tumor-specific, lasting immunity that has both the effector functions sufficient for the clearance of tumor without induction of autoimmunity, and the long-term memory to the mucin antigen. Some strategies employed so far in animal models and in humans primarily in Phase-I clinical trials, were effective at eliciting antibodies and delayed-type hypersensitivity (DTH) responses but were unable to elicit CTL responses, others have succeeded in developing cytolytic responses to mucin but clearance of tumor was not achieved. The challenge in developing a vaccine to mucin expressed by tumor cells is to target presentation of the mucin antigens to the appropriate location within the antigen-presenting cell and within the lymphatic system to obtain a full range of immune responses including cellular and humoral immunity that will result in elimination of tumor, and not precipitate autoimmunity.

4.1. Model Systems for Development of MUC1 Vaccines

4.1.1. Preclinical Studies

The development of mucin-vaccine protocols is complicated by the need for an appropriate animal model. Unfortunately, the mouse is not an ideal model to investigate immune responses to human mucin. Human MUC1 bears little homology to mouse MUC1 *(3)*, and is therefore recognized as a foreign antigen that is highly immunogenic in this model. A more relevant mouse model, MUC1 transgenic mouse, is now being bred for use in studies involving immune responses to human mucin expressed as a self-antigen *(24)*. This model will be particularly worthwhile because the expression of the human mucin within the mouse correlates precisely with the expression of MUC1 in human tissues. This will enable the observation of any potential problems related to tolerance or autoimmunity that could affect the result of immunization to mucin. Until vaccine trials involving these transgenic animals are conducted, the current studies employing conventional mice immunized with various forms of human mucin have proven very useful for the purposes of evaluating the most effective vaccine formulations to stimulate the desired mucin-specific immune responses within the limitations of this model.

The chimpanzee represents another, more relevant animal model for the study of mucin-specific immunity *(25)*. Chimpanzee MUC1 is virtually identical to the human molecule, and importantly, the immunodominant tandem-repeat region is completely identical. Immune responses stimulated by immunization against mucin in this animal model would therefore closely resemble the expected immune responses in humans. This animal model has been used for the evaluation of several vaccine formulations against mucin *(26–29)* and holds much promise for future studies.

4.1.2. Clinical Studies

Ultimately, the most critical evaluation of MUC1 vaccines will have to be derived from Phase I clinical trials with cancer patients. Clinical trials of several MUC1 vaccines have been initiated over the last several years and have yielded marginal but informative results *(30–32)*. It is very difficult to perform well-controlled immunologic studies in human subjects because they are an outbred population and patients with the same disease often undergo different treatment regimens that may impact on the vaccination outcome. It is also difficult to evaluate immunologic data obtained in Phase-I vaccine trials because for the most part they are designed primarily to test the toxicity of the vaccine and only secondarily its immunogenic potential. The patients entered into these Phase-I trials are often immunocompromised owing to either chemotherapeutic treatment or late stage of disease. Still, these studies must be done after the thorough investigation in appropriate animal models in order to gain further insight, if possible, into vaccine formulations and specific vaccination protocols that are likely to work well so that those can then be tested under optimal conditions. These include vaccinating patients early in disease before neither the disease nor other treatments have had a chance to adversely affect the immune system.

4.2. Design and Outcome of MUC1 Vaccines

Vaccines against MUC1 have been designed in many forms. The whole protein has been used as an immunogen, as have peptides derived from its amino-acid sequence. Carbohydrate moieties mimicking those exposed on the tumor mucin owing to its aberrant glycosylation have also been used in numerous forms to stimulate anti-tumor immunity. These antigenic preparations have been expressed in bacterial or viral vectors as fusion proteins, expressed in or pulsed onto several cell types, and have been used in conjunction with different adjuvants.

4.2.1. Peptide Vaccines

There are several difficulties associated with designing a peptide-based vaccine to induce recognition of mucin on tumor cells. As previously stated, there is currently only one tumor-specific peptide epitope identified, the immunodominant sequence PDTRP present at the beginning of each tandem repeat, recognized by MHC-unrestricted CTL (18–20). Recognition of this epitope by the CTL depends on the presence of at least several tandem repeats. To use this epitope as a synthetic vaccine that could boost MHC-unrestricted CTL has required synthesis of very long peptides. There have been reports of other MUC1 peptides that bind specific human major histocompatibility (HLA) class I molecules and could potentially serve as a vaccine to induce MUC1-specific MHC-restricted CTL. For example, one class-I MHC-binding epitope that has been reported is located in the MUC1 tandem-repeat sequence, between residues 9 and 17. It binds to HLA-A11 with high enough affinity to prime CTL that can kill HLA-A11[+] tumor cells (22). Some of the peptides from the same tandem-repeat region have been found to bind HLA-A2. The problem with these peptides is that there is no compelling reason to expect that they will elicit a tumor-specific response. Normal ductal epithelial cells in various organs express MUC1 as well as HLA class-I molecules and would be expected to present these MUC1 peptides equally well or perhaps better than the tumor cells. This would also make them susceptible targets to the immune-effector mechanisms induced by the peptide vaccination.

Inasmuch as all these questions can only be answered by designing appropriate experiments, several groups have continued to test peptide-based vaccines. One such vaccine study used a 20 amino-acid long peptide, corresponding to one MUC1 tandem repeat, which was coupled to a protein-carrier keyhole limpet hemocyanine (KLH), emulsified in RIBI® adjuvant, and administered to mice. This immunization was able to elicit a strong DTH reactions to peptides containing the immunodominant peptide PDTRP *(33)* but there was no induction of cytolytic T-cell responses. The immune responses generated through this vaccination were sufficient to slow the growth of tumor upon challenge, but not for tumor protection.

In another study in mice, stronger antibody responses against MUC1 were elicited by immunization with soluble peptides coupled to diptheria toxin and emulsified in Freund's adjuvant than by immunization with tumor cells *(34)*. Again, there was no evidence of CTL responses generated through this immunization, but some DTH responses were elicited. These studies demonstrate the effective induction of antibody and DTH responses to mucin when peptides are administered with adjuvants, but there is no evidence that these responses are sufficient to effect tumor rejection. These results are to be expected inasmuch as the preferred route of antigen presentation of soluble peptides is by MHC class-II molecules. This preferentially stimulates helper T-cells (DTH) and antibody production. The cytotoxic T-cells that are still considered the primary effector cell in tumor destruction are not readily stimulated by soluble antigens.

A peptide-vaccine strategy is currently being tested that could facilitate presentation of the peptides by both MHC class-I and class-II molecules. This is being attempted by conjugating a MUC1 peptide sequence to mannan (polymannose), which is expected to target this conjugate to the mannose receptors on antigen-presenting cells, in particular macrophages and dendritic cells. When one such conjugate containing five MUC1 tandem repeats was administered to mice intraperitoneally at weekly intervals for 3 wk, strong CTL responses developed. Interestingly, antibody responses that were also expected, were not elicited *(35)*. Still, the immunized mice were significantly protected against tumor challenge, confirming the need for CTL.

Success in generating a tumor-rejection CTL response in the mouse with this form of a peptide vaccine provided a basis for a clinical trial in patients with metastatic breast cancer. Twenty-five patients were immunized subcutaneously 8 times over a 13-wk period with the MUC1-mannan conjugate. Antibody, DTH, and CTL responses were monitored. Unlike the results in the mouse model, this treatment resulted in the development of antibody responses of the IgG isotype, T helper cell-proliferative responses to MUC1 peptides, and in a small number of patients, development of a CTL response. Though it could not be conclusively shown that these CTL responses were MHC restricted (owing to small sample size), there was a strong correlation with HLA-A2 expression and development of the CTL response. This group of investigators has previously described HLA-A2 restricted CTL responses to two mucin peptides (STAPPAHGV and APDTRPA) in HLA-A2 transgenic mice immunized with the same conjugate (I.F.C. McKenzie, personal communication) and these same epitopes may be involved in eliciting CTL in humans. These results collectively suggest that this vaccine protocol may serve as a powerful method to enhance uptake of peptide antigens and to induce strong CTL responses to class-I and class-II MUC1 epitopes. No specific epitopes on the MUC1 molecule have been defined to date that can be presented in human class II. Only a sporadic activation of helper T-cells following some immunization protocols, suggests that it might be possible to identify such epitopes and use them in vaccine preparations to generate helper T-cell responses more reproducibly. These responses are critically important for the amplification of both CTL and antibody responses.

The potential of a peptide-based vaccine to elicit or boost the MUC1-specific CTL responses to the MHC-unrestricted immunodominant epitope on the polyproline-rich knob, the only tumor-specific MUC1 epitope, is also being explored. After many years of in vitro experimentation, a phase-I clinical trial was performed using a 105 amino-acid synthetic MUC1 peptide (containing 5 tandem-repeat segments) admixed with BCG as an adjuvant *(30)*. In this clinical protocol, patients were immunized three times. Antibody, CTL, and DTH responses were monitored. As expected, this vaccine was best at boosting CTL immunity. There was no change in DTH or antibody responses *(30)*. The CTL numbers, although increased over the preimmunization samples, were still too low to be therapeutic. For the CTL to expand to higher numbers following activation, concurrent activation of tumor-specific helper cells must take place. For that reason, these and other investigators are trying to identify MUC1 helper epitopes that can be used in conjunction with epitopes designed to stimulate either MHC-unrestricted or MHC-restricted CTL.

4.2.2. Carbohydrate Vaccines

There have been several attempts to target-immune responses to tumor cells by immunizing with carbohydrate-based vaccines that mimic aberrant (tumor-specific) carbohydrates expressed on the MUC1 molecule. A great advantage of this vaccine is the exquisite tumor specificity of these epitopes. However, as immunogens they have many limitations, the main one being that they are expected to elicit only antibody responses. Moreover, the carbohydrate is recognized by B-cells as a hapten, which must be conjugated to a carrier protein in order to elicit helper T-cells needed for the full activation and antibody production by the B-cells. The helper T-cells generated are carrier-protein specific and not tumor-specific. Consequently, helper T-cell memory is also carrier-specific and not tumor-specific. This would not provide any long-term immune protection against potentially recurring tumor. Nevertheless, these vaccines have been tested in animal models and in clinical trials.

One such formulation incorporated the synthetic tumor associated glycoprotein antigen TF. The TF antigen was conjugated to a carrier protein, KLH, and mixed with the RIBI adjuvant *(36)* for injection into mice. This vaccination scheme was able to stimulate both DTH responses and antibody responses specific for carbohydrate determinants expressed on tumor cells (a T/Tn+ mammary adencarcinoma) or on a tumor-associated glycoprotein, epiglycanin. There was also some protection of these immunized mice against tumor challenge. A more recent study employed a similar protocol in which sialyl-Tn antigens coupled to KLH were admixed with RIBI adjuvant and administered to mice or patients with metastatic breast cancer. This protocol elicited strong IgG responses in mice, but weaker antibody responses in breast-cancer patients *(37)*. There was some evidence of DTH responses in these immunized patients, but only when immunized with small doses of antigen.

Some success in preventing recurrence of human breast adenocarcinoma has been achieved through repeated immunizations with the T/Tn antigen preparation derived from red blood cells *(38)*. This T/Tn antigen preparation was repeatedly administered to patients intradermally in Freund's adjuvant over the course of many years. This vaccination resulted in a strong DTH response at the site of immunization and a statistically significant reduction in the number of patients with recurrent disease.

4.2.3. Recombinant Viral Vectors and Naked DNA Vaccines

The use of viral vectors to elicit mucin-specific immunity is quite an attractive strategy, considering that the cDNA for this antigen has been isolated and it is possible to clone it into various vectors and take advantage of this new form of a vaccine that has been effective at eliciting both cellular and humoral immune responses to many other antigens. Antigens expressed in viral vectors also have the added benefit of being made inside an antigen-presenting cell and being available for presentation via class-I MHC to CTL.

There are also several problems associated with this vaccine approach. MUC1 mucin is a very unusual cDNA and difficult to stably incorporate into viral or other gene vectors owing to its numerous tandem repeats. These tandemly repeated segments are highly susceptible to homologous recombination and there is continuous loss of tandem repeats in cells infected with these vectors. This also leads to the loss of MUC1 immunogenicity. In spite of these theoretical and practical problems, there has been some progress in this area as demonstrated in several mouse models using a recombinant vaccinia *(39–42)*. These studies have confirmed the reproducible capacity of such vaccines to develop cellular immune responses to mucin. The most recent study employed a vaccine combining vaccinia virus that was engineered to express 10 tandem repeats of MUC1 with another vaccinia expressing the murine B-7 costimulatory molecule *(40)*. Mice immunized with the MUC1 recombinant vaccinia virus alone demonstrated CTL responses to mucin that were much enhanced in mice co-immunized with the recombinant vaccinia expressing the B-7 molecule. Two inoculations of the mucin expressing vaccinia were sufficient to prevent pulmonary metastasis in mice, but even three inoculations were not sufficient to protect the mice from succumbing to established tumor *(40)*.

A clinical trial is currently in progress using a vaccinia virus coexpressing MUC1 and IL-2 (VV-MUC1-IL-2). Nine patients with cutaneous metastasis of breast cancer were vaccinated. Serum analysis showed increased titer of IgG antibodies specific for the vaccinia virus and a slight rise in MUC1 specific IgM antibodies. One patient mounted a transient proliferative in vitro response to MUC1 tandem-repeat peptide 28 d after injection (stimulation index of 7). This patient was given a boost with the same dose of the VV-MUC1-IL-2 whereupon she mounted a more vigorous in vitro proliferative response to the MUC1 peptide (stimulation index of 14) at d 14 after the boost. This response also proved to be transient. Disease in all patients eventually progressed and they were put back on chemotherapy (B. Acres, personal communication).

A potentially useful approach for eliciting mucin-specific immunity in vivo is the use of naked MUC1 cDNA as an immunogen. In a single study reported so far, mice were immunized with varying doses of cDNA four times at 3-wk intervals. This method of immunization provided some protection against tumor challenge, in a dose-dependent manner with 100 μg DNA providing optimal protection (80% survival) *(42)*. Although both DTH and antibody responses were generated through this immunization, no CTL activity was elicited through injection of naked DNA alone.

4.2.4. Cellular Vaccines

The use of cellular vaccines for the development of mucin-specific immunity is based on the expectation that these types of vaccines will be able to present not only the correct antigen for tumor-specific immunity, but also provide the correct costimulatory signals required for the development of a strong, lasting immune response. One advantage of this immunization scheme is that antigens can be presented or expressed in specified locations based on whether the cell is pulsed with exogenous antigen, or engineered to express the antigen within the cell via any number of expression vectors. This enables the targeting of antigen to either MHC class I or class II for presentation. Numerous types of antigen-presenting cells have been used in these studies including tumor cells, B-cells, and dendritic cells. In attempts to develop tumor-specific immunity, autologous tumor cells have been used in several protocols by transfecting them with defined antigens and/or irradiating them in order to render them more immunogenic. In one such study, the human MUC1 gene was transfected into the mouse mammary-tumor cell line and the transfected cells used to immunize mice *(42)*. Such immunization resulted in a reduction in tumor incidence after challenge with the same MUC1+ tumor. Another such study compared immunization with mucin-tranfected 3T3 tumor cells with synthetic-peptide immunization *(34)*. This report demonstrated that only the immunization with tumor cells (MUC1+ 3T3 cells) was able to stimulate anti-mucin CTL activity and provide some protection against tumor challenge.

Another example of a cellular vaccine strategy that has been tested is using Epstein-Barr virus (EBV)-immortalized B-cells transfected with the MUC1 gene. This vaccine was designed to present MUC1 on the surface of a cell that also expresses costimulatory molecules *(79)*. In this study, the chimpanzee animal model was employed. Autologous EBV B-cells were transfected with cDNA encoding the human MUC1 gene. These B-cells were then treated with an inhibitor of glycosylation (to mimic the underglycosylated mucin expressed on tumor cells) and injected into chimpanzees four times, at three week intervals. This vaccine elicited a high frequency of CTL specific for the underglycosylated mucin, as well as helper T-cells. No antibody response was generated *(29)*.

A better outcome may be expected if instead of B-cells as antigen presenting cells (APC), a MUC1 vaccine were to use dendritic cells (DC) as APC. This cell type is thought to stimulate the greatest degree of T-cell activation and is the only cell type capable of priming naive T-cells *(43)*. With the recently improved techniques for the growth and culture of DC in vitro *(44,45)*, this cell type has become available for use in vaccines. DC can be derived from several sources, the easiest being peripheral blood monocytes cultured in granulocyte/macrophage colony stimulating factor (GM-CSF) and interleukin 4 (IL-4). Through this culture regimen, blood progenitors become terminally differentiated into DC and express high levels of both class-I and class-II MHC molecules as well as B7-1 and B7-2, the critical costimulatory molecules necessary for priming T-cells.

Recently, DC have been stably genetically engineered to express MUC1, using a retroviral vector *(46)*. This was accomplished by transducing progenitor CD34+ cells with a retroviral vector containing MUC1 cDNA and then differentiating the transduced progenitor cells in culture into DC using GM-CSF and IL-4. Mature DC expressed a full-length, highly glycosylated MUC1 on the cell surface. The same retroviral vector was also used to transduce an immortalized murine dendritic cell line, which was then used as a vaccine in a mouse model of mucin-specific immunity *(47)*.

This is the only vaccine approach so far that induced all the effector components of the immune response, cytolytic and proliferative T-cell responses as well as antibodies. DC-based MUC1 vaccines in which MUC1 is either expressed by the DC or MUC1 proteins and peptides are loaded onto the DCs are currently being tested in the chimpanzee model *(26,27)*.

Another type of DC vaccine has recently been utilized by Gong et al. They have fused MUC1$^+$ carcinoma cells to DC and used the hybrids to immunize mice in vivo *(48)*. The rationale for this method was to combine many putative antigens present on the tumor cell with the T-cell-activating potential of the DC to elicit strong and lasting tumor-specific immunity. Immunization of mice with such hybrids elicited the development of strong anti-tumor responses. Both CD4$^+$ and CD8$^+$ T-cells were required for protection against challenge with the same adeno-carcinoma. There was also the rejection of established metastases in mice immunized with these fused cells *(48)*.

5. CONCLUDING REMARKS AND PERSPECTIVES

Immunotherapy of breast cancer is an attractive idea whose time has come. Not only has immunologic knowledge advanced to the point where the failures from previous attempts at immunotherapy are fully understood, the new approaches based on the new knowledge are technologically within our reach. There are several molecules expressed in breast cancer that are candidates for breast-cancer vaccines. In addition to MUC1, immune responses have been documented to Her2/neu, p53, and carcino-embryonic antigen (CEA). Efforts are ongoing to identify others. Vaccine approaches based on individual antigens are currently being tested in animal models and in clinical trials. These studies will show the relative potential of different antigens as well as different vaccine formulations. It is conceivable that they will also show that combinations of these antigens, rather than each alone, will be needed for an effective tumor-rejection response. The next several years will see an increased use of these vaccines as therapy, preferably in the setting of minimal residual disease. The greatest benefit of cancer vaccines will ultimately be derived from using these prophylactically. Genetic studies have already focused on cancer-causing genes, two important ones, BRCA1 and BRCA2, have been identified in breast cancer. Epidemiological studies have also identified populations at risk for developing cancer owing to exposure to cancer-causing agents. One can foresee a rewarding future when cancer incidence will be lowered in these populations simply by the administration of an effective vaccine.

REFERENCES

1. Brockhausen, I., J.-M. Yang, J. Burchell, C. Whitehouse, and J. Taylor-Papadimitriou. 1995. Mechanisms underlying abberrant glycosyation of MUC1 mucin in breast cancer cells. *Eur. J. Biochem.* **233:** 606–617.
2. Shankar, V., P. Pichan, R. L. J. Eddy, V. Tonk, N. Nowak, S. N. Sait, T. B. Shows, R. E. Schultz, G. Gotway, R. C. Elkins, M. S. Gilmore, and G. P. Sachdev. 1997. Chromosomal localization of a human mucin gene (MUC–8) and cloning of the cDNA corresponding to the carboxy terminus. *Am. J. Respir. Cell Mol. Biol.* **16:** 232–241.
3. Gendler, S. J. and A. P. Spicer. 1995. Epithelial cell mucins. *Ann. Rev. Physiol.* **57:** 607–634.

4. Baruch, A., M. Hartman, S. Zrihan-Licht, S. Greenstein, M. Burstein, I. Keydar, M. Weiss, N. Smorodinsky, and D. H. Wreschner. 1997. Preferential expression of novel MUC1 tumor antigen isoforms in human epithelial tumors and their tumor-potentiating function. *Int. J. Cancer* **71:** 741–749.

5. Fontenot, J. D., N. Tjandra, D. Bu, C. Ho, R. C. Montelaro, and O. J. Finn. 1993. Biophysical characterization of one-, two-, and three -tandem repeats of human mucin (MUC1) protein core. *Cancer Res.* **53:** 5386–5394.

6. Fontenot, J. S., S. Mariappan, S. V. Catasti, N. Domenech, O. J. Finn, and G. Gupta. 1994. Structure of a tumor associated antigen containing a tandemly repeated immunodominant epitope. *J. Biomol. Str. Dyn.* **13:** 245–260.

7. Ligtenberg, M. J. L., L. Kruijshaar, F. Bujis, M. van Meijer, and S. V. Litvinov. 1992. Cell associated episialin is a complex containing two proteins derived from a common precursor. *J. Biol. Chem.* **267:** 6171–6177.

8. Hilkens, J. and F. Bujis. 1988. Biosynthesis of MAM–6, an epithelial sialomucin. *J. Biol. Chem.* **263:** 4215–4222.

9. Linsley, P. S., J. C. Kallestad, and D. Horn. 1988. Biosynthesis of high molecular weight breast cancer associated mucin glycoproteins. *J. Biol. Chem.* **263:** 8390–8397.

10. Litvinov, S. V. and J. Hilkens. 1993. The epithelial sialomucin, episialin, is sialylated during recycling. *J. Biol. Chem.* **268:** 21,364–21,271.

11. Pimental, R. A., J. Julian, S. J. Gendler, and D. D. Carson. 1996. Synthesis and intracellular trafficking of MUC1 and mucins by polarized mouse uterine epithelial cells. *J. Biol. Chem.* **271:** 28,128–28,137.

12. Nishimori, I., N. R. Johnson, S. D. Sanderson, F. Perini, K. Mountjoy, R. L. Cerny, M. I. Gross, and M. A. Hollingsworth. 1994. Influence of acceptor substrate primary amino acid sequence on the activity of human UDP-acetylgalactosamine:polypeptide N-acetylgalactosaminyltransferase. *J. Biol. Chem.* **269:** 16,123–16,130.

13. Stadie, T. R. E., W. Chai, A. M. Lawson, P. G. H. Byfield, and F.-G. Hanish. 1995. Studies on the order and site specificity of GalNAc transfer to MUC1 tandem repeats by UDP-GalNac:polypeptide N-acetylgalactosaminlyltransferase from milk of mammary carcinoma cells. *Eur. J. Biochem.* **229:** 140–147.

14. Hareuveni, M., C. Gautier, M.-P. Kienv, D. Wreschner, P. Chambon, and R. Lathe. 1990. Vaccination against tumor cells expressing breast cancer epithelial tumor antigen. *Proc. Natl. Acad. Sci. USA* **87:** 9498–9502.

15. Burchell, J., S. Gendler, J. Taylor-Papadimitriou, A. Girling, A. Lewis, R. Millis, and D. Lamport. 1987. Development and characterization of breast cancer reactive monoclonal antibodies directed to the core protein of the human milk mucin. *Cancer Res.* **47:** 5476–5482.

16. Burchell, J., J. Taylor-Papadimitriou, M. Boschell, and T. Duhig. 1989. A short sequence within the amino acid tandem repeat of a cancer-associated mucin contains immunodominant epitopes. *Int. J. Cancer* **44:** 691–696.

17. Xing, P. X., J. J. Tjandra, S. A. Stacker, J. G. The, C. H. Thompson, P. J. McLaughlin, and I. F. C. McKenzie. 1989. Monoclonal antibodies reactive with mucin in breast cancer. *Immuno. Cell Biol.* **67:** 183–195.

18. Barnd, D. L., M. S. Lan, R. S. Metzgar, and O. J. Finn. 1989. Specific, major histocompatibility complex-unrestricted recognition of tumor-associated mucins by human cytotoxic T cells. Proc. *Natl. Acad. Sci. USA* **86:** 7159–7163.

19. Jerome, K. R., D. L. Barnd, K. M. Bendt, C. M. Boyer, J. Taylor-Papadimitriou, I. F. C. McKenzie, J. R. C. Bast, and O. J. Finn. 1991. Cytotoxic T lymphocytes derived from patients with breast adenocarcinoma recognize an epitope present on the protein core of a mucin molecule preferentially expressed by malignant cells. *Cancer Res.* **51:** 2908–2916.

20. Ioannides, C. G., B. Fisk, K. R. Jerome, T. Irimura, J. T. Wharton, and O. J. Finn. 1993. Cytotoxic T cells from ovarian malignant tumors can recognize polymorphic epithelial mucin core peptides. *J. Immunol.* **151:** 3693–3703.

21. Jerome, K. R., N. Domenech, and O. J. Finn. 1993. Tumor-specific cytotoxic T cell clones from patients with breast and pancreatic adenocarcinoma recognize EBV-immortalized B cells transfected with polymorphic epithelial cell mucin complimentary DNA. *J. Immunol.* **151:** 1654–1662.

22. Domenech, N., R. A. Henderson, and O. J. Finn. 1995. Identification of an HLA-A11-restricted epitope from the tandem repeat domain of the epithelial tumor antigen mucin. *J. Immunol.* **155:** 4766–4774.

23. Longenecker, B. M., M. Reddish, R. Koganty, and G. D. MacLean. 1994. Specificity of the IgG response in mice and human breast cancer patients following immunization against synthetic sialyl-Tn, an epitope with possible functional significance in metastasis, in *Antigen and Antibody Molecular Engineering in Breast Cancer Diagnosis* (Ceriani, R. L., ed.), Plenum, New York, pp. 105–124.

24. Peat, N., S. J. Gendler, E.-N. Lalani, T. Duhig, and J. Taylor-Papadimitriou. 1992. Tissue-specific expression of a human polymorphic epithelial mucin (MUC1) in transgenic mice. *Cancer Res.* **52:** 1954–1960.

25. Barratt-Boyes, S. M. 1996. Making the most of mucin: a novel target for immunotherapy. *Cancer Immunol. Immunother.*

26. Barratt-Boyes, S. M., R. A. Henderson, and O. J. Finn. 1996. Chimpanzee dendritic cells with potent immunostimulatory function can be propagated from peripheral blood. *Immunology* **87:** 528–534.

27. Barratt-Boyes, S. M., H. Kao, and O. J. Finn. 1998. Chimpanzee dendritic cells derived in vitro from blood monocytes and pulsed with antigen elicit specific immune responses in vivo. *J. Immunother.* **21:** 142–148.

28. Barratt-Boyes, S. M., S. C. Watkins, and O. J. Finn. 1997. In vivo migration of dendritic cells generated in vitro. *J. Immunol.* **158:** 4543–4547.

29. Pecher, G. and O. J. Finn. 1996. Induction of cellular immunity in chimpanzees to human tumor-associated antigen mucin by vaccination with MUC1 cDNA-transfected Epstein-Barr virus immortlized autologous B cells. *Proc. Natl. Acad. Sci. USA* **93:** 1699–1704.

30. Goydos, J. S., E. Elder, T. L. Whiteside, O. J. Finn, and M. T. Lotze. 1996. A phase I clinical trial of a synthetic mucin peptide vaccine. *J. Surg. Res.* **63:** 289–304.

31. MacLean, D. G., M. Redidsh, R. Koganty, S. Gandhi, M. Smolnski, J. Samuel, J. M. Nabholtz, and B. M. Longenecker. 1993. Immunization of breast cancer patients using a synthetic sialyl-Tn glycoconjugate plus Detox adjuvant. *Cancer Immunol. Immunother.* **36:** 215–222.

32. Kjeldsen, T., H. Clausen, S. Hirohashi, T. Ogawa, H. Iijima, and S. Hakamori. 1988. Preparation and characterization of monoclonal antibodies directed to the tumor-associated O-linked sialosyl-2-6α N-acetyl-galactosaminyl (sialosyl-Tn) epitope. *Cancer Res.* **48:** 2214–2220.

32. McKenzie, I. F. C. 1998. Antibody and T cell responses of patients with adenocarcinomas immunized with mannan-MUC1 fusion protein. *J. Clin. Invest.* **100:** 2783–2795.

33. Ding, L., E. N. Lalani, M. Reddish, R. Kaganty, T. Wong, J. Samuel, M. B. Yacshyn, A. Miekle, P. Y. S. Fung, J. Taylor-Papadimitriou, and B. M. Longenecker. 1993. Immunogenicity of synthetic peptides related to the core peptide sequence encoded by the human MUC1 gene: effects of immunization of the growth of murine mammary adenocarcinoma cells transfected with the human MUC1 gene. *Cancer Immunol. Immunother.* **36:** 9–17.

34. Apostolopulous, V., P.-X. Xing, and I. F. C. McKenzie. 1994. Murine immune reponse to cells transfected with the human MUC1: immunization with cellular and synthetic antigens. *Cancer Res.* **54:** 5186–5193.

35. Apostolopoulos, V., G. A. Pietersz, and I. F. C. Mckenzie. 1996. Cell mediated immune reponse to MUC1 fusion protein coupled to mannan. *Vaccine* **14:** 930–938.

36. Henningson, C. M., S. Selvaraj, G. D. MacLean, M. R. Suresh, A. A. Noujaim, and B. M. Longenecker. 1987. T cell recognition of a tumor-associated glycoprotein and its synthetic carbohydrate epitopes: stimulation of anti-cancer T cell immunity in vivo. *Cancer Immunol. Immunother.* **25:** 231–241.

37. Longenecker, B. M., M. Reddish, R. Koganty, and G. D. MacLean. 1993. Immune responses of mice and human breast cancer patients following immunization with synthetic sialyl-Tn conjugated to KLH plus detox adjuvant. *Ann. NY Acad. Sci.* **690:** 276–291.

38. Springer, G. F., P. R. Desai, H. Tegtmeyer, S. C. Carlstedt, and E. F. Scanlon. 1994. T/Tn antigen vaccine is effective and safe in preventing recurrence of human advanced breast carcinoma. *Cancer Biother.* **9:** 7–15.

39. Acres, R. B., M. Hareuveni, J.-M. Balloul, and M.-P. Kieny. 1993. Vaccinia virus MUC1 Immunization of mice: immune response and protection against the growth of murine tumors bearing the MUC1 antigen. *J. Immunother.* **14:** 136–143.

40. Akagi, J., J. W. Hodge, J. P. McLaughlin, L. Gritz, G. Mazzara, D. Kufe, J. Schlom, and J. A. Kantor. 1997. Therapeutic antitumor response after immunization with an admixture of recombinant vaccinia viruses expressing a modified MUC1 gene and the murine costimulatory molecule B-7. *J. Immunother.* **20:** 38–47.

41. Bu, D., N. Domenech, J. Lewis, J. Taylor-Papamadimitriou, and O. J. Finn. 1993. Recombinant vaccina mucin vector: in vitro analysis of tumor-associated epitopes for antibody and human cytoxic T cell function. *J. Immunother.* **14:** 127–135.

42. Graham, R. A., J. M. Burchell, P. Beverly, and J. Taylor-Papadimitriou. 1996. Intramuscular immunization with MUC1 cDNA can protect C57 mice challenged with MUC1-expressing syngeneic mouse tumor cells. *Int. J. Cancer* **65:** 664–670.

43. Steinman, R. M. 1991. The dendritic cell system and its role in immunogenicity. *Ann. Rev. Immunol.* **9:** 217–296.

44. Caux, C., C. Dezutter-Dambuyant, D. Schmitt, and J. Banchereau. 1992. GM-CSF and TNF-α cooperate in the generation of dendritic Langerhan cells. *Nature* **360:** 258–261.

45. Sallusto, F. and A. Lanzavecchia. 1994. Efficient presentation of soluble antigen by cultured human dendritic cells is maintained by granulocyte/macrophage colony-stimulating factor plus interleukin 4 and downregulated by tumor necrosis factor α. *J. Exp. Med.* **179:** 1109–1118.

46. Henderson, R. A., M. T. Nimgaonkar, S. C. Watkins, P. D. Robbins, E. D. Ball, and O. J. Finn. 1996. Human dendritic cells genetically engineered to express high levels of human epithelial tumor antigen mucin (MUC1). *Cancer Res.* **56:** 3763–3770.

47. Henderson, R. A., W. M. Konitsky, S. M. Barratt-Boyes, M. Soares, P. D. Robbins, and O. J. Finn. 1997. Retroviral expression of MUC1 human tumor antigen with intact tandem repeat structure and capacity to elicit immunity in vivo. *J. Immunother.*, in press.

48. Gong, J., D. Chen, M. Kashiwaba, and D. Kufe. 1997. Induction of antitumor activity by immunization with fusions of dendritic and carcinoma cells. *Nature Med.* **3:** 558–561.

22

Aromatase Inhibitors and the Role
of Hormonal Therapy in Breast Cancer

Kendall E. Donaldson Herschler and Angela Brodie

1. INTRODUCTION

Breast cancer is the second leading cause of cancer death among American women, afflicting one in eight women and killing more than 46,000 women each year *(1,2)*. In the United States, a woman has a 10.2% cumulative lifetime probability of developing breast cancer with a 3.0% probability of the affliction culminating in death *(2)*. A disease of such prevalence and devastating consequences places imminent demands on researchers and clinicians to elucidate the optimal treatment strategies for various patient populations. This challenge has also opened the door to continued efforts in the search for further treatment options with hopes to increase patient longevity and quality of life.

2. ETIOLOGY OF BREAST CANCER

An effective evaluation of various treatment strategies for breast cancer requires a preliminary consideration of the epidemiology and risk factors associated with the disease. The development and progression of breast cancer appears to be owing to a complex interplay between genetic, environmental and endocrine factors. The elucidation of these factors through epidemiological studies allows us to target particular high-risk populations for screening and primary prevention programs. The difficulty with designing such programs, is that 70–80% of breast cancer patients do not have any presently determined risk factors *(3)*.

Some of the risk factors found to be highly associated with breast cancer include family history of breast cancer, duration of exposure to estrogens (early menarche and late menopause increase risk), late first pregnancy, and exposure to radiation *(4,5)*. Some factors have shown weak association including some types of fibrocystic breast changes (with atypical hyperplasia), hormone replacement therapy, and use of diethylstilbestrol during pregnancy. Whereas, other factors once hypothesized to have been associated with the disease have not been substantiated, including dietary fat intake and oral contraceptives as currently used.

There are three primary genetic risk factors that have been associated with breast cancer. Having a first degree relative (including a sister, mother, or child) with breast

From: Breast Cancer: *Molecular Genetics, Pathogenesis, and Therapeutics*
Edited by: A. M. Bowcock © Humana Press Inc., Totowa, NJ

cancer increases the risk by two to three fold, relative to the general population *(4,6)*. The risk is further increased if the relative was premenopausal at the onset of the disease or if the cancer was bilateral. Aside from this nonspecific propensity toward the disease, two genetic mutations have also been associated with breast cancer. Approximately five percent of breast cancer patients have a point mutation in the p53 tumor suppressor gene on chromosome 17 *(7)*. This mutation has been linked to a variety of cancers including: breast, colon, cervical, brain, bladder, ovarian, and lung cancer. In total, the p53 gene has now been implicated in 52 varieties of human cancer and could also provide us with some insights into a potential treatment strategy for cancer as a single entity *(7,8)*. A second genetic association, also localized to chromosome 17 is the loss of heterozygosity at the BRCA1 gene found on the long arm of the chromosome *(9,10)*. The penetrance of this mutation is estimated to be as high as 85% *(9,10)*. Estimates of the mutation's prevalence range from 1 in 200 to 1 in 400 American woman who are carriers for the trait *(9,10)*. Similarly, a gene known as BRCA2 has been localized to chromosome 13 and has also been associated with a susceptibility to breast cancer *(11)*. However, these two mutations account for only a fraction of the total cases of breast cancer. Some of these genetic risk factors are discussed in greater detail in other chapters.

Women with fibrocystic breast changes with severe or atypical hyperplasia are at increased risk of progression to breast cancer *(12)*. Fibrocystic breast changes characterize a benign condition of nonspecific proliferation of epithelial and mesenchymal tissue and the presence of macroscopic, fluid-filled cysts throughout the breast. Women biopsied and found to have this condition with evidence of ductal or lobar cell proliferation (without atypical hyperplasia) have a 1.9 relative risk of proceeding to develop breast cancer, whereas women with atypical hyperplasia have a 5.3 relative risk (95% CI = 3.1–8.8) of developing cancer *(13)*. If a woman has both atypic fibrocystic changes and a first degree relative with breast cancer, her risk of cancer is increased approx 11-fold (95% CI = 5.5–24) *(13)*.

Endocrine factors associated with breast cancer may provide answers regarding both etiology of and treatment strategies for the disease. Early menarche, nulliparity, late age of first pregnancy and late onset of menopause are independently associated with breast cancer incidence *(4)*. It has been hypothesized that diet and exercise may be indirectly associated with the disease through their effects on age of menarche and regularity of menses. The higher incidence of breast cancer in Westernized societies has been attributed to differences in dietary fat intake *(16)*. However, studies investigating the relationship between diet, obesity and breast cancer are difficult to perform and easily confounded, and well-controlled trials are still needed to establish the importance of diet and dietary fat in breast cancer. Further discussion of these issues is provided in Chapter 25. Early pregnancy (prior to age 18) appears to be protective while late pregnancy (after age 30) appears to promote development of the disease *(4)*. Estrogen clearly has the single most important role in breast cancer, as the disease rarely occurs in ovariectomized individuals. However, only recently has a mechanism which might increase endogenous estrogen production been proposed. Breast cancer risk was found to be associated with polymorphism of the CYP 17 gene that encodes for 17α-hydroxylase-$C_{17,20}$-lyase which mediate the synthesis of estrogen precursor steroids and could result in a lifetime increase in estrogen exposure *(14)*. In recent studies, we identified expression of aromatase in both normal breast epithelium and stromal cells in breast cancer, suggesting that local production of estrogen may have a role in promoting breast cancer *(15)*. Despite the strong association of hormonal regulation with breast cancer, use of oral contraceptives and hormone replacement therapy appear to play only a minor (if any) role in the etiology of breast cancer. Use of estrogen replacement therapy (ERT) for less than ten years does not increase disease risk, however prolonged use of estrogen (exceeding 10 yr) has been reported to yield a relative risk between 1.3 and 2.2 *(3)*. Romieu et al. conducted a meta-analysis of the literature to determine the association between oral contraceptives and breast cancer incidence. They found no association except in premenopausal women who had used oral contraceptives for at least four years prior to their first pregnancy (RR = 1.72, 95% CI = 1.36–2.19) *(17)*. Most studies that have observed a strong association between contraceptive use and breast cancer were conducted prior to the introduction of pills containing lower doses of hormones (1970s and 1980s). In addition, the use of oral contraceptives for more than four years prior to the first pregnancy has been reported to increase the relative risk for breast cancer to 1.7 *(2)*. The benefits with regard to cardiovascular health of ERT and prevention of unwanted pregnancies by the oral contraceptive pill outweigh the equivocal or minor elevations of relative risk in most cases.

It is difficult to estimate an individual's risk for breast cancer since most of the etiological factors elucidated thus far probably do not exert their effects independently and may function additively or synergistically in many cases. However, the greatest difficulty still remains the fact that 70–80% of breast cancer cases emerge with no known underlying risk factors. Ongoing efforts to uncover the basis of the disease will hopefully expose new interventions and treatment strategies for breast cancer.

3. TREATMENT

Over the past hundred years since the discovery of the hormone dependency of breast cancer, major advances have been made in development of new treatment modalities, particularly in the area of endocrine therapy and in the promotion of more conservative surgical interventions. Treatment options are subdivided into curative and palliative therapy and are issued according to disease stage and prognosis. A wide variety of prognostic factors are used in determining treatment options for patients with early stage breast cancer, including: tumor size, extent of lymph node involvement, hormone receptor status (estrogen and progesterone receptors present/absent), histologic and nuclear grade of tumor (polyploidy/ aneuploidy, number of mitotic figures per high power field, degree of differentiation), C-erbB-2 oncoprotein expression, and the presence of metastasis.

3.1. Chemotherapy

Based on measurements of estrogen and progesterone concentrations in the tumor, patients with low levels of steroid receptors are treated with cytotoxic agents. These include about 60% of premenopausal patients, whereas among postmenopausal patients a higher proportion are likely to respond to hormonal therapy, as only approx 30% are ER negative *(18)*. Although breast cancer responds to several types of cytotoxic agents, it responds preferentially to adriamycin. Substantial response also occurs with cyclophosphamide (C), methotrexate (M), and 5-fluorouracil (F). Recently, taxol derivatives, paclitaxol and taxotere, have also been found to produce an impressive response rate. Combinations of these drugs, such as CA, CAF, or CMF, have been shown to be more effective than individual agents. These drugs have maximum benefit when administered for periods of four to six months. Treatment with all of these agents are accompanied by substantial toxicities. Over the past 10 yr, high dose chemotherapy with autologous stem cell support has been performed in patients with refractory or responsive metastatic breast cancer and in patients with high-risk primary breast cancer in phase I and II trials. Results thus far are promising but inconclusive as phase III trials need to be conducted before this therapy is offered to patients outside the confines of an organized clinical trial. Unresolved questions include which patient populations will most benefit from this therapy, whether the benefits outweigh the toxicities, and whether patients will enjoy long-term quality of life as a result of this intervention.

3.2. Endocrine Therapy

In 1896, Beatson surgically removed the ovaries of premenopausal patients and found that this led to regression of breast cancer in most cases *(19)*. Later, adrenalectomy/hypophysectomy which induces estrogen deprivation, yielded similar results indicating a primary role for estrogen in the growth and development of breast cancer. These studies provided the rationale for endocrine therapy. As indicated above, not all malignant tumors of the breast are responsive to endocrine therapy. However, there is an age related increase in dependence of tumors on hormones *(18)*. Thus, tumors of postmenopausal patients are more likely to be dependent on estrogen for their progression. Estrogen receptor positive tumors are more common in older women and are generally more differentiated, slower growing, and carry a more positive prognosis. Following menopause, when the ovary is no longer the main source of estrogen, production is increased in peripheral tissue, such as adipose and muscle which compose most of the body mass. Thus, systemic approaches to treatment, rather than surgical removal of adrenals or the pituitary, have been proving effective in blocking the effects of estrogens, are well tolerated and are associated with less morbidity and mortality. Patients who have soft tissue and bone involvement are more likely to respond to endocrine therapy as compared to those with visceral involvement. The only option for patients with metastatic disease who are nonresponsive to endocrine therapy and/or are estrogen receptor negative is systemic chemotherapy.

One of the main advantages of endocrine therapy is the low incidence of side effects in comparison with chemotherapy. A number of endocrine therapies are now available. LHRH analogs can be used as alternatives to ovariectomy for premenopausal patients. They function to modify the adrenal/pituitary axis, thus reducing circulating estrogen. LHRH analogs cause initial stimulation of pituitary LH release followed by inhibition of LH secretion. This inhibition is thought to be owing to a down-regulation of LHRH receptors in the pituitary. The lack of LHRH stimulation of the pituitary causes a decreased release of gonadotrophin and therefore a decrease in estrogen synthesis, but it does not affect peripheral conversion of adrenal androgens to estrogens. Therefore, LHRH analogs are useful only in the treatment of premenopausal breast cancer. Their use in conjunction with an aromatase inhibitor appears to be an effective strategy *(see below) (20)*. High dose progestins, androgens, corticosteroids, have been used to treat postmenopausal patients but are associated with notable side effects. Antiestrogens, and more recently aromatase inhibitors are specifically targeted for blocking the effects of estrogen and are better tolerated than high dose progestins, androgens or corticosteroids. These agents are discussed in more detail below.

3.2.1. Antiestrogens

Antiestrogens, such as tamoxifen, were designed to block the action of estrogens by binding with high affinity to the estrogen receptor. Aromatase inhibitors reduce the amount of available estrogen by blocking its synthesis. Both agents deprive the tumor of its stimulus for proliferation. Although less well defined, it is believed that other agents such as progestins and androgens, also provide an antiproliferative effect by inhibiting the physiologic stimulus through their hormonal receptors (when present) in the tumor and by alterations in circulating hormone levels.

The use of tamoxifen for estrogen receptor positive tumors has been an important therapeutic advance in breast cancer treatment. The efficacy of tamoxifen in the treatment of breast cancer was first reported by Cole et al. in 1971, and has since become the most widely used endocrine therapy in breast cancer *(21)*. The Early Breast Cancer Trialists' Collaborative Group established the efficacy of tamoxifen over chemotherapy as the treatment of postmenopausal breast cancer *(22)*. This group reviewed 40 randomized clinical trials of tamoxifen with more than 30,000 patients, 22,000 of whom had been taking tamoxifen for at least two years and 8,000 who had been taking tamoxifen for at least one year. The analysis compared the use of tamoxifen, with or without chemotherapy, with placebo. All of the trials in this analysis began prior to 1985 and have been analyzed to determine the 10-yr relapse and mortality rates. The meta-analysis yielded three conclusions regarding the efficacy of tamoxifen treatment. Results of the trials showed that a greater decrease in relapse and mortality rates was achieved during extended duration of therapy (at least 2 yr) with tamoxifen. The overall 10 year mortality for node-negative patients was 26.5% for patients receiving tamoxifen and 29% for patients in the placebo group ($p < 0.001$). For node positive patients, the 10-yr mortality rate was 49.6% for the tamoxifen group and 57.8% for the placebo group ($p < 0.001$). The effects of tamoxifen were most pronounced in postmenopausal women over the age of sixty. The analysis predictably revealed tamoxifen to be most effective in cases of estrogen receptor positive tumors as compared with receptor-poor tumors (<10 fmols/mg cytosolic protein). The differences in mortality rates may appear meager, however the absolute number of patients surviving for a longer duration after diagnosis provides these findings with clinical significance.

Although the use of tamoxifen in node positive disease is widely accepted and recommended by the National Institutes of Health Consensus Development Panel on Adjuvant Chemotherapy and Endocrine Therapy, its efficacy has been debated in node-negative patients with estrogen-receptor positive tumors. Fisher et al. (1989) conducted a double-blind randomized placebo-controlled clinical trial of postoperative therapy with tamoxifen (10 mg twice a day) in 2644 patients with early stage breast cancer *(23)*. During a four year follow-up period, no survival advantage was observed (92% in the placebo group vs 93% in the treatment group). However, a significant increase in disease-free survival was observed in the women who were treated with tamoxifen (83% vs 77%; $p < 0.001$). This observation was consistent among premenopausal and postmenopausal patients. Additionally, the rate of treatment failure was reduced by

44% in patients under the age of 50. Few side effects were observed. These included nausea, vomiting, and hot flashes and resulted in a similar number of patients withdrawing from the tamoxifen and control groups. In addition, the drug significantly reduced the rate of treatment failure at local and distant sites, reduced tumor recurrence in the same location after lumpectomy and breast irradiation, and reduced recurrence in the opposite breast as compared with placebo. This study, as well as others, supports the premise that tamoxifen therapy may have an overall advantage independent of menopausal, nodal, or estrogen-receptor status. Multivariate analyses on the data failed to identify any subgroup of patients who would not benefit from tamoxifen therapy. The moderate benefit of tamoxifen in node-negative patients may outweigh the minimal side effects in many patients. However, patients must still be considered on an individual basis, at least until further trials have substantiated the findings of this study.

Most breast cancer patients with metastatic disease experience at least a trial with tamoxifen during management of their disease. A patient's response to tamoxifen is determined by four factors including estrogen receptor status, age of the patient, dominant site of the disease and previous exposure to endocrine therapy. Tamoxifen has been compared with other endocrine therapies and has been found to be equally effective and extremely well-tolerated by patients with very few side effects. Unfortunately, the antiestrogenic activity of tamoxifen is limited to the tumor cells and tamoxifen may actually function as an estrogen agonist in other regions of the body occasionally leading to secondary tumors of the liver and uterus (24). Several studies have documented the role of tamoxifen in the development of hepatic tumors in rats receiving high-dose exposure, although this finding has not been substantiated in humans (24–26). Other studies have noted a threefold increased incidence of endometrial carcinoma in tamoxifen treated patients (27,28). However, the beneficial effects of its estrogenic action on preventing osteoporosis and decreasing the risk of cardiovascular disease could prove helpful in long-term management. Other research efforts have focused on the development of new antiestrogen agents that are free of the peripheral estrogenic activities of tamoxifen (such as is evident on the endometrium) with hopes of reducing the incidence of secondary tumors. Alternatively, these agents may be useful following treatment failure with other agents. Two of these "pure" antiestogens are roloxifene and toremifene which are presently undergoing clinical trials. Studies evaluating tamoxifen combined with one or two other endocrine therapies administered simultaneously have not shown any advantage of the combination therapy to date (29). By administering endocrine therapies individually and sequentially, it is more likely that a longer therapeutic effect will be achieved by using a second agent following treatment failure or development of resistance to the initial agent. Tamoxifen in conjunction with systemic chemotherapy also has been shown to provide the patient with no additional benefit over chemotherapy alone (30).

Despite its success in reducing tumor size and lessening recurrences, resistance ultimately develops to tamoxifen leaving the tumor to flourish unabated. Following prolonged exposure to tamoxifen a selection process may occur favoring cells which have mutations of the estrogen receptor which allow cells to use tamoxifen to stimulate proliferation or increase its estrogenicity (31). There now appears to be little evidence to support intracellular tamoxifen metabolism as a mechanism of tamoxifen resistance (32). However, several other speculations have been made to explain the development of resistance to tamoxifen, such as an alteration in receptor proteins (33).

3.2.2. Aromatase Inhibitors

Although originally designed in part as a non-estrogenic alternative to antiestrogen such as tamoxifen by Schwarzel et al. *(34),* aromatase inhibitors are presently proving useful in tamoxifen treatment failures. These compounds function effectively to halt estrogen synthesis by inhibiting aromatase (cytochrome $P450_{arom}$). Following the publication of a pioneering paper from our group in 1973, development of aromatase inhibitors has progressed over the last 23 yr. Today, aromatase inhibitors are the latest addition to breast cancer treatment. These inhibitors include steroidal substrate analogs and nonsteroidal compounds and are classified as competitive inhibitors (type II), affinity labels, and mechanism-based inhibitors (suicide inactivators or irreversible type I inhibitors). Summaries of research studies (basic and clinical aspects) on aromatase inhibitors have been published from three international conferences *(35–37)* and a number of reviews on aromatase inhibitors have also appeared. *(38–40).*

Steroidal aromatase inhibitors, such as 4-hydroxyandrostenedione (formestane) shown in Fig. 1, are substrate analogs and also "suicide" inactivators of the enzyme, while the nonsteroidal compounds are type II inhibitors. Suicide inactivators are thought to compete with the natural substrate and subsequently interact with the active site of the enzyme. They bind either very tightly or irreversibly to the enzyme, thus causing its inactivation *(41).* Because they bind irreversibly to the active site, these inhibitors are quite specific and have lasting effects in vivo. Thus, the continued presence of the drug to maintain inhibition is not necessary when using type I (suicide) inhibitors, and the chance of toxic side effects will therefore be reduced.

The nonsteroidal inhibitors possess a heteroatom as a common feature that interferes with steroidal hydroxylation by binding with the heme iron of cytochrome P-450 $_{arom}$. Although nonsteroidal type II inhibitors were developed from antifungal agents which inhibit multiple cytochrome P-450-mediated hydroxylations they are quite specific for aromatase. The two nonsteroidal aromatase inhibitors now available for clinical use in the US are anastrozole and letrozole *(40)* and are shown in Fig. 1. These are very selective, can achieve a high degree of suppression of peripheral aromatization and are therapeutically effective in postmenopausal patients with advanced breast cancer. In premenopausal women, estrogen suppression is most effectively achieved through the additive effects of an aromatase inhibitor in conjunction with an LHRH agonist *(42).*

The first clinical trial of 4-OHA was published in 1984 by Coombes et al. This potent aromatase inhibitor was administered to postmenopausal patients with advanced metastatic breast cancer who had been heavily pretreated with multiple agents *(43).* The aromatase inhibitor yielded a reduction in serum estradiol which persisted for at least two weeks following a single IM injection. Follow-up phase II reports revealed supporting evidence for the efficacy of 4-OHA in the management of postmenopausal breast cancer patients with advanced disease and estrogen receptor positive or unknown receptor type tumors while yielding few systemic side effects or toxicities *(44).* Plasma estradiol levels were significantly suppressed throughout the four months of monitoring yielding a baseline plasma estradiol level of 7.2 ± 0.8 pg/mL, which declined to 2.6 ± 0.2, 2.7 ± 0.2 and 2.8 ± 0.3 pg/mL at 1, 2, and 4 mo after study initiation. Therefore, they were able to demonstrate a sustained depression of plasma estradiol levels of

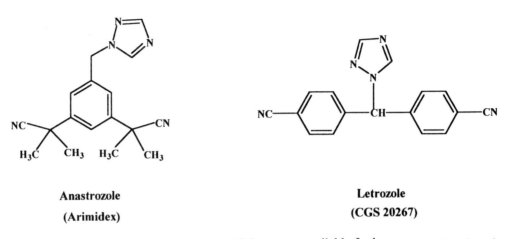

Anastrozole

(Arimidex)

Letrozole

(CGS 20267)

Fig. 1. The two non-steroidal aromatase inhibitors now available for breast cancer treatment.

greater than a 50% reduction from baseline. A response rate of 27% was achieved while 19% experienced disease stabilization and 54% experienced disease progression. Although all patients studied showed estrogen suppression, this response rate may be related to the fact that these patients had become resistant to other endocrine treatments. In addition, 42% of the subjects were initially estrogen receptor positive and 6% were estrogen receptor negative, whereas a larger proportion were of unknown estrogen receptor status (52%) and may have included some estrogen receptor negative patients. This study provided the first strong support that the selective inhibition of estradiol synthesis is influential in the treatment of breast cancer.

A comparison of the efficacy of 4-hydroxyandrostenedione (4-OHA) with that of tamoxifen was performed by Perez et al. (1994) *(45)*. Four hundred and nine patients with steroid receptor positive or unknown receptor status having metastatic disease were divided into two balanced groups (according to extent of metastasis, duration of disease, prior therapy and disease-free interval) that received either 250 mg 4-OHA IM biweekly or 30 mg/d oral tamoxifen. Response rates were similar, 31% and 28%, for tamoxifen and 4-OHA, respectively ($p = 0.51$). Median survival times were also similar between the groups, at 38 and 35 mo for tamoxifen and 4-OHA, respectively ($p = 0.73$). However, time to progression (199 d—4-OHA; 269 d—tamoxifen; $p = 0.01$) and time to treatment failure (176 d—4-OHA; 247 d—tamoxifen; $p < 0.001$) were significantly longer for the tamoxifen group. Both of these therapies were extremely well tolerated with the most common side effect in each group being flushing seen in 8% of the 4-OHA patients and 7% of the tamoxifen patients. Other minor side effects included rash and nausea in both groups and local irritation owing to the IM injection in 7% of the 4-OHA patients.

More recently, we have witnessed the emergence and approval of two nonsteroidal (achiral triazole derivatives), selective, orally-dosed aromatase inhibitors, anastrozole and new letrozole, that show efficacy against breast cancer in postmenopausal patients *(46–48)*. Two recent studies have compared the efficacy of anastozole (1 mg and 10 mg oral doses, administered daily) with the progestin, megestrol acetate (megace), in post-menopausal patients with advanced metastatic cancer *(49,50)*. No significant difference was observed between the two dosages in a comparison of toxicity and efficacy. A complete or partial response to therapy was observed in 10.3, 8.9, and 7.9% of the 1 mg and 10 mg daily anastrozole groups and megestrol acetate groups, respectively. In addition, the disease failed to progress in 25.1, 22.6, and 26.1% of patients, respectively. However, after 31 mo, there was significantly longer survival among patients receiving 1 mg anastrozole (26.7 mo) compared to megace. *(51)*. Administration of megestrol acetate was accompanied by significant weight gain in 64% of the patients. In contrast, anastrozole was extremely well-tolerated by patients with occasional complaints of gastrointestinal disturbances resulting in a 3% incidence of withdrawal. Anastrozole's favorable pharmacodynamic profile, low incidence of side effects and increased survival of patients make it a feasible alternative for endocrine treatment of postmenopausal breast cancer.

Letrozole is another selective, nonsteroidal (triazole derivative) aromatase inhibitor which has recently been approved. In patients administered oral letrozole in dosages of 0.1, 0.5, or 2.5 mg/d, estradiol levels were markedly suppressed in all three groups and achieved undetectable levels in many patients *(52–54)*. Response to treatment was observed in 33% of patients while an additional 23.8% of patients achieved disease stabilization for at least 3 mo.

A phase II study of letrozole involving 63 postmenopausal Japanese women with advanced disease yielded response to treatment in 28% of patients receiving 0.5 mg/d and a greater response of 39% in patients receiving 1 mg/d *(55)*. In addition, a large proportion of patients (40%) benefited by stabilization of their disease. A double-blind multicenter trial comparing letrozole with megestrol acetate has been conducted with 551 postmenopausal women with advanced disease previously treated with antiestogens *(56)*. Patients were divided into three groups to receive 0.5 mg letrozole daily, 2.5 mg letrozole daily or 160 mg megestrol acetate once daily. Letrozole was found to be significantly more effective at the higher dosage and was found to yield a greater tumor response rate and longer time to treatment failure compared with megestrol acetate. Additionally, letrozole was associated with fewer side effects, notably significant weight gain which occurs with megestrol acetate.

In conclusion, aromatase inhibitors, although they have been studied mainly as second line therapy to date, are beginning to show important benefits in terms of objective response rates, stabilization of disease and longer survival of patients. Additional considerations include their excellent tolerability that may substantially alter quality of life for the patient. Aromatase inhibitors appear to be important new contributors to the treatment of breast cancer. Further studies of their effects in combination or in sequence with antiestrogens may provide strategies for optimizing their efficacy.

REFERENCES

1. Mayer, R. J. 1990. *Breast Cancer*, vol. 1 (Reprints from the New England Journal of Medicine—introduction). NEJM Books, Waltham, MA.
2. Last, J. M. 1983. *A Dictionary of Epideniology*, 1st ed. Oxford University Press, New York.
3. Henderson, I. C. 1994. Breast cancer, in *Harrison's Principles of Internal Medicine*, 13th ed. McGraw-Hill. New York, pp. 1840–1850.
4. Shapiro, S., P. Strax, L. Venet, et. al. 1968. The search for risk factors in breast cancer. *Am. J. Public Health* **58**: 820.

5. Hildreth, N. G., R. E. Shore, and P. M. Dvoretsky. 1989. The risk of breast cancer after irradiation of the thymus in infancy. *N. Engl. J. Med.* **321**: 1281–1284.

6. Ottman, R., M. King, M. C. Pike, et. al. 1983. Practical guide for estimating risk for familial breast cancer. *Lancet* **ii**: 556.

7. Minden, M. D. and A. J. Pawson. 1992. *The Basic Science of Oncology*, 2nd ed. (Tannock, I. F. and R. P. Hill, eds.), McGraw-Hill, New York, pp. 61–87.

8. Begley S. The cancer killer. *Newsweek* 42–47; December 23, 1996.

9. Futreal, P. A., Q. Liu, D. Shattuck-Eidens, et. al. 1994. *BRCA1* mutations in primary breast and ovarian carcinomas. *Science* **266**: 120–122.

10. Miki, Y., J. Swensen, D. Shattuck-Eidens, et. al. 1994. A strong candidate for the breast and ovarian cancer susceptibility gene *BRCA1*. *Science* **266**: 66–71.

11. Reynolds, T. 1994. Questions and answers. The *BRCA1* breast cancer susceptibility gene. National Cancer Institute Office of Cancer Communications. National Institutes of Health, Bethesda MD.

12. Love, S. M., R. S. Gelman, and W. Silen. 1982. Fibrocystic "disease" of the breast—a nondisease? *N. Engl. J. Med.* **307**: 1010–1014.

13. Dupont, W. D. and D. L. Page. 1985. Risk factors for breast cancer in women with proliferative breast disease. *N. Engl. J. Med.* **312**: 146.

14. Feigelson, H. S., G. A. Coetzee, L. N. Kolonel, et. al. 1997. A polymorphism in the CYP 17 gene increases the risk of breast cancer. *Cancer Res.* **57**: 1063–1065.

15. Lu, Q., J. Nakamura, A. Savinov et. al. 1996. Expression of aromatase protein and messenger ribonucleic acid in tumor epithelial cells and evidence of functional significance of locally produced estrogen in human breast cancers. *Endocrinology* **137**: 3061–3068.

16. Buell, P. 1972. Changing incidence of breast cancer in Japanese women. *J. Natl. Cancer Inst.* **51**: 1479–1483.

17. Romieu, I., J. A. Berlin, and G. Colditz. 1990. Oral contraceptives and breast cancer: review and meta-analysis. *Cancer* **66**: 2253.

18. McGuire, W. L. 1980. An update on estrogen and progesterone receptors in prognosis for primary and advanced breast cancer, in *Hormones and Cancer*, vol. 15 (Iacobelli, S., et. al.) Raven Press, New York, pp. 337–344.

19. Beatson, G. T. 1896. On the treatment of inoperable cases of carcinoma of the mamma: suggestions for a new method of treatment with illustrative cases. *Lancet* **ii**: 104–107.

20. Lonning E. and E. A. Lien. 1995. Mechanisms of action of endocrine treatment in breast cancer. Critical Rev. Oncology-Hematology **21(1–3)**: 158–193.

21. Cole, M. P, C. T. A. Jones, and I. D. H. Todd. 1971. A new antiestrogenic agent in late breast cancer. An early appraisal of ICI 46,474. *Br. J. Cancer* **25**: 270–275.

22. Early Breast Cancer Trialists' Collaborative Group: Systemic treatment of early breast cancer by hormonal cytotoxic or immune therapy: 133 randomized trials involving 31,000 recurrences and 24,000 deaths among 75,000 women. *Lancet* **339**: 1–15, 71–85, 1992.

23. Fisher, B., J. Costantino, C. Redmond, R. Poisson, et. al. 1989. A randomized clinical trial evaluating tamoxifen in the treatment of patients with node-negative breast cancer who have estrogen-receptor-positive tumors. *N. Engl. J. Med.* **320**: 479–484.

24. Jordan, V. C. 1995. Tamoxifen: toxicities and drug resistance during the treatment and prevention of breast cancer. *Ann. Rev. Pharmacol. Toxicol.* **35**: 195–211.

25. Williams, G. M., M. J. Iatropoulos, M. V. Djordjevic, O. P. Kaltenberg. 1993. The triphenylethylene drug tamoxifen is a strong liver carcinogen in the rat. *Carcinogenesis* **14**: 315–317.

26. Greaves, P., R. Goonetillebe, G. Nunn, J. Topham, and T. Orton. 1993. Two year carcinogenicity study of tamoxifen in Alderley Park Wistar-derived rats. *Cancer Res* **53**: 3919–3924.

27. Fornander, T., L. E. Rutqvist, B. Cedermark, U. Glass, A. Mattson, et. al. 1989. Adjuvant tamoxifen in early breast cancer: occurrence of new primary cancer *Lancet* **1**: 117–120.

28. Fornander, T., A. C. Hellstrom, and B. Moberger. 1993. Descriptive clinicopathologic study of 17 patients with endometrial cancer during or after adjuvant tamoxifen in early breast cancer. *J. Natl. Cancer Inst.* **815:** 1850–1855.

29. Powles, T. J. and I. E. Smith. 1991. *Medical management of breast cancer.* J.B. Lippincott, Philadelphia, PA.

30. Early breast cancer trialists' collaborative group. Effects of adjuvant tamoxifen and cytotoxic therapy on mortality in early breast cancer. An overview of 61 randomized trials among 28,896 women. *N. Engl. J. Med.* **319:** 1681–1692, 1988.

31. Catherino, W. H. and V. C. Jordan. 1995. A naturally occurring estrogen receptor mutation results in increased estrogenicity of a tamoxifen analogue. *Mol. Endocrinol.* **9:** 153–163

32. Osborn, C. K., M. Jarman, R. McCague, E. B. Coronado, S. G. Hilsenbeck, and A. E. Wakeling AE. 1994. The importance of tamoxifen metabolism in tamoxifen-stimulated breast tumor growth. *Cancer Chemother Pharm* **34:** 89–95.

33. Fuqua, S. A. W., C. Wiltschke, C. Castles, D. Wolf, and D. C. Allred. 1995. A role for estrogen-receptor variants in endocrine resistance. *Endocrine-related Cancer* **2:** 19–25.

34. Schwarzel, W. C., W. Kruggel, and A. Brodie. 1973. Studies on the mechanism of estrogen biosynthesis. VII. The development of inhibitors of the enzyme system in human placenta. *Endocrinology* **92:** 866–880.

35. Santen, R. J. , S. Santner, and A. Lipton. 1982. Aromatase: new perspectives for breast cancer. *Cancer Res.* **42(Suppl.):** 3267s–3468s.

36. Santen, R. J. 1987. Aromatase: future perspective. *Steroids* **50:** 1–665.

37. Brodie, A, H. R. Brodie, G. Callard, C. H. Robinson, C. Roselli, and R. Santen. 1993. Recent advances in steroid biochemistry and molecular biology. Proceedings of the third international aromatase conference-basic and clinical aspects of aromatase. *J. Steroid Biochem. Mol. Biol.* **44:** 321–693.

38. Cole, P. A. and C. H. Robinson. 1990. Mechanism and inhibition of cytochrome P–450 aromatase. *J. Med. Chem.* **33:** 2933–2944.

39. Brueggemeier, R. W. 1990. Biochemical and Molecular aspects of aromatase. *J. Enzym. Inhib.* **4:** 101–111.

40. Brodie, A. M. H. and B. C. O. Njar. 1996. Aromatase inhibitors and breast cancer. *Semin. Oncol.* **23(Suppl.):**10–20.

41. Sjoerdsma, A. 1981. Suicide inhibitors as potential drugs. *Clin. Pharmacol. Ther.* **30:** 3–22.

42. Dowsett, M., R. C. Stein, R. C., and Coombes. 1992. Aromatization inhibition alone or in combination with GnRH agonists for the treatment of premenopausal breast cancer patients. *J Steroid Biochem* **43:** 155–159.

43. Coombes, R. C., P. Goss, M. Dowsett, J. C. Gazet, and A. Brodie. 1984. 4-hydroxy-androstenedione in treatment of postmenopausal patients with advanced breast cancer. *The Lancet* **ii:** 1237–1239.

44. Goss, P. E., T. J. Powles, M. Dowsett, Hutchinson, et. al. 1986. Treatment of advanced breast cancer with an aromatase inhibitor, 4-hydroxyandrostenedione: Phase II Report. *Cancer Res.* **46:** 4823–4826.

45. Perez, C. R., C. V. Alberola, F. Calabresi, et. al. 1994. Comparison of the selective aromatase inhibitor formestane with tamoxifen as first-line hormonal therapy in postmenopausal women with advanced breast cancer. *Ann. Oncol.* **5(Suppl. 7):** S19–S24.

46. Plourde, P. V., M. Dyroff, and M. Dukes. 1994. Arimidex: a potent and selective fourth-generation aromatase inhibitor. *Breast Cancer Res. Treat.* **30:** 103–111.

47. Plourde, P. V., M. Dyroff, M. Dowsett, L. Demers, et. al. 1995. Arimidex: a new oral, once-a-day aromatase inhibitor. *J. Steriod Biochem. Mol. Biol.* **53:** 175–179.

48. Yates, R. A., M. Dowsett, G. V. Fisher, A. Selen, and P. J. Wyld. 1996. Arimidex (ZD 1033): a selective, potent inhibitor of aromatase in postmenopausal female volunteers. *Br. J. Cancer* **73:** 543–548.

49. Buzdar, A., W. Jonat, A. Howell, S. E. Jones, et. al. 1996. Anastrozole (Arimidex), a potent and selective aromatase inhibitor versus megestrol acetate (Megace) in postmenopausal women with advanced breast cancer: results of an overview analysis of two phase III trials. *J. Clin. Oncol.* **14**: 2000–2011.

50. Jonat, W., A. Howell, C. Blomqvist, W. Eiermann, et. al. 1996. A randomized trial comparing two doses of the new selective aromatase inhibitor anastrozole (Arimidex) with megestrol acetate in postmenopausal patients with advanced breast cancer. *Eur. J .Cancer* **32A**: 404–412.

51. Buzdar, A., W. Jonat, A. Howell, H. Yin, and D. Lee. 1997. Significant improved survival with Arimidex (anastrozole) versus megestrol acetate in postmenopausal advanced breast cancer update: results of two randomized trials. The Aromatize International study Group, Houston, TX, Keel, Germany, Manchester, UK, Wilmington, DE, Macclesfield, UK, (Aromatize is a trademark, property of Zeneca Limited). *Proceed. Am. Soc. Clin. Oncol.* **16**: 156am.

52. Bhatnagar, A. S., A. Hausler, P. Trunet, K. Schieweck, et. al. 1990. Highly selective inhibition of estrogen biosynthesis by CGS 20267, a new non-steroidal aromatase inhibitor. *J. Steroid Biochem. Mol. Biol.* **37**: 1021–1027.

53. Iverson, T. J., I. E. Smith, J. Ahern, D. A. Smithers, P. F. Trunet, and M. Dowsett. 1993. Phase I study of the oral non- steroidal aromatase inhibitor CGS 20267 in healthy postmenopausal women. *J. Clin. Endocr. Metab.* **77**: 324–331.

54. Smith, I. E. 1996. Letrozole: creating a new standard, in *Advanced Breast Cancer. Reassessing Hormonal Therapy—Ciba International Symposium Series*, vol. 2, Parthenon, New York, pp. 45–55.

55. Tominaga. T. Phase II trial of letrozole in postmenopausal patients with advanced or recurrent breast cancer, in *Advanced Breast Cancer. Reassessing Hormonal Therapy—Ciba International Symposium Series*, vol. 2, Parthenon, New York, pp. 57–63.

56. Letrozole International Trial Group (AR/BC2).

23

Drug Resistance in Breast Cancer

Devchand Paul and Kenneth H. Cowan

1. INTRODUCTION

Breast cancer is a disease that responds to a wide variety of antineoplastic agents as well as to hormonal therapy (for review, *see* refs. *1* and *2*). Unfortunately, although patients with metastatic breast cancer may respond initially to chemotherapy or hormonal therapy, progressive disease invariably occurs within a few months to a few years. Patients may respond again to other agents, however, response rates and the duration of response to second line therapy are generally less than that of initial therapy, a phenomenon attributed to the development of drug resistance.

The mechanisms of resistance to antineoplastic agents have been extensively studied in an effort to elucidate potential targets for reversal or circumvention of drug resistance. Studies in tumor cell lines selected for drug resistance in vitro have identified many mechanisms whereby tumor cells can become insensitive to the cytotoxic effects of antineoplastic agents. Some of these mechanisms result in specific resistance to a single class of agents with a common mechanism of cytotoxicity. Other mechanisms of resistance lead to broad spectrum resistance to a wide variety of structurally dissimilar drugs with disparate mechanisms of action. This phenotype of pleiotropic resistance is commonly referred to as multidrug resistance.

In this chapter, we shall explore various mechanisms of antineoplastic drug resistance identified in tissue culture and animal models. We shall also review studies on the development of clinical drug resistance in breast cancers and various experimental approaches to drug resistance in breast cancer patients.

2. GENERAL MECHANISMS OF DRUG RESISTANCE

As previously noted, studies from many laboratories have identified a wide range of mechanisms of resistance to antineoplastic agents. The general mechanisms used by tumor cells to become resistant to antineoplastic agents are listed in Table 1. It is important to recognize that within a given tumor, multiple mechanisms for the emergence of drug resistance may be working concurrently. Specific pathways that apply to the agents commonly used to treat breast cancer will be discussed.

2.1. Decreased Drug Accumulation

Tumor cells that are able to reduce the intracellular burden of anticancer drugs will obviously become refractory to the cytotoxic effects of anticancer drugs. Decreased

From: Breast Cancer: *Molecular Genetics, Pathogenesis, and Therapeutics*
Edited by: A. M. Bowcock © Humana Press Inc., Totowa, NJ

Table 1
General Mechanisms of Drug Resistance

I. Cellular and Biochemical Mechanisms
Decreased Drug Accumulation
Decreased drug influx
Increased drug efflux
Altered intracellular trafficking of drug
Altered Drug Metabolism
Decreased drug activation
Increased inactivation of drug/toxic intermediate
Increased Repair of Drug Induced Damage
DNA, proteins, membranes
Altered Drug Targets, qualitative or quantitative
Altered Cofactor or Metabolite Levels
Decreased Apoptosis
II. Mechanisms Relevant in Vivo
Host-Drug Interactions
Increased drug inactivation by normal tissues
Decreased drug activation by normal tissues
Relative increase in normal tissue drug sensitivity/toxicity
Host-Tumor Interactions

(Modified from ref. *311.*)

intracellular accumulation of drugs may occur through each of the following mechanisms: decreased drug influx, increased drug efflux, altered intracellular trafficking of drugs, and increased drug sequestration or binding within tumor cells.

Some chemotherapy agents enter cells via specific transport systems and defects in these transporters can lead to drug resistance. For example, antifolates such as methotrexate enter cells via two pathways: a low-affinity, high-capacity transporter (reduced folate carrier) and a high-affinity binding protein (folate receptors) (for review, *see* ref. *3*). Studies in methotrexate resistant cell lines have shown that decreased influx is a common mechanisms of resistance to antifolates. Decreased influx of methotrexate via alterations in either the reduced folate carrier *(4–13)* or folate receptors can result in methotrexate resistance *(14–18)*.

Increased drug efflux is a common mechanism of resistance in cells that develop a multidrug-resistance (MDR) phenotype. Indeed, multidrug resistant cell lines are readily obtained following exposure in vitro to step-wise, increasing exposure to a single antineoplastic agent, generally an anthracycline or a tubulin binding agent. In many instances, the drug-resistant cells are not only resistant to the selecting agent, but also demonstrate cross resistance to other classes of chemotherapy drugs with different cytotoxic mechanisms of action. As previously noted, this phenotype has been commonly called multidrug resistance or MDR. The MDR phenotype is commonly seen following exposure of cells to one of the "naturally occurring" anticancer drugs, including doxorubicin, vincristine, vinblastine, etoposide, Actinomycin D, paclitaxel, colchicine, vinorelbine, topotecan, and irinotecan (CPT-11) *(19–22*, and for review, *see* ref. *23)*. The cytotoxic substrates of MDR1 are listed in Table 2. Although

Table 2
Cytotoxic Substrates of MDR1

Anthracyclines	Taxanes
Doxorubicin	Paclitaxel
Daunorubicin	Docetaxel
Vinca Alkaloids	Camptothecins
Vincristine	Topotecan
Vinblastine	Irinotecan (CPT-11)
Vinorelbine	
Epipodophyllotoxins	Antitumor antibiotic
Etoposide	Actinomycin D
Teniposide	

Modified from ref. *312*.

many of these MDR-related drugs are derived from plants or micro-organisms, they are structurally dissimilar and have different intracellular targets. However, they do share some features in that they are all preferentially soluble in lipids, enter the cell by passive diffusion, and are all relatively large in size (300–900 Mr) *(24)*.

Thus far, at least three distinct classes of MDR phenotypes have been characterized and each of them is associated with alterations in different gene products: classical MDR (P-glycoprotein), non-P-glycoprotein MDR (MRP), and atypical MDR (topoisomerase II) (for review, *see* ref. *24*).

2.2. Classical MDR

Riordan and Ling *(25)* identified that MDR in hamster cells selected for resistance to colchicine was associated with reduced intracellular drug accumulation and over-expression of a high molecular weight (170 kDa) membrane protein referred to as P-glycoprotein (Pgp). Subsequent studies have shown that Pgp is an energy-dependent unidirectional drug-efflux pump with broad substrate specificity and encoded in human cells by the MDR1 gene *(26–28)*. Pgp is composed of two homologous halves each consisting of six predicted transmembrane domains and an intracellular loop with consensus ATP binding motif *(27–29)* (*see* Fig. 1). Post-translational glycosylation of Pgp apparently contributes to correct folding, proper routing, and stabilization of the molecule *(30)*. Drug efflux through Pgp is an energy-dependent process requiring ATP *(31,32)*. The role of this gene in the development of MDR has been clearly established by transfection studies in which expression of full-length human MDR1 cDNA in a drug sensitive cell line conferred a complete MDR phenotype *(33)*.

One proposed model for the function of the Pgp drug pump *(23)* suggests that the major function of the multidrug transporter is to extrude drugs directly from the plasma membrane. Uncharged drug molecules entering the lipid bilayer of the cell by passive diffusion, are removed from the membrane, before they can enter the cytoplasm. Another important feature of this model is that transport presumably occurs through a single chamber of the transporter following aggregation of both halves of one or more p170 subunits to form a single transport channel.

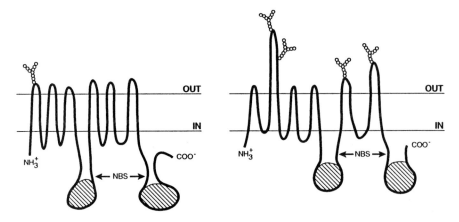

Fig. 1. Proposed models of P-glycoprotein (Pgp) and the multidrug resistance-associated protein (MRP) in the cell membrane. Both proteins span the membrane 12 times, have major glycosylation sites (open circles), and two potential ATP (nucleotide)-binding cites (NBS). From ref. *313.*

Pgp is found in a variety of tumors as well as in normal tissues, where it may play a role in detoxification of xenobiotic substances *(24)*. High levels of MDR mRNA have been found in the medulla of the adrenal gland and in kidney; intermediate levels in colon, rectum, lung, and liver; and low levels in ovary, stomach, renal cortex, esophagus, heart, muscle, and skin *(34)*.

MDR1 expression has been examined in both primary untreated breast cancers as well as in cancers from patients who have relapsed following chemotherapy. Some investigators have detected high levels of MDR1 expression in untreated primary breast cancer with 30–90% of breast-cancer cells staining positive for Pgp expression by immunohistochemistry *(35–46)*. In contrast, some studies have reported low levels of MDR1 expression in primary breast tumors *(47–50)*. Differences in techniques for quantitating MDR1 expression may account for some of these apparent differences. Increased MDR1 expression is commonly seen in breast tumors of patients following treatment with neoadjuvant chemotherapy as compared to primary untreated breast tumors *(35,51)* and in breast tumors following relapse *(34)*.

Of the two prospective studies assessing the prognostic role of the MDR1 gene in breast carcinomas, one found MDR1 RNA levels in primary breast carcinomas to be negative in 54% of cancers, low positive in 29%, and highly positive in 17% *(37)*. No differences in age, menopausal status, estrogen and progesterone receptor levels, tumor size, lymph-node involvement, and c-erbB-2 gene expression was seen between MDR1 RNA negative patients and MDR1 RNA positive patients. The other prospective study employed an immunohistochemical analysis and found that strong Pgp staining in a majority of breast-cancer cells in patients with locally advanced or metastatic breast cancer was associated with a lack of initial response to chemotherapy and shorter progression-free survival *(42)*. Given the differences in the clinical studies to date and the difficulty in quantitating MDR1 expression in breast-cancer cells, additional prospective studies are needed in order to assess the prognostic influence of MDR1 expression in breast-cancer cells.

Table 3
Chemotherapeutic Agents Demonstrating
MRP-Mediated Drug Resistance

Anthracyclines	Camptothecins
Doxorubicin	Topotecan
Daunorubicin	
Epirubicin	
Vinca Alkaloids	Antitumor antibiotic
Vincristine	Actinomycin D
Vinblastine	
Epipodophyllotoxins	
Etoposide	
Teniposide	

2.3. MRP

Another MDR phenotype in the absence of MDR1 expression was noted by several laboratories *(52,53)*. Subsequent studies identified another high molecular-weight membrane protein in MDR1 negative drug-resistant cell lines which was called MDR-associated protein (MRP) or P-190 *(52–55)*. The MRP gene product has striking homology to MDR and other members of ATP-binding cassette transmembrane transporter proteins *(52,53)* (*see* Fig. 1) and the ability of MRP to confer MDR has been demonstrated via gene transfer studies *(56–58)*.

The biochemical mechanism responsible for MRP-mediated multidrug resistance remains speculative (*56–60*, and reviewed in ref. *61*). MRP can pump glutathione, glutathione conjugates, glucuronate, and sulfated conjugates. Natural-product cytotoxic drug-resistance in some MRP-overexpressing cell lines can be reversed by a glutathione-depleting agent. This might suggest that MRP confers natural-product drug resistance by transporting either drug glutathione conjugates or anionic drug metabolites *(62)*. A recent study has demonstrated that MRP is an ATP-dependent pump that transports both anionic products of glutathione conjugation and weakly cationic, unaltered lipophilic natural-product cytotoxic drugs *(63)*. In this model, the location of the transporter to plasma *(52)* and cytoplasmic *(64)* membranes would be consistent with decreased accumulation and/or increased efflux of lipophilic cytotoxic drugs. MRP located in the plasma membrane would transport drug out of the cell; resulting in decreased intracellular drug concentration and MRP localized to cytoplasmic membranes could transport drug into enclosed cytoplasmic structures. It is unknown whether drug accumulation into cytoplasmic structures contributes to resistance.

Although there are similarities between MDR1 and MRP, cells overexpressing MRP have defects in drug accumulation which, in general, are quantitatively less than that observed in MDR1 overexpressing cells *(65,66)*. Chemotherapeutic agents demonstrating MRP-mediated drug resistance are listed in Table 3.

MRP expression, in contrast to MDR1, is detectable in all cell lines and tissues studied thus far *(9,59,67)*. Clinical studies have shown that MRP and not MDR1 overexpression is frequently observed in lung cancers *(68–72)*. Overexpression of MRP has been observed in patients with relapsed acute leukemia *(67,73,74)*. Other studies in patients with neuroblastoma have noted that overexpression of MRP portends a poorer prognosis *(75,76)*. The only studies thus far of MRP expression in breast cancer has been done in drug-resistant cell lines. Schneider et al. *(67)* found MRP gene overexpression in a human breast-carcinoma cell line (MCF7/VP) selected for etoposide resistance. In addition, reversal of MRP mediated resistance to doxorubicin was reported in breast-cancer cells (MCF-7) treated with ansamycin *(77)*.

2.4. Multidrug Resistance Associated with Topoisomerase Poisons

The third mechanism of MDR involves alterations in topoisomerases, which are nuclear enzymes that catalyze the formation of transient single- or double-stranded DNA breaks. By relieving torsional stress on DNA, topoisomerases facilitate the passage of DNA strands through these breaks *(78–80)*, and promote subsequent rejoining of the DNA strands *(81,82)*. These enzymes are thought to play critical roles in DNA replication, transcription, repair, and recombination. There are two classes of mammalian DNA topoisomerases, topoisomerase I and II, and defects in both can lead to anticancer drug resistance.

Topoisomerase II catalyzes both single- and double-stranded DNA breaks, ATP-dependent relaxation, knotting-unknotting, and catenation-decatination reactions (for review, *see* ref. *83)*. Topoisomerase II may also play a role in the elongation and termination stages of DNA replication *(84)*. Chen and Liu *(83)* have proposed a model for the ATP-dependent strand-passing activity of topoisomerase II. Topoisomerase II can cleave both single- and double-stranded DNA and rejoin the double helix by forming an equilibrium mixture of noncleavable and cleavable complexes. During the cleavage reactions, exposure to topoisomerase II poisons, can lead to the formation of stable DNA topoisomerase drug complexes, which can block strand religation. The formation of these stabilized DNA complexes is believed to initiate the production of lethal DNA strand breaks. Topoisomerase II poisons, which include nonintercalators such as etoposide and teniposide, as well as DNA intercalators including doxorubicin, daunorubicin, amsacrine, mitoxantrone, and actinomycin D, induce sister chromatid exchange, chromosomal aberrations, increased levels of recombinant chromosomes, and illegitimate recombination.

Studies in cell lines have demonstrated a number of different mechanisms involving changes in topoisomerases that can lead to the emergence of drug resistance. Because the formation of drug-induced DNA strand breaks is the principle mechanism of cytotoxicity of this class of anticancer drugs, alterations in either the level of topoisomerase II expression or the expression of mutant forms (point mutations) of topoisomerase II with reduced drug sensitivity may lead to drug resistance secondary to reduced cleavable complex formation *(86–91,144)*. Indeed, laboratory studies have shown that decreased levels of topoisomerase II activity result in decreased drug-induced DNA strand breaks and decreased drug cytotoxicity *(92,93)*. Furthermore, studies by Gudkov et al. *(94)* have shown that the expression in cells of a dominant-negative genetic-suppressor element (GSE) specifically targeting topoisomerase II gene expression can decrease the cellular levels of functional topoisomerase II activity and lead to resistance to topoisomerase II inhibitors. Decreased nuclear matrix-associated topoisomerase II *(95)*, expression of a truncated form of topoisomerase II *(96)*, or alterations in various cytoplasmic or membrane components *(97)* have also been shown to result in the emergence of resistance to topoisomerase II inhibitors.

Type I topoisomerases are ATP independent and function to make a transient single-stranded nick in DNA, pass another single-strand of DNA through the nick, and then religate the DNA. This serves to decrease the torsional strain on DNA and allows replication, transcription, recombination, and repair to proceed *(98,99)*. Topoisomerase I-mediated-cleavable complexes are DNA single-stranded breaks with the enzyme linked to the 3' phosphoryl end of the DNA via a phosphotyrosine linkage. Camptothecins, which include CPT-11, topotecan, 9-amino-camptothecin (9AC), and 7-N-methyl-piperazinomethyl-10,11-ethylene dioxy-20-S-camptothecin, are topoisomerase I inhibitors. These agents and their derivatives inhibit topoisomerase I by stabilizing the covalent topoisomerase I-DNA cleavable complex and preventing DNA religation *(85,100)*. Inhibition of both DNA relaxation and induction of DNA single-strand breaks resulting in fork arrest occurs following treatment with CPT-11 *(101)*. CPT-11 treatment inhibits RNA synthesis *(102)* and results in prolonged S phase or G2 arrest of the cell cycle *(103,104)*. It also induces sister chromatid exchange *(105)* and recombinations that occur during the process of repair, which can lead to mutations *(106)* and/or apoptosis *(107)*.

Drug resistance to camptothecins can occur by several different mechanisms. Overexpression of Pgp in lung and colon cancers can lead to reduced drug accumulation and cytotoxicity of topotecan *(45,108–110)*. Resistance to CPT-11 may also be owing to decreased total activity of topoisomerase I and reduced levels of SN-38, the active metabolite of CPT-11 *(111)*. Furthermore, mutations in the topoisomerase I gene can lead to a reduced ability of camptothecins to stabilize the cleavable complexes and contribute to the development of drug resistance (for review, *see* ref. *99*). Rearrangements, deletions, and hypermethylation can also lead to loss of topoisomerase I activity *(112–114)*. Camptothecin resistance in a human breast-cancer cell line has been reported in which normal topoisomerase I activity was found and the resistant cells had increased DNA repair *(115)*.

Although topoisomerase I inhibitors have activity against colon and lung cancers, their role in the treatment of breast cancer is not yet known. A phase II study of the topoisomerase I inhibitor CPT-11 or irinotecan in patients with advanced or recurrent breast cancer has shown an overall response rate of 23% *(116)*. In this study, the response rate of patients with prior endocrine therapy and prior chemotherapy, including adriamycin, was 27% and estrogen-receptor negative and premenopausal patients had 32% and 27% response rates, respectively. However, a preliminary report from another phase II trial of CPT-11 in patients with previously treated metastatic breast cancer noted only one response (complete response) out of 12 evaluable patients *(117)*. Currently the role of camptothecins in the treatment of advanced breast cancer remains promising, but unknown and further trials are underway.

Another model of MDR has been described in cells selected for resistance to mitoxantrone *(67,118)*. In one example, MCF-7 cells selected for resistance to mitoxantrone, a topoisomerase II inhibitor, were also noted to develop cross-resistance to camptothecins, which are topoisomerase I inhibitors *(67,119)*. Resistance in mitoxantrone resistant MCF-7 cells is not associated with any alterations in either topoisomerase I or II, but rather involves decreased drug accumulation in the absence of either MDR1 or MRP overexpression. The gene(s) responsible for this mechanism of MDR has not yet been identified.

2.5. Alterations in Programed Cell Death

Because many cytotoxic drugs can induce apoptosis, or programmed cell death, cellular resistance to apoptosis may play an important role in refractoriness of tumors to cancer chemotherapy *(120)*. In breast-cancer cells, apoptosis can be induced by a variety of treatments including chemotherapy, hormonal manipulation, and treatment with polypeptides (tumor necrosis factor [TNF], epidermal growth factor [EGF]) *(121–126)*. The tumor-suppressor gene p53 has been shown to play a critical role in inducing apoptosis in cells resulting from exposure to cytotoxic drugs such as doxorubicin and 5-fluorouracil *(127)*. Mutations in the p53 gene in murine sarcoma have been associated with resistance to anthracyclines *(128)* and to cisplatin in nonsmall cell lung-cancer cells *(129)*. Presumably this is related to the inability of the chemotherapy-induced cellular damage to induce apoptosis in p53 mutant tumor cells.

Mutations in p53 generally result in a nonfunctional protein that accumulates in tumor-cell nuclei *(130)*. Although mutant forms of P53 are generally less active as transcriptional enhancers, some studies have suggested that certain forms of mutant p53 can stimulate transcription of the MDR1 promoter *(138)*. Furthermore, loss of wild-type p53 function results in genetic instability in cells and subsequent amplification and overexpression of drug-resistance genes such as MDR1 *(46)*.

Clinical studies have indicated that mutations in the p53 gene in breast cancers predict a poor prognosis *(130,132–135)*, yet a better response overall to radiotherapy *(136)* or chemotherapy *(137)*. A recent report has linked specific p53 gene mutations with primary resistance to doxorubicin therapy and early relapse in breast-cancer patients *(138)*. Nuclear accumulation of mutant p53 has been associated with shorter disease-free and overall survival in node-negative *(130,139)* and node-positive *(139)* breast cancer as well as in hereditary breast cancer *(139)*. Nuclear mutant p53 accumulation has also been shown to be associated with Pgp expression in primary breast cancer and the simultaneous expression of mutant p53 and P-glycoprotein is associated with decreased survival in patients with locally advanced breast cancer *(140)*. Although some breast-cancer cell lines selected for drug resistance have developed mutations in the p53 gene during the selection for drug resistance, other drug-resistant breast-cancer cell lines retain wild type p53 protein *(141,142)*. Thus, although p53 mutations may be sufficient for the development of drug resistance, they are certainly not necessary.

Other studies have shown that overexpression of the bcl-2 proto-oncogene may play an important role in preventing programmed cell death following exposure of cells to various chemotherapeutic agents including doxorubicin, taxol, methotrexate, hydroperoxy-cyclophosphamide, 5-fluorodeoxyuridine (FUDR), camptothecin, nitrogen mustard, etoposide, cisplatin, vincristine, and AraC *(143,145–147,315)*. The bcl-2 protein exerts its inhibitory effects on apoptosis by a mechanism that includes a shift in the redox potential of the cell to a more reduced state *(148,149)*. An increase in the nonprotein sulfhydryl content of cells is felt to be important to this mechanism *(148–150)*. Overexpression of a dominant negative inhibitor of bcl-2 in MCF-7 breast-cancer cells increase their sensitivity to VP-16 or taxol *(147)*. In contrast, other studies have reported that despite downregulation of bcl-2 protein in an adriamycin-resistant human breast-cancer cell line (MCF/Adr), these cells are still highly resistant to apoptosis *(151)*.

Bax is a cellular protein that binds to bcl-2 and promotes apoptosis *(152,153)*. Changes in the relative levels of bcl-2 and bax can influence the sensitivity of cells to apoptosis. Thus, treatment of human breast-cancer cells with estrogen increases the level of bcl-2 relative to bax resulting in resistance to taxol-mediated cytotoxicity and apoptosis *(154)*. Conversely, decreased bcl-2 expression in MCF-7 cells transfected with antisense bcl-2 constructs results in increased sensitivity to doxorubicin *(155)*. Bax-alpha gene (a splice variant of bax) expression in breast-cancer cells induces apoptosis, possibly owing to its ability to form homodimers that antagonize the anti-apoptotic function of bcl-2, and in doing so increases sensitivity to epirubicin *(166)*. Bax-alpha is expressed in high amounts in normal cell lines and breast tissue (which are susceptible to apoptosis), where little or no expression of bax-alpha can be detected in cancer-cell lines and malignant breast tissues resistant to apoptosis *(159)*. In addition, transfected bax-alpha gene into breast-cancer cell lines restores sensitivity towards both serum starvation and APO-1/Fas-triggered apoptosis and significantly reduce tumor growth in (SCID) mice *(161)*. Overexpression of bax, by stable transfection, can also sensitize human breast-cancer cells to radiation-induced apoptosis *(167)*.

The effects of bcl-2 and bax expression in clinical breast cancer is unclear. One study noted a significantly lower relapse-free and distant metastasis-free survival at 5 yr in estrogen receptor-positive, node-positive, postmenopausal women with breast cancers that expressed high levels of mutant p53 and low levels of bcl-2 *(135)*. Another study suggested that reduced expression of bax is associated with a poor response to chemotherapy and shorter survival in women with metastatic breast cancer *(168)*. Further studies are needed to better understand the role of p53, bcl-2, and bax in the emergence of drug resistance in human breast cancer.

Fas antigen, also known as APO-1 and CD95, is a cell-surface protein which belongs to the family of tumor-necrosis factor/nerve growth factor receptors, and is capable of triggering apoptosis when bound by a monoclonal antibody (MAb) (anti-Fas antibody) *(156,243)*. Anti-Fas antibody does not kill cells via an immune-mediated mechanism, but rather induces apoptosis as a receptor agonist *(156,157)*. In all known instances of apoptosis, a family of cysteine proteases related to interleukin-1B-converting enzyme (ICE) becomes activated and induces apoptosis through specific cleavage of substrates (for review, *see* ref. *158*). In addition, overexpression of death domain-containing proteins, such as FADD/MORT1, TRADD, and RIB also induce apoptosis. Although the death domain is required for interaction with Fas, a separate domain DED may actually signal apoptosis in the case of Fas-mediated apoptosis.

Fas-mediated apoptosis has been described in human breast-cancer cells by several investigators *(159,164)*. Keane et al. *(167)* recently examined Fas expression and function in normal and malignant breast-cancer cell lines. These workers found that although nontransformed mammary epithelial cell lines expressed high levels of Fas mRNA and protein, only 1/7 breast-cancer cell lines (T47D) expressed high levels of Fas. Furthermore, all breast-cancer cell lines examined, except T47D, were resistant to Fas-mediated apoptosis.

Several laboratories have examined the possible interaction of drug-induced cyto-toxicity with the Fas-mediated apoptosis pathway. Mizutani et al. *(165)* found that treatment of human bladder-cancer cells with doxorubicin enhanced their expression of Fas and sensitized the cells to Fas-mediated cytotoxicity. Other studies suggested that apoptosis induced by methotrexate in hepatoma cells was *(169)* mediated at least in part by a p53-dependent stimulation of the Fas receptor/ligand system *(169)*.

Other studies have investigated the role of Fas expression and function in the development of drug resistance. For example, ovarian-cancer cell lines selected for resistance to doxorubicin had decreased expression of Fas and were resistant to anti-Fas antibody induced apoptosis *(170)*. Weller et al. *(171)* reported that bcl-2 overexpression in human malignant glioma cells conferred resistance to chemotherapeutic drugs and therapeutic irradiation and that these cells were also resistant to Fas/APO-1 antibody-mediated apoptosis. Landowski et al. *(172)* examined Fas-mediated apoptosis in myeloma and T-cell leukemia cell lines selected for drug resistance. These workers found a correlation between the level of resistance to doxorubicin and mitoxantrone and the degree of resistance to Fas-mediated apoptosis. Clinical studies in acute myeloid leukemia found that low expression of Fas was associated with a low completes remission rate after induction chemotherapy *(173)*. Although these studies suggest a role for changes in fas expression and/or function in some models of drug resistance, the role of Fas-mediated drug resistance in breast-cancer cells is still under investigation.

2.6. erbB-2 Receptors and Drug Resistance

The c-erbB-2/neu oncogene encodes a 185kd transmembrane glycoprotein (P185), which has significant sequence homology to the epidermal growth factor receptor (EGFR) *(174,175*, and *see* ref. *176* for review) and has intrinsic tyrosine-kinase activity *(177–179)*. Amplification/overexpression of the c-erbB-2/neu occurs in 20–30% of breast cancers *(180)* and is associated with an increase rate of relapse and decreased overall survival *(116,181,182)*. A possible role for erbB-2 in the development of hormone and drug resistance has been suggested in studies in cell lines. Amplification of erbB-2 in steroid-receptor positive breast cancer has been shown to be associated with tamoxifen resistance *(183)*. The transfection of c-Ha-ras and c-erbB-2 oncogenes can induce multidrug resistance in MCF-10A human breast-cancer cells *(184)*. In addition, overexpression of c-erbB-2/neu in breast-cancer cells has been shown to increase resistance to paclitaxel via mechanisms independent from MDR-1 *(185)*. In one clinical study, c-erbB-2 expression was prognostically significant for node-positive breast cancer patients and tumors displaying overexpression of the c-erbB-2 oncogene were less responsive to cyclophosphamide, methotrexate, and 5-flurouracil (CMF) adjuvant chemotherapy than those with a normal amount of gene product *(186)*.

2.7. DNA Repair

Resistance to chemotherapy as a result of increased DNA repair is best seen following exposure to nitrosoureas. Mechanisms of resistance to these agents include expression of the DNA repair enzyme O^6-alkylguanine-DNA alkyltransferase. This enzyme can remove alkyl adducts at the O^6 position of guanine before cross-link formation can occur and thus prevent nitrosourea-induced cytotoxic DNA damage *(187)*. Another mechanism of resistance to nitrosoureas may involve decreased cellular accumulation of the drug *(188)*. The cytotoxic effects of platinum analogs also involve binding to DNA. Resistance to platinum compounds involves a number of mechanisms including decreased drug accumulation, enhanced drug inactivation, the extent of platinum-DNA adduct formation, and the rate at which DNA damage is repaired (reviewed in *(189)*. DNA mismatch-repair defects in cells result in microsatellite instability in tumors (274). Tumor cells with defects in mismatch repair are resistant to methylating agents *(191,192)* and show low-level resistance to cisplatin *(193–195)*. Other studies suggest that mismatch repair deficiency may play a role in adriamycin resistance in ovarian-tumor cell lines *(196)*.

2.8. Altered Drug Metabolism or Metabolite Levels

Resistance to chemotherapeutic agents can also occur as a result of decreased drug activation or increased inactivation of a drug or its toxic intermediate. For example, 5-fluorouracil (5FU) must first be converted to its active metabolite FUDR in order to inhibit thymidylate synthase and subsequent DNA synthesis. Insufficient inhibition of thymidylate synthase resulting from decreased activation of 5FU, and increased inactivation of 5FU or 5FU-nucleotides are frequent mechanisms of resistance to 5FU *(197)*. Inhibition of thymidylate synthase by 5FU requires formation of the active intermediate fdUMP as well as optimal levels of 5,10 methylene-terahydrofolate, which is required for ternary complex formation with thymidylate synthase *(198)*. Cells may become resistant to 5FU by reducing their intracellular levels of reduced folates.

Electrophilic alkylating agents used in the treatment of breast cancer, such as cyclophosphamide, mediate cytotoxicity via the formation of interstrand DNA cross-links *(199)*. Glutathione plays an important role in inactivation or detoxification of alkylators and platinum and elevated intracellular levels of glutathione are associated with resistance to these agents *(200*, and for review *see 201)*. Conversely, buthionine sulfoximine (BSO), an inhibitor of glutathione synthesis, can increase the sensitivity of cells to alkylating agents and platinum. Alkylators can react spontaneously with reduced glutathione, resulting in metabolites that have increased solubility in water and are less toxic. Glutathione-S-transferases (GSTs) are a superfamily of isozymes that catalyze the conjugation of electrophillic agents with glutathione *(202–206)*. Studies using purified enzymes indicate that some isozymes of GSTs can enhance the catalytic conjugation of alkylating agents with glutathione *(207)*. Although increased expression of GST isozymes can lead to resistance to alkylators *(208)*, their role in resistance to anticancer drugs is less clear *(206,209,210)*.

Cyclophosphamide detoxification can also be mediated by aldehyde dehydrogenase, an enzyme that catalyzes the conversion of aldophosphamide (an activated species of cyclophosphamide) to carboxyphosphamide, an inactive form of cyclophosphamide *(211)*. Human breast-adenocarcinoma MCF-7 cells selected for resistance to mafosfamide exhibit elevated levels of aldehyde dehydrogenase *(212)* and transfection of a variety of cell types, including MCF-7 cells with vectors that overexpress aldehyde dehydrogenase, can increase the levels of resistance of these cells to alkylating agents including cyclophosphamide *(213–217)*.

Doxorubicin cytotoxicity has been linked in part to the generation of free radicals by metabolites of this agent *(218–220)*. Increased scavenging of reactive species by glutathione or glutathione peroxidases, may also be associated with the development of resistance to doxorubicin *(221)*.

2.9. Altered Drug Targets

Both quantitative or qualitative alterations or changes in the target proteins of antineoplastic drugs can contribute to the development of antineoplastic drug resistance. As previously described, changes in DNA topoisomerase II or topoisomerase I activity have been associated with resistance to topoisomerase inhibitors *(222)*. Other examples include quantitative and/or qualitative changes in dihydrofolate reductase, the target enzyme of methotrexate, resulting in resistance to methotrexate *(223)*. Paclitaxel can stabilize microtubules by blocking their depolymerization, resulting in metaphase arrest *(224,225)*. In addition to overexpression of MDR1, alterations or mutations in tubulins can lead to paclitaxel resistance *(226–228)*.

Tamoxifen, a nonsteroidal anti-estrogen agent, is an effective treatment for all stages of breast cancer. Although a favorable response to tamoxifen can be expected in 70–80% of patients with metastatic breast cancer that are estrogen- and progesterone-receptor positive, most tumors will eventually develop tamoxifen resistance, resulting in disease recurrence or progression. In some cases, tamoxifen resistance occurs as a result of loss of estrogen-receptor positive tumor cells *(229)*. However, other changes can result in tamoxifen resistance in breast cancer (reviewed in ref. *230*). These include changes in ligand metabolism and availability, defects in estrogen-receptor post-translational modification, alterations in the estrogen response element, and mutations in estrogen receptors.

2.10. Genetic vs Epigenetic Alterations and Drug Resistance

Enhanced genetic diversity or genomic instability in tumor cell populations *(231)* are most likely a result of the higher rate of mutation seen in malignant cells as opposed to normal cells *(232,233)*. The development of drug resistance, tumor progression, and metastasis is believed to result from genetic instability inherent to cancer cells. Epigenetic diversity (changes which influence the phenotype without altering the genotype) may also play a role in tumor progression and the development of drug resistance *(234,235)*. Nyce *(236)* has recently reviewed drug-induced DNA hypermethylation and its role in acquired drug resistance during cancer chemotherapy and has noted several important findings. Extensive DNA hypermethylation is seen following exposure of tumor cells to certain antineoplastic agents and is felt to be important with respect to drug-induced toxicity. Inhibition of expression of genes being synthesized during the period of drug-induced toxicity and the emergence of drug resistance by randomly inactivating genes whose products are required to activate certain chemotherapy agents may possibly result from DNA hypermethylation. Furthermore, drug-induced DNA hypermethylation can occur in patients undergoing chemotherapy for leukemia and can be inhibited by various agents in vitro as well as in vivo in these same patients. Lastly, drug-induced hyper or hypomethylation contributes to tumor-cell epigenetic and genetic instability.

Topoisomerase II inhibitors can induce DNA hypomethylation *(237,238)* and may render large stretches of DNA methylation-resistant as a result of DNA conformational changes. It has been postulated that the ability of topoisomerase inhibitors to activate

Table 4
Relevant Pathways of Drug Resistance in Human Breast Cancer

Drug	Mechanism
Doxorubicin	MDR1/MRP overexpression
	Altered levels of topoisomerase II expression
	Expression of mutated forms of topoisomerase II
	Increased glutathione or glutathione peroxidase levels
	DNA mismatch repair deficits
	Cellular resistance to apoptosis
Paclitaxel	MDR1 overexpression
	Alterations/mutations in expression of tubulin
	Cellular resistance to apoptosis
	erbB-2/neu amplification
Vinblastine,	MDR1/MRP overexpression
Vincristine	Alterations in tubulin
Cyclophosphamide	Elevated glutathione levels
	Glutathione-S-transferases with enhanced conjugation
	Elevated levels of aldehyde dehydrogenase
	Cellular resistance to apoptosis
5-Flourouracil	Decreased drug activation
	Increased drug intermediate inactivation
	Decreased reduced folate levels
	Cellular resistance to apoptosis
Methotrexate	Decreased influx by altered reduced folate carrier or receptors
	Increased activity of dihydrofolate reductase (DHFR)
	Impaired polyglutamination
	Mutations in DHFR gene affecting binding to DHFR
Mitoxantrone	Decreased drug accumulation in the absence of MDR1/MRP
	Cellular resistance to apoptosis
Topotecan	MDR1/MRP (topotecan) overexpression
Irinotecan (CPT-11)	Decreased metabolic activation
	Topoisomerase I mutation affecting cleavable complex formation
	Increased DNA repair
Tamoxifen	Quantitative or qualitative changes in estrogen receptors
	Changes in ligand availability and metabolism
	Defects in estrogen receptor post-translational modification

gene expression may be related to their ability to inhibit DNA methylation *(238)*. Increased topoisomerase II enzyme levels in tumor cells may be linked to ectopic gene expression in malignant cells, induction of polyploidy, and DNA hypomethylation, all markers for genetic instability in malignant cells *(239,240)*. Relevant pathways of drug resistance in human breast cancer are summarized in Table 4.

2.11. Host-Tumor-Drug Interactions

In the previous sections, we have primarily discussed genetic and/or epigenetic changes that may occur in tumor cells that may render them insensitive to anticancer agents. It is also clear that failure to achieve a therapeutic response to anticancer drugs may involve mechanisms that are not mediated by alterations in tumor cells. For example, it is well-known that diminished drug delivery into anatomic sanctuary sites, such as brain and testes, may result in high rates of relapse in patients with acute lymphoblastic leukemia *(241)*. In these relapses, the leukemic cells themselves may still be sensitive to cytotoxic agents and failure of therapy results from failure to achieve tumoricidal levels of drugs in these sites. Recent studies have indicated that the mechanism of decreased drug delivery into sanctuary sites involve drug-resistance genes. For example, the MDR gene MDR1 is overexpressed in endothelial cells in the central nervous system (CNS) and testes *(242,244,245)* and gene-knockout studies in mice demonstrate that elimination of the MDR-1a and MDR-1b genes in mice results in increased delivery of anticancer genes into the CNS *(245–248)*.

Large tumor masses may be refractory to chemotherapy in part because the relatively diminished blood supply can result in decreased drug delivery to tumor cells within the mass. The development of acidosis and hypoxia in poorly perfused areas of a tumor mass may also interfere with the cytotoxicity of certain drugs. Teicher and coworkers *(249)* have hypothesized that tumors may become refractory to chemotherapy by altering blood supply to the tumor or by changing the clearance or metabolism of a drug by the host. Under these circumstances, drug testing of the tumor cells in vitro will indicate that the tumor cells are sensitive to chemotherapy; however, tumors in vivo will be refractory to chemotherapy.

3. CLINICAL APPROACHES TO DRUG RESISTANCE

3.1. Dose-Intensive Chemotherapy to Circumvent Drug Resistance

One approach to the treatment of drug resistance in breast cancer is the use of increased doses of chemotherapy and or increased dose intensity (the amount of drug delivered per unit time). Increasing dose intensity can be accomplished by either increasing drug doses or decreasing the interval between drug treatments. The use of high-dose chemotherapy with autologous bone marrow or peripheral stem-cell support has been extensively explored in the treatment of breast cancer. Theoretically, the very high levels of the chemotherapeutic agents used in these regimens may be cytotoxic to cancer cells resistant to standard doses.

Initial interest in dose intensity in breast cancer resulted from a retrospective analysis of an early adjuvant chemotherapy trial, which suggested that patients who received at least 85% of their planned CMF dose benefited from adjuvant chemotherapy, whereas patients receiving less than 65% of the planned dose had the same disease-free survival and overall survival as the control group treated with surgery alone *(250)*. Another retrospective study of several trials also suggested that CMF dose intensity correlated with 3-yr disease free survival in breast-cancer patients *(251)*.

Several studies were subsequently designed to prospectively investigate the value of increased dose intensity in the adjuvant therapy of breast cancer. In one randomized study (CALGB 8541) of adjuvant chemotherapy for stage II, node-positive breast cancer, patients were randomized to receive different doses of the same adjuvant chemotherapy *(252)*. The first group was treated with six cycles of cyclophosphamide 400 mg/m^2 and doxorubicin 40 mg/m^2 once every 28 d and fluorouracil 400 mg/m^2 twice every 28 d. The second group received 50% higher doses (600, 60, 600, respectively) for only 4 cycles so that the total dose was identical to the first group, but the dose intensity was higher. The third group received 4 cycles of cyclophosphamide 300 mg/m^2 and doxorubicin 30 mg/m^2 once every 28 d and fluorouracil 300 mg/m^2 (CAF) twice every 28 d, which is half the total dose used in the other two groups and at half the dose intensity used in the second group. After a median follow-up of 3.4 yr, women treated with higher- (Group 2) or moderate-dose intensity (Group 1) had significantly longer median disease free-survival (74% and 70% vs 63% at 3 yr) and overall survival (92% and 90% vs 84% at 3 years) than those treated with low-dose intensity CAF. However, it was not possible to differentiate between a dose-intensity effect as opposed to a total cumulative dose effect in this study, because no difference in survival between the high- and moderate-dose intensity groups were seen. In addition, by current standards, the doses used in this trial are not considered high-dose chemotherapy and hematopoietic growth factor support was not instituted.

Muss et al. *(253)* examined c-erbB-2 expression and the response to adjuvant chemotherapy in women with node-positive early breast cancer, taken from the same CALGB 8541 trial discussed previously. In this analysis, the benefit from the "high-dose" CAF treatment occured only in patients whose tumors expressed high erbB-2 receptor levels. Thus, patients randomly assigned to the high-dose regimen as compared to the moderate- and low-dose CAF regimens had significantly longer disease-free (80%, 50%, and 25%, respectively) and overall (85%, 55%, and 40%, respectively) survival at 60 mo, only if their tumors manifested high c-erbB-2-overexpression. There was no difference in disease-free survival and overall survival among the three treatment groups in patients who had low levels of erbB-2 expression. The authors suggest that overexpression of c-erbB-2 may be a useful marker to identify breast-cancer patients who are most likely to benefit from high doses of adjuvant chemotherapy. The mechanism of this possible relationship between erbB-2 overexpression and clinical drug resistance is not known.

Other prospective clinical studies in the use of increased dose intensity and total dose of adjuvant chemotherapy have recently been reported. In NSABP B22, node-positive breast-cancer patients received adriamycin 60 mg/m^2 in combination with either standard-dose cyclophosphamide (600 mg/m^2) for 4 cycles (group 1), high dose cyclophosphamide (1200 mg/m^2) for 2 cycles (group 2), or high-dose cyclophosphamide (1200 mg/m^2) for 4 cycles (group 3). There was no difference in the 3-yr disease-free survival or the overall survival in any of the three treatment groups in this study *(73)*, *(92)*). Increasing the dose of cyclophosphamide in the AC regimen still further (1200 mg/m^2 vs 2400 mg/m^2) through the use of hematopoietic growth factors is currently being studied in the NSABP B25 trial. In addition, increasing the dose or dose intensity of doxorubicin while keeping the cyclophosphamide dose constant in the AC regimen is currently being evaluated in an Intergroup adjuvant chemotherapy trial *(256)*.

Very high-dose chemotherapy can be given to patients using autologous hematopioetic stem cell (HSC) support. Pilot studies exploring the use of high-dose chemotherapy with HSC support in patients with metastatic breast cancer have shown that this therapy is associated with high overall response rates and complete response rates up to 50%. Although the median time to recur following high-dose chemotherapy with HSC support is approximately 9 mo, 15–30% of patients receiving this therapy remain disease-free for greater than 1 yr.

One randomized trial of high-dose chemotherapy with autologous bone-marrow transplant in patients with metastatic breast cancer has shown promising results *(257)*. In this trial, patients were treated with either 2 cycles of high-dose cyclophosphamide, mitoxantrone, and etoposide (HD-CNV) with autologous bone-marrow or stem-cell rescue, or 6–8 cycles of conventional doses of cyclophosphamide, mitoxantrone, vincristine (CNV) as first-line treatment for metastatic breast cancer. The overall response rate in patients treated with HD-CNV was 95% (vs 53% in the conventional-dose CNV arm) and with a complete response rate of 53% in the HD-CNV arm (vs 4% in the conventional-dose CNV arm). Both duration of response (80 vs 34 wk) and duration of survival (90 vs 45 wk) were significantly longer for patients who received HD-CNV.

High-dose chemotherapy with HSC has also been studied as adjuvant chemotherapy in high-risk stage-II breast-cancer patients with greater than 10 positive axillary nodes. A pilot study of high-dose chemotherapy (cyclophosphamide, cisplatin, carmustine) with autologous bone-marrow transplantation as consolidation after standard-dose adjuvant chemotherapy CAF reported an actuarial event-free survival of 72% (median follow-up of 2.5 yr), which was superior to a historical series of high-risk stage II breast-cancer patients. Based on these results, two randomized trials of high-dose chemotherapy with autologous bone-marrow support are currently underway in the U.S. in high-risk stage II breast-cancer patients ($\geq$10 positive axillary nodes). In one trial, patients receive standard CAF followed by either low-dose cyclophosphamide, cisplatin, and carmustine or high doses of the same drugs with bone-marrow support *(258)*. Another trial randomizes patients to receive CAF followed by tamoxifen or CAF followed by high-dose cyclophosphamide plus thiotepa with bone-marrow rescue. These clinical studies should provide valuable information on the usefulness of high-dose chemotherapy in the treatment of high-risk stage-II breast cancer.

3.2. Pgp Reversing Agents

Laboratory studies identifying specific mechanisms of drug resistance have also led to pharmacological approaches to drug resistance. For example, once Pgp (mdr1 gene product) was identified as an energy-dependent, drug-efflux pump, a large number of nonanticancer drugs were subsequently identified that could inhibit or modulate the function of Pgp (for review, *see* ref. *259*). These agents have been collectively termed MDR modulators or chemosensitizers and include verapamil, cyclosporin A, quinidine, quinine, and tamoxifen as first generation Pgp inhibitors. Many of these compounds (e.g., verapamil, a potent calcium-channel blocker) have significant toxicities that would preclude their use clinically in cancer patients. A series of second-generation Pgp inhibitors have therefore been identified that have fewer associated toxicities. These second-generation compounds include dexverapamil (R-verapamil), dexniguldipine (also a calcium-channel blocker), and S9788 (a triazionoaminoperdine derivative). However, both the first- and second-generation MDR inhibitors have relatively low affinity for Pgp. Thus, a third generation of Pgp inhibitors have been identified that are characterized by increased potency for inhibition of Pgp activity in vitro. These compounds include PSC 833 (a nonimmunosuppressive analog of cyclosporin), CGP41251 (a derivative of staurosporine), and GF120918 or GG918 (an acridonecarboxamide). Selected pharmacological agents with the ability to reverse MDR are listed in Table 5.

Table 5
Selected Pharmacological Agents with Ability
to Reverse Multidrug Resistance (MDR)

Calcium channel blockers	Cyclic peptides
R-Verapamil (5–10 μM)	Cyclosporin A (0.8–2 μM)
Dexniguldipine (0.1-1 μM)	SDZ PSC 833 (0.1–1 μM)
Gallopamil (5 μM)	SDZ 280-466 (0.1–1 μM)
Ro11-2933 (2-6 μM)	FK506 (3 μM)
PAK-200 (5 μM)	Rapamycin (3 μM)
Calmodulin antagonists	Vinca alkyloid analogues
Trifluoperazine (3–5 μM)	Vindoline (20–50 μM)
Fluphenazine (3 μM)	Thaliblastine (2 μM)
Trans-Flupenthixol (3 μM)	Miscellaneous compounds
Protein kinase C inhibitors	S 9788 (1–3 μM)
Calphostin C (250 nM)	GF120918 (0.02-0.1 μM)
Staurosporine (200 nM)	Tolyporphin (0.1–0.5 μM)
CGP 41251 (150 nM)	Dipyridamole (5-10 μM)
NPC 15437 (60 μM)	BIBW 22 (1 μM)
Safingol (20–50 μM)	Quinidine (10 μM)
Steroidal agents	Terfenadine (3-6 μM)
Progesterone (2 μM)	Reserpine (5 μM)
Tamoxifen (2–10 μM)	Amiodarone (4 μM)
Toremifene (5–10 μM)	Methadone (75 μM)
Megestrol acetate (5 μM)	

Concentrations in parentheses are those shown to have effect in reversing MDR in vitro. From ref. *314*.

Several MDR-reversing agents have been evaluated in phase-I trials in combination with various chemotherapy regimens *(260–281)* and some have been evaluated in phase-II trials with single-agent or combination chemotherapy in the treatment of a number of different malignancies including nonHodgkins lymphoma *(282–285)*, small-cell lung cancer *(286)*, myeloma *(287,288)*, renal-cell carcinoma *(289–295)*, colon cancer *(296)*, and acute leukemia *(297,298)*. Results from these phase-II trials have indicated that many of the MDR reversing agents alter the pharmacokinetics of anticancer drugs. Thus the analysis of the effects of these agents on toxicity and antitumor efficacy should include an assessment of their effects on the pharmacokinetics of anticancer drugs. Although results from some phase-II trials suggest a possible benefit of MDR-reversing agents, a recent randomized phase-III trial of oral verapamil in refractory myeloma patients treated with vincristine, doxorubicin, and dexamethasone (VAD) showed no beneficial effects *(118)*.

Studies in human breast-cancer cell lines suggested that MDR-reversing compounds might be useful. For example, resistance to taxol and doxorubicin in breast-cancer cells grown as multicellular tumor spheroids was almost completely reversed by the addition of PSC 833 *(299)*. Another study indicated that thaliblastine, a Pgp inhibitor, could partially reverse resistance in MDR breast-cancer cells (MCF/ADR), and fully reverse resistance to taxol in these cells *(300)*.

To date there have been few clinical trials evaluating the usefulness of MDR-reversing agents in breast cancer. The addition of dexverapamil to epirubicin in patients with advanced breast cancer with stable or progressive disease on epirubicin alone yielded some partial responses and temporarily stabilized progressive disease *(301)*. In one randomized trial *(302)*, 223 breast-cancer patients were given epirubicin and prednisolone bolus or epirubicin/prednisolone plus oral quinidine prior to undergoing breast-cancer surgery. No differences in survival or toxicity were seen. Two points bear consideration with regards to this study. First, corticosteroids have been shown to increase Pgp expression in vitro *(303)*, and second, tumor biopsies for Pgp expression were not obtained *(259)*. Another clinical trial explored the use of amiodarone as a Pgp antagonist given in combination with infusional doxorubicin or vinblastine in refractory breast cancer. In this trial, 9/33 patients had a partial response *(304)*. However, significant toxicities were noted in this study and the authors concluded that amiodarone was associated with too many untoward effects to be utilized as a drug resistance-reversing agent.

Another trial investigated the addition of R-verapamil to paclitaxel in patients with metastatic breast cancer who developed stable disease or disease progression following treatment with paclitaxel alone. In 29 patients who crossed over to receive R-verapamil with paclitaxel after achieving stable or progressive disease, 2 had minor responses to the combination therapy *(305)*. Both patients demonstrated positive staining for Pgp on fine-needle aspirates. However, the area under the concentration x time curve (AUC) of paclitaxel increased 2-fold following the addition of R-verapamil, thus complicating the interpretation of the results *(305,306)*. In this study, 19% of biopsies obtained from patients prior to treatment with paclitaxel showed Pgp staining, and this number increased to 76% following paclitaxel treatment.

Yet another study investigated the activity of cyclophosphamide, vincristine, adriamycin, and dexamethasone (CVAD) in combination with two MDR-reversing agents, quinine and verapamil, in patients with advanced breast cancer that failed to respond or progressed on CVAD *(307)*. In this trial, CVAD treatment alone resulted in a partial response rate of 11% with no complete responses, lasting approximately 5–10 mo. The addition of verapamil and quinine to the CVAD regime resulted in one complete response of approximately 12 mo duration and a 15% partial-response rate lasting 3–40 mo duration. The overall rate of CVAD sensitization by verapamil and quinine was 19%. Pgp expression was not analyzed in this study. Additional studies examining the effects of second- and third-generation MDR-reversing agents are currently underway and will ultimately determine whether these agents have a role in the treatment of breast cancer.

3.3. Transferring Drug-Resistance Genes into HSC

Another approach to increasing dose intensity and decreasing host toxicity is to increase the expression of drug resistance genes in bone-marrow cells. Studies by Mickisch et al. *(308)* have shown that increasing MDR1 expression in bone marrow cells of transgenic animals resulted in decreased hematopoietic toxicity from anticancer drugs that were MDR1 substrates. Further studies by Sorrentino et al. *(309)* demonstrated that mouse hematopoietic cells transduced with a retroviral vector containing the MDR1 gene could be expanded in vivo following treatment of animals with paclitaxel, an MDR substrate. Based on these preclinical studies, several clinical studies are exploring the ability to transfer MDR genes into hematopoietic progenitor cells in breast-cancer patients undergoing high-dose chemotherapy with HSC support *(85)*.

In addition to the numerous mechanisms of drug resistance discussed in this chapter, it has been predicted that several hundred additional ABC transporters (to which MDR and MRP belong) are present in the human genome *(310)*. Thus the potential of breast-cancer cells to develop anticancer drug resistance remains enormous and the circumvention of this resistance may appear daunting at this time. However, the fact that some types of cancers at even advanced stages can be cured with chemotherapy is encouraging. Future studies examining new mechanisms of drug resistance may ultimately provide for better treatment of patients with recurrent or refractory breast cancer.

REFERENCES

1. Piccart, M. J., L. Biganzoli, and J. A. Roy. 1996. Adjuvant systemic therapy for breast cancer. *Curr. Opin. Oncol.* **8:** 478–484.
2. Robert, N. J. 1997. Clinical efficacy of tamoxifen. *Oncology* (Huntingt). **11(2 Suppl 1):** 15–20.
3. Banerjee, D., E. Ercikan-Abali, M. Waltham, B. Schnieders, D. Hochhauser, W. W. Li, J. Fan, R. Gorlick, E. Goker, and J. R. Bertino. 1995. Molecular mechanisms of resistance to antifolates, a review. *Acta Biochim. Pol.* **42:** 457–464.
4. Goldman, I. D., N. S. Lichtenstein, and V. T. Oliverio. 1968. Carrier-mediated transport of the folic acid analogue, methotrexate, in L1210 leukemia cells. *J. Biol. Chem.* **243:** 5007.
5. Kessel, D., T. C. Hall, D. Roberts, et al. 1965. Uptake as a determinant of methotrexate resistance in mouse leukemias. *Science* **150:** 752.
6. Dixon, K. H., B. C. Lanpher, J. Chiu, K. Kelly, and K. H. Cowan. 1994. A novel cDNA restores reduced folate carrier activity and methotrexate sensitivity to transport deficient cells. *J. Biol. Chem.* **269:** 17–20.
7. Moscow, J. A., P. G. Johnston, D. Cole, D. G. Poplack, and K. H. Cowan. 1995. Characterization of cross-resistance to methotrexate in a human breast cancer cell line selected for resistance to melphalan. *Biochem. Pharmacol.* **49:** 1069–1078.
8. Moscow, J. A., M. Gong, R. He, M. K. Sgagias, K. H. Dixon, S. L. Anzick, P. S. Meltzer, and K. H. Cowan. 1995. Isolation of a gene encoding a human reduced folate carrier (RFC1) and analysis of its expression in transport deficient methotrexate-resistant human breast cancer cells. *Cancer Res.* **55:** 3790–3794.
9. Moscow, J. A., E. Schneider, and K. H. Cowan. 1996. Multidrug resistance. *Cancer Dhemother. Biol. Response Mod. Ann.* **16:** 111–131.
10. Gong, M., J. Yess, T. Connolly, S. P. Ivy, T. Ohnuma, K. H. Cowan, and J. A. Moscow. 1997. Molecular mechanism of antifolate transport-deficiency in a methotrexate-resistant MOLT–3 human leukemia cell line. *Blood* **89:** 2494–2499.
11. Sierra, E. E., K. E. Brigle, M. J. Spinella, and I. D. Goldman. 1997. pH dependence of methotrexate transport by the reduced folate carrier and the folate receptor in L1210 leukemia cells. *Biochem. Pharmacol.* **53:** 223–231.
12. Spinella, M. J., K. E. Brigle, S. J. Freemantle, E. E. Sierra, and I. D. Goldman. 1996. Comparison of methotrexate polyglutamylation in L1210 leukemia cells when influx is mediated by the reduced folate carrier or the folate receptor. Lack of evidence for influx route-specific effects. *Biochem. Pharmacol.* **52:** 703–712.
13. Brigle, K. E., M. J. Spinella, E. E. Sierra, and I. D. Goldman. 1995. Characterization of a mutation in the reduced folate carrier in a transport defective L1210 murine leukemia cell line. *J. Biol. Chem.* **270:** 22,974–22,979.

14. Hill, B. T., B. D. Bailey, J. C. White, and I. D. Goldman. 1979. Characteristics of transport of 4-amino antifolates and folate compounds by two cell lines of LY5178Y lymphoblasts, one with impared transport of methotrexate. *Cancer Res.* **39:** 2440.

15. Sirotnak, F. M., D. M. Moccio, L. E. Kelleher, and L. J. Goutsas. 1981. Relative frequency and kinetic properties of transport defective phenotypes among methotrexate-resistant L1210 clonal cell lines derived in vivo. *Cancer Res.* **41:** 4447.

16. Anthony, A. C., M. A. Kare, R. M. Portillo, P. C. Elwood, and J. F. Kolhouse. 1985. Studies of the role of a particulate folate-binding protein in the uptake of 5-methytetrahydrofolate by cultured human KB cells. *J. Biol. Chem.* **260:** 14,911.

17. Saikawa, Y., C. B. Knight, T. Saikawa, S. T. Page, B. A. Chabner, and P. C. Elwood. 1993. Decreased expression of the human folate receptor mediates transport-defective methotrexate resistance in KB cells. *J. Biol. Chem.* **268:** 5293–5301.

18. Chung, K. N., Y. Saikawa, T. H. Paik, K. H. Dixon, T. Mulligan, K. H. Cowan, and P. C. Elwood. 1993. Stable transfectants of human MCF-7 breast cancer cells with increased levels of the human folate receptor exhibit an increased sensitivity to antifolates. *J. Clin. Invest.* **91:** 1289–1294.

19. Hill, B. T. 1993. Differing patterns of cross-resistance resulting from exposure to specific antitumor drugs or to radiation in vitro. *Cytotechnology* **12:** 265–288.

20. Nielsen, D., and T. Skovsgaard. 1992. P-glycoprotein as multidrug transporter: a critical review of current multidrug resistant cell lines. *Biochem. Biophys. Acta.* **1139:** 169–183.

21. Adams, D. J., and V. C. Knick. 1992. MDR and non-MDR forms of cellular resistance to 5'-noranhydrovinblastine (Navelbine). *Proc. Annu. Mgt. Am. Assoc. Cancer Res.* **33:** A2760.

22. Mattern, M. R., G. A. Hofmann, R. M. Polsky, L. R. Funk, F. L. McCabe, and R. K. Johnson. 1993. In vitro and in vivo effects of clinically important campthecin analogues on multidrug-resistant cells. *Oncol. Res.* **5:** 467–474.

23. Gottesman, M. M. and I. Pastan. 1993. Biochemistry of multidrug resistance mediated by the multidrug transporter. *Annu. Rev. Biochem.* **62:** 385–427.

24. Nooter, K. and G. Stoter. 1996. Molecular mechanisms of multidrug resistance in cancer chemotherapy. *Path. Res. Pract.* **192:** 768–780.

25. Riordan, J. R., and V. Ling. 1979. Purification of P-glycoprotein from plasma membrane vesicles of Chinese hamster ovary cell mutants with reduced colchicine permeability. *J. Biol. Chem.* **254:** 12,701–12,705.

26. Chen, C., J. E. Chin, K. Ueda, D. P. Clark, I. Pastan, M. M. Gottesman, and I. B. Roninson. 1986. Internal duplication and homology with bacterial transport proteins in the mdr1 (P-glycoprotein) gene from multidrug-resistant human cells. *Cell* **47:** 381–389.

27. Gerlach, J. H., J. A. Endicott, P. F. Juranka, G. Henderson, F. Sarangi, K. L. Deuchars, and V. Ling. 1986. Homology between P-glycoprotein and a bacterial haemolysin transport protein suggests a model for multidrug-resistance. *Nature* **324:** 485—489.

28. Gros, P., J. Croop, and D. Housman. 1986. Mammalian multidrug resistance gene; complete cDNA sequence indicates strong homology to bacterial transport proteins. *Cell* **47:** 371–380.

29. Cole, S. P. C., E. R. Chanda, F. P. Dicke, J. H. Gerlach, and S. E. L. Mirski. 1991. Non-P-glycoprotein-mediated multidrug resistance in a small lung cancer cell line: evidence for decreased susceptibility to drug-induced DNA damage and reduced levels of topoisomerase II. *Cancer Res.* **51:** 3345–3352.

30. Schinkel, A., S. Kemp, M. Dolle, G. Rudenko, and E. Wagenaar. 1993. N-glycosylation and deletion mutants of the human MDR1 P-glycoprotein. *J. Biol. Chem.* **268:** 7474–7481.

31. Hamada, H. and T. Tsuruo. 1988. Characterization of the ATPase activity of the Mr 170,000 to 180,000 membrane glycoprotein (P-glycoprotein) associated with multidrug resistance in K562/ADM cells. *Cancer Res.* **48:** 4926–4932.

32. Horio, M., M. M. Gottesman, and I. Pastan. 1988. ATP-dependent transport of vinblastine in vesicles from human multidrug-resistant cells. *Proc. Natl. Acad. Sci. USA* **85:** 3580–3584.

33. Fairchild, C. R., S. P. Ivy, T. Rushmore, G. Lee, P. Koo, M. E. Goldsmith, C. E. Myers, E. Farber, and K. H. Cowan. 1987. Carcinogen-induced mdr overexpression is associated with xenobiotic resistance in rat preneoplastic liver nodules and hepatocellular carcinomas. *Proc. Natl. Acad. Sci. USA* **84:** 7701–7705.

34. Giai, M., N. Biglia, and P. Sismondi. 1991. Chemo resistance in breast cancer. *Eur. J. Gynaec. Oncol.* **12:** 359–373.

35. Sanfilippo, O., E. Ronchi, C. DeMarco, G. Difronzo, and R. Silvestrini. 1991. Expression of P-glycoprotein in breast cancer tissue and in vitro resistance to doxorubicin and vincristine. *Eur. J. Cancer* **27:** 155–158.

36. Correnti, M., M. E. Cavazza, N. Guedez, O. Herrera, and N. R. Suarez-Chacon. 1995. Expression of the multidrug-resistance (mdr) gene in breast cancer. *J. Chemother.* **7:** 449–451.

37. Wallner, J., D. Depisch, M. Hopfner, K. Haider, J. Spong, H. Ludwig, and R. Pirker. 1991. MDR 1 gene expression and prognostic factors in primary breast carcinomas. *Eur. J. Cancer* **27:** 1352–1355.

38. Charpin, C., P. Vielh, F. Duffaud, B. Devictor, L. Andrac, M. N. Lavaut, C. Allasia, N. Horschowski, and L. Piana. 1994. Quantitative immunocytochemical assays of P-glycoprotein in breast carcinomas: correlation to messenger RNA expression and to immunohistochemical prognostic indicators. *J. Natl. Cancer Inst.* **86:** 1539–1545.

39. Veneroni, S., N. Zaffaroni, M. G. Daidone, E. Benini, R. Villa, and R. Silvestrini. 1994. Expression of P-glycoprotein and in vitro or in vivo resistance to doxorubicin and cisplatin in breast and ovarian cancers. *Eur. J. Cancer* **30A:** 1002–1007.

40. Kacinski, B. M., L. D. Yee, and D. Carter. 1989. Quantitation of tumor cell expression of the P-glycoprotein (mdr1) gene in human breast carcinoma clinical specimens. *Cancer Bull.* **41:** 44–48.

41. Keith, W. N., S. Stallard, and R. Brown. 1990. Expression of mdr1 and gst-p in human breast tumors: comparison to in vitro chemosensitivity. *Br. J. Cancer.* **61:** 712.

42. Verrelle, P., F. Meissonnier, Y. Fonck, V. Feillel, C. Dionet, F. Kwiatkowski, R. Plagne, and J. Chassagne. 1991. Clinical relevance of immunohistochemical detection of multidrug resistance of P-glycoprotein in breast carcinoma. *J. Natl. Cancer Inst.* **3:** 111–116.

43. Wishart, G. C., J. A. Plumb, J. J. Going, A. M. McNicol, C. S. McArdle, T. Tsuruo, and S. B. Kaye. 1990. P-glycoprotein expression in primary breast cancer detected by immunochemistry with two monoclonal antibodies. *Br. J. Cancer.* **62:** 758–761.

44. Salmon, S. E., T. M. Grogan, T. Miller, R. Scheper, and W. S. Dalton. 1989. Prediction of doxorubicin resistance in vitro in myeloma, lymphoma, and breast cancer by P-glycoprotein staining. *J. Natl. Cancer Inst.* **81:** 696–701.

45. Goldstein, L. J., H. Galski, A. Fojo, M. Willingham, S. L. Lai, A. Gazdar, R. Pirker, A. Green, W. Crist, G. M. Brodeur, et al. 1989. Expression of a multidrug resistance gene in human cancers. *J. Natl. Cancer Inst.* **81:** 116–124.

46. Bodey, B., B. J. Bodey, A. M. Groger, J. V. Luck, S. E. Siegel, C. R. Taylor, and H. E. Kaiser. 1997. Immunocytochemical detection of the p170 multidrug resistance (MDR) and the p53 tumor suppressor gene proteins in human breast cancer cells: clinical and therapeutical significance. *Anticancer Res.* **17(2B):** 1311–1318.

47. Merkel, D. E., S. A. Fuqua, A. K. Tandon, S. M. Hill, A. U. Buzdar, and W. L. McGuire. 1989. Electrophoretic analysis of 248 clinical breast cancer specimens for P-glycoprotein overexpression or gene amplification. *J. Clin. Oncol.* **7:** 1129–1136.

48. Schneider, J., M. Bak, T. Efferth, M. Kaufmann, J. Mattern, and M. Volm. 1989. P-glycoprotein expression in treated and untreated human breast cancer. *Br. J. Cancer.* **60:** 815–818.

49. Moretti, J., H. Azaloux, D. Boisseran, J. Kouyoumdjian, and J. Vilcoq. 1996. Primary breast cancer imaging with Technetium–99m sestamibi and its relation with P-glycoprotein overexpression. *Eur. J. Nucl. Med.* **23:** 980–986.

50. DeLa Torre, M., R. Larsson, P. Nygren, A. Lindgren, and J. Bergh. 1994. Expression of the multidrug-resistance gene product in untreated human breast cancer and its relationship to prognostic markers. *Acta Oncol.* **33:** 773–777.

51. Ro, J., A. Sahin, J. Y. Ro, H. Fritsche, G. Hortobagyi, and M. Blick. 1990. Immunohistochemical analysis of P-glycoprotein expression correlated with chemotherapy resistance in locally advanced breast cancer. *Hum. Pathol.* **21:** 787–791.

52. Krishnamachary, N. and M. S. Center. 1993. The MRP gene associated with a non-P-glycoprotein multidrug resistance encoded a 190-kDa membrane bound glycoprotein. *Cancer Res.* **53:** 3658–3661.

53. Cole, S. P. C., G. Bhardwaj, and J. H. Gerlach. 1992. Overexpression of a transporter gene in a multidrug-resistant human lung cancer cell line. *Science* **258:** 1650–1654.

54. Barrand, M. A., A. C. Heppell-Parton, K. A. Wright, P. H. Rabbitts, and P. R. Twentyman. 1994. A 190-kilodalton protein overexpressed in non-P-glycoprotein-containing multidrug-resistance cells and its relationship to the MRP gene. *J. Natl. Cancer Inst.* **(86):** 110–117.

55. Hipfner, D. R., S. D. Gauldie, R. G. Deeley, and S. P. C. Cole. 1994. Detection of the Mr 190,000 multidrug resistance protein, MRP, with monoclonal antibodies. *Cancer Res.* **54:** 5788–5792.

56. Zaman, G. J. R., C. H. M. Versantvoort, S. J.J.M, W. H. M. Eijdems, M. deHaas, M. De Hass, A. J. Smith, H. J. Broxterman, N. H. Mulder, E. G. E. De Vries, F. Baas, and P. Borst. 1993. Analysis of the expression of MRP, the gene for a new putative transmembrane drug transporter in human multidrug resistant lung cancer cell lines. *Cancer Res.* **53:** 1747–1750.

57. Kruh, G. D., A. Chan, K. Myers, K. Gaughon, T. Miki, and S. A. Aaronson. 1994. Expression complementary DNA library transfer establishes mrp as a multidrug resistance gene. *Cancer Res.* **54:** 1649–1652.

58. Grant, A. V., G. Valdimarsson, D. R. Hipfner, K. C. Almquist, S. P. Cole, and R. G. Deeley. 1994. Overexpression of multidrug resistance-associated protein (MRP) increase resistance to natural product drugs. *Cancer Res.* **54:** 357–361.

59. Zaman, G. J., M. J. Flens, M. R. Van Leusden, M. de Haas, H. S. Mulder, J. Lankelma, H. M. Pinedo, R. J. Scheper, F. Baas, H. J. Broxterman, and others. 1994. The human multidrug resistance-associated protein MRP is a plasma membrane drug-efflux pump. *Proc. Natl. Acad. Sci. USA* **13:** 8822–8826.

60. Leier, I., G. Jedlitschky, U. Buchholz, S. P. Cole, R. G. Deeley, and D. Keppler. 1994. The MRP gene encodes an ATP-dependent export pump for leukotriene C4 and structurally related conjugates. *J. Biol. Chem.* **269:** 27,807–27,810.

61. Kavallaris, M. 1997. The role of multidrug resistance-associated protein (MRP) expression in multidrug resistance. *Anti-Cancer Drugs* **8:** 17–25.

62. Ishikawa, T., K. Akimaru, M. T. Kuo, W. Priebe, and M. Suzuki. 1995. How does the MRP/GS-X pump export doxorubicin? *J. Natl. Cancer Inst.* **87:** 1639–1640.

63. Paul, S., L. M. Breuninger, K. D. Tew, H. Shen, and G. D. Kruh. 1996. ATP-dependent uptake of natural product cytotoxic drugs by membrane vesicles establishes MRP as a broad specificity transporter. *Proc. Natl. Acad. Sci. USA* **93:** 6929–6934.

64. Flens, M. J., M. A. Izquierdo, G. L. Scheffer, J. M. Fritz, C. J. Meijer, R. J. Scheper, and G. J. Zaman. 1994. Immunochemical detection of the multidrug resistance-associated protein MRP in human multidrug-resistant tumor cells by monoclonal antibodies. *Cancer Res.* **54:** 4557–4563.

65. Cole, S. P. C., K. E. Sparks, K. Fraser, D. W. Loe, C. E. Grant, G. M. Wilson, and R. G. Deeley. 1994. Pharmacological characterization of multidrug resistant MRP-transfected human tumor cells. *Cancer Res.* **54:** 5902–5910.

66. Almquist, K. C., D. W. Low, and D. R. Hipfner. 1995. Characterization of the MR 190,000 multidrug resistance protein (MRP) in drug-selected and transfected human tumor cells. *Cancer Res.* **55:** 102–110.

67. Schneider, E., J. K. Horton, C. H. Yang, M. Nakagawa, and K. H. Cowan. 1994. Multidrug resistance-associated protein gene overexpression and reduced drug sensitivity of topoisomerase II in a human breast carcinoma MCF-7 cell line selected for etoposide resistance. *Cancer Res.* **54:** 152–158.

68. Eijems, E. W. H. M., M. DeHaas, and J. M. Coco-Martin. 1995. Mechanisms of MRP overexpression in four human lung-cancer cell lines and analysis of the MRP amplicon. *Int. J. Cancer* **60:** 676–684.

69. Sugawara, I. 1995. Multidrug resistance: role of multidrug resistance-associated protein (MRP). *Cancer J.* **8:** 59–61.

70. Binaschi, M., R. Supino, and R. A. Gambetta. 1995. MRP gene over-expression in a human doxorubicin-resistant SCLC cell line: alterations in cellular pharmacokinetics and in a pattern of cross-resistance. *Int. J. Cancer* **62:** 84–89.

71. Sugawara, I., H. Yamada, H. Nakamura, A. Sumizawa, S. Akiyama, A. Masunaga, and S. Itoyama. 1995. Preferential expression of the multidrug resistance associated protein MRP in adenocarinoma of the lung. *Int. J. Cancer* **64:** 322–325.

72. Narasaki, F., I. Matsuo, N. Ikuno, M. Fukuda, H. Soda, and M. Oka. 1996. Multidrug resistance-associated protein (MRP) gene expression in human lung cancer. *Anticancer Res.* **16:** 2079–2082.

73. Hart, S. M., K. Ganeshaguru, A. V. Hoftbrand, H. G. Prentice, and A. B. Mehta. 1994. Expression of the multidrug resistance-associated protein (mrp) in acute leukemia. *Leukemia* **8:** 2162–2168.

74. Beck, J., R. Handgreinger, R. Dopfer, T. Klingebiel, D. Niethammer, and V. Gekeler. 1995. Expression of mdr1, mrp, topoisomerase II a/b and cycline A in primary or relapsed states of acute lymphoblastic leukemias. *Brit. J. Haematol.* **89:** 356–363.

75. Norris, M. D., S. B. Bordow, and G. M. Marshall. 1996. Expression of the gene for multidrug-resistance-associated protein and outcome in patients with neuroblastoma. *N. Engl. J. Med.* **334:** 231-238.

76. Bordow, S. B., M. Haber, and J. Madafiglio. 1994. Expression of the multidrug resistance-associated protein (MRP) gene correlates with amplification and overexpression of the N-myc oncogene in childhood neuroblastoma. *Cancer Res.* **54:** 5036–5040.

77. Perez-Soler, R., N. Neamati, Y. Zou, E. Schneider, L. A. Doyle, M. Andreeff, W. Priebe, and Y. H. Ling. 1997. Annamycin circumvents resistance mediated by the multidrug resistance-associated protein (MRP) in breast MCF-7 and small-cell lung UMCC-1 cancer cell lines selected for resistance to exposide. *Int. J. Cancer* **71:** 35–41.

78. Vosberg, H. P. 1985. DNA topoisomerases: enzymes that control DNA conformation. *Curr. Top. Microbiol. Immunol.* **114:** 19.

79. Wang, J. C. 1985. DNA topoisomerases. *Annu. Rev. Biochem.* **54:** 665.

80. Maxell, G. and M. Gellert. 1986. Mechanistic aspects of DNA topoisomerases. *Adv. Protein Chem.* **38:** 69.

81. Zhang, H., P. D'Arpa, and L. F. Liu. 1990. A model for tumor cell killing by topoisomerase poisons. *Cancer Cells* **2:** 23.

82. Liu, L. 1989. DNA topoisomerase poisons as antitumor drugs. *Annu. Rev. Biochem.* **58:** 351.

83. Chen, A. Y. and L. F. Liu. 1994. DNA topoisomerases: essential enzymes and lethal targets. Annu. Rev. Pharmacol. Toxicol. **94:** 194–218.

84. Yang, L., L. F. Liu, J. J. Li, M. S. Wold, and T. J. Kelly. 1986. The roles of DNA topoisomerase in SV40 DNA replication. *UCLA Symp. Mol. Cell Biol.* **47:** 315–325.

85. Moscow, J., J. Zujewski, H. Huang, B. Sorrentino, Y. Chiang, W. Wilson, E. Cullen, N. McAtee, M. Gottesman, I. Pastan, C. Dunbar, N. A., and K. Cowan. 1997. Hematopoietic

reconstitution with CD34-selected cells transduced with a retroviral vector containing the MDR1 gene in patients with metastatic breast cancer. *Proceed. AACR* **38**: 343.

86. Hochhauser, D. and A. L. Harris. 1993. The role of topoisomerase II alpha and beta in drug resistance. *Cancer Treat. Rev.* **19**: 181–194.

87. Bugg, B. Y., M. K. Danks, W. T. Beck, and D. P. Suttle. 1991. Expression of a mutant DNA topoisomerase II in CCRF-CEM human leukemic cells selected for resistance to teniposide. *Proc. Natl. Acad. Sci. USA* **88**: 7654–7658.

88. Chan, V. T. W., S. W. Ng, J. P. Eder, and L. E. Schnipper. 1993. Molecular cloning and idenfication of a point mutation in the topoisomerase II cDNA from an etoposide-resistant chinese hamster ovary cell line. *J. Biol. Chem.* **268**: 2160–2165.

89. Danks, M. K., M. R. Warmoth, E. Friche, B. Granzen, B. Y. Bugg, W. G. Harker, L. A. Zwelling, B. W. Futscher, D. P. Suttle, and W. T. Beck. 1993. Single-strand conformational polymorphism analysis of the Mr 170,000 isozyme of DNA topoisomerase II in human tumor cells. *Cancer Res.* **53**: 1373–1379.

90. Hinds, M., K. Deisseroth, J. Mayes, E. Altschuler, R. Jansen, F. D. Ledley, and L. A. Zwelling. 1991. Identification of a point mutation in the topoisomeras II gene from a human leukemia cell line containing an amsacrine-resistant form of topoisomerase II. *Cancer Res.* **51**: 4729–4731.

91. Lee, M. S., J. C. Wang, and M. Beran. 1992. Two independent amsacrine-resistant human myeloid leukemia cell lines share an identical point mutation in the 170-kDa form of human topoisomerase II. *J. Mol. Biol.* **223**: 837–843.

92. Deffie, A. M., J. K. Batra, and G. J. Goldenberg. 1989. Direct correlation between DNA topoisomerase II activity and cytotoxicity in adriamycin-sensitive and resistant p388 leukemic cell lines. *Cancer Res.* **49**: 58.

93. Per, S. R., M. R. Mattern, and C. K. Mirabelli. 1987. Characterization of a subline of p388 leukemia resistant to amsacrine: evidence of altered topoisomerase II function. *Mol. Pharmacol.* **32**: 17.

94. Gudkov, A. V., C. R. Zelnick, A. R. Kazarov, R. Thimmapaya, D. P. Suttle, W. T. Beck, and I. B. Roninson. 1993. Isolation of genetic suppressor elements, inducing resistance to topoisomerase II-interactive cytotoxic drugs, from human topoisomerase II cDNA. *Proc. Natl. Acad. Sci. USA* **90**: 3231–3235.

95. Fernandez, D. J., D. M.J., and W. T. Beck. 1990. Decreased nuclear matrix DNA topoisomerase II in human leukemic cells resistant to UM-26 and m-AMSA. *Biochemistry* **29**: 4235–4241.

96. Mirski, S. E. L., C. D. Evans, K. C. Almquist, M. L. Slovak, and S. P. Cole. 1993. Altered topoisomerase II alpha in a drug-resistant small cell lung cancer cell line selected in VP-16. *Cancer Res.* **53**: 4866–4873.

97. Campain, J. A., R. Padmanabhan, J. Hwang, M. M. Gottesman, and I. Pastan. 1993. Characterization of an unusual mutant of human melanoma cells resistant to anticancer drugs that inhibit topoisomerase II. *J. Cell Physiol.* **155**: 414–425.

98. Meirno, A., K. R. Madden, W. S. Lane, J. J. Champoux, and D. Reinberg. 1993. DNA topoisomerase I is involved in both repression and activation of transcription. *Nature* **365**: 227.

99. Gupta, M., A. Fujimori, and Y. Pommier. 1995. Eukaryotic DNA topoisomerases I. *Biochem. Biophys. Acta.* **1262**: 1–14.

100. Pommier, Y. and A. Tanizawa. 1994. Camptothecins: mechanism of action and resistance. *Cancer Invest.* **11**: 3–6.

101. Hsiang, Y. H., R. Hertzberg, S. Hecht, and L. F. Liu. 1985. Camptothecin induces protein-linked DNA breaks via mammalian DNA topoisomerase I. *J. Biol. Chem.* **260**: 14,873–14,878.

102. Bendixen, C., B. Thomsen, J. Alsner, and O. Westergaard. 1990. Camptothecin-stabilized topoisomerase I-DNA adducts cause premature termination of transcription. *Biochemistry* **29**: 5613–5619.

103. Covey, J. M., C. Jaxel, K. W. Kohn, and Y. Pommier. 1989. Protein-linked DNA strand breaks induced in mammalian cells by camptothecin, an inhibitor of topoisomerase I. *Cancer Res.* **49:** 5016–5022.

104. Tsao, Y. P., A. Russo, G. Nyamuswa, R. Silber, and L. F. Liu. 1993. Interaction between replication forks and topoisomerase I DNA cleavable complexes: studies in a cell-free SV40 DNA replication system. *Cancer Res.* **53:** 5908–5914.

105. Chatterjee, S., M.-F. Cheng, D. Trived, S. J. Petzold, and N. A. Berger. 1989. Campto-thecin hypersensitivity in poly (adenosine diphosphate-ribose) polymerase-deficient cell lines. *Cancer Commun.* **1:** 389–394.

106. Bullock, P., J. J. Champoux, and M. Botchan. 1985. Association of crossover points with topoisomerase I cleavage sites: a model for nonhomologous recombination. *Science* **230:** 954–958.

107. Bertrand, R., E. Solary, J. Jenkins, and Y. Pommier. 1993. Apoptosis and its modulation in human promyelocytic HL-60 cells treated with DNA toposomerase I and II inhibitors. *Exp. Cell Res.* **207:** 388–397.

108. Chen, A. Y., C. Yu, M. Potmesil, M. E. Wall, M. C. Wani, and L. F. Liu. 1991. Camptothecin overcomes MDR1-mediated resistance in human KB carcinoma cells. *Cancer Res.* **51:** 6039–6044.

109. Hendricks, C. B., E. K. Rowinsky, L. B. Grochow, R. C. Donehower, and S. H. Kaufmann. 1992. Effect of p-glycoprotein expression on the accumulation and cyto-toxicity of topotecan (SK alpha F 104864), a new camptothecin analogue. *Cancer Res.* **52:** 2268–2278.

110. Lai, S. L., L. Goldstein, M. M. Gottesman, I. Pastan, C. M. Tsai, B. E. Johnson, J. L. Mulshine, D. C. Ihde, K. Kayser, and A. F. Gazdar. 1989. MDR1 gene expression in lung cancer. *J. Natl. Cancer Inst.* **81:** 1144–1150.

111. Kanzawa, F., Y. Sugimoto, K. Minato, K. Kasahara, M. Bungo, K. Nakagawa, Y. Fujiwara, L. F. Liu, and N. Saigo. 1990. Establishment of a camptothecin analogue (CPT-11)-resistant cell line of human non-small cell lung cancer: characterization and mecha-nism of resistance. *Cancer Res.* **50:** 5919–5924.

112. Sugimoto, Y., S. Tsukahara, T. Oh-hara, L. F. Liu, and T. Tsuruo. 1990. Elevated expres-sion of DNA topisomerase II in camptothecin-resistant human tumor cell lines. *Cancer Res.* **50:** 7962–7965.

113. Tan, K. B., M. R. Mattern, W.-K. Eng, F. L. McCabe, and R. K. Johnson. 1989. Nonpro-ductive rearrangement of DNA topoisomerase I and II genes: correlation with resistance to topoisomerase inhibitors. *J. Natl. Cancer Inst.* **81:** 1732–1735.

114. Madelaine, I., S. Prost, A. Naudin, G. Riou, F. Lavelle, and J.-F. Riou. 1993. Sequential modifications of topoisomerase I activity in a camptothecin-resistant cell line established by progressive adaptation. *Biochem. Pharmacol.* **45:** 339–348.

115. Fujimori, A., G. Malini, Y. Hoki, and Y. Pommier. 1996. Acquired camptothecin resis-tance of human breast cancer MCF-7/C4 cells with normal topoisomerase I and elevated DNA repair. *Mol. Pharmacol.* **50:** 1472–1478.

116. Taguchi, T., T. Tominaga, M. Ogawa, T. Ishida, K. Morimoto, and N. Ogawa. 1994. A late phase II study of CPT-11 (irinotecan) in advanced breast cancer. CPT-11 Study Group on Breast Cancer. *Gan to Kagaku Ryoho* **21:** 1017–1124.

117. Bonneterre, J., J. M. Pion, A. Adenis, M. Tubiana-Hulin, T. Tursz, M. Marty, and A. Mathieu-Boue. 1993. A phase II study of a new camptothecin analogue CPT-11 in previ-ously treated advanced breast cancer patients. *Proc. Am. Soc. Clin. Oncol.* **12:** 94.

118. Dalton, W. S., J. J. Crowley, S. S. Salmon, T. M. Grogan, L. R. Laufman, G. R. Weiss, and J. D. Bonnet. 1995. A phase III randomized study of oral verapamil as a chemosensitizer to reverse drug resistance in patients with refractory myeloma. *Cancer* **75:** 815–820.

119. Yang, C. J., J. K. Horton, K. H. Cowan, and E. Schneider. 1995. Cross-resistance to camptothecin analogues in a mitoxantrone-resistant human breast carcinoma cell line is not due to DNA topoisomerase I alterations. *Cancer Res.* **55:** 4004–4009.

120. Kerr, J. F. R., C. M. Winterford, and B. V. Harmon. 1994. Apoptosis: Its significance in cancer and cancer therapy. *Cancer* **73:** 2013–2026.

121. Warri, A. M., R. L. Huovinen, A. M. Laine, P. M. Martikainen, and P. L. Harkoner. 1993. Apoptosis in toremifene-induced growth inhibition of human breast cancer cells in vivo and in vitro. *J. Natl. Cancer Inst.* **85:** 1412–1418.

122. Pagliacci, M. C., R. Tognellini, F. Grignani, and I. Nicoletti. 1991. Inhibition of human breast cancer cell (MCF-7) growth in vitro by the stomatostatin analog SMS 201-995: effects on cell cycle parameters and apoptotic cell death. *Endocrinology.* **129:** 2555–2562.

123. Kyprianou, N., H. F. English, N. E. Davidson, and J. T. Isaacs. 1991. Programmed cell death during regression of the MCF-7 human breast cancer following estrogen ablation. *Cancer Res.* **51:** 162–166.

124. Bitonti, A. J., J. A. Dumont, T. L. Bush, E. A. Cashman, D. D. Cross, P. S. Wright, D. P. Matthews, J. R. McCarthy, and D. A. Kaplan. 1994. Regression of human breast tumor xenografts in response to (E)-2'-deoxy–2'-(fluoromethylene) cytidine, an inhibitor of ribonucleoside diphosphate reductase. *Cancer Res.* **54:** 1485–1490.

125. Bellomo, G., M. Perotti, F. Taddei, F. Mirabelli, G. Finardi, P. Nicotera, and S. Orrenius. 1992. Tumor necrosis factor alpha induces apoptosis in mammary adenocarcinoma cells by an increase in intranuclear free Ca^{2+} concentration and DNA fragmentation. *Cancer Res.* **52:** 1342–1346.

126. Armstrong, D. K., S. H. Kaufmann, Y. L. Ottaviano, Y. Furuya, J. A. Buckley, J. T. Isaacs, and N. E. Davidson. 1994. Epidermal growth factor-mediated apoptosis of MDA-MB-468 human breast cancer cells. *Cancer Res.* **54:** 5280–5283.

127. Lowe, S. W., H. E. Ruley, T. Jacks, and D. E. Housman. 1993. P53-dependent apoptosis modulates the cytotoxicity of anticancer agents. *Cell* **74:** 957–967.

128. Lowe, S. W., S. Bodis, A. McClatchey, L. Remington, H. E. Ruley, D. E. Fisher, D. E. Housman, and T. Jacks. 1994. P53 status and the efficacy of cancer therapy in vivo. *Science* **226:** 807–810.

129. Rusch, V., D. Klimstra, E. Venkatraman, J. Oliver, N. Martini, R. Gralla, M. Kris, and E. Dimitrovsky. 1995. Aberrant p53 expression predicts clinical resistance to cisplatin-based chemotherapy in locally advanced non-small cell lung cancer. *Cancer Res.* **55:** 5038–5042.

130. Allred, D. C., G. M. Clark, R. Elledge, S. A. Fuqua, R. W. Brown, G. C. Chamness, C. K. Osborne, and W. L. McGuire. 1993. Association of p53 protein expression with tumor cell proliferation rate and clinical outcome in node-negative breast cancer. *J. Natl. Cancer Inst.* **85:** 200–206.

131. Chin, K.-U., K. Ueda, I. Pastan, and M. M. Gottesman. 1992. Modulation of activity of the promoter of the human mdr1 gene by Ras and p53. *Science* **255:** 459–462.

132. Bergh, J., T. Norberg, S. Sjogren, A. Lindgren, and L. Holmberg. 1995. Complete sequencing of the p53 gene provides prognostic information in breast cancer patients, particularly in relation to adjuvant systemic therapy and radiotherapy. *Nature Med.* **1:** 1029–1034.

133. Borresen, A. L., T. I. Andersen, J. E. Eyfjord, R. S. Cornelis, S. Thorlacius, A. Borg, U. Johansson, C. Theillet, S. Scherneck, S. Hartman, and others. 1995. TP53 mutations and breast cancer prognosis: particularly poor survival rates for cases with mutations in the zinc-binding domains. *Genes Chromosom. Cancer* **14:** 71–75.

134. Kovach, J. S., A. Hartmann, H. Blaszyk, J. Cunningham, D. Schaid, and S. S. Sommer. 1996. Mutation detection by highly sensitive methods indicates that p53 gene mutations in breast cancer can have important prognostic value. *Proc. Natl. Acad. Sci. USA* **93:** 1093–1096.

135. Silvestrini, R., E. Benini, S. Veneroni, M. G. Daidone, G. Tomasic, P. Squicciarini, and B. Salvadori. 1996. P53 and Bcl-2 expression correlates with clinical outcome in a series of node-positive breast cancer patients. *J. Clin. Oncol.* **14:** 1604–1610.

136. Jansson, T., M. Inganas, S. Sjogren, T. Norberg, A. Lindgren, L. Holmberg, and J. Bergh. 1995. P53 status predicts survival in breast cancer patients treated with/without postoperative radiotherapy: A novel hypothesis based on clinical findings. *J. Clin. Oncol.* **13:** 2745–2751.

137. Stal, O., M. Stenmark-Askmalm, S. Wingren, L. E. Rutqvist, L. Skoog, L. Ferraud, S. Sullivan, J. Carstensen, and B. Nordenskjold. 1995. P53 expression and the result of adjuvant therapy of breast cancer. *Acta Oncol.* **34:** 767–770.

138. Aas, T., A. L. Borresen, S. Geisler, B. Smith-Sorensen, H. Johnsen, J. E. Varhaug, L. A. Akslen, and P. E. Lonning. 1996. Specific p53 mutations are associated with de novo resistance to doxorubicin in breast cancer patients. *Nat. Med.* **2:** 811–814.

139. Thor, A. D., D. H. Moore II, S. M. Edgerton, E. S. Kawasaki, E. Reihsaus, H. T. Lynch, J. N. Marcus, L. Schwartz, L.-C. Chen, B. H. Mayall, and H. S. Smith. 1992. Accumulation of p53 tumor suppressor gene protein: an independent marker of prognosis in breast cancer. *J. Natl. Cancer Inst.* **84:** 845–55.

140. Linn, S. C., A. H. Honkoop, K. Hoekman, P. Van der Valk, H. M. Pinedo, and G. Giaccone. 1996. P53 and P-glycoprotein are often co-expressed and are associated with poor prognosis in breast cancer. *Br. J. Cancer.* **74:** 63–68.

141. Wosikowski, K., J. T. Regis, R. W. Robey, M. Alvarez, J. T. Buters, J. M. Gudas, and S. E. Bates. 1995. Normal p53 status and function despite the development of drug resistance in human breast cancer cells. *Cell Growth Differ.* **6:** 1395–1403.

142. Gudas, J. M., H. Nguyen, T. Li, and L. Sadzewicz. 1996. Drug-resistant breast cancer cells frequently retain expression of a functional wild-type p53 protein. *Carcinogenesis* **17:** 1417–1427.

143. Walton, M. I., D. Whysong, P. M. O'Connor, D. Hockenbery, S. J. Korsmeyer, and K. W. Kohn. 1993. Constitutive expression of human bcl-2 modulates nitrogen mustard and camptothecin induced apoptosis. *Cancer Res.* **53:** 1853–1861.

144. Harker, W. G., D. L. Slade, F. H. Drake, and R. L. Parr. 1991. Mitoxantrone resistance in HL-60 leukemia cells: reduced nuclear topoisomerase II catalytic activity and drug-induced DNA cleavage in association with reduced expression of the topoisomerase-IIB-isoform. *Biochemistry* **30:** 9953–9961.

145. Fisher, T. L., A. E. Milner, C. D. Gregory, A. L. Jackman, G. W. Aherne, J. A. Hartley, C. Dive, and J. A. Hickman. 1993. Bcl–2 modulation of apoptosis induced by anticancer drugs: resistance to thymidylate stress is independent of classical resistance pathways. *Cancer Res.* **53:** 3321–3326.

146. Dole, M., G. Nunez, A. K. Merchant, J. Maybaum, C. K. Rode, C. A. Bloch, and V. P. Castle. 1994. Bcl–2 inhibits chemotherapy-induced apoptosis in neuroblastoma. *Cancer Res.* **54(12):** 3253–3259.

147. Sumantran, V. N., M. W. Ealovega, G. Nunez, M. F. Clarke, and M. S. Wicha. 1995. Overexpression of Bcl-Xs sensitizes MCF-7 cells to chemotherapy-induced apoptosis. *Cancer Res.* **55:** 2507–2510.

148. Kane, D. J., T. A. Sarafian, R. Anton, H. Hahn, E. B. Gralla, J. S. Valentine, T. Ord, and D. E. Bredesen. 1993. Bcl-2 inhibition of neural death: decreased generation of reactive oxygen species. *Science* **262:** 1274–1277.

149. Albrecht, H., J. Tschopp, and C. V. Jongeneel. 1994. Bcl–2 protects from oxidative damage and apoptotic cell death without interfering with activation of NF-KB by TNF. *FEBS Lett.* **351:** 45–48.

150. Cortazzo, M. and N. F. Schor. 1996. Potentiation of enediyne-induced apoptosis and differentiation by bcl-2. *Cancer Res.* **56:** 1199–1203.

151. Ogretmen, B. and A. R. Safa. 1996. Down-regulation of apoptosis-related bcl-2 but not bcl-xl or bax proteins in multidrug-resistant MCF-7/Adr human breast cancer cells. *Int. J. Cancer* **67**: 608–614.

152. Bafy, G., T. Miyashita, J. R. Williamson, and J. C. Reed. 1993. Apoptosis induced by withdrawal of Interleukin-3 (IL-3) from an IL-3 dependant hematopoetic cell line is associated with repartitioning of intracellular calcium and is blocked by enforced Bcl2 oncoprotein production. *J. Biol. Chem.* **268**: 6511–6519.

153. Oltvai, Z. N., C. L. Millimann, and S. J. Korsmeyer. 1994. BH1 and BH2 domains of Bcl-2 are required for inhibition of apoptosis and heterodimerization with bax. *Nature* **359**: 321–323.

154. Huang, Y., S. Ray, J. L. Reed, A. M. Ibrado, C. Tang, A. Nawabi, and K. Bhalla. 1997. Estrogen increases intracellular p26 bcl-2 to p21 bax ratios and inhibits taxol-induced apoptosis of human breast cancer MCF-7 cells. *Breast Cancer Res. Treat.* **42**: 73–81.

155. Teixeira, C., J. C. Reed, and C. M. A. Pratt. 1995. Estrogen promotes chemotherapeutic drug resistance by a mechanism involving bcl-2 proto-oncogene expression in human breast cancer cells. *Cancer Res.* **55**: 3902–3907.

156. Trauth, B. C., C. Klas, A. M. Peters, S. Matzku, P. Moller, W. Falk, K. M. Debatin, and P. H. Krammer. 1989. Monoclonal antibody-mediated tumor regression by induction of apoptosis. *Science* **245**: 301–305.

157. Dhein, J., P. T. Daniel, B. C. Trauth, A. Oehm, P. Moller, and P. H. Krammer. 1992. Induction of apoptosis by monoclonal antibody anti-APO-1 class switch variants is dependant on cross-linking of APO-1 cell surface antigens. *J. Immunol.* **149**: 3166–3173.

158. Rowan, S., and D. E. Fisher. 1997. Mechanisms of apoptotic cell death. *Leukemia* **11**: 457–465.

159. Bargou, R. C., P. T. Daniel, M. Y. Mapara, K. Bommert, C. Wagener, B. Kallinich, M. D. Royer, and B. Dorken. 1995. Expression of the bcl-2 gene family in normal and malignant breast tissue: low bax-alpha expression on tumor cells correlates with resistance towards apoptosis. *Int. J. Cancer* **60**: 854–859.

160. Jaattela, M., M. Benedict, M. Tewari, J. A. Shayman, and V. M. Dixit. 1995. Bcl-x and Bcl-2 inhibit TNF and Fas-induced apoptosis and activation of phospholipase A2 in breast carcinoma cells. *Oncogene* **10**: 2297–2305.

161. Bargou, R. C., C. Wagener, K. Bommert, M. Y. Mapara, P. T. Daniel, W. Arnold, M. Dietel, H. Guski, A. Feller, H. D. Royer, and B. Dorken. 1996. Overexpression of the death-promoting gene bax-alpha which is down regulated in breast cancer restores sensitivity to different apoptotic stimuli and reduces tumor growth in SCID mice. *J. Clin. Invest.* **97**: 2403–2404.

162. Keane, M. M., S. A. Ettenburg, G. A. Lowrey, E. K. Russell, and S. Lipkowitz. 1996. Fas expression and function in normal and malignant breast cell lines. *Cancer Res.* **56**: 4791–4798.

163. Turley, J. M., T. Fu, F. W. Ruscetti, J. A. Mikovits, D. C. Bertolette, III, and M. C. Birchenall-Roberts. 1997. Vitamin E succinate induces Fas-mediated apoptosis in estrogen receptor-negative human breast cancer cells. *Cancer Res.* **57**: 881–890.

164. Shen, K. and R. F. Novak. 1997. Fas-signaling and effects on receptor tyrosine kinase signal transduction in human breast epithelial cells. *Biochem. Biophys. Res. Commun.* **230**: 89–93.

165. Mizutani, Y., Y. Okada, O. Yoshida, M. Fukumoto, and B. Bonavida. 1997. Doxorubicin sensitizes human bladder carcinoma cells to Fas-mediated cytotoxicity. *Cancer* **79**: 1180–1189.

166. Wagener, C., R. C. Bargou, P. T. Daniel, K. Bommert, M. Y. Mapara, H. D. Royer, and B. Dorken. 1996. Induction of the death-promoting gene bax-alpha sensitizes cultured breast-cancer cells to drug-induced apoptosis. *Int. J. Cancer* **67**: 138–141.

167. Sakakura, C., E. A. Sweeney, T. Shirahama, Y. Igarashi, S. Hakomori, H. Nakatani, H. Tsujimoto, T. Imanishi, M. Ohgaki, T. Ohyama, J. Yamazaki, A. Hagiwara, T. Yamaguchi, K. Sawai, and T. Takahashi. 1996. Overexpression of bax senstizes human breast cancer MCF-7 cells to radiation-induced apoptosis. *Int. J. Cancer* **67**: 101–105.

168. Krajewski, S., C. Blomqvist, K. Franssila, M. Krajewski, U.-M. Wasenius, E. Niskanen, S. Nordling, and J. C. Reed. 1995. Reduced expression of pro-apoptotic gene bax is associated with poor response rates to combination chemotherapy and shorter survival in women with metastatic breast adenocarcinoma. *Cancer Res.* **55**: 4471–4478.

169. Muller, M., S. Strand, H. Hug, E. M. Heinemann, H. Walczak, W. J. Hofmann, W. Stremmel, P. H. Krammer, and P. R. Galle. 1997. Drug-induced apoptosis in hepatoma cells is mediated by the CD 95 (APO-1/Fas) receptor/ligand system and involves activation of wild-type p53. *J. Clin. Invest.* **99**: 403–413.

170. Wakahara, Y., A. Nawa, T. Okamoto, A. Hayakawa, F. Kikkawa, N. Suganama, F. Wakahara, and Y. Tomoda. 1997. Combination effect of anti-Fas antibody and chemotherapeutic drugs in ovarian cancer cells in vitro. *Oncology.* **54**: 48–54.

171. Weller, M., U. Malipiero, A. Aguzzi, J. C. Reed, and A. Fontana. 1995. Proto oncogene bcl-2 gene transfer abrogates Fas/APO-1 antibody-mediated apoptosis of human malignant glioma cells and confers resistance to chemotherapeutic drugs and therapeutic irradiation. *J. Clin. Invest.* **95**: 2633–2643.

172. Landowski, T. H., M. C. Gleason-Guzman, and W. S. Dalton. 1997. Selection for drug resistance results in resistance to Fas-mediated apoptosis. *Blood* **89**: 1854–1861.

173. Min, Y. H., S. Lee, J. W. Lee, S. Y. Chong, J. S. Hahn, and Y. W. Ko. 1996. Expression of Fas antigen in acute myeloid leukemia is associated with therapeutic response to chemotherapy. *Br. J. Haematol.* **93**: 928–930.

174. Bargmann, C. I., M.-C. Hung, and R. A. Weinberg. 1986. The neu oncogene encodes an epidermal growth factor receptor-related protein. *Nature* **319**: 226–230.

175. Yamamoto, T., S. Ikawa, T. Akiyama, K. Semba, N. Nomura, N. Miyajima, T. Saito, and K. Toyoshima. 1986. Similarity of protein encoded by the human c-erb-B-2 gene to epidermal growth factor receptor. *Nature* **319**: 230–234.

176. Lupu, R., M. Cardillo, C. Cho, L. Harris, M. Hijazi, C. Perez, K. Rosenburg, D. Yang, and C. Tang. 1996. The significance of heregulin in breast cancer tumor progression and drug resistance. *Breast Cancer Res. Treat.* **38**: 57–66.

177. Akiyama, T., C. Sudo, H. Ogawar, K. Toyoshima, and T. Yamaoto. 1986. The product of the human c-erbB–2 gene: a 185-kilodalton glycoprotein with tyrosine kinase activity. *Science* **232**: 1644–1646.

178. Coussens, L., T. L. Yang-Feng, Y.-C. Liao, E. Chen, A. Gray, J. McGrath, P. H. Seeburg, T. A. Liberman, J. Schlessinger, U. Francke, A. Levinson, and A. Ullrich. 1985. Tyrosine kinase receptor with extensive homology to EGF receptor shares chromosomal location with neu oncogene. *Science* **230**: 1132–1139.

179. Stern, D. F., P. A. Heffernan, and R. A. Weinberg. 1986. P185, a product of the neu proto-oncogene is a receptor-like protein associated with tyrosine kinase activity. *Mol. Cell Biol.* **6**: 1729–1740.

180. Slamon, D. J., W. Godolphin, L. A. Jones, J. A. Holt, S. G. Wong, D. E. Keith, W. J. Levin, S. G. Stuart, J. Udove, A. Ullrich, and W. L. McGuire. 1989. Studies of the HER-2/neu proto-oncogene in human breast and ovarian cancer. *Science* **244**: 707–712.

181. Lacroix, H., J. D. Iglehart, M. A. Skinner, and M. H. Kraus. 1989. Overexpression of erbB-2 or EGF receptor proteins present in early stage mammary carcinoma is detected simultaneously in matched primary tumors and regional metastases. *Oncogene* **4**: 145–151.

182. Slamon, D. J., G. M. Clark, S. G. Wong, W. J. Levin, A. Ullrich, and W. L. McGuire. 1987. Human breast cancer: correlation of relapse and survival with amplification of the HER-2/neu oncogene. *Science* **235**: 177–182.

183. Borg, A., B. Baldetorp, M. Ferno, D. Killander, H. Olsson, S. Ryden, and H. Sigurdsson. 1994. ErbB-2 amplification is associated with tamoxifen resistance in steroid-receptor positive breast cancer. *Cancer Lett.* **81:** 137–144.

184. Sabbatini, A. R., F. Basolo, P. Valentini, L. Mattii, S. Calvo, L. Fiore, F. Ciardiello, and M. Petrini. 1994. Induction of multidrug resistance (MDR) by transfection of MCF–10A cell line with C-Ha-ras and C-erbB-2 oncogenes. *Int. J. Cancer* **59:** 208–211.

185. Yu, D., B. Liu, M. Tan, J. Li, S. S. Wang, and M. C. Hung. 1996. Overexpression of c-erbB-2/neu in breast cancer cells confers increased resistance to Taxol via mdr-1-independent mechanisms. *Oncogene* **13:** 1359–1365.

186. Gusterson, B. A., R. D. Gelber, A. Goldhirsch, K. N. Price, J. Save-Soderborgh, R. Anbazhagan, J. Styles, C.-M. Rudenstam, R. Golouh, R. Reed, F. Martinez-Tello, A. Tiltman, J. Torhorst, P. Grigolato, R. Bettelheim, A. M. Neville, K. Burki, M. Castillione, J. Collins, J. Lindtner, H.-J. Senn, and I. B. C. S. G. Ludwig. 1992. Prognostic importance of c-erbB-2 expression in breast cancer. *J. Clin. Oncol.* **10:** 1049–1056.

187. Pegg, A. E. 1990. Mammalian 06-alkylguanine-DNA alkyltransferase: regulation and importance in response to alkylating carcinogenic and therapeutic agents. *Cancer Res.* **50:** 6119.

188. Colvin, O. M. 1994. *Mechanisms of resistance to alkylating agents.* Kluwer Academic Publishers, Boston.

189. Van der Zee, A. G. J., H. H. Hollema, H. W. A. DeBruijn, P. H. B. Willemse, H. Boonstra, N. H. Mulder, J. G. Aalders, and E. G. E. De Vries. 1995. Cell biology markers of drug resistance in ovarian carcinoma. *Gynecologic Oncol.* **58:** 165–178.

190. Thibodeau, S. N., A. J. French, P. C. Roche, J. M. Cunningham, D. J. Tester, N. M. Lindor, G. Moslein, S. M. Baker, R. M. Liskay, L. J. Burgart, R. Honchel, and K. C. Halling. 1996. Altered expression of hMSH2 and hMLH1 in tumors with microsatellite instability and genetic alterations in mismatch repair genes. *Cancer Res.* **56:** 4836–4840.

191. Liu, L., S. Markowitz, and S. L. Gerson. 1996. Mismatch repair mutations override alkyltransferase in conferring resistance to temozolomide but not to 1,3 -Bis (2chloroethyl) nitrosourea. *Cancer Res.* **56:** 5375–5379.

192. Carethers, J. M., M. T. Hawn, D. P. Chauhan, M. C. Luce, G. Marra, M. Koi, and C. R. Boland. 1996. Competency in mismatch repair prohibits clonal expansion of cancer cells treated with N-Methyl-N Nitro-N-Nitrosoguanidine. *J. Clin. Invest.* **98(1):** 199–206.

193. Aebi, S., B. Kurdi-Haidar, R. Gordan, B. Cenni, M. Zheng, D. Fink, R. D. Christen, C. R. Boland, M. Koi, R. Fishel, and S. B. Howell. 1996. Loss of DNA mismatch repair in acquired resistance to cisplatin. *Cancer Res.* **56(13):** 3087–3090.

194. Fink, D., S. Nebel, S. Aebi, H. Zheng, B. Cenni, A. Nehme, R. D. Christen, and S. B. Howell. 1996. The role of DNA mismatch repair in platinum drug resistance. *Cancer Res.* **56:** 4881–4886.

195. Fink, D., H. Zheng, S. Nebel, P. S. Norris, S. Aebi, T. P. Lin, A. Nehme, R. D. Christen, M. Haas, E. L. Macleod, and S. B. Howell. 1997. In vitro and in vivo resistance to cisplatin in cells that have lost DNA mismatch repair. *Cancer Res.* **57:** 1841–1845.

196. Drummond, J. T., A. Anthoney, R. Brown, and P. Modrich. 1996. Cisplatin and adriamycin resistance are associated with mutalpha and mismatch repair deficiency in an ovarian tumor cell line. *J. Biol. Chem.* **27:** 19,645–19,648.

197. Pinedo, H. M. and G. J. Peters. 1988. 5-Fluorouracil: biochemistry and pharmacology. *J. Clin. Oncol.* **6:** 1653–1664.

198. Houghton, J. A., S. J. Maroda, J. O. Phillips, and P. J. Houghton. 1981. Biochemical determinants of responsiveness to 5-fluorouracil and its derivatives in xenografts of human colorectal adenocarcinomas in mice. *Cancer Res.* **41:** 144–149.

199. Epstein, R. J. 1990. Drug-induced DNA damage and tumor chemosensitivity. *J. Clin. Oncol.* **8:** 2062–2084.

200. Tew, K. D. 1994. Glutathione-associated enzymes in anticancer drug resistance. *Cancer Res.* **54**: 4313.
201. Morrow, C. S., and K. H. Cowan. 1990. Glutathione S-transferases and drug resistance. *Cancer Cells* **1**: 15–22.
202. McGown, A. T. and B. W. Fox. 1986. A proposed mechanism of resistance to cyclophosphamide and phosphoramide mustard in a Yoshida cell line in vitro. *Cancer Chemother. Pharmacol.* **17**: 223–226.
203. Tew, K. D. and M. L. Clapper. 1988. *Glutathione-S-transferases and anticancer drug resistance.* Academic Press, San Diego, CA.
204. Butler, A. L., M. L. Clapper, and K. D. Tew. 1987. Glutatuione-S-transferases in nitrogen mustard-resistant and sensitive cell lines. *Mol. Pharmacol.* **31**: 575.
205. Bellamy, W. T., W. S. Dalton, M. C. Gleason, T. M. Grogan, and J. M. Trent. 1991. Development and characterization of a melphalan-resistant human multiple myeloma cell line. *Cancer Res.* **51**: 995.
206. Moscow, J. A., A. J. Townsend, and K. H. Cowan. 1989. Elevation of TT class glutathione S-transferase activity in human breast cancer cells by transfection of the GST TT gene and its affect on sensitivity to toxins. *Mol. Pharmacol.* **36**: 22–28.
207. Yuan, Z. M., C. Fenselau, D. M. Dulik, W. Martin, W. B. Emary, R. B. Brundrett, O. M. Colvin, and R. J. Cotter. 1990. Laser desorption electron impact: application to a study of the mechanism of conjugation of glutathione and cyclophosphamide. *Anal. Chem.* **62**: 868–870.
208. Fields, W. R., Y. Li, and A. J. Townsend. 1994. Protection by transfected glutathione S-transferase isozymes against carcinogen-induced alkylation of cellular macromolecules in human MCF-7 cells. *Carcinogenesis* **15**: 1155–1160.
209. Leyland-Jones, B. R., A. J. Townsend, C. D. Tu, K. H. Cowan, and M. E. Goldsmith. 1991. Antineoplastic drug sensitivity of human MCF-7 breast cancer cells stably transfected with a human alpha class glutathione-S-transferase gene. *Cancer Res.* **51**: 587–594.
210. Townsend, A. J., C. P. Tu, and K. H. Cowan. 1992. Expression of human mu or alpha class glutathione S-transferase in stably transfected human MCF-7 breast cancer cells: effect on cellular sensitivity to toxins. *Mol. Pharmacol.* **41**: 230–236.
211. Sladek, N. E. 1994. *Metabolism and pharmacokinetic behavior of cyclophosphamide and related oxazaphosphorines.* Pergamon, Oxford, UK.
212. Sreerama, L. and N. E. Sladek. 1994. Identification of a methylcholantrene-induced aldehyde dehydrogenase in a human breast adenocarcinoma cell line exhibiting oxazaphosphorine-specific acquired resistance. *Cancer Res.* **54**: 2176–85.
213. Bunting, K. D., R. Lindahl, and A. J. Townsend. 1994. Oxazaphosphorine-specific resistance in human MCF-7 breast carcinoma cell lines expressing transfected rat class 3 aldehyde dehydrogenase. *J. Biol. Chem.* **269**: 23,197–23,203.
214. Moreb, J., M. Schweder, A. Suresh, and J. R. Zucali. 1996. Overexpression of the human aldehyde dehydrogenase class I results in increased resistance to 4-hydroperoxycyclophosphamide. *Cancer Gene Ther.* **3**: 24–30.
215. Bunting, K. D. and A. J. Townsend. 1996. Protection by transfected rat or human class 3 aldehyde dehydrogenase against the cytotoxic effects of oxazaphorine alkylating agents in hamster V79 cell lines. Demonstration of aldophosphamide metabolism by the human cytosolic class 3 isozyme. *J. Biol. Chem.* **271**: 11,891–11,896.
216. Koc, O. N., J. A. Allay, K. Lee, B. M. Davis, J. S. Reese, and S. L. Gerson. 1996. Transfer of drug resistance genes into hematopoietic progenitors to improve chemotherapy tolerance. *Semin. Oncol.* **23**: 46–65.
217. Magni, M., S. Shammah, R. Schiro, W. Mellado, R. Dalla-Favera, and A. M. Gianni. 1996. Induction of cyclophosphamide-resistance by aldehyde-dehydrogenase gene transfer. *Blood* **87**: 1097–1103.

218. Benchekroun, M. N., B. K. Sinha, and J. Robert. 1993. Doxorubicin-induced oxygen free radicle formation in sensitive and doxorubicin-resistant variants of rat glioblastoma cell lines. *FEBS Lett.* **326:** 302–305.

219. Sinha, B. K., and E. C. Mimnaugh. 1990. Free radicals and anticancer drug resistance: oxygen free radicals in the mechanisms of drug cytotoxicity and resistance by certain tumors. *Free Radic. Biol. Med.* **8:** 567–581.

220. Myers, C. 1991. Anthracyclines. *Cancer Chemother. Biol. Response Modif.* **12:** 43–49.

221. Lee, F. Y. F., D. W. Sieman, and R. M. Sutherland. 1989. Changes in cellular glutathione content during adriamycin treatment in human ovarian cancer: a possible indicator of chemosensitivity. *Br. J. Cancer.* **60:** 291–298.

222. Pommier, Y., D. Kerrizan, R. E. Schwartz, J. A. Swack, and A. McCurdy. 1986. Altered DNA topoisomerase II activity in chinese hamster cells resistant to topoisomerase II inhibitor. *Cancer Res.* **46:** 3075–3081.

223. Haber, D. A., S. M. Beverley, M. L. Kiely, and R. T. Schimke. 1981. Properties of an altered dihydrofolate reductase encoded by amplified genes in cultured mouse fibroblasts. *J. Biol. Chem.* **256:** 9501–9510.

224. Schiff, P. B., J. Fant, and S. B. Horowitz. 1979. *Nature* **227:** 665–667.

225. Grover, S., J. R. Rimoldi, A. A. Molinero, A. G. Chaudhary, D. G. I. Kingston, and E. Hamel. 1995. *Biochemistry* **34:** 3927–3934.

226. Haber, M., C. A. Burkhart, D. L. Regl, J. Madafiglio, M. D. Norris, and S. B. Horwitz. 1995. Altered expression of M beta 2, the class II beta-tubulin isotype, in a murine 5774.2 cell line with a high level of taxol resistance. *J. Biol. Chem.* **270:** 31,269–31,275.

227. Minotti, A. M., S. B. Barlow, and F. Cabral. 1991. Resistance to antimitotic drugs in chinese hamster ovary cells correlates with changes in the level of polymerized tubulin. *J. Biol. Chem.* **266:** 3987–3994.

228. Casazza, A. M. and C. R. Fairchild. 1996. Paclitaxel (Taxol): mechanisms of resistance. *Cancer Treat. Res.* **87:** 149–71.

229. Encarnation, C. A., D. R. Ciocca, W. L. McGuire, G. M. Clark, S. A. Fuqua, and C. K. Osborne. 1993. Measurement of steroid hormone receptors in breast cancer patients on tamoxifen. *Breast Cancer Res. Treat.* **26:** 237–246.

230. Tonetti, D. A. and V. C. Jordan. 1995. Possible mechanisms in the emergence of tamoxifen-resistant breast cancer. *Anti-Cancer Drugs* **6:** 498–507.

231. Usmani, B. A. 1993. Genomic instability and metastatic progression. *Pathobiology* **61:** 109–116.

232. Sweezy, M. A. and A. Fishel. 1994. Multiple pathways leading to genomic instabilities and tumorigenesis. *Ann. NY Acad. Sci.* **726:** 165–177.

233. Cheng, K. C. and L. Loeb. 1993. Genomic instability and tumor progression: mechanistic considerations. *Adv. Cancer Res.* **60:** 121–156.

234. Nyce, J., D. Mylott, S. Lenard, L. Willis, and A. Kataria. 1989. Detection of drug-induced DNA hypermethylation in human cells exposed to cancer chemotherapy agents. *J. Liq. Chrom.* **12:** 1313–1321.

235. Nyce, J. W. 1989. Drug-induced DNA hypermethylation and drug resistance in human tumors. *Cancer Res.* **49:** 5829–5836.

236. Nyce, J. W. 1997. Drug-induced DNA hypermethylation: a potential mediator of acqired drug resistance during cancer chemotherapy. *Mutat. Res.* **386:** 153–161.

237. Nyce, J., L. Liu, and P. A. Jones. 1986. Variable effects of DNA synthesis inhibitors upon DNA methylation in mammalian cells. *Nucleic Acids Res.* **14:** 4353–4367.

238. Schonfeld, S., S. Schulz, and J. W. Nyce. 1992. Effects of inhibitors of topoisomerases I and II on DNA methylation and DNA synthesis in human colonic adenocarcinoma cells in vitro. *Int. J. Oncology.* **1:** 807–814.

239. Holden, J. A., D. H. Rolfson, and C. T. Wittwer. 1990. Human DNA topoisomerase II: evaluation of enzyme activity in normal and neoplastic tissues. *Biochemistry* **29:** 2127–2134.

240. Hsiang, Y. H., H. Y. Wu, and L. F. Liu. 1988. Proliferation-dependent regulation of DNA topoisomerase II in cultured cells. *Cancer Res.* **48:** 3230–3235.

241. Poplack, D. G. and G. Reaman. 1988. Acute lymphoblastic leukemia in childhood. *Pediatr. Clin. North AM.* **35:** 903.

242. Lum, B. L. and M. P. Gosland. 1995. MDR expression in normal tissues. Pharmacologic implications for the clinical use of P-glycoprotein inhibitors. *Hematol. Oncol. Clin. North Am.* **9:** 319–336.

243. Yonehara, S., A. Ishii, and M. Yonehara. 1989. A cell-killing monoclonal antibody (anti-Fas) to a cell surface antigen co-down regulated with the receptor of tumor necrosis factor. *J. Exp. Med.* **169:** 1747–1756.

244. Toth, K., M. M. Vaughan, N. S. Peress, H. K. Slocum, and Y. M. Rustum. 1996. MDR1 P-glycoprotein is expressed by endothelial cells of newly formed capillaries in human gliomas but is not expressed in the neovasculature of other primary tumors. *Am. J. Pathol.* **149:** 853–858.

245. Schinkel, A. M., C. A. Mol, E. Wagenaar, L. Van Deemter, J. J. Smit, and P. Borst. 1995. Multidrug resistance and the role of P-glycoprotein knockout mice. *Eur. J. Cancer* **31A:** 1295–1298.

246. Schinkel, A. H., E. Wagenaar, L. Van Deemter, C. A. Mol, and P. Borst. 1995. Absence of the mdr1a P-glycoprotein in mice affects tissue distribution and pharmacokinetics of dexamethasone, digoxin, and cyclosporin A. *J. Clin. Invest.* **96:** 1698–1705.

247. Schinkel, A. H., E. Wagenaar, C. A. Mol, and L. Van Deemter. 1996. P-glycoprotein in the blood-brain barrier of mice influences the brain penetration and pharmacological activity of many drugs. *J. Clin. Invest.* **97:** 2517–2524.

248. Schinkel, A. H., U. Mayer, E. Wagenaar, C. A. Mol, L. Van Deemter, J. J. Smit, M. A. Van der Valk, A. C. Voordouw, H. Spits, O. Van Tellingen, J. M. Zijlmans, W. E. Fibbe, and P. Borst. 1997. Normal viability and altered pharmacokinetics in mice lacking mdr1-type (drug-transporting) P-glycoproteins. *Proc. Natl. Acad. Sci. USA* **94:** 4028–4033.

249. Teicher, B. A., T. S. Herman, S. A. Holden, Y. Y. Wang, M. R. Pfeffer, J. W. Crawford, and E. d. Frei. 1990. Tumor resistance to alkylating agents conferred by mechanisms operative only in vivo. *Science* **247:** 1457–1461.

250. Bonadonna, G., and P. Valagussa. 1981. Dose-response effect of adjuvant chemotherapy in breast cancer. *N. Engl. J. Med.* **304:** 10.

251. Hryniuk, W. and M. N. Levine. 1986. Analysis of dose intensity for adjuvant chemotherapy trials in stage II breast cancer. *J. Clin. Oncol.* **4:** 1162.

252. Wood, W. C., D. R. Budman, A. H. Korzun, M. R. Cooper, J. Younger, R. D. Hart, A. Moore, J. A. Ellerton, L. Norton, C. R. Ferree, A. C. Ballow, E. I. Frei, and I. C. Henderson. 1994. Dose and dose intensity of adjuvant chemotherapy for stage II, node positive breast carcinoma. *N. Engl. J. Med.* **330:** 1253–1259.

253. Muss, H. B., A. D. Thor, D. A. Berry, T. Kute, E. T. Liu, F. Koerner, C. T. Cirrincione, D. R. Budman, W. C. Wood, M. Barcos, and I. C. Henderson. 1994. C-erbB-2 expression and response to adjuvant therapy in women with node-positive early breast cancer. *N. Engl. J. Med.* **330:** 1260–1266.

254. Dimitrov, N., S. Anderson, B. Fisher, C. Redmond, D. L. Wickerham, R. Pugh, C. Spurr, J. Goodnight, N. Abramson, and J. Wolter. 1994. Dose intensification and increased total dose of adjuvant chemotherapy for breast cancer (BC): finding from NSABP B-22. *Proc. ASCO.* **13:** 64.

255. Fisher, B., S. Anderson, L. Wickerham, A. DeCillis, N. Dimitrov, E. Mamounas, N. Wolmark, R. Pugh, J. N. Atkins, F. Meyers, N. Abramson, J. Wolter, R. S. Bornstein, L. Levy, E. H. Romond, V. Caggiano, M. Grimaldi, P. Jochimsen, and P. Deckers. 1997. Increased intensification and total dose of cyclophosphamide in a doxorubicin-cyclophosphamide regimen for the treatment of primary breast cancer: findings from National Surgical Adjuvant Breast and Bowel Project B-22. *J. Clin. Oncol.* **15:** 1858–1869.

256. Jones, R. B., J. F. Holland, S. Bhardwaj, L. Norton, C. Wilfinger, and A. Strashun. 1987. A phase I-II study of intensive-dose adriamycin for advanced breast cancer. *J. Clin. Oncol.* **5:** 172–177.

257. Bezwoda, W. R., L. Seymour, and R. D. Dansey. 1995. High-dose chemotherapy with hematopoietic rescue as primary treatment for metastatic breast cancer: a randomized trial. *J. Clin. Oncol.* **13:** 2483–2489.

258. Hurd, D. D., and W. P. Peters. 1995. Randomized, comparative study of high dose (with autologous bone marrow support) versus low-dose cyclophosphamide, cisplatin, carmustine as consolidation to adjuvant cyclophosphamide, doxorubicin, and fluorouracil for patients with operable stage II or III breast cancer involving 10 or more axillary lymph nodes (CALGB Protocol 9082). Cancer and leukemia group B. *J. Natl. Cancer Inst. Monogr.* **19:** 41–44.

259. Ferry, D. R., H. Traunecker, and D. J. Kerr. 1996. Clinical trials of P-glycoprotein reversal in solid tumors. *Eur. J. Cancer* **32A:** 1070–1081.

260. Cantwell, B., P. Buamah, and A. L. Harris. 1985. Phase I and II study of oral verapamil and intravenous vindesine. *Proc. Am. Soc. Clin. Oncol.* **42:** 161.

261. Saltz, L., B. Murphy, N. Kemeny, J. Bertino, W. Tong, D. Keefe, Y. Tzy-Jun, Y. Tao, D. Kelsen, and J. P. O'Brien. 1994. A Phase I trial of intrahepatic verapamil and doxorubicin. Regional therapy to overcome multidrug resistance. *Cancer* **74:** 2757–2764.

262. Kronbach, T., V. Fischer, and V. A. Meyer. 1988. Cyclosporin metabolism in human liver: identification of a cytochrome P-450 gene family as the major cyclosporin metabolizing enzyme explains interactions of cyclosporin with other drugs. *Clin. Pharmacol. Ther.* **43:** 630–635.

263. Bartlett, N. L., B. L. Lum, G. A. Fisher, N. A. Brophy, M. N. Ehsan, J. Halsey, and B. I. Sikic. 1994. Phase I trial of doxorubicin with cyclosporine as a modulator of multidrug resistance. *J. Clin. Oncol.* **12:** 835–842.

264. Erlichman, C., M. Moore, J. J. Thiessen, I. G. Kerr, S. Walker, P. Goodman, G. Bjarnason, C. DeAngelis, and P. Bunting. 1993. Phase I pharmacokinetic study of cyclosporine A combined with doxorubicin. *Cancer Res.* **35:** 4837–4842.

265. List, A. F., C. Spier, J. Greer, S. Wolff, J. Hutter, R. Dorr, S. Salmon, B. Futscher, M. Baier, and W. Dalton. 1993. Phase I/II trial of cyclosporine as a chemotherapy-resistance modifier in acute leukemia. *J. Clin. Oncol.* **11:** 1652–1660.

266. Stuart, N. S., P. Philip, A. L. Harris, K. Tonkin, S. Houlbrook, J. Kirk, E. A. Lien, and J. Carmichael. 1992. High-dose tamoxifen as an enhancer of etoposide cytotoxicity. Clinical effects and in vitro assessment in P-glycoprotein expressing cell lines. *Br. J. Cancer.* **66:** 833–839.

267. Bissett, D., D. J. Kerr, J. Cassidy, P. Meredith, U. Traugott, and S. B. Kaye. 1991. Phase I and pharmacokinetic study of D-verapamil and doxorubicin. *Br. J. Cancer.* **64:** 1168–1171.

268. Panella, T. J., J. J. Costanzi, F. Rathgeb, H. Schuller, and P. A. Bunn. 1993. A phase I trial of oral dexniguldipine (B8509-035) (dNIG) in patients with refractory solid tumors. *Proc. Ann. Mtg. Am. Soc. Clin. Oncol.* **12:** A404.

269. Scheulen, M., V. Nussler, M. Kriegmair, and others. 1994. Phase I study of iv dexniguldipine plus vinblastine. *Proc. Ann. Mtg. Am. Soc. Clin. Oncol.* **13:** A419.

270. Awada, A., O. Pagani, M. Piccart, and others. 1993. Phase I clinical and pharmacokinetic trials of S9788 alone and in combination with adriamycin (ADM). *Proc. Ann. Mgt. Am. Assoc. Cancer Res.* **34:** A1274.

271. Fisher, G. A., J. Hausdorff, B. L. Lum, and others. 1994. Phase I trial of etoposide with the cyclosporin SDZ PSC 833, a modulation of multidrug resistance (MDR). Proc. Ann. Mgt. Am. Soc. Clin. Oncol. **13:** A368.

272. Giaccone, G., S. C. Linn, G. Catimel, and others. 1994. Phase I and pharmacokinetic study of SD2 PSC 833 po in combination with doxorubicin in patients with solid tumors. *Proc. Ann. Mtg. Am. Soc. Clin. Oncol.* **13:** A364.

273. Erlichman, G., M. Moore, J. Thiessen, A. C. De, P. Goodman, and J. Manzo. 1994. A phase I trial of doxorubicin (D) and PSC 833: A modulator of multidrug resistance (MDR). *Proc. Ann. Mtg. Am. Soc. Clin. Oncol.* **13:** A326.

274. Sonneveld, P., J. P. Marie, C. Laburte, and M. Schoester. 1994. Phase I study of SDZ PSC 833, a multidrug resistance modulating agent, in refractory multiple myeloma. *Proc. Ann. Mtg. Am. Assoc. Cancer Res.* **35:** A2141.

275. Duran, G. E., M. P. Gosland, A. L. Ho, and B. I. Sikic. 1994. In vitro modulation of multidrug resistance (MDR) using human patient serum from EP–1: a phase I clinical trial of etoposide (VP–16) and SDZ PSC 833. *Proc. Ann. Mtg. Am. Assoc. Cancer Res.* **35:** A2093.

276. Nuessler, V., M. E. Scheulen, R. Oberneder, M. Kriegmair, K. J. Goebel, F. Rathgeb, W. Wurst, K. Zech, and W. Wilmanns. 1997. Phase I and pharmacokinetic study of the P-glycoprotein modulator dexniguldipine-HCl. *Eur. J. Med. Res.* **2:** 55–61.

277. Agarwala, S. S., R. R. Bahnson, J. W. Wilson, J. Szumowski, and M. S. Ernstoff. 1995. Evaluation of the combination of vinblastine and quinidine in patients with metastatic renal cell carcinoma. A phase I study. *Am. J. Clin. Oncol.* **18:** 211–215.

278. Brandes, L. J., K. J. Simons, S. P. Bracken, and R. C. Warrington. 1994. Results of a clinical trial in humans with refractory cancer of the intracellular histamine antagonist, N,N-diethyl-2-[4-(phenylmethyl) phenoxy] ethanamine-HCl, in combination with various single antineoplastic agents. *J. Clin. Oncol.* **12:** 1281–1290.

279. Smith, D. C. and D. L. Trump. 1995. A phase I trial of high-dose oral tamoxifen and CHOPE. *Cancer Chemother. Pharmacol.* **36:** 65–68.

280. Wilson, W. H., C. Jamis-Dow, G. Bryant, F. M. Balis, R. W. Klecker, S. E. Bates, B. A. Chabner, S. M. Steinberg, D. R. Kohler, and R. E. Wittes. 1995. Phase I and pharmacokinetic study of the multidrug resistance modulator dexverapamil with EPOCH chemotherapy. *J. Clin. Oncol.* **13:** 1985–1994.

281. Kornblau, S. M., E. Estey, T. Madden, H. T. Tran, S. Zhoa, V. Consoli, V. Snell, G. Sanchez-Williams, H. Kantarjian, M. Keating, R. A. Newman, and M. Andreeff. 1997. Phase I study of mitoxantrone plus etoposide with multidrug blockade by SDZ PSC-833 in replapsed or refractory acute myelogenous leukemia. *J. Clin. Oncol.* **15:** 1796–802.

282. Pennock, G. D., W. S. Dalton, W. R. Roeske, C. P. Appleton, K. Mosley, P. Plezia, T. P. Miller, and S. E. Salmon. 1991. Systemic toxic effects associated with high dose verapamil infusion and chemotherapy administration. *J. Natl. Cancer Inst.* **83:** 105–110.

283. Miller, T. P., T. M. Grogan, W. S. Dalton, C. M. Spier, R. J. Scheper, and S. E. Salmon. 1991. P-glycoprotein expression in malignant lymphoma and reversal of clinical drug resistance with chemotherapy plus high dose verapamil. *J. Clin. Oncol.* **9:** 17–24.

284. Mross, K., D. Hamm, and K. Hossfeld. 1993. Effects of verapamil on pharmacokinetics and metabolism of epirubicin. *Cancer Chemother. Pharmacol.* **31:** 369–375.

285. Wilson, W. H., S. E. Bates, A. Fojo, G. Bryant, Z. Zhan, J. Regis, R. E. Wittes, E. S. Jaffe, S. M. Steinberg, J. Herdt, and others. 1995. Controlled trial of dexverapamil, a modulator of multidrug resistance in lymphomas refractory to EPOCH chemotherapy. *J. Clin. Oncol.* **13:** 1995–2004.

286. Milroy, R. 1993. A randomized clinical study of verapamil in addition to combination chemotherapy in small cell lung cancer. West of Scotland Lung Cancer Research Group and the Aberdeen Oncology Group. *Br. J. Cancer.* **68:** 813–818.

287. Sonneveld, P., B. G. M. Durie, H. M. Lokhorst, J. P. Marie, G. Solbu, S. Suciu, R. Zittoun, B. Lowenberg, and K. Nooter. 1992. Modulation of multidrug resistant myeloma by cyclosporin. *Lancet* **340:** 255–259.

288. Sonneveld, P., J. P. Marie, C. Huisman, A. Vekhoff, M. Schoester, A. M. Faussat, J. van Kapel, A. Groenewegen, S. Charnick, R. Zittoun, and B. Lowenberg. 1996. Reversal of multidrug resistance by SD2 PSC 833, combined with VAD (vincristine, doxorubicin, dexamethasone) in refractory multiple myeloma. A phase I study. *Leukemia* **10:** 1741–1750.

289. Rodenburg, C. J., K. Nooter, H. Herweijer, R. Seynaeve, G. Stoter, and J. Verweij. 1991. Phase II study combining vinblastine and cyclosporin A to circumvent multidrug resistance in renal cell cancer. *Ann. Oncol.* **2:** 305–306.

290. Samuels, B. L., D. L. Trump, G. Rosner, and others. 1994. Multidrug resistance (MDR) modulation in renal cell carcinoma (RCC) using cyclosporine A (CSA) or tamoxifen (TAM) (CALGB 9163). *Proc. Ann. Mtg. Am. Soc. Clin. Oncol.* **13:** A793.

291. Lyn, P. A., R. J. Motzer, J. O'Brien, L. T. Murray, P. Fisher, and M. J. Ochoa. 1994. Phase I/II trial of velban (VLB) + dexverapamil (DEX) for patients (Pts) with advanced renal cell carcinoma (RCC). *Proc. Ann. Mtg. Am. Soc. Clin. Oncol.* **13:** A760.

292. Mickisch, G. H. 1994. Chemoresistance of renal cell carcinoma: 1986–1994. *World J. Urol.* **12:** 214–223.

293. Motzer, R. J., P. Lyn, P. Fischer, P. Lianes, R. L. Ngo, C. Cordon-Cardo, and J. P. O'Brien. 1995. Phase I/II trial of dexverapamil plus vinblastine for patients with advanced renal cell carcinoma. *J. Clin. Oncol.* **13:** 1958–1965.

294. Warner, E., S. W. Tobe, I. L. Andrulis, Y. Pei, J. Trachtenberg, and K. L. Skorecki. 1995. Phase I-II study of vinblastine and oral cyclosporin A in metastatic renal cell carcinoma. *Am. J. Clin. Oncol.* **18:** 251–256.

295. Murphy, B. R., S. M. Rynard, K. L. Pennington, W. Grosh, and P. J. Loehrer. 1994. A phase II trial of vinblastine plus dipyridamole in advanced renal cell carcinoma. A Hoosier *Oncology* Group study. *Am. J. Clin. Oncol.* **17:** 10–13.

296. Eckardt, J. R., E. Campbell, H. A. Burris, G. R. Weiss, G. I. Rodriguez, S. M. Fields, A. M. Thurman, N. W. Peacock, P. Cobb, M. L. Rothenberg, and others. 1994. A phase II trial of Daunoxome, liposome-encapsulated daunorubicin, in patients with metastatic adenocarcinoma of the colon. *Am. J. Clin. Oncol.* **17:** 498–501.

297. Solary, E., D. Caillot, B. Chauffert, R. O. Casasnovas, M. Dumas, M. Maynadie, and H. Guy. 1992. Feasibility of using quinine, a potential multidrug resistance-reversing agent, in combination with mitoxantrone and cytarabine for the treatment of acute leukemia. *J. Clin. Oncol.* **10:** 1730–1736.

298. Berman, E., M. McBride, S. Lin, C. Menedez-Botet, and W. Tong. 1995. Phase I trial of high-dose tamoxifen as a modulator of drug resistance in combination with daunorubicin in patients with relapsed or refractory acute leukemia. *Leukemia* **9:** 1631–1637.

299. Ehrlich, P. H., Z. A. Moustafa, A. E. Archinal-Mattheis, M. J. Newman, K. W. Bair, and D. Cohen. 1997. The reversal of multidrug resistance in multicellular tumor spheroids by SDZ PSC 833. *Anticancer Res.* **17:** 129–133.

300. Chen, G., B. A. Teicher, and E. I. Frei. 1996. Differential interactions of Pgp inhibitor thaliblastine with adriamycin, etoposide, taxol and anthrapyrazole CI 941 in sensitive and multidrug-resistant human MCF-7 breast cancer cells. *Anticancer Res.* **16:** 3499–3505.

301. Thurlimann, B., N. Kroger, J. Greiner, K. Mross, J. Schuller, E. Schernhammer, K. Schumacher, G. Gastl, J. Hartlapp, H. Kupper, and others. 1995. Dexverapamil to overcome epirubicin resistance in advanced breast cancer. *J. Cancer Res. Clin. Oncol.* **121(Suppl. 3):** R3–6.

302. Wishart, G. C., J. A. Plumb, J. G. Morrison, T. G. Hamilton, and S. B. Kaye. 1992. Adequate tumor quinidine levels for multidrug resistance modulation can be achieved in vivo. *Eur. J. Cancer* **28:** 28–31.

303. Fardel, O., V. Lecureur, and A. Guillouzo. 1993. Regulation by dexamethasone of P-glycoprotein expression in cultural rat hepatocytes. *FEBS Lett.* **327:** 189–193.

304. Bates, S. E., B. Meadows, B. R. Goldspiel, A. Denicoff, T. B. Le, E. Tucker, S. M. Steinberg, and L. J. Elwood. 1995. *Cancer Chemother. Pharmacol.* **35:** 457–463.

305. Tolcher, A. W., K. H. Cowan, D. Solomon, F. Ognibene, B. Goldspiel, R. Chang, M. H. Noone, A. M. Denicott, C. S. Barnes, M. R. Gossard, P. A. Fetsch, S. L. Berg, F. M. Balis, D. J. Venzon, and J. A. O'Shaughnessy. 1996. Phase I crossover study of paclitaxel with r-verapamil in patients with metastatic breast cancer. *J. Clin. Oncol.* **14:** 1173–1184.

306. Berg, S. L., A. Tolcher, J. A. O'Shaughnessy, A. M. Denicoff, M. Noone, F. P. Ognibene, K. H. Cowan, and F. M. Balis. 1995. Effect of R-verapamil on the pharmacokinetics of paclitaxel in women with breast cancer. *J. Clin. Oncol.* **13**: 2039–2042.

307. Taylor, C. W., W. S. Dalton, K. Mosley, R. T. Dorr, and S. E. Salmon. 1997. Combination chemotherapy with cyclophosphamide, vincristine, adriamycin, and dexamethasone (CVAD) plus oral quinine and verapamil in patients with advanced breast cancer. *Breast Cancer Res. Treat.* **42**: 7–14.

308. Mickisch, G. H., I. Aksentijevich, P. V. Schoenlein, L. J. Goldstein, H. Galski, C. Stahle, D. H. Sachs, I. Pastan, and M. M. Gottesman. 1992. Transplantation of bone marrow cells from transgenic mice expressing the human MDR1 gene results in long-term protection against the myelosuppressive effects of chemotherapy in mice. *Blood* **79**: 1087–1093.

309. Sorrentino, B. P., K. T. McDonagh, D. Woods, and D. Orlic. 1995. Expression of retroviral vectors containing the human multidrug resistance 1 cDNA in hematopoietic cells of transplanted mice. *Blood* **86**: 491–501.

310. Ling, V. 1997. Multidrug resistance: molecular mechanisms and clinical relevance. *Cancer Chemother. Pharmacol.* **40(Suppl.)**: S3–S8.

311. Morrow, C. S. and K. H. Cowan. 1997. Drug resistance and its clinical circumvention, in *Cancer Medicine*, 4th ed. (Holland, J. F., E. Frei, III, R. C. Bast, Jr., D. W. Kufe, D. L. Morton, and R. R. Weichselbaum, eds.), Williams & Wilkins, Baltimore, pp. 799–815.

312. Goldstein, L. J. 1995. Clinical reversal of drug resistance. *Curr. Probl. Cancer* **19(2)**: 65–124.

313. Beck, W. T., C. E. Cass, and P. J. Houghton. 1997. Anticancer drugs from plants: Vinca alkyloids and taxanes, in *Cancer Medicine*, 4th ed. (Holland, J. F., E. Frei, III, R. C. J. R. Bast, D. W. Kufe, D. L. Morton, and R. R. Weichselbaum, eds.), Williams & Wilkins, Baltimore, pp. 1005–1025.

314. Ford, J. M. 1996. Experimental reversal of P-glycoprotein-mediated multidrug resistance by pharmacological chemosensitisers. *Eur. J. Cancer* **32A(6)**: 991–1001.

315. Miyashita, T. and J. C. Reed. 1993. Bcl-2 oncoprotein blocks chemotherapy-induced apoptosis in a human leukemia cell line. *Blood* **81**: 151–157.

III

Therapeutics and Diagnostics

Environmental Risk Factors

24

Smoking as a Risk Factor for Breast Cancer

Christine B. Ambrosone and Peter G. Shields

1. INTRODUCTION

Breast cancer is the most commonly occurring cancer among women in the United States, except for nonmelanotic skin cancer, and is second only to lung cancer as a cause of cancer death in women *(1)*. The incidence of breast cancer has increased dramatically over the last 10 yr, so that now it is estimated that approx 1 in 8 American women will develop breast cancer sometime in their life *(2)*.

For the most part, the etiology of breast cancer remains unknown. Some risk factors for breast cancer have been elucidated, which are mostly related to hormonal status or family history. Yet, these risk factors explain only a portion of the variability in disease incidence *(3)*. Environmental causes are suspected of playing a role in breast cancer, because there is a disparity in breast cancer rates between geographic regions. In this country, the incidence is highest in the northeast, especially in urban areas *(4)*. Differences also exist between countries, where there can be a five- to 10-fold difference in incidence *(5)*. Migrant studies also have shown that breast cancer incidence rates increase as women move from low-risk countries to those with higher rates *(6)*. Underdeveloped countries with traditionally low incidence rates are also experiencing a rise in breast cancer incidence *(7)*. Although variations in dietary, socioeconomic, and reproductive factors may partially explain geographic differences in breast cancer incidence rates, they do not appear to fully account for geographic and temporal disparities. It is plausible that environmental contaminants and dietary carcinogens that are associated with a more westernized lifestyle (i.e., tobacco smoking) may be related to breast cancer risk. Some suspect chemical exposures include aryl and heterocyclic aromatic amines, nitro- and polycyclic aromatic hydrocarbons, and N-nitroso compounds.

Although epidemiological studies generally have not implicated specific nonhormonally related environmental or chemical etiologies, the hypothesis is that these exposures can contribute to human breast cancer risk. It is well known that there is a wide interindividual variation *(8)* in cancer risk related to carcinogen metabolism. Given this, and data showing that carcinogenesis is a multistage complex process, the authors believe that there are subgroups of women who are susceptible to particular carcinogens, based on specific heritable susceptibilities. When these subgroups are grouped together, however, as in population-based studies, the effects of a particular exposure may not be observable above the background of other exposures and suscep-

From: Breast Cancer: *Molecular Genetics, Pathogenesis, and Therapeutics*
Edited by: A. M. Bowcock © Humana Press Inc., Totowa, NJ

tibilities. In this case, the effects may be diluted and, thus, are not statistically significant. Molecular epidemiological approaches that stratify women on the basis of carcinogen-metabolizing capacity, for example, is one method that can categorize susceptible groups of women. An analogy for studying at-risk subgroups, assuming the presence of a priori hypotheses, is a traffic safety study, in which cars driving on a highway do not pose a risk to pedestrians, and pedestrians walking in a mall are not at risk, but pedestrians walking on a highway have an increased risk of being hit. The basis of our hypothesis, which focuses on tobacco use, and the use of molecular epidemiological methods, is detailed below.

2. BIOLOGICAL BASIS FOR CHEMICAL CARCINOGENS AND BREAST CANCER IN HUMANS

Laboratory animal, in vitro, and human breast cancer studies are consistent with the conclusion that nonhormonal chemical carcinogens can play a role in human breast cancer. Examinations of the mutational spectrum of the p53 tumor-suppressor gene in breast cancer indicate that racial and geographic differences in the spectrum might be a result of heritable and environmental factors *(9–12)*. The mutational spectrum also supports a role for chemical carcinogens, because the pattern of mutations in breast cancer is quite similar to that found in lung cancer, in which chemical carcinogens are known to be etiologically related *(13)*. In laboratory animals, numerous chemical carcinogen models of breast cancer are available *(14)*. Also, it is known that chemical carcinogens can reach the breast in laboratory animals and humans, and because of lipophilicity, they are stored in breast adipose tissue *(15,16)*. Ductal epithelial cells are directly exposed to nicotine *(17)* and mutagenic compounds *(18)*. Heterocyclic amines administered to nursing rat dams were found at high levels in the breast tissue, and were excreted in the milk *(19)*. Other lines of evidence indicate that breast tissues can metabolically activate chemical carcinogens, and increase the biologically effective dose. Three studies have identified DNA adducts in normal breast tissue from women with and without breast cancer *(20–22)*, some of which were putatively related to tobacco smoking. Endogenously produced chemicals also may play a role in DNA adduct formation *(23)*. Therefore, the breast is certainly exposed to chemical carcinogens, and can be susceptible to the carcinogenic process.

Tobacco smoke would logically be a breast cancer risk factor through multiple pathways. Cigarettes contain about 3600 chemicals, some of which may affect the metabolism, mutagenicity of hormones and/or other carcinogens in breast cancer tissue *(24)*. Other agents in tobacco smoke have antiestrogenic effects, which would preclude the adverse effects of chemical carcinogens in the breast *(25)*. For example, cigarette smoking induces CYP1A2, which decreases the level of circulating estradiol. Because of these competing effects, the epidemiological assessment of breast cancer patients may be clouded, because genetic differences in metabolism and detoxification may make some women more susceptible than others. It is hypothesized here that genetic variability in metabolism of aromatic and heterocyclic amines, polycyclic aromatic hydrocarbons, and N-nitroso compounds from dietary sources or cigarette smoking might be breast cancer risk factors. Specifically, it is proposed that women who have certain alleles of polymorphic genes that may result in greater activation or lesser detoxification of aryl aromatic and heterocyclic amines (NAT1, NAT2, CYP1A2), PAHs (GSTM1, CYP1A1), and N-nitroso compounds (CYP2E1) may be at greater risk for breast cancer, if they have exposure to the substrates for these enzymes. Among women with wild-type alleles for these genes, an hypothesized antiestrogenic effect of tobacco smoke may overwhelm tobacco smoke's carcinogenic potential.

2.1. Specific Chemical Carcinogens

2.1.1. Polycyclic Aromatic Hydrocarbons

Polycyclic aromatic hydrocarbons (PAHs) are products of incomplete combustion in the burning of fossil fuels, and are emitted in automobile exhaust and industrial waste output. They contaminate air, water, and foods. Human PAH exposure from foods relates to the grilling of meats, fish, and poultry. Descriptive evidence implicates PAHs in human breast cancer. Morris and Seifter *(15)* plotted the geographic distribution of hydrocarbon residues in relation to the geographic distribution of breast cancer in the United States. Hydrocarbon combustion byproducts are consistently higher in urban than in rural areas, clustering with the distribution of breast cancer cases, and suggesting that the higher risk ratio for urban to rural women with breast cancer may be, in part, the result of exposure to higher levels of hydrocarbons.

Laboratory animal studies provide evidence that PAHs are breast carcinogens. In experimental models, mammary tumors have been induced by PAHs in rodents by various routes of administration, including gavage, intravenous injection, and application to the organ itself *(26–28)*, and PAHs are mutagenic to breast cell lines *(29)*. PAHs are lipophilic, and are stored in adipose tissue, including that of the breast *(15)*. Metabolism of PAHs by mammary epithelial cells (MEC) has been noted in cell lines derived from rats, and these cells were found to activate 7,12-dimethyl-benz[a]anthracene (DMBA) to mutagenic metabolites in a dose-response fashion *(30)*. Studies with human mammary epithelial cells (HMEC) have shown that PAHs are metabolized and activated by these cells *(31)*, and treatment with benzo(a)pyrene, a common PAH, causes more DNA adduct formation *(22,32)*. When compared with human fibroblasts from the same breast specimens, HMEC showed adduct formation more quickly, and at lower concentrations of PAHs. Benzo(g)chrysene also has been shown to be activated by MCF-7 mammary human cancer cell line *(33)*. Thus, the metabolic events leading to formation of adducts can take place entirely within the mammary epithelial cells, where 99% of all human breast cancers occur.

2.1.2. Aryl Aromatic Amines

The role of aryl aromatic amines in carcinogenesis has been suspected since the nineteenth century, when an association was observed between exposure in aniline dye workers and bladder cancer *(34)*. Women may be exposed to aromatic amines from mainstream and sidestream tobacco smoke, synthetic fuels, or as the result of metabolic reduction of polycyclic nitroaromatic hydrocarbons, which are ubiquitous in diesel exhaust and in airborne particulates *(34)*. Experimental evidence indicates that some aromatic amines, such as 4-aminobiphenyl and b-naphthylamine, are potentially mutagenic and carcinogenic to human breast cells. In vivo, activated aromatic amine metabolites have been shown to cause DNA damage in rodents *(35–37)*, to transform mouse mammary glands *(28)*, and to induce rodent mammary tumors *(38,39)*. Amines and nitroaromatic hydrocarbons demonstrate organotropism, and mammary tissue is a target in female rats for several such compounds. Certain dinitropyrenes found in diesel exhaust also have been shown to target the mammary gland in rodent carcinogenicity studies *(36)*. In vitro, aromatic amines form DNA adducts in cultured human mammary epithelial cells *(40)*, and cause unscheduled DNA synthesis *(41)*, indicating a capacity of breast epithelial cells to bioactivate these compounds. Human breast tissue also has been shown to possess N-acetyltransferase (NAT) 1 activity, but not NAT2, indicating one pathway for the activation of aromatic amines *(42,43)*. The activation of NATs in the breast might also be related to estrogen receptor activity, suggesting a specific role for postmenopausal breast cancer *(44)*.

2.2.3. Heterocyclic Amines

Mutagenic heterocyclic aromatic amines (HAAs) are formed when meat is cooked, but also are present in tobacco smoke at lower levels. Identified as risk factors for colon cancer *(45)*, some HAAs are powerful mammary carcinogens in rodents, and may be breast cancer risk factors in humans. Certain HAAs are distributed to the mammary gland and form DNA adducts in rats *(46)*. Specifically, 2-amino-1-methyl-6-phenylimidazo[4,5]pyridine (PhIP), 2-amino-3- methylimidazo[4,5-f]quinoline (IQ), and 2-amino-3,8-dimethylimidazo[4,5-f]quinoxaline (MeIQx) cause mammary cancer in rodents *(47,48)*. In male rats, administration of both PhIP and IQ resulted in colon cancer, but females fed IQ and PhIP supplements developed mammary, rather than colon, cancer *(29,49,50)*. HAAs are activated and form DNA adducts in cultured HMEC *(51)*; PhIP has been demonstrated to be more mutagenic than other heterocyclic amines in cultured mammalian cells *(52,53)*.

2.2.4. N-Nitrosamines

Human exposure to N-nitrosamines occurs through diet, endogenous formation in the stomach, tobacco smoke, and occupation and medical therapies *(54)*. N-nitrosamines cause DNA damage *(55)*, such as the promutagenic O6-methyldeoxyguanosine adducts *(56)*. Exposures to these compounds result in decreasing levels of the repair enzyme O6-alkylguanine-DNA alkyl transferase *(56)*, perhaps increasing the susceptibility to nitroso compounds. N-nitrosamines also have been shown to cause rodent mammary tumors *(57–60)*, which are histologically similar to human cancers *(55,61)* and can metastasize *(59,61)*. They can transform cultured mouse mammary cells *(55,62)*, and cultured HMECs undergo unscheduled DNA synthesis *(41)*. Although it was originally believed that N-nitrosamine exposure induced a specific GGA/EGAA transition in the twelfth codon of the HRAS1 oncogene *(60,63)*, it is more likely that the observed mutation is a result of cell selection for pre-existing mutations *(64)*.

3. CIGARETTE SMOKING AND BREAST CANCER RISK: THE EPIDEMIOLOGICAL EVIDENCE

Given the laboratory evidence for a role of N-nitroso compounds, PAHs, and aromatic and heterocyclic amines in mammary carcinogenesis, one would expect to see an association between cigarette smoking and breast cancer risk in epidemiologic studies. This topic has been thoroughly investigated in the past few decades, with inconsistent results. In 1993, Palmer and Rosenberg evaluated the epidemiologic evidence for a causal relationship between cigarette smoking and breast cancer risk *(65)*. Weighing the evidence from numerous case-control and cohort studies, the authors concluded that it was unlikely that cigarette smoking had either a net effect of reducing the risk of breast cancer or of materially increasing risk. Studies published since that time are summarized in Table 1. Of these studies, there also did not appear to be an effect of smoking on breast cancer risk, except in Japanese populations. In both of the published studies from Japan, one composed of 607 premenopausal cases and 15,084 controls, cigarette smoking significantly increased risk.

A number of studies have evaluated possible effects of smoking within various subgroups of women, or by different aspects of smoking behavior. Some studies have found an increased risk of breast cancer with age at which smoking began. In a study of hospital patients and controls, Palmer et al. found that smoking slightly increased risk (OR = 1.3, CI, 1.1–1.6), particularly among women who began smoking before age 16 (OR = 1.8, CI, 1.0–3.4) *(66)*. Similar associations were observed in another study that used neighborhood controls *(66)*. A slight increased risk for beginning smoking at an early age was also observed in large studies by Brinton (OR = 1.3, CI, 1.0–1.6) *(67)* and by Chu (OR = 1.1, CI, 1.0–1.2) *(68)*. Others have not observed this phenomenon, however *(69–74)*. Some investigators also have evaluated the intensity of smoking, that is, number of cigarettes smoked per day. In studies that found significantly increased risk associated with heavier smoking (>15 cigarettes/d), estimates of risk were, for the most part, small. With more than 5000 cases, Stockwell et al. found that current smoking significantly increased risk, although this estimate was only 1.2 *(75)*. In studies by Chu *(68)* and by Hiatt *(76)*, similar weak increases in risk with heavy smoking were observed, as well as in a study of breast cancer in African-American women *(77)*, but a number of studies have not supported these findings on intensity of smoking and breast cancer risk.

Previous studies investigating the link between exposure to passive smoke and breast cancer risk have indicated an increased risk *(78–80)*. In these studies, women who were passive smokers were compared to those with no active or passive exposure. Morabia et al. applied this model to active smoking, and used an innovative methodologic approach to study cigarette smoking and breast cancer risk *(78)*. Because exposure to passive smoke has been found to be associated with breast cancer risk to a greater degree than active smoking, Morabia hypothesized that inclusion of passive smokers in the reference category of nonsmokers would dilute estimates of risk associated with active smoking. In a large case-control study of breast cancer, with a reference category only of women exposed to neither active nor passive cigarette smoke, a clear dose–response association was observed between lifetime smoking and breast cancer risk, with an odds ratio of 4.6 (95% confidence interval 2.2–9.7) in the highest quartile of use. It is possible that previous studies, by not allowing for passive smokers in the reference category, were biased by misclassification of never-smokers.

4. VARIABILITY IN HUMAN CARCINOGEN METABOLISM AND BREAST CANCER RISK

Functional genetic polymorphisms for carcinogen metabolism might affect breast cancer risk related to smoking. For example, persons with an increased ability to metabolically activate a tobacco smoke mutagen, or a decreased ability to detoxify a reactive metabolite, might have a greater likelihood of DNA damage. Metabolism varies

Table 1
Tobacco Smoking and Breast Cancer

Reference number	Geographic location	Type of study	Cases	Controls	Level of smoking	Odds ratio for tobacco smoking	
						Active smoking	Passive smoking
(25)	Italy	Case-control	2569	2588	>Cigarettes/d	1.18	
(38)	CASH study	Case-control	4720	4682	>25 Cigarettes/d	1.2*	
(46)	Denmark	Case-control	1480	1332	>25 Cigarettes/d	0.75	
					Smoking ≤ age 15	0.83	
(136)	UK	Case-control	755	755	>16 Cigarettes/d	1.10	
		Premenopausal	205	199	>400 Cigarette yr		2.73*
(66)	Japan	Case-control					
		Premenopausal	607	15,084	>Cigarettes/d	1.31*	
		Postmenopausal	445	6215			1.30*
(44)	Norway	Cohort	603		Current smoking	1.0	
					Former smoking	1.1	
(15)	Denmark	Mammography	230		>30 yr	1.6*	
(69)	Japan	Case-control	157	369	Ex-or current	2.31*	
(127)	Sweden	Case-control					
		Premenopausal	177	195	>11 Cigarettes/d	1.2	
		Postmenopausal	216	254	>Cigarettes/d	0.8	
(30)	US	Cohort-fatal	880	604,412	>40 Cigarettes/d	1.74*	
(57)	US	Case-control	144	232	>20 Pack/yr	1.0	
		Bilateral					
		Sister controls					
		Premenopausal					

*Odds ratio is statistically significant.

524

among individuals, because of inheritance (i.e., coded by genetic polymorphisms) and acquired factors (i.e., induction of a protein).

Metabolic metabolism of most carcinogens occurs primarily in the liver. However, activation or detoxification of tobacco smoke carcinogens could also occur in breast epithelial cells, depending on the substrate, so that there is a combined effect by the liver (remote from the breast) and in the breast (local). An analogy for remote and local metabolism for breast cancer risk can be found in the model for aryl aromatic amines and bladder cancer risk. It is believed that aryl aromatic amines undergo oxidative activation by cytochrome P4501A2 to form corresponding N-hydroxy metabolites, and are then detoxified by NAT2. But some of these metabolites escape detoxification and freely circulate in the blood. The N-hydroxy metabolites reaching the bladder can be further activated by bladder NAT1, NAT2, sulfotransferases, and ATP-dependent kinase(s) *(81)*. The resultant reactive esters may bind to DNA, forming adducts that are promutagenic, and, if not repaired, are likely to participate in the multiple stages of human carcinogenesis. Of additional importance is the concept that, in the liver, there are multiple detoxification pathways for the metabolism of aromatic amines and their metabolites, including reaction with glutathione and conjugation with glucuronic or sulfuric acid. Detoxified conjugates may be excreted in the urine, but the activated N-hydroxy metabolites can be further detoxified in the circulation by absorption into the erythrocyte and formation of covalent hemoglobin adducts *(82)*. In the bladder, the electrophilic N-acetoxy amine product can be detoxified by conjugation to glutathione via the action of GST, or by conversion of the acetoxy form to the parent compound by a glutathione peroxidase reaction *(83)*. However, the presence of enzymes involved in the activation and detoxification of specific carcinogens in the target tissue may ultimately determine the mutagenic potential of these components. For breast cancer, the circulating reactive aryl aromatic amine metabolites also might cause DNA damage, as described above.

4.1. Aryl Aromatic and Heterocyclic Amines

Using the bladder model for breast cancer, interindividual variation in several metabolizing enzymes might increase risk. There are several polymorphic sites at the NAT2 locus that result in decreased NAT activity *(84,85)*, and slow NAT2 acetylation is associated with bladder cancer *(86,87)*. Also, cigarette smoking has been found to be a major risk factor for bladder cancer *(88)*, and studies have shown that smokers with the slow acetylator phenotype have higher circulating levels of 4-aminobiphenyl-hemoglobin adducts, reflecting higher levels of reactive arylamine metabolites *(89–91)*. Several studies have been conducted to evaluate the possible association between NAT2 phenotype and breast cancer risk. In most of these studies, there was either no association observed, or rapid acetylators were found to be at increased risk *(92–96)*. Recently, it was found that, although NAT2 genotype did not affect breast cancer risk, postmenopausal slow acetylators who smoked more than a pack of cigarettes a day had four times the risk of nonsmokers *(97)*. Either null or inverse associations between smoking and risk were noted among rapid acetylators. This association between smoking, NAT2, and breast cancer risk was also observed in a recent study in Taiwan *(98)*. There is a possibility that phenotype could be affected by disease status or treatment, but it is more likely that inconsistent results between studies is, again, related to the importance of exposure misclassification and the need to study gene–environment interactions. Thus, if aromatic amines are both related to breast carcinogenesis, risk associated with NAT2 polymorphism would be dependent on exposures in the study population.

Although NAT2 has high hepatic activity, NAT1 is poorly expressed in the liver; however, depending on the substrate, NAT1 appears to bioactivate aromatic amine metabolites by O-acetylation in the breast. A recently identified polymorphism in NAT1 has been shown to result in a two- to threefold increase in NAT1 activity in the bladder (84). Additionally, there is a linear correlation between NAT1 phenotype and adduct levels in the bladder (99). The genetic polymorphism matches the rapid phenotype in activity, and individuals with the rapid genotype have NAT1 tissue activity and adduct levels that are two to three times higher than those with the NAT1 slow genotype. Individuals with slow NAT2 and rapid NAT1 polymorphisms have been found to have highest adduct levels (99). To date, studies of NAT1 and breast cancer have not been published.

Another pathway for the bioactivation of HAA and AA involves sulfonation by phenol sulfotransferases to form reactive electrophiles that can form DNA adducts (100). This activation appears to correlate with the extent of p-nitrophenol conjugation, which has been shown to be primarily dependent on a thermostable isoform of phenol sulfotransferase (ST1A3) (101). This enzyme demonstrates genetic polymorphism, with wide interindividual variability (102). Since ST1A3 polymorphisms may affect an individual's ability to detoxify environmental carcinogens, the ST1A3 phenotype is a potentially important human risk factor, particularly if combined with exposure and other phenotype and genotype data. In addition, this activation pathway has important ramifications, because the sulfoxy metabolite does not appear to be detoxified by GST (103). To date, there have been no molecular epidemiologic studies evaluating sulfotransferase variability and breast cancer risk.

4.2. Polycyclic Aromatic Hydrocarbons

PAHs are metabolized to reactive intermediates by polymorphic cytochrome P4501A1 (CYP1A1), and detoxified by enzymes such as glutathione S-transferases (104,105). Cytochrome P4501A1 activates PAHs, and polymorphisms in CYP1A1 are known to affect levels of activity. An amino acid exchange (isoleucine to valine) in exon 7 of CYP1A1 has been linked to increased inducible activity of the enzyme (106), and a polymorphism has also been identified at the MspI restriction site. CYP1A1 mRNA has been identified in the breast (107), and activity has been identified using immunohistochemical staining (108). The presence of these enzymes in the breast suggest that PAHs may undergo local activation in the target tissue. In the Western New York Breast Cancer Study, evaluation of the CYP1A1 exon 7 substitution indicated that the polymorphism was weakly associated with increased breast cancer risk, and that this risk was highest among light smokers (109). In the Nurses' Health Study, no association was found with either the exon 7 or the MspI polymorphism (110), and in a study by Taioli et al., neither the exon 7 nor the MspI polymorphism increased risk among Caucasian women. African-American women with breast cancer, however, were more likely to carry the polymorphic allele (111).

4.3. Glutathione-S-transferases

The human GSTs are a multigene, isoenzyme family, and have been classified into four major families, GST alpha (GSTA), GST mu (GSTM), GST pi (GSTP), and GST theta (GSTT). Isoenzymes from the first three classes have been identified in both normal and malignant breast tissue *(108,112,113)*. Known to have a number of agents as substrates, GSTs also deal with oxidative stress within the cell *(114,115)*. Genetic polymorphisms have been identified in GSTM1, GSTT1, and GSTP1. In the first two, the polymorphism is a gene deletion, and, for GSTP1, it is an isoleucine to valine substitution in exon 5. This results in altered activity, depending on the substrate. Studies of GSTs have shown that enzyme activity is not normally distributed; however, the basis is not yet known. Some research groups have evaluated possible associations between genetic polymorphisms in GSTs and breast cancer risk. In the authors' case-control study of postmenopausal breast cancer *(109)*, it was found that the GSTM1 null genotype did not increase overall breast cancer risk, nor modify risk associated with smoking. Among younger women, however, the null genotype appeared to be associated with increased risk. Kelsey, in analysis from the Nurses' Health Study *(116)*, found that, although GSTM1 null was not associated with incident breast cancer risk, it did appear to confer improved survival. Zhong et al. also found no association between GSTM1 polymorphisms and breast cancer risk *(72)*, and this was supported by studies in Taiwan *(117)* and Japan *(118)*.

4.4. N-Nitrosamines

Cytochrome P450IIE1 is one of several enzymes responsible for the metabolic activation of N-nitrosamines (including tobacco-specific nitrosamines) and other low mol wt compounds *(119–122)*. The activity of this enzyme varies widely among individuals *(123–125)*. One specific genetic polymorphism is revealed through a *Dra*I restriction enzyme digestion *(125)*. Although clear in vitro data are lacking for evidence that the polymorphic alleles affect function, this polymorphism has been associated with altered protein levels in human liver samples *(126)* and increased 7-methyl-2'-deoxyguanosine adduct levels in human lung *(127)*. Moreover, this polymorphism has been associated with lung cancer in a Japanese study *(125)*, including a modification of smoking-related risk *(126)*, although no effect has been observed in studies of Caucasians in Europe *(128–130)* and the United States *(129)*, or African-Americans in the United States *(129)*. The polymorphism, however, has not been shown to be associated with either gastric *(126)* or nasopharyngeal carcinoma *(131)*. In the authors' case-control study of breast cancer *(132)*, there was no statistically significant association for the CYP2E1 and breast cancer risk for pre- or postmenopausal women. However, when women were categorized as nonsmokers vs smokers, premenopausal women with one or two C alleles, who had a history of smoking, were found be at increased risk, although the number of study subjects with this genotype was small. Similar findings were not revealed for postmenopausal women. There are no other known studies of polymorphisms in CYP2E1 and breast cancer risk.

Cytochrome P450 2D6 is another metabolizing enzyme that might be related to breast cancer through a tobacco-smoking etiology. This enzyme metabolically activates a tobacco- specific N-nitrosamine (NNK) *(133,134)*, and a relationship to lung cancer and smoking for extensive metabolizers has been reported *(135–137)*. CYP2D6 activity has been measured phenotypically in breast cancer case-control studies. Some studies suggest a risk for poor-metabolizer postmenopausal women *(138)*, and, in one study, when compared to women with benign breast lesions *(139)*, although another study that used subjects with benign breast lesions *(140)* did not find an association. CYP2D6 polymorphisms predicting the poor metabolizer phenotype, measured by PCR, have also been found to be related to breast cancer risk in one study *(141)*, although not in another *(142)*, which had a poorly defined control group, and another that used volunteers responding to posters *(143)*.

REFERENCES

1. Boring, C. C., T. S. Squires, and T. Tong. 1992. Cancer statistics, 1992. *CA Cancer J. Clin.* **42**: 19–38.
2. Feuer, E. J., L. M. Wun, C. C. Boring, W. D. Flanders, M. J. Timmel, and T. Tong. 1993. The lifetime risk of developing breast cancer. *J. Natl. Cancer Inst.* **85**: 892–897.
3. Madigan, M. P., R. G. Ziegler, J. Benichou, C. Byrne, and R. N. Hoover. 1996. Proportion of breast cancer cases in the United States explained by well-established risk factors. *J. Natl. Cancer Inst.* **87**: 1681–1685.
4. Marshall, E. 1993. The politics of breast cancer. *Science* **259**: 616–617.
5. Willett, W. 1989. The search for the causes of breast and colon cancer. *Nature* **338**: 389–394.
6. Buell, P. 1973. Changing incidence of breast cancer in Japanese-American women. *J. Natl. Cancer Inst.* **51**: 1479–1483.
7. Boyle, P. and R. Leake. 1988. Progress in understanding breast cancer: epidemiological and biological interactions. Breast. *Cancer Res. Treatment* **11**: 91–112.
8. Harris, C. C. 1989. Interindividual variation among humans in carcinogen metabolism, DNA adduct formation and DNA repair. *Carcinogenesis* **10**: 1563–1566.
9. Hartmann, A., H. Blaszyk, J. S. Kovach, and S. S. Sommer. 1997. The molecular epidemiology of p53 gene mutations in human breast cancer. *Trends Genet.* **13**: 27–33.
10. Blaszyk, H., A. Hartmann, Y. Tamura, S. Saitoh, J. M. Cunningham, R. M. McGovern, et al. 1996. Molecular epidemiology of breast cancers in northern and southern Japan: the frequency, clustering, and patterns of p53 gene mutations differ among these two low-risk populations. *Oncogene* **13**: 2159–2166.
11. Shiao, Y. H., V. W. Chen, W. D. Scheer, X. C. Wu, and P. Correa. 1995. Racial disparity in the association of p53 gene alterations with breast cancer survival. *Cancer Res.* **55**: 1485–1490.
12. Blaszyk, H., C. B. Vaughn, A. Hartmann, R. M. McGovern, J. J. Schroeder, J. Cunningham, et al. 1994. Novel pattern of p53 gene mutations in an American black cohort with high mortality from breast cancer. *Lancet* **343**: 1195–1197.
13. Biggs, P. J., W. Warren, S. Venitt, and M. R. Stratton. 1993. Does a genotoxic carcinogen contribute to human breast cancer? The value of mutational spectra in unravelling the aetiology of cancer. *Mutagenesis* **8**: 275–283.
14. Gould, M. N. 1995. Rodent models for the study of etiology, prevention and treatment of breast cancer. *Semin. Cancer Biol.* **6**: 147–152.
15. Obana, H., S. Hori, T. Kashimoto, and N. Kunita. 1981. Polycyclic aromatic hydrocarbons in human fat and liver. *Bull. Environ. Contam. Toxicol.* **27**: 23–27.
16. Morris, J. J. and E. Seifter. 1992. The role of aromatic hydrocarbons in the genesis of breast cancer. *Med. Hypotheses* **38**: 177–184.
17. Petrakis, N. L., L. D. Gruenke, T. C. Beelen, N. Castagnoli, Jr., and J. C. Craig. 1978. Nicotine in breast fluid of nonlactating women. *Science* **199**: 303–305.

18. Petrakis, N. L., C. A. Maack, R. E. Lee, and M. Lyon. 1980. Mutagenic activity in nipple aspirates of human breast fluid [letter]. *Cancer Res.* **40:** 188–189.

19. Ghoshal, A. and E. G. Snyderwine. 1993. Excretion of food-derived heterocyclic amine carcinogens into breast milk of lactating rats and formation of DNA adducts in the newborn. *Carcinogenesis* **14:** 2199–2203.

20. Perera, F. P., A. Estabrook, A. Hewer, K. Channing, A. Rundle, L. A. Mooney, R. Whyatt, and D. H. Phillips. 1995. Carcinogen-DNA adducts in human breast tissue. *Cancer Epidemiol. Biomarkers Prev.* **4:** 233–238.

21. Li, D., M. Wang, K. Dhingra, and W. N. Hittelman. 1996. Aromatic DNA adducts in adjacent tissues of breast cancer patients: clues to breast cancer etiology. *Cancer Res.* **56:** 287–293.

22. Seidman, L. A., C. J. Moore, and M. N. Gould. 1988. 32P-postlabeling analysis of DNA adducts in human and rat mammary epithelial cells. *Carcinogenesis* **9:** 1071–1077.

23. Vaca, C. E., J. L. Fang, M. Mutanen, and L. Valsta. 1995. 32P-postlabelling determination of DNA adducts of malonaldehyde in humans: total white blood cells and breast tissue. *Carcinogenesis* **16:** 1847–1851.

24. Office on Smoking and Health. 1996. Smoking and Health. A report to the Surgeon General of the Public Health Services. (Abstract)

25. MacMahon, B., D. Trichopoulos, P. Cole, and J. Brown. 1982. Cigarette smoking and urinary estrogens. *N. Engl. J. Med.* **307:** 1062–1065.

26. Cavalieri, E., E. Rogan, and D. Sinha. 1988. Carcinogenicity of aromatic hydrocarbons directly applied to rat mammary gland. *J. Cancer Res. Clin. Oncol.* **114:** 3–9.

27. Tonelli, Q. J., R. P. Custer, and S. Sorof. 1979. Transformation of cultured mouse mammary glands by aromatic amines and amides and their derivatives. *Cancer Res.* **39:** 1784–1792.

28. Chatterjee, M. and M. R. Banerjee. 1982. Selenium mediated dose-inhibition of 7,12-dimethylbenz[a] anthracene-induced transformation of mammary cells in organ culture. *Cancer Lett.* **17:** 187–195.

29. Reddy, B. S. and A. Rivenson. 1993. Inhibitory effect of Bifidobacterium longum on colon, mammary, and liver carcinogenesis induced by 2-amino-3-methylimidazo[4,5-f]quinoline, a food mutagen. *Cancer Res.* **53:** 3914–3918.

30. Gould, M. N. 1982. Chemical carcinogen activation in the rat mammary gland: intra-organ cell specificity. *Carcinogenesis* **3:** 667–669.

31. MacNicoll, A. D., G. C. Easty, A. M. Neville, P. L. Grover, and P. Sims. 1980. Metabolism and activation of carcinogenic polycyclic hydrocarbons by human mammary cells. *Biochem. Biophys. Res. Commun.* **95:** 1599–1606.

32. Stampfer, M. R., J. C. Bartholomew, H. S. Smith, and J. C. Bartley. 1981. Metabolism of benzo[a]pyrene by human mammary epithelial cells: toxity and DNA adduct formation. *Proc. Natl. Acad. Sci USA* **78:** 6251–6255.

33. Agarwal, R., S. L. Coffing, W. M. Baird, A. S. Kiselyov, R. G. Harvey, and A. Dipple. 1997. Metabolic activation of benzo[g]chrysene in the human mammary carcinoma cell line MCF-7. *Cancer Res.* **57:** 415–419.

34. Hein, D. W. 1988. Acetylator genotype and arylamine-induced carcinogenesis. *Biochim. Biophys. Acta* **948:** 37–66.

35. King, C. M., N. R. Traub, Z. M. Lortz, and M. R. Thissen. 1979. Metabolic activation of arylhydroxamic acids by N-O-acyltransferase of rat mammary gland. *Cancer Res.* **39:** 3369–3372.

36. Allaben, W. T., C. C. Weis, N. F. Fullerton, and F. A. Beland. 1983. Formation and persistence of DNA adducts from the carcinogen N-hydroxy-2-acetylaminofluorene in rat mammary gland in vivo. *Carcinogenesis* **4:** 1067–1070.

37. Wang, C. Y., H. Yamada, K. C. Morton, K. Zukowski, M. S. Lee, and C. M. King. 1988. Induction of repair synthesis of DNA in mammary and urinary bladder epithelial cells by N-hydroxy derivatives of carcinogenic arylamines. *Cancer Res.* **48:** 4227–4232.

38. Shirai, T., J. M. Fysh, M. S. Lee, J. B. Vaught, and C. M. King. 1981. Relationship of metabolic activation of N-hydroxy-N-acylarylamines to biological response in the liver and mammary gland of the female CD rat. *Cancer Res.* **41:** 4346–4353.

39. Allaben, W. T., C. E. Weeks, C. C. Weis, G. T. Burger, and C. M. King. 1982. Rat mammary gland carcinogenesis after local injection of N-hydroxy-N-acyl-2-aminofluorenes: relationship to metabolic activation. *Carcinogenesis* **3:** 233–240.

40. Swaminathan, S., S. M. Frederickson, and J. F. Hatcher. 1994. Metabolic activation of N-hydroxy-4-acetylaminobiphenyl by cultured human breast epithelial cell line MCF 10A. *Carcinogenesis* **15:** 611–617.

41. Eldridge, S. R., M. N. Gould, and B. E. Butterworth. 1992. Genotoxicity of environmental agents in human mammary epithelial cells. Chemical Industry Institute of Toxicology, Research Triangle Park, North Carolina 27709. *Cancer Res.* **52:** 5617–5620.

42. Debiec-Rychter, M., S. J. Land, and C. M. King. 1996. Tissue-specific expression of human acetyltransferase 1 and 2 detected by non-isotopic in situ hybridization. *Proc. Am. Assoc. Cancer Res.* **37:** 133(Abstract).

43. Sadrieh, N., C. D. Davis, and E. G. Snyderwine. 1996. N-Acetyltransferase expression and metabolic activation of the food-derived heterocyclic amines in the human mammary gland. *Cancer Res.* **56:** 2683–2687.

44. Lee, J. H., J. G. Chung, J. M. Lai, G. N. Levy, and W. W. Weber. 1997. Kinetics of arylamine N-acetyltransferase in tissues from human breast cancer. *Cancer Lett.* **111:** 39–50.

45. Lang, N. P., M. A. Butler, J. Massengill, M. Lawson, R. C. Stotts, M. Hauer-Jensen, and F. F. Kadlubar. 1994. Rapid metabolic phenotypes for acetyltransferase and cytochrome P4501A2 and putative exposure to food-borne heterocyclic amines increase the risk for colorectal cancer or polyps. *Cancer Epidemiol. Biomarkers Prev.* **3:** 675–682.

46. Snyderwine, E. G. 1994. Some perspectives on the nutritional aspects of breast cancer research. Food-derived heterocyclic amines as etiologic agents in human mammary cancer. *Cancer* **74:** 1070–1077.

47. Kato, T., H. Migita, H. Ohgaki, S. Sato, S. Takayama, and T. Sugimura. 1989. Induction of tumors in the Zymbal gland, oral cavity, colon, skin and mammary gland of F344 rats by a mutagenic compound, 2-amino-3,4-dimethylimidazo[4,5-f]quinoline. *Carcinogenesis* **10:** 601–603.

48. Tanaka, T., W. S. Barnes, G. M. Williams, and J. H. Weisburger. 1985. Multipotential carcinogenicity of the fried food mutagen 2-amino-3-methylimidazo[4,5-f]quinoline in rats. *Jpn. J. Cancer Res.* **76:** 570–576.

49. Ito, N., R. Hasegawa, M. Sano, S. Tamano, H. Esumi, S. Takayama, and T. Sugimura. 1991. A new colon and mammary carcinogen in cooked food, 2-amino-1-methyl-6-phenylimidazo[4,5-b]pyridine (PhIP). *Carcinogenesis* **12:** 1503–1506.

50. Hasegawa, R., M. Sano, S. Tamano, K. Imaida, T. Shirai, M. Nagao, T. Sugimura, and N. Ito. 1993. Dose-dependence of 2-amino-1-methyl-6-phenylimidazo[4,5-b]-pyridine (PhIP) carcinogenicity in rats. *Carcinogenesis* **14:** 2553–2557.

51. Pfau, W., M. J. O'Hare, P. L. Grover, and D. H. Phillips. 1992. Metabolic activation of the food mutagens 2-amino-3-methylimidazo[4,5-f]quinoline (IQ) and 2-amino-3,4-dimethyl-imidazo[4,5-f]quinoline (MeIQ) to DNA binding species in human mammary epithelial cells. *Carcinogenesis* **13:** 907–909.

52. Thompson, L. H., J. D. Tucker, S. A. Stewart, M. L. Christensen, E. P. Salazar, A. V. Carrano, and J. S. Felton. 1987. Genotoxicity of compounds from cooked beef in repair-deficient CHO cells versus Salmonella mutagenicity. *Mutagenesis* **2:** 483–487.

53. Holme, J. A., H. Wallin, G. Brunborg, E. J. Soderlund, J. K. Hongslo, and J. Alexander. 1989. Genotoxicity of the food mutagen 2-amino-1-methyl-6-phenylimidazo[4,5-b]pyridine (PhIP): formation of 2-hydroxamino-PhIP, a directly acting genotoxic metabolite. *Carcinogenesis* **10:** 1389–1396.

54. Bartsch, H. and R. Montesano. 1984. Relevance of nitrosamines to human cancer. *Carcinogenesis* **5:** 1381–1393.

55. Delp, C. R., J. S. Treves, and M. R. Banerjee. 1990. Neoplastic transformation and DNA damage of mouse mammary epithelial cells by N-methyl-N'-nitrosourea in organ culture. *Cancer Lett.* **55:** 31–37.

56. Fong, L. Y., D. E. Jensen, and P. N. Magee. 1990. DNA methyl-adduct dosimetry and O6-alkylguanine-DNA alkyl transferase activity determinations in rat mammary carcinogenesis by procarbazine and N-methylnitrosourea. *Carcinogenesis* **11:** 411–417.

57. Rivera, E. S., N. Andrade, G. Martin, G. Melito, G. Cricco, N. Mohamad, et al. 1994. Induction of mammary tumors in rat by intraperitoneal injection of NMU: histopathology and estral cycle influence. *Cancer Lett.* **86:** 223–228.

58. Zarbl, H., S. Sukumar, A. V. Arthur, D. Martin-Zanca, and M. Barbacid. 1985. Direct mutagenesis of Ha-ras-1 oncogenes by N-nitroso-N-methylurea during initiation of mammary carcinogenesis in rats. *Nature* **315:** 382–385.

59. Huggins, C. B., N. Ueda, and M. Wiessler. 1981. N-Nitroso-N-methylurea elicits mammary cancer in resistant and sensitive rat strains. *Proc. Natl. Acad. Sci USA* **78:** 1185–1188.

60. el-Bayoumy, K. 1992. Environmental carcinogens that may be involved in human breast cancer etiology. *Chem. Res. Toxicol.* **5:** 585–590.

61. Thompson, H. J., H. Adlakha, and M. Singh. 1992. Effect of carcinogen dose and age at administration on induction of mammary carcinogenesis by 1-methyl-1-nitrosourea. *Carcinogenesis* **13:** 1535–1539.

62. Miyamoto, S., R. C. Guzman, R. C. Osborn, and S. Nandi. 1988. Neoplastic transformation of mouse mammary epithelial cells by in vitro exposure to N-methyl-N-nitrosourea. *Proc. Natl. Acad. Sci. USA* **85:** 477–481.

63. Sukumar, S., V. Notario, D. Martin-Zanca, and M. Barbacid. 1983. Induction of mammary carcinomas in rats by nitroso-methylurea involves malignant activation of H-ras-1 locus by single point mutations. *Nature* **306:** 658–661.

64. Cha, R. S., W. G. Thilly, and H. Zarbl. 1994. N-nitroso-N-methylurea-induced rat mammary tumors arise from cells with pre-existing oncogenic Ha-ras-1 gene mutations. *Proc. Natl. Acad. Sci. USA* **91:** 3749–3753.

65. Palmer, J. R. and L. Rosenberg. 1993. Cigarette smoking and the risk of breast cancer. *Epidemiol. Rev.* **15:** 145–156.

66. Palmer, J. R., L. Rosenberg, E. A. Clarke, P. D. Stolley, M. E. Warshauer, A. G. Zauber, and S. Shapiro. 1991. Breast cancer and cigarette smoking: a hypothesis [see comments]. *Am. J. Epidemiol.* **134:** 1–13.

67. Brinton, L. A., C. Schairer, J. L. Stanford, and R. N. Hoover. 1986. Cigarette smoking and breast cancer. *Am. J. Epidemiol.* **123:** 614–622.

68. Chu, S. Y., N. E. Stroup, P. A. Wingo, N. C. Lee, H. B. Peterson, and M. L. Gwinn. 1990. Cigarette smoking and the risk of breast cancer. *Am. J. Epidemiol.* **131:** 244–253.

69. Adami, H. O., E. Lund, R. Bergstrom, and O. Meirik. 1988. Cigarette smoking, alcohol consumption and risk of breast cancer in young women. *Br. J. Cancer* **58:** 832–837.

70. Braga, C., E. Negri, C. La Vecchia, R. Filiberti, and S. Franceschi. 1996. Cigarette smoking and the risk of breast cancer. *Eur. J. Cancer Prev.* **5:** 159–164.

71. Ewertz, M. 1990. Smoking and breast cancer risk in Denmark. *Cancer Causes Control* **1:** 31–37.

72. Field, N. A., M. S. Baptiste, P. C. Nasca, and B. B. Metzger. 1992. Cigarette smoking and breast cancer. *Int. J. Epidemiol.* **21:** 842–848.

73. London, S. J., G. A. Colditz, M. J. Stampfer, W. C. Willett, B. A. Rosner, and F. E. Speizer. 1989. Prospective study of smoking and the risk of breast cancer. *J. Natl. Cancer Inst.* **81:** 1625–1631.

74. Hu, Y. H., C. Nagata, H. Shimizu, N. Kaneda, and Y. Kashiki. 1997. Association of body mass index, physical activity, and reproductive histories with breast cancer: a case-control study in Gifu, Japan. *Breast Cancer Res. Treatment* **43**: 65–72.

75. Stockwell, H. G. and G. H. Lyman. 1987. Cigarette smoking and the risk of female reproductive cancer. *Am. J. Obstet. Gynecol.* **157**: 35–40.

76. Hiatt, R. A. and B. H. Fireman. 1986. Smoking, menopause, and breast cancer. *J. Natl. Cancer Inst.* **76**: 833–838.

77. Mayberry, R. M. and C. Stoddard-Wright. 1992. Breast cancer risk factors among black women and white women: similarities and differences. *Am. J. Epidemiol.* **136**: 1445–1456.

78. Morabia, A., M. Bernstein, S. Heritier, and N. Khatchatrian. 1996. Relation of breast cancer with passive and active exposure to tobacco smoke. *Am. J. Epidemiol.* **143**: 918–928.

79. Smith, S. J., J. M. Deacon, and C. E. Chilvers. 1994. Alcohol, smoking, passive smoking and caffeine in relation to breast cancer risk in young women. UK National Case-Control Study Group. *Br. J. Cancer* **70**: 112–119.

80. Wells, A. J. 1991. Breast cancer, cigarette smoking, and passive smoking [letter] [see comments]. *Am. J. Epidemiol.* **133**: 208–210.

81. Lin, D. X., N. P. Lang, and F. F. Kadlubar. 1995. Species differences in the biotransformation of the food-borne carcinogen 2-amino-1-methyl-6-phenylimidazo[4,5-b]pyridine by hepatic microsomes and cytosols from humans, rats, and mice. *Drug Metab. Dispos.* **23**: 518–524.

82. Kadlubar, F. F., K. L. Dooley, C. H. Teitel, D. W. Roberts, R. W. Benson, M. A. Butler, et al. 1991. Frequency of urination and its effects on metabolism, pharmacokinetics, blood hemoglobin adduct formation, and liver and urinary bladder DNA adduct levels in beagle dogs given the carcinogen 4-aminobiphenyl. *Cancer Res.* **51**: 4371–4377.

83. Spitz, M. R., J. J. Fueger, S. Halabi, S. P. Schantz, D. Sample, and T. C. Hsu. 1993. Mutagen sensitivity in upper aerodigestive tract cancer: a case-control analysis. *Cancer Epidemiol. Biomarkers Prev.* **2**: 329–333.

84. Bell, D. A., E. A. Stephens, T. Castranio, D. M. Umbach, M. Watson, M. Deakin, et al. 1995. Polyadenylation polymorphism in the acetyltransferase 1 gene (NAT1) increases risk of colorectal cancer. *Cancer Res.* **55**: 3537–3542.

85. Blum, M., A. Demierre, D. M. Grant, M. Heim, and U. A. Meyer. 1991. Molecular mechanism of slow acetylation of drugs and carcinogens in humans. *Proc. Natl. Acad. Sci. USA* **88**: 5237–5241.

86. Tsuda, H. and S. Hirohashi. 1994. Association among p53 gene mutation, nuclear accumulation of the p53 protein and aggressive phenotypes in breast cancer. *Int. J. Cancer* **57**: 498–503.

87. Hanssen, H. P., D. P. Agarwal, H. W. Goedde, H. Bucher, H. Huland, W. Brachmann, and R. Ovenbeck. 1985. Association of N-acetyltransferase polymorphism and environmental factors with bladder carcinogenesis. Study in a north German population. *Eur. Urol.* **11**: 263–266.

88. Mommsen, S. and J. Aagard. 1983. Tobacco as a risk factor in bladder cancer. *Carcinogenesis* **4**: 335–338.

89. Yu, M. C., P. L. Skipper, K. Taghizadeh, S. R. Tannenbaum, K. K. Chan, B. E. Henderson, and R. K. Ross. 1994. Acetylator phenotype, aminobiphenyl-hemoglobin adduct levels, and bladder cancer risk in white, black, and Asian men in Los Angeles, California. *J. Natl. Cancer Inst.* **86**: 712–716.

90. Vineis, P., H. Bartsch, N. Caporaso, A. M. Harrington, F. F. Kadlubar, M. T. Landi, et al. 1994. Genetically based N-acetyltransferase metabolic polymorphism and low-level environmental exposure to carcinogens. *Nature* **369**: 154–156.

91. Vineis, P., N. Caporaso, S. R. Tannenbaum, P. L. Skipper, J. Glogowski, H. Bartsch, et al. 1990. Acetylation phenotype, carcinogen-hemoglobin adducts, and cigarette smoking. *Cancer Res.* **50:** 3002–3004.

92. Agundez, J. A., J. M. Ladero, M. Olivera, R. Abildua, J. M. Roman, and J. Benitez. 1995. Genetic analysis of the arylamine N-acetyltransferase polymorphism in breast cancer patients. *Oncology* **52:** 7–11.

93. Bulovskaya, L. N., R. G. Krupkin, T. A. Bochina, A. A. Shipkova, and M. V. Pavlova. 1978. Acetylator phenotype in patients with breast cancer. *Oncology* **35:** 185–188.

94. Evans, D. A. 1986. *Ethnic Differences in Reactions to Drugs and Xenobiotics.* Progress in Clinical and Biological Research. A.R. Liss, New York.

95. Greiner, J. W., A. H. Bryan, L. B. Malan-Shibley, and D. H. Janss. 1980. Aryl hydrocarbon hydroxylase and epoxide hydratase activities: age effects in mammary epithelial cells of Sprague-Dawley rats. *J. Natl. Cancer Inst.* **64:** 1127–1133.

96. Sardas, S., I. Cok, O. S. Sardas, O. Ilhan, and A. E. Karakaya. 1990. Polymorphic N-acetylation capacity in breast cancer patients [letter]. *Int. J. Cancer* **46:** 1138–1139.

97. Ambrosone, C. B., J. L. Freudenheim, S. Graham, J. R. Marshall, J. E. Vena, J. R. Brasure, et al. 1996. Cigarette smoking, N-acetyltransferase 2 genetic polymorphisms, and breast cancer risk. *JAMA* **276:** 1494–1501.

98. Chern, H. D., C. S. Huang, C. Y. Wang, C. Y. Shen, and K. J. Chang. 1997. Association of N-acetyltransferase polymorphism with the susceptibility of breast cancer in Taiwan. *Proc. Am. Assoc. Cancer Res.* **38:** 214(Abstract).

99. Badawi, A. F., A. Hirvonen, D. A. Bell, N. P. Lang, and F. F. Kadlubar. 1995. Role of aromatic amine acetyltransferases, NAT1 and NAT2, in carcinogen-DNA adduct formation in the human urinary bladder. *Cancer Res.* **55:** 5230–5237.

100. Abu-Zeid, M., Y. Yamazoe, and R. Kato. 1992. Sulfotransferase-mediated DNA binding of N-hydroxyarylamines(amide) in liver cytosols from human experimental animals. *Carcinogenesis* **13:** 1307–1314.

101. Chou, H. C., N. P. Lang, and F. F. Kadlubar. 1995. Metabolic activation of N-hydroxy arylamines and N-hydroxy heterocyclic amines by human sulfotransferase(s). *Cancer Res.* **55:** 525–529.

102. Price, R. A., R. S. Spielman, A. L. Lucena, J. A. Van Loon, B. L. Maidak, and R. M. Weinshilboum. 1989. Genetic polymorphism for human platelet thermostable phenol sulfotransferase (TS PST) activity. *Genetics* **122:** 905–914.

103. Kadlubar, F. F., M. A. Butler, K. R. Kaderlik, H. C. Chou, and N. P. Lang. 1992. Polymorphisms for aromatic amine metabolism in humans: relevance for human carcinogenesis. *Environ. Health Perspectives* **98:** 69–74.

104. Nebert, D. W. 1991. Role of genetics and drug metabolism in human cancer risk. *Mutat. Res.* **247:** 267–281.

105. Mannervik, B. and U. H. Danielson. 1988. Glutathione transferases: structure and catalytic activity. *CRC Crit. Rev. Biochem.* **23:** 283–337.

106. Kawajiri, K., K. Nakachi, K. Imai, J. Watanabe, and S. Hayashi. 1993. The CYP1A1 gene and cancer susceptibility. *Crit. Rev. Oncol. Hematol.* **14:** 77–87.

107. Huang, Z., M. J. Fasco, H. L. Figge, K. Keyomarsi, and L. S. Kaminsky. 1996. Expression of cytochromes P450 in human breast tissue and tumors. *Drug Metab. Dispos.* **24:** 899–905.

108. Murray, G. I., R. J. Weaver, P. J. Paterson, S. W. Ewen, W. T. Melvin, and M. D. Burke. 1993. Expression of xenobiotic metabolizing enzymes in breast cancer. *J. Pathol.* **169:** 347–353.

109. Ambrosone, C. B., J. L. Freudenheim, S. Graham, J. R. Marshall, J. E. Vena, J. R. Brasure, et al. 1995. Cytochrome P4501A1 and glutathione S-transferase (M1) genetic polymorphisms and postmenopausal breast cancer risk. *Cancer Res.* **55:** 3483–3485.

110. Ishibe, N., K. Kelsey, S. Hankinson, and D. Hunter. 1996. Genetic polymorphisms in the cytochrome P450 1A1 gene and breast cancer risk. *Proc. Am. Assoc. Cancer Res.* **37:** 261(Abstract).

111. Taioli, E., J. Trachman, X. Chen, P. Toniolo, and S. J. Garte. 1995. A CYP1A1 restriction fragment length polymorphism is associated with breast cancer in African-American women. *Cancer Res.* **55:** 3757–3758.

112. Albin, N., L. Massaad, C. Toussaint, M. C. Mathieu, J. Morizet, O. Parise, A. Gouyette, and G. G. Chabot. 1993. Main drug-metabolizing enzyme systems in human breast tumors and peritumoral tissues. *Cancer Res.* **53:** 3541–3546.

113. Forrester, L. M., J. D. Hayes, R. Millis, D. Barnes, A. L. Harris, J. J. Schlager, G. Powis, and C. R. Wolf. 1990. Expression of glutathione S-transferases and cytochrome P450 in normal and tumor breast tissue. *Carcinogenesis* **11:** 2163–2170.

114. Mitchell, J. B. and A. Russo. 1987. The role of glutathione in radiation and drug induced cytotoxicity. *Br. J. Cancer* Suppl. **8:** 96–104.

115. Arrick, B. A. and C. F. Nathan. 1984. Glutathione metabolism as a determinant of therapeutic efficacy: a review. *Cancer Res.* **44:** 4224–4232.

116. Kelsey, K. T., S. E. Hankinson, G. A. Colditz, K. Springer, M. Garcia-Closas, D. Spiegelman, et al. 1997. Glutathione S-transferase class mu deletion polymorphism and breast cancer: results from prevalent versus incident cases. *Cancer Epidemiol. Biomarkers Prev.* **6:** 511–515.

117. Chern, H. D., C. S. Huang, H. J. Wang, M. Wang, and K. T. Chang. 1996. Glutathione S-transferase M1 and T1 polymorphisms: susceptibility of breast cancer in Taiwan. *Proc. Am. Assoc. Cancer Res.* **37:** 106(Abstract).

118. Kato, S., M. Onda, N. Matsukura, A. Tokunaga, N. Matsuda, K. Furukawa, K. Yamashita, and P. G. Shields. 1996. Cytochrome P450 1A1 (CYP1A1) and glutathione-S-transferase M1 (GSTM1) genetic polymorphisms for gastric and breast cancer risk. *Proc. Am. Assoc. Cancer Res.* **37:** 259(Abstract).

119. Yamazaki, H., Y. Inui, C. H. Yun, F. P. Guengerich, and T. Shimada. 1995. Cytochrome P450 2E1 and 2A6 enzymes as major catalysts for metabolic activation of N-nitrosodialkylamines and tobacco-related nitrosamines in human liver microsomes. *Carcinogenesis* **13:** 1789–1794.

120. Guengerich, F. P., D. H. Kim, and M. Iwasaki. 1991. Role of human cytochrome P-450 IIE1 in the oxidation of many low molecular weight cancer suspects. *Chem. Res. Toxicol.* **4:** 168–179.

121. Yang, C. S., J. S. Yoo, H. Ishizaki, and J. Y. Hong. 1990. Cytochrome P450IIE1: roles in nitrosamine metabolism and mechanisms of regulation. *Drug Metab. Rev.* **22:** 147–159.

122. Nouso, K., S. S. Thorgeirsson, and N. Battula. 1992. Stable expression of human cytochrome P450IIE1 in mammalian cells: metabolic activation of nitrosodimethylamine and formation of adducts with cellular DNA. *Cancer Res.* **52:** 1796–1800.

123. Hayashi, S., J. Watanabe, and K. Kawajiri. 1991. Genetic polymorphisms in the 5'-flanking region change transcriptional regulation of the human cytochrome P450IIE1 gene. *J. Biochem.* (Tokyo) **110:** 559–565.

124. Uematsu, F., S. Ikawa, H. Kikuchi, I. Sagami, R. Kanamaru, T. Abe, et al. 1994. Restriction fragment length polymorphism of the human CYP2E1 (cytochrome P450IIE1) gene and susceptibility to lung cancer: possible relevance to low smoking exposure. *Pharmacogenetics* **4:** 58–63.

125. Peter, R., R. Bocker, P. H. Beaune, M. Iwasaki, F. P. Guengerich, and C. S. Yang. 1990. Hydroxylation of chlorzoxazone as a specific probe for human liver cytochrome P-450IIE1. *Chem. Res. Toxicol.* **3:** 566–573.

126. Uematsu, F., H. Kikuchi, M. Motomiya, T. Abe, I. Sagami, T. Ohmachi, et al. 1991. Association between restriction fragment length polymorphism of the human cytochrome P450IIE1 gene and susceptibility to lung cancer. *Jpn. J. Cancer Res.* **82:** 254–256.

127. Kato, S., E. D. Bowman, A. M. Harrington, B. Blomeke, and P. G. Shields. 1995. Human lung carcinogen-DNA adduct levels mediated by genetic polymorphisms in vivo. *J. Natl. Cancer Inst.* **87:** 902–907.

128. Persson, I., I. Johansson, H. Bergling, M. L. Dahl, J. Seidegard, R. Rylander, et al. 1993. Genetic polymorphism of cytochrome P4502E1 in a Swedish population. Relationship to incidence of lung cancer. *FEBS Lett.* **319:** 207–211.

129. Hirvonen, A., K. Husgafvel-Pursiainen, S. Anttila, A. Karjalainen, and H. Vainio. 1993. The human CYP2E1 gene and lung cancer: DraI and RsaI restriction fragment length polymorphisms in a Finnish study population. *Carcinogenesis* **14:** 85–88.

130. Kato, S., P. G. Shields, N. E. Caporaso, H. Sugimura, G. E. Trivers, M. A. Tucker, et al. 1994. Analysis of cytochrome P450 2E1 genetic polymorphisms in relation to human lung cancer. *Cancer Epidemiol. Biomarkers Prev.* **3:** 515–518.

131. Hildesheim, A., C.-J. Chen, N. E. Caporaso, Y.-J. Cheng, R. N. Hoover, M.-M. Hsu, et al. 1995. *Cytochrome* P4502E1 genetic polymorphisms and risk of nasopharyngeal carcinoma: results from a case-control study conducted in Taiwan. *CEBP* **4:** 607–610.

132. Shields, P. G., C. B. Ambrosone, S. Graham, E. D. Bowman, A. M. Harrington, K. A. Gillenwater, et al. 1996. A cytochrome P450IIE1 genetic polymorphism (CYP2E1) and tobacco smoking in breast cancer. *Mol. Carcinog.* **17:** 144–150.

133. Crespi, C. L., B. W. Penman, H. V. Gelboin, and F. J. Gonzalez. 1991. A tobacco smoke-derived nitrosamine, 4-(methylnitrosamino)-1-(3-pyridyl)-1-butanone, is activated by multiple human cytochrome P450s including the polymorphic human cytochrome P4502D6. *Carcinogenesis* **12:** 1197–1201.

134. Penman, B. W., J. Reece, T. Smith, C. S. Yang, H. V. Gelboin, F. J. Gonzalez, and C. L. Crespi. 1993. Characterization of a human cell line expressing high levels of cDNA-derived CYP2D6. *Pharmacogenetics* **3:** 28–39.

135. Caporaso, N. E., M. A. Tucker, R. Hoover, R. B. Hayes, L. W. Pickle, H. Issaq, et al. 1990. Lung cancer and the debrisoquine metabolic phenotype. *J. Natl. Cancer Inst.* **85:** 1264–1272.

136. Ayesh, R., J. R. Idle, J. C. Ritchie, M. J. Crothers, and M. R. Hetzel. 1984. Metabolic oxidation phenotypes as markers for susceptibility to lung cancer. *Nature* **312:** 169–170.

137. Bouchardy, C., S. Benhamou, and P. Dayer. 1996. The effect of tobacco on lung cancer risk depends on CYP2D6 activity. *Cancer Res.* **56:** 251–253.

138. Ladero, J. M., J. Benitez, C. Jara, A. Llerena, M. J. Valdivielso, J. J. Munoz, and E. Vargas. 1991. Polymorphic oxidation of debrisoquine in women with breast cancer. *Oncology* **48:** 107–110.

139. Pontin, J. E., H. Hamed, I. S. Fentiman, and J. R. Idle. 1990. Cytochrome P450dbl phenotypes in malignant and benign breast disease. *Eur. J. Cancer* **26:** 790–792.

140. Huober, J., B. Bertram, E. Petru, M. Kaufmann, and D. Schmahl. 1991. Metabolism of debrisoquine and susceptibility to breast cancer. *Breast Cancer Res Treatment* **18:** 43–48.

141. Ladona, M. G., R. E. Abildua, J. M. Ladero, J. M. Roman, M. A. Plaza, J. A. Agundez, J. J. Munoz, and J. Benitez. 1996. CYP2D6 genotypes in Spanish women with breast cancer. *Cancer Lett.* **99:** 23–28.

142. Wolf, C. R., C. A. Smith, A. C. Gough, J. E. Moss, K. A. Vallis, G. Howard, et al. 1992. Relationship between the debrisoquine hydroxylase polymorphism and cancer susceptibility. *Carcinogenesis* **13:** 1035–1038.

143. Buchert, E. T., R. L. Woosley, S. M. Swain, S. J. Oliver, S. S. Coughlin, L. Pickle, B. Trock, and A. T. Riegel. 1993. Relationship of CYP2D6 (debrisoquine hydroxylase) genotype to breast cancer susceptibility. *Pharmacogenetics* **3:** 322–327.

144. Martucci, C. P. and J. Fishman. 1993. P450 enzymes of estrogen metabolism. *Pharmacol. Ther.* **57:** 237–257.

145. Michnovicz, J. J. and H. L. Bradlow. 1990. Dietary and pharmacological control of estradiol metabolism in humans. *Ann. NY Acad. Sci.* **595:** 291–299.

146. Nelson, D. R., T. Kamataki, D. J. Waxman, F. P. Guengerich, R. W. Estabrook, R. Feyereisen, et al. 1993. The P450 superfamily: update on new sequences, gene mapping, accession numbers, early trivial names of enzymes, and nomenclature. *DNA Cell. Biol.* **12:** 1–51.

147. Osborne, M. P., H. L. Bradlow, G. Y. Wong, and N. T. Telang. 1993. Upregulation of estradiol C16 alpha-hydroxylation in human breast tissue: a potential biomarker of breast cancer risk [see comments]. *J. Natl. Cancer Inst.* **85:** 1917–1920.

148. Bradlow, H. L., R. Hershcopf, C. Martucci, and J. Fishman. 1986. 16 alpha-hydroxylation of estradiol: a possible risk marker for breast cancer. *Ann. N. Y. Acad. Sci.* **464:** 138–151.

149. Sutter, T. R., Y. M. Tang, C. L. Hayes, Y. Y. Wo, E. W. Jabs, X. Li, et al. 1994. Complete cDNA sequence of a human dioxin-inducible mRNA identifies a new gene subfamily of cytochrome P450 that maps to chromosome 2. *J. Biol. Chem.* **269:** 13,092–13,099.

150. Liehr, J. G., M. J. Ricci, C. R. Jefcoate, E. V. Hannigan, J. A. Hokanson, and B. T. Zhu. 1995. 4-Hydroxylation of estradiol by human uterine myometrium and myoma microsomes: implications for the mechanism of uterine tumorigenesis. *Proc. Natl. Acad. Sci USA* **92:** 9220–9224.

151. Bhattacharyya, K. K., P. B. Brake, S. E. Eltom, S. A. Otto, and C. R. Jefcoate. 1995. Identification of a rat adrenal cytochrome P450 active in polycyclic hydrocarbon metabolism as rat CYP1B1. Demonstration of a unique tissue-specific pattern of hormonal and aryl hydrocarbon receptor-linked regulation. *J. Biol. Chem.* **270:** 11,595–11,602.

152. Kerlan, V., Y. Dreano, J. P. Bercovici, P. H. Beaune, H. H. Floch, and F. Berthou. 1992. Nature of cytochromes P450 involved in the 2-/4-hydroxylations of estradiol in human liver microsomes. *Biochem. Pharmacol.* **44:** 1745–1756.

153. Kataoka, A., T. Nishida, T. Sugiyama, N. Hirakawa, T. Maruuchi, K. Imaishi, and M. Yakushiji. 1992. [Immunohistochemical studies of recessive oncogene p53 and N-myc oncogene expression in 7, 12 dimethylbenz (a) anthracene-induced rat ovarian tumors]. *Nippon Sanka. Fujinka. Gakkai Zasshi* **44:** 391–396.

154. Kataoka, A., N. Hirakawa, T. Sugiyama, T. Higashijima, T. Nishida, and M. Yakushiji. 1991. [Immunohistochemical studies of ras oncogene product p21 in 7,12 dimethylbenz (a) anthracene-induced rat ovarian tumors]. *Nippon Sanka. Fujinka. Gakkai Zasshi* **43:** 1209–1213.

155. Guldberg, H. C. and C. A. Marsden. 1975. Catechol-O-methyl transferase: pharmacological aspects and physiological role. *Pharmacol. Rev.* **27:** 135–206.

156. Lavigne, J. A., K. J. Helzlsouer, H. Y. Huang, P. T. Strickland, D. A. Bell, O. Selmin, et al. 1997. An association between the allele coding for a low activity variant of catechol-O-methyltransferase and the risk for breast cancer. *Cancer Res.* **57:** 5493–5497.

157. Hirose, K., K. Tajima, N. Hamajima, M. Inoue, T. Takezaki, T. Kuroishi, M. Yoshida, and S. Tokudome. 1995. A large-scale, hospital-based case-control study of risk factors of breast cancer according to menopausal status. *Jpn. J. Cancer Res.* **86:** 146–154.

158. Engeland, A., A. Andersen, T. Haldorsen, and S. Tretli. 1996. Smoking habits and risk of cancers other than lung cancer: 28 years' follow-up of 26,000 Norwegian men and women. *Cancer Causes Control* **7:** 497–506.

159. Bennicke, K., C. Conrad, S. Sabroe, and H. T. Sorensen. 1995. Cigarette smoking and breast cancer. *Br. Med. J.* **310:** 1431–1433.

160. Ranstam, J. and H. Olsson. 1995. Alcohol, cigarette smoking, and the risk of breast cancer. *Cancer Detect. Prev.* **19:** 487–493.

161. Calle, E. E., H. L. Miracle-McMahill, M. J. Thun, and C. W. Heath,Jr. 1994. Cigarette smoking and risk of fatal breast cancer. *Am. J. Epidemiol.* **139:** 1001–1007.

162. Haile, R. W., J. S. Witte, G. Ursin, J. Siemiatycki, J. Bertolli, W. D. Thompson, and A. Paganini-Hill. 1996. A case-control study of reproductive variables, alcohol, and smoking in premenopausal bilateral breast cancer. *Breast Cancer Res. Treatment* **37:** 49–56.

25

The Estrogenicity of Selected Nutrients, Phytochemicals, Pesticides, and Pollutants

Their Potential Roles in Breast Cancer

Leena Hilakivi-Clarke, Bruce Trock, and Robert Clarke

1. INTRODUCTION

Breast cancer remains one of the leading causes of mortality among women in westernized societies. Although the mortality rates for this disease have been markedly lower in many Oriental countries, immigrants to the West rapidly acquire the increased incidence of their adopted country. This has led to the hypothesis that the increased incidence seen in the West is not a result of genetic differences, but rather of environmental exposures. One of the most obvious differences between Eastern and Western societies has been diet, although countries like Japan are now exhibiting a clear trend toward consumption of a more Western diet. Among the dietary differences are the lower consumption of high-fat foods and total caloric intake in the East, and the higher consumption of dietary fiber and soy-based food products. In experimental animal models, each of these differences, when studied alone, can significantly influence mammary carcinogenesis. Exposure to specific pesticides and pollutants also has been suggested to contribute to breast cancer risk. However, it is often difficult to assess relative differences in exposure to these compounds in such international studies.

Estrogenicity is a common thread in the implication of these dietary and environmental exposures. In general, it appears that serum estrogen levels are lower in Oriental populations, compared with the United States or Western Europe *(5)*. Consumption of a high-fat diet is associated with increased serum estrogen levels; a high-fiber diet can reduce these levels. It is often difficult, in human studies, to tease such effects apart, since populations eating a high-fat diet generally do so in the context of a low-fiber diet. In animal studies, each can affect serum estrogen levels when the effects of the other are adequately and appropriately controlled. Many soy-based foods contain high levels of isoflavone, which are compounds that can function as effective estrogens in some animal models.

Estrogens are widely implicated as effectors in mediating altered breast cancer risk *(39)*. This is apparent from the endocrinologic associations with risk, including ages at menarche, menopause, and first birth *(92)*. Breast cancer risk is increased in postmenopausal women taking estrogen replacement therapy *(71)*, and estrogens induce potent

From: Breast Cancer: Molecular Genetics, Pathogenesis, and Therapeutics
Edited by: A. M. Bowcock © Humana Press Inc., Totowa, NJ

mitogenic effects in some human breast cancer cells growing both in vitro and in immunodeficient rodents *(35,37,38)*. However, the timing of exposure may be critical. Obesity is associated with increased serum estrogen levels and increased breast cancer risk in postmenopausal women. In marked contrast, there is evidence of an association between obesity and reduced risk in premenopausal women, in whom this may reflect effects on the hypothalamic–pituitary–gonadal axis, since some obese women become amenorrheic. This would ultimately reduce the number of lifetime menstrual cycles, an effect that could reduce premenopausal breast cancer risk.

This chapter will review recent evidence linking nutrition, pesticides, and pollutants to breast cancer. Rather than attempt an encyclopedic approach, the chapter illustrates the controversies by reference to specific examples. From a nutritional perspective, it focuses on the effects of a high-fat diet and the consumption of selected phytoestrogenic compounds found either in soy-based foods, or as contaminants in grains and cereals. However, there is not sufficient time or space to discuss other compounds with potent estrogenic activities, e.g., the naturally occurring lignans, or the industrial byproduct bisphenol A, which is found in the diet, probably as a result of the plastic used to wrap food *(165)*. The chapter will also review the conflicting evidence implicating exposure to selected environmental compounds in affecting breast cancer risk, an area in which there is considerable debate, but little consistent epidemiologic data.

2. HIGH-FAT DIET

2.1. Dietary Fat: Human Studies

A diet containing high levels of fat appears detrimental to human health. It clearly contributes to the development of cardiovascular diseases, diabetes, and various other diseases. Some evidence indicates that consumption of a high-fat diet also is associated with increased risk of cancers of the prostate *(65)*, colon *(186)*, and breast *(86,139)*. The initial evidence linking fat intake to breast cancer was obtained through studies showing that the national fat intake correlates with breast cancer incidence in a given country *(28)*. Americans both consume high levels of dietary fats and have a high breast cancer incidence; Asians consume a low-fat diet and have a low breast cancer risk *(139)*.

Many case-control studies have been performed to test the hypothesis that a high-fat intake increases breast cancer risk. Pooled and meta-analysis of the case-control studies suggest that a high total fat intake increases the risk of developing breast cancer *(22,86)*. The studies further indicate that some fats, such as monounsaturated, saturated fats, and polyunsaturated fatty acids (PUFAs), increase breast cancer risk. PUFAs consist both of n-6 and n-3 fatty acids. There is some evidence that n-6 PUFA may increase the risk of recurrence of breast cancer *(82)*. Fish and other marine oils that contain high levels of n-3 PUFAs, on the other hand, may reduce breast cancer risk *(31)*. In marked contrast to the case-control studies, most cohort studies have not confirmed the adverse association with a high-fat diet. Although some cohort studies do report this association *(16,85)*, the majority are negative *(174)*. Furthermore, a meta-analysis of these studies, most of which have been performed in the United States, found no correlation between dietary fat intake and breast cancer *(94)*.

Despite the animal data supporting the role of dietary factors in the etiology of breast cancer, the presence of some apparently contradictory cohort and case-control studies, and the lack of a well-defined and tested mechanism of action, remain problematic (28,29,85,185). These problems partly reflect differences in study design, energy adjustment methods, population size and demography, inaccuracies in dietary assessment, the narrow range of diets consumed in some studies, and the statistical power of the data analysis to actually identify significant risk *(20,84,108,143)*. Nevertheless, no compelling conclusion can be drawn either way as to the precise effect of consumption of a high-fat diet on breast cancer risk in humans.

2.2. Dietary Fat: Animal Studies

Many animal studies have been performed to explore the possible link between dietary fat and breast cancer. Most of these studies suggest that a high-fat intake promotes carcinogen- or viral-induced mammary tumorigenesis in rodents *(62,181)*. The n-6 PUFA, e.g., the linoleic acid present in high levels in corn oil, soybean oil, safflower-seed oil, and sunflower-seed oil, have been strongly implicated as promotional agents in both carcinogen-induced rat mammary tumor models *(24,32)* and in models of tumor metastasis in nude mice *(154)*. However, saturated fats of animal origin, e.g., lard and beef tallow, and of plant origin, e.g., coconut oil and palm oil, can inhibit promotion of carcinogen-induced mammary tumorigenesis in rats *(181)*. Similar to the human data, the n-3 PUFAs present in fish oils inhibit both breast tumor growth *(2,31,144)* and metastasis *(154)*. The role of n-3 PUFAs was recently reviewed, and a meta-analysis of the animal studies also was recently published *(58)*.

The effect of dietary fat on mammary tumorigenesis, before initiation has occurred, is not clear. In animal models, high levels of saturated fats consumed from puberty through adulthood, until the time when carcinogen is administered, stimulate the subsequent development of mammary tumors (168). At this same period of administration, n-6 PUFA is relatively ineffective. However, *in utero* exposure to a diet high in n-6 PUFA through the pregnant mother, increases mammary tumorigenesis in rats *(74)* and mice *(177)*.

2.3. Are There Sensitive Periods for Dietary Fat Intake to Affect Breast Cancer?

The animal data suggest that the timing of dietary fat exposure may be of critical importance in determining risk *(73)*. Since it is not known when the initiation of breast cancer occurs in humans, it is difficult to directly assess the role of dietary fats in the timing of this process in the human disease. However, the incidence of breast cancer is several-fold higher for Caucasian women living in the United States than in Oriental women living in Asian countries *(137)*. This difference eventually disappears in Oriental women who move to the West. Breast cancer rates increase over succeeding generations in women migrating from Asia to the United States, eventually reaching that in Caucasian populations *(53,101,113,169)*. Breast cancer risk among Asians is already 80% higher after a decade of living in the United States, compared with the risk of Asian women remaining in the East *(195)*. The most dramatic difference in risk occurs between Asian-Americans born in the West and those born in the East *(195)*. A higher dietary fat intake during pregnancy in the West than in the East may contribute to the transition toward higher breast cancer risk between Asian generations living in the West.

More direct evidence that *in utero* fat intake may be responsible for the elevated breast cancer risk in women whose mothers consumed a high-fat diet during pregnancy can be obtained from some epidemiological studies. For example, high intake of n-6 PUFAs during pregnancy increases birth weight *(123,167)*, and a high birth weight is associated with an increased breast cancer risk in women *(127,157)*. The opposite also appears true. Women exposed to a fetal environment low in PUFAs, e.g., their mothers suffered from pregnancy-dependent pre-eclampsia *(55)*, have a significantly reduced breast cancer risk. Our animal studies further support the association between a maternal high-fat diet and increased breast cancer risk among female offspring. Female rats whose mothers consumed a diet high in n-6 PUFA (46% calories from corn oil) during pregnancy have a twofold higher incidence of carcinogen-induced mammary tumors than the female offspring of mothers that consumed a low-fat diet (12% calories from corn oil) during pregnancy *(74)*. After birth, both the high- and low-fat offspring were maintained on the same diet. Similar data have been obtained in mice that develop spontaneous mammary tumors at a relatively old age *(177)*.

In addition to fetal life, there may be other sensitive periods when the mammary gland is particularly vulnerable to the effects of dietary fats. These periods are probably characterized by the rapid proliferation of mammary epithelial cells, e.g., the proliferation that occurs during puberty and pregnancy. The authors' animal studies indicate that a high-fat intake, when limited to pregnancy, increases both circulating estrogen levels and breast cancer risk in the mothers *(75)*.

The same may be true for humans. It already is known that some pregnancy complications affect breast cancer risk. Women who suffer from pregnancy-induced hypertension, and have low circulating PUFA levels *(175)*, subsequently exhibit a significantly reduced incidence of breast cancer *(88)*. Increased risk is reported in women who suffer from severe nausea during pregnancy *(56)*. The relationship between nausea and serum PUFA levels is not known. Since serum estrogen levels are elevated in pregnancy nausea *(50)*, and a high PUFA intake increases circulating estrogens *(74,75)*, it is possible that women experiencing severe nausea during pregnancy have altered serum PUFA levels.

2.4. Mechanism of Action of Dietary Fat on the Breast

Some of the controversy in human studies probably could be resolved by identifying the mechanisms mediating the effects of dietary fat on the breast. Currently, several different pathways for the action of fat have been proposed. These include changes in lipid peroxidation *(19)* or fatty acid metabolism *(147,154)*, which then alter the composition of the cell membranes (96), and probably affect several signal transduction pathways. For example, a high-fat intake can influence protein kinase C (PKC) activity in the skin (34), colon (149), and mammary gland (76). The PKC family of genes mediates events triggered at the cell surface, which lead to a variety of intracellular responses. At least 10 different isoenzymes of the PKC family have been identified; their activity and biological functions vary in different tissues *(12,49,91)*. These isoenzymes are activated by diacylglycerol *(132)*, a product of membrane phospholipids cleaved by phospholipases. The activity of phospholipases, in turn, is regulated by various hormones and growth factors, including E2 *(39)*, linking PKC activity to the estrogenic regulation of cell proliferation and differentiation.

2.4.1. Estrogens

Dietary fat also may affect mammary tumorigenesis by altering circulating estrogen levels. Human studies indicate that a high-fat intake increases *(5)*, and restriction of fat intake reduces, plasma estrogen levels *(17,21,142,153)*. Data from animal studies are less clear *(42,152,168)*, possibly because animals effectively regulate their feed intake. For example, animals kept on a high-fat–high-caloric diet voluntarily reduce food intake. In studies in which the caloric intake is kept the same between animals consuming a high- or low-fat diet, a high-fat intake increases serum estrogens *(33,74,75,95)*.

Several alternative mechanisms exist for a high-fat diet to increase circulating estrogens. Fat intake often leads to accumulation of adipose tissue, which is an important site for the conversion of adrenally derived androstenedione to estrone *(63)*. The fatty acid metabolite arachidonic acid activates the P450 aromatase, which increases conversion of androstenedione to estrone *(133)*. Additionally, PUFAs can reduce the binding of serum estrogens to both sex-hormone-binding globulin (SHBG) and albumin, thereby increasing the circulating levels of biologically potent free estrogens *(23)*. This latter mechanism does not operate in rodents, since they do not have SHBG.

2.4.2. Estrogen Receptors

The biological effects of estrogens are mediated chiefly through the estrogen receptor (ER). In vivo and in vitro studies indicate that estrogens generally downregulate ER *(69,148)*. Since a high-fat diet often increases circulating levels of estrogens, this could lead to reduced ER. However, indirect evidence in humans indicates that a high-fat consumption elevates ER protein levels. For example, a high-fat intake and obesity increase the risk for developing ER-positive (but not ER-negative) mammary tumors in some postmenopausal women *(141)*. Women with ER-positive tumors also have a significantly increased risk for recurrence, if they consume a diet high in PUFA and saturated fats *(82)*. This increased risk does not appear to apply to patients with ER-negative tumors.

The authors have explored the effect of a high-fat intake on mammary ER content. In female mice, consumption of a diet high in n-6 PUFA increases the mammary ER levels by sixfold *(76)*. Thus, it is possible that a fat-induced promotion of tumor growth, in ER-positive rodent breast cancer models *(155)*, may occur through ER. This could contribute to the lack of effect of fat in some cohort studies, since approx 30–40% of women have ER-negative tumors. These would be unaffected by an indirect estrogenic stimulus mediated through a high fat intake.

3. PHYTOESTROGENS AND BREAST CANCER

Phytoestrogens are plant-derived compounds that exhibit estrogenic activities *(40)*. There are several groups of plant estrogens, including lignans, flavones, isoflavones (e.g., genistein: 4',5,7-trihydroxyisoflavone), and mycotoxins derived from fungal molds (e.g., zearalenone: 2,4-dihydroxy-6-[10-hydroxy-6-oxo-trans-1-undecenyl]-β-resorcyclic acid-μ lactone). The estrogenic activity of these compounds has been described both in vitro and in vivo (*see* recent reviews in refs. *7* and *40*). Isoflavonoids are often considered "good" phytoestrogens, being occasionally associated with a reduced breast cancer risk *(7)* and an ability to inhibit the growth of some experimental tumors *(7)*. Several synthetic and naturally occurring flavonoids inhibit in vitro growth of MCF-7 and ZR- 75-1 cells, when given in pharmacological doses *(77,182)*. However, at physiological concentrations, lignans and isoflavones stimulate the growth of breast cancer cell lines *(117,182)*.

3.1. The Epidemiology of Soy and Breast Cancer Risk

Genistein and the related compound daidzein are among the major phytoestrogenic compounds present in soy *(4,15)*. Although the United States is one of the world's major producers of soy, most is exported and consumed abroad. Soybean-based foods are typical for diets of Asian countries, but not for American *(15)*. Several of those countries with a high intake of soy products also appear to have a relatively low incidence of breast cancer *(3)*.

Americans are exposed to 1–3 mg/d of isoflavones (0.02–0.06 mg/kg/d); in Oriental countries, the exposure varies between 25 and 100 mg/d *(124,125)*. The level of genistein exposure is 1.5–4 mg/person/day in Asia and about twenty times less in the US. Approximately 50% of the daily isoflavone exposure in Orientals is composed of genistein (0.25–1 mg/kg/d) *(125)*. Thus, it is not surprising that international studies, comparing the low incidence of breast cancer with the higher incidence in Western countries, have been used to support the possible association between soy intake and breast cancer risk *(3)*. These international studies are difficult to interpret, being potentially confounded by other dietary and environmental variables, e.g., differences in the patterns of soy consumption and the relative amounts of caloric and fat intake. Previously, these types of international studies have been used to show an association between breast cancer risk and several other dietary components, including dietary fat, different sources of dietary fat, and caloric intake, interpretations that are still hotly disputed *(22,36)*. Many of the factors that have confounded an assessment of the validity of these observations also may apply to interpretations regarding soy/isoflavone intake and breast cancer risk.

Case-control studies represent the most widely used study design to explore the soy/ breast cancer hypothesis *(79,80,112,134,188,193,194)*. Four of eight studies find no statistically significant association (Table 1). The smallest case-control study found an association for Japanese soup, but not for tofu *(134)*, despite both foods probably having comparable genistein/isoflavone levels *(44,54)*. The lack of an association with tofu consumption was subsequently contradicted by Wu et al. *(193)*, who found a significant effect in both premenopausal and postmenopausal women. However, the study by Lee et al. failed to find any association with soy protein intake and breast cancer risk in postmenopausal patients, reporting a negative association only in premenopausal women *(112)*. Thus, significant inconsistencies are apparent among studies reporting the possible protective effects of soy consumption. Some studies report increased risk associated with soy consumption, but the odds ratios (OR) are not significant. For example, in the study by Yuan et al. (194), the OR = 1.4 (95% CI = 0.7, 3.0) for soy protein and OR = 1.4 (95% CI = 0.8, 2.6) for soy/total protein intakes in Tianjin. Hirose et al. *(80)* reported increased risks that approached statistical significance of OR = 1.16 (95% CI = 0.98, 1.37) for miso soup consumption in premenopausal women, and OR =

Table 1
Epidemiologic Studies Comparing the Intake of Soy
with Breast Cancer Risk in Studies Identified to Date

Population	Exposure	Association	Citation
212 Patients 212 Hospital (ctr) 212 Community (ctr)	Total Soybean Producrs	None	(79)
534 Patients 534 Community (ctr)	Total soy protein	None	(194)[+]
300 Patients 300 Community (ctr)	Total Soy Protein	None	(194)[+]
86 Spouses of patients	Weekly intakes	Tofu^: none Soup: -ve*	(134)
222 Patients 222 Sisters	Tofu^ intake	None[#]	(188)
200 Cases 420 Hospital (ctr)	Soy protein	Postmen: none Pretmen: none	(112)
597 Cases 996 Community (ctr)	Tofu intake	-ve*	(193)
1,186 Cases 23,163 Hospital (ctr)	Miso soup	Postmen: none Pretmen: none	(80)
	Bean curd (multivariate analysis)	Postmen: -ve* Premen: none	

[#]Borderline for a negative (OR = 0.5; 0.2–1.1);
*Negative association (higher consumption associated with lower breast cancer risk);
^Tofu has a higher isoflavone content than soy drink (54), and levels comparable to, or slightly lower than miso and other japanese soups (44);
[+]Two independent studies in two different cities/populations reported together in the one paper;
Ctr = Control population.

1.17 (95% CI = 0.92, 1.49) for bean curd consumption 13 times/wk in postmenopausal women.

Although no studies have been found that show significantly increased breast cancer risk, there are studies showing an increased risk associated with those cancers that are more prevalent in Eastern countries (45,78,83,90), e.g., cancers of the stomach. However, it is likely that these increases reflect the nature of the way soy foods are processed. Where a high salt content is produced, the isoflavones in soy appear unable to prevent the carcinogenic process in the stomach.

3.2. Soy, Genistein, and Breast Cancer Risk in Animal Studies

Among 31 animal studies containing 11 different tumor sites, 23 (74%) reported that consumption of soy had a tumor-inhibiting effect (125). The multiplicity of carcinogen-induced mammary tumors in rats can be reduced by a consumption of a high soybean diet (14,70). However, others have failed to find a difference in carcinogen-induced mammary tumorigenesis in rats fed soy protein (27,89). In one report, soy

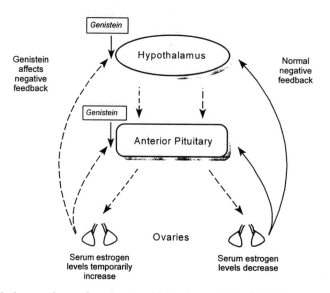

Fig. 1. Possible interactions of genistein with the hypothalamic-pituitary-gonadal axis. The prescence of genistein could initially produce a weaker estrogenic response (ER occupied by the weaker genistein rather than E2). This would result in increased gonadotropin secretion and "hyper"-stimulation of the ovaries, as is seen in premenopausal women receiving Tamoxifen (reviewed in *[37]*). However, as ovarian estrogen production increases, sufficient E2 levels would eventually be reached to override the effects of genistein and suppresss gonadotropin secretion, with a subsequent drop in serum E2 levels. Thus, the overall effect could be to "detune" the axis and prolong an otherwise normal cycle.

intake increased spontaneous mammary tumorigenesis in mice, although latency was increased *(67)*. Many of the studies showing reduced breast cancer risk used pharmacologic, not physiologic, doses. Thus, these studies cannot be used directly to either support or contradict the epidemiologic data.

3.3. Estrogenic Properties of Soy in Humans

There is clear evidence that soy is estrogenic in humans. Several studies have shown that the administration of soy-based foods significantly perturb function of the hypothalamic–pituitary–gonadal axis in premenopausal *(30,115,138)*, but not postmenopausal, women *(13)*. The presence of sufficient genistein could initially produce a weaker estrogenic response, which would result in increased gonadotropin secretion and hyperstimulation of the ovaries, as is seen in premenopausal women receiving the weak partial estrogen agonist tamoxifen (reviewed in ref. *37*). However, as ovarian estrogen production increases, sufficient E2 levels would eventually be reached to override the effects of genistein (weaker estrogen than E2) and suppress gonadotropin secretion, with a subsequent drop in serum E2 levels. Thus, the overall effect could be to detune the axis, temporarily increase serum estrogen levels, and prolong an otherwise normal cycle (Fig. 1.). This hypothesis would require the tissue concentrations of bioavailable genistein in the brain to reach levels sufficient to effectively compete with the available E2.

3.4. Early Genistein Exposure and Breast Cancer Risk

The reported connection between perinatal estrogen exposure and breast cancer risk strongly suggests that an early exposure to dietary phytoestrogens can influence breast cancer risk. Neonatal treatment with pharmacological doses of genistein (equivalent to approx 500 mg/kg; exposure among Orientals is 0.25–1 mg/kg) lengthens the latency to the appearance of DMBA-induced mammary tumors, and reduces tumor incidence *(110,128)*. The authors have been studying the effects of physiological doses of genistein, following either reduced tumor multiplicity, or reduced tumor growth rates (Hilakivi-Clarke et al., unpublished data). However, DMBA-induced mammary tumor incidence was not affected by postnatal administration of physiological doses of genistein. No changes in tumor latency, multiplicity (number of tumors per animal), or growth were noted. These findings suggest that genistein acts as an estrogen during the fetal period, and increases subsequent breast cancer risk. Currently being explored is the possibility that a lifetime exposure of genistein is required for the protective effects to be seen. Genistein intake is reduced in Asian women migrating to the West *(193)*, and, simultaneously, breast cancer risk is elevated *(195)*.

The authors also have treated pregnant rats with 1 mg/kg genistein (Hilakivi-Clarke et al., unpublished data). The data indicate that *in utero* exposure to genistein increases subsequent breast cancer risk.

3.5. Potential Mechanisms of Action of Genistein: Interactions with ERs

Several phytoestrogens bear a striking structural similarity to the major naturally occurring estrogens *(40)*. Consequently, it is not surprising that one potential mechanism of action is through activation of ER, and the subsequent regulation of gene expression *(40,120)*. Genistein interacts with both the classical ERα and the recently described ERβ form *(105)*. The relative binding affinities (relative to E2 = 100) for binding genistein have been reported as ERα = 5, ERβ = 36 *(104)*. Thus, genistein is likely to be more biologically active (perhaps up to fivefold) through its interactions with ERβ. Ultimately, the biological response will depend upon the relative levels of expression of each ER form, any differences in transcriptional regulation between these forms, and the concurrent presence and concentration of other estrogenic compounds.

Although genistein inhibits the uterovaginal action of E2 *(59,163)*, this does not indicate that genistein acts as an antiestrogen. Sufficient concentrations of any weak agonist should produce this effect, since the probability is increased that ER will be occupied by the weaker compound. This can dilute the potency of E2, and appear antagonistic relative to E2, while the occupied receptors are still producing a weak agonist effect.

3.6. Alternative Mechanisms of Action of Genistein and Other Soy Isoflavones

There are targets for phytoestrogens independent of direct ER interactions (Table 2; *8,43,60,61,99,180*). Isoflavones stimulate the synthesis of SHBG (for review, *see* ref. 7). Increased levels of SHBG affect the metabolic clearance rate for estradiol and uptake of sex hormones, thereby reducing the concentration of free (bioavailable) hormone. Genistein is a potent inhibitor of tyrosine kinase *(8)* and topoisomerase II activities *(135)*. It also arrests cell-cycle progression at G_2-M *(119)*, and inhibits in vitro angio-

Table 2
Some Activities of Genistein and Their Approximate IC$_{50}$s*

Endpoint	IC$_{50}$	Citation
Angiogenesis	150 μM	(61)
Serine-threonine kinase (PKC)	111 μM	(8)
Antioxidant	30 μM	(180)
Cell growth in vitro	25–40 μM	(14)
Topoisomerase II	111 μM	(43)
Tyrosine kinase (EGF-receptor)	3 μM	(8)

*Data are from different cell models. Some activities may have different IC$_{50}$s in mammary cells.

genesis *(61)*. These diverse effects, alone or in combination, may be responsible for its ability to inhibit tumor cell growth. Isoflavones also inhibit the human aromatase that catalyzes the conversion of androgens to estrogens *(98)*, and reduce the expression of EGFR mRNA. Each of these actions could contribute to the effects of genistein on mammary glands, but most other molecular targets will likely be affected by pharmacologic (not physiologic) exposures (Table 2).

Not all of these activities would be expected to be beneficial in normal tissues. For example, an inhibition of topoisomerase II activity might induce DNA strand breaks, since the torsional forces in DNA that are corrected by this enzyme would be inhibited. Other topoisomerase II inhibitors include cytotoxic drugs, such as doxorubicin, many of which are mutagenic in normal tissues. Estrogenic effects on cell-mediated immunity also would be expected to be detrimental. Estrogens inhibit natural-killer-cell activity, producing a degree of immune suppression *(35)*.

When considered together, the estrogenic activity of genistein is readily apparent. This includes estrogenic effects in breast cancer cells, e.g., proliferation and regulation of ERE-reporter expression in transcription assays, in the mammary gland and reproductive endocrinology of human subjects fed soy products *(138,192)*, and in the development of the normal rodent mammary gland. However, given the potential for several mechanisms to operate simultaneously, it is likely that the biological responses seen to genistein reflect the sum of each of these effects. This cumulative dose–response relationship will reflect the consequences of several concurrent effects, each with its own individual dose–response curve. A similar effect was previously suggested for the antiestrogen tamoxifen, which also exhibits several potentially overlapping mechanisms of action *(41)*.

3.6. Zearalenone

The resorcyclic acid lactone zearalenone is mostly produced by the mold *Fusarium graminearum (68)*, and is found in a variety of host plants and debris from soil in the United States *(25)*. It is present as a contaminant in stored cereals, e.g., barley, wheat, corn, corn flakes, rice, and maize, at concentrations from 35 to 115 g/kg *(66,68,116,120,160)*. The affinity of zearalenone for SHBG is low (5 vs 100% for E2) *(117)*, implying elevated free (unbound) concentrations in serum, and potentially increasing its ability to activate estrogenic pathways. Individuals living in the United

States are exposed to 1–5 mg/d (0.02–0.1 mg/kg/d) of zearalenone *(106)*, a level comparable to the exposure to genistein in Asian countries.

Zearalenone is used as an anabolic agent to enhance growth in cattle and lambs *(145,184)*, as an estrogen replacement therapy in postmenopausal women *(158,173)*, and as a contraceptive *(72)*. However, zearalenone can influence reproductive functions, and may increase breast cancer risk. Female mice treated with zearalenone during the neonatal period exhibit ovarian dysfunction and preneoplastic and/or neoplastic changes in the cervicovaginal epithelium *(187)*. The United States Public Health Service National Toxicology Program (USPHS NTP) report on feeding high-dose zearalenone to rodents describes the induction of uterine fibrosis and cystic ducts in the mammary glands of female mice. Zearalenone stimulates the growth of the MCF-7 human breast cancer cells *(117)*, increases the proportion of cells in S and G_2/M, and increases transcription in ERE-promoter-reporter assays (Hilakivi-Clarke et al., unpublished data). It also has been reported to enlarge the mammary gland, and, at pharmacologic doses, to induce spontaneous mammary tumors in both mice *(159)* and rats *(160)*.

3.7. Zearalenone Binds to Both ERα and ERβ

Data from ER binding, promoter–reporter, and cell proliferation assays supports the estrogenic properties of zearalenone (*see* recent review in ref. *7*). Zearalenone is a more potent estrogen than genistein in all assays the authors have used to date in MCF-7 cells (preferentially express ERα). However, zearalenone probably has a lower affinity for ERβ than genistein, since the relative binding affinities for its major metabolite, zearalenol, are reported as ERα = 16, ERβ = 14 *(104)*.

3.8. Effects of Zearalenone on Breast Cancer Risk

Since zearalenone exhibits many of the estrogenic properties seen with the soy isoflavones, we also have begun to investigate its ability to influence breast cancer risk in rodents. While a maternal exposure to zearalenone produces early estrogenic effects in the female offsprings' mammary glands, the gland completes appropriate differentiation. In genistein (or E2)-exposed offspring, the proliferative effects of estrogens are not followed by appropriate differentiation of the terminal end bud structures into lobuloalveolar units. When challenged with a mammary carcinogen, the genistein- but not zearalenone-exposed offspring exhibit an increased breast cancer incidence (Hilakivi-Clarke et al., in preparation).

If both compounds are functioning as estrogens, why do their respective treatments have different effects on carcinogenesis? One possibility is that proliferation and differentiation are differentially regulated through interactions with ERα and/or ERβ. Genistein is likely to be a more effective estrogen through ERβ, and zearalenone is likely to be more effective through ERα *(104)*. Estradiol is equally effective through both receptor isoforms. The proliferative responses may be induced through both receptor forms, with the differentiation functions primarily mediated by ERα. A potent activation of ERβ by either E2 or genistein may induce a phenotype characterized by a dominance of proliferation over differentiation. Activation primarily of ERα, as occurs with zearalenone, could produce an initial proliferative phenotype that is either primed for, or responsive to, subsequent differentiation stimuli. Whether the primary changes occur in the mammary gland or elsewhere is unknown. However, the authors have observed that *in utero* zearalenone-exposed offspring often exhibit a persistent estrus, something that does not occur with offspring comparably exposed to either genistein or E2. This persistent estrus, which could reflect perturbations at almost any point in the hypothalamic–pituitary–gonadal axis, could either directly affect the differentiation of the mammary gland (through the associated changes in serum estrogens), or simply reflect critical changes that occur elsewhere.

4. ORGANOCHLORINE COMPOUNDS AND BREAST CANCER RISK

Organochlorine compounds are ubiquitous in the environment and as contaminants in water and some foods. Although there are approximately 15,000 such compounds extant, attention has recently focused on a relatively small number that have been shown to mimic some properties of estrogen, so-called *xenoestrogens*. Because these organochlorines are lipophilic, slow to metabolize, and persistent in bodily tissues, they accumulate up the food chain, and it is through food that human exposure most commonly occurs. The widespread occurrence of organochlorines, and their tendency to bioaccumulate, has raised concern that they may produce chronic low-level estrogenic stimulation, resulting in increased risk of breast cancer. Increasing exposure and accumulation of organochlorines in the environment has been put forward as an explanation for long-term trends of increasing breast cancer incidence in many countries worldwide *(81,100)*. A wide range of in vitro and in vivo studies have demonstrated multiple biologic activities of the organochlorines, including both estrogenic and antiestrogenic effects, and tumor promotion. Relatively few human studies have examined the association between organochlorine compounds and breast cancer risk, and some of these exhibit significant limitations of study design that complicate their interpretation. This review will describe the biological evidence for estrogenic activity of the most prominently studied organochlorines, and examine the epidemiologic evidence that these compounds contribute to breast cancer risk. In fact, this is but one facet of a larger concern that organochlorine contaminants in the environment contribute to more pervasive alterations of normal endocrine pathways, resulting in reproductive and developmental anomalies in animals as well as humans. This review will focus only on breast cancer, as the larger issue of endocrine disruptors is beyond the scope of this chapter.

4.1. Organochlorines Implicated as Xenoestrogens

Three groups of organochlorines have been most thoroughly studied for estrogenic effects, the chlorinated pesticides, chiefly DDT [1,1,1-trichloro-2-2-bis(4-chlorophenyl)ethane] and its metabolites, the polychlorinated biphenyls, and the polychlorinated dibenzo compounds. Although surveys conducted during the 1970s and 1980s showed that detectable levels of these compounds could be found in most of the population of the US, levels have steadily decreased over the last two decades *(109,150)*. The properties of each of these groups will be briefly discussed.

4.1.1. Chlorinated Pesticides

The most well known of these is DDT, which was first produced as an insecticide more than 50 years ago. While banned in the US in 1972, DDT is still commonly used in many developing countries. Other widely used chlorinated pesticides include kepone (chlordecone), methoxychlor, hexachlorobenzene, hexachlorocyclohexane (lindane), chlordane and related compounds, toxaphene, aldrin and dieldrin, several of which are no longer used in the US. DDT is readily metabolized to a more stable lipophilic compound DDE [1,1-dichloro-2,2-bis(p-chlorophenyl) ethylene], which has more commonly been measured in biological studies *(171)*. DDT and DDE have been found in breast milk, serum and adipose tissue *(51,52,87,111,114)*.

4.1.2. Polychlorinated Biphenyls (PCBs)

The PCBs have been produced commercially for more than 60 years for use as flame retardants, insecticides, fungicides *(1)*, lubricants, plasticizers and in cutting oils *(103)*. Once widely used as electrical insulators, their production in the U.S. was discontinued in 1977. PCB contamination of the environment continued to occur through incineration, waste disposal (particularly leaching and runoff from landfill dumps), and industrial leakage. As with the PCDs (below), the PCBs exhibit structural differences in activity and toxicity, influenced by the number of chlorine substituents in the ortho position on the two benzene rings. Those with two or fewer chlorines exhibit properties similar to the dioxins, while more highly substituted congeners lose this activity *(171)*. PCBs have been found in breast milk, serum and adipose tissue *(120,151,191)*.

4.1.3. Polychorinated dibenzo compounds (PCDs)

This group is comprised of a large number of chlorinated tricyclic aromatic hydrocarbons, broadly classified as either polychlorinated dibenzo-p-dioxins (PCDDs) or polychlorinated dibenzofurans (PCDFs). These compounds are not manufactured commercially, but occur as contaminants and byproducts in a number of production and combustion processes. Most of these PCDs are found at only low levels in human tissue or blood. Only those congeners with chlorine in the 2,3,7 and 8 positions in the benzene rings appear to have the stability and lipophilicity to build up in biological material *(171)*.

4.2. Estrogenic and Antiestrogenic Effects of Organochlorines

4.2.1 Estrogenic Effects

DDT binds to the estrogen receptor (ER) and competitively inhibits estradiol binding in vitro in both human and rat mammary tumor cells *(107,118)* and in vivo *(121)*. A recent study showed that DDT increased cyclin-dependent kinase 2 and stimulated ER-positive breast cancer cells (MCF-7 and T47D) to enter the cell cycle, an effect inhibited by the antiestrogen ICI 182,780 *(48)*. DDT and PCBs were shown to shown to stimulate ER-positive preneoplastic mammary epithelial cells (MCF10AT) and malignant cells (MCF-7), as well as increasing expression of a plasmid reporter construct and the pS2 gene. The study suggested (but did not rigorously quantify) synergism between different DDT enantiomers or between DDT and estradiol *(196)*. DDT also stimulated proliferation of ER-positive (MCF-7 and T47D) but not ER-negative (MDA-MB-231, MDA-MB-486, HS578T) breast cancer cell lines *(166)*. Most of these estrogenic effects of DDT are structure-dependent, with the most pronounced activity seen for the o,p' enantiomer. However, the effects of DDT are 1–3 orders of magnitude less potent than estradiol. DDT has also been associated with enhancement of mammary cancer induced in the rat by 2-acetamidophenanthrene *(161)*. However, this study only used male rats. DDE levels in human milk have been shown to correlate inversely with duration of lactation *(151)*. Furthermore, DDE levels in adipose tissue from breast cancer patients were significantly correlated with ER levels, but HCH did not show such a correlation *(130)*.

PCBs have exhibited a number of estrogenic effects, including induction of precocious uterine growth and puberty in weanling rats and ovariectomized mice *(64,102)*. As with DDT, the estrogenic activity of the various PCB congeners is structure-dependent, with the most potent being 1–2 orders of magnitude less potent than estradiol. It is important to note that the laboratory studies have tended to use commercial mixtures of PCB that differ from the compounds or mixtures of compounds encountered in most human exposures, which makes etiologic inferences more difficult *(171)*.

β-hexachlorocyclohexane (HCH) also has exhibited estrogenic effects, stimulating proliferation of ER-positive but not ER-negative breast cancer cells, effects that were inhibited by the antiestrogen ICI 164,384. This effect was of equal magnitude to estradiol, but in a competitive binding assay, HCH was more than four orders of magnitude less potent than estradiol *(166)*. Kepone bound to the ER in chicken oviduct, stimulated increased progesterone and protein synthesis. Only the latter effect was blocked by tamoxifen *(136)*.

A recent study seemed to provide evidence to explain how xenoestrogens, which typically have much lower activity than estradiol, could produce biological effects on hormonally sensitive tissues. Arnold and colleagues used yeast cells transformed with human ER to show that combinations of pesticides appeared to demonstrate synergy in the form of enhanced inhibition of estradiol binding to ER. In combination, the organochlorines were up to 1000 times more potent than any of the compounds singly *(10)*. However, a subsequent study utilizing mouse uterus, MCF-7 breast cancer cells, and a yeast-based reporter gene failed to demonstrate any synergy among the pesticides *(146)*. The authors of the original study were also unable to repeat their earlier results and withdrew the original report *(197)*.

4.2.2. Antiestrogenic Effects

The most well-studied of the PCDs, TCDD (2,3,7,8-tetrachlorodibenzo-p-dioxin) has been shown to have anti-estrogenic activities. Estradiol binding to ER and its activation of an ERE in MCF-7 cells was decreased by TCDD, an effect that was partially blocked by inhibition of the aryl hydrocarbon receptor (AhR) *(178)*. Estradiol-induced secretion of procathepsin D and cathepsin D was inhibited by TCDD in MCF-7 cells but not in MDA-MB-231 cells *(18,156)*. In immature female rats, TCDD inhibited estradiol-induced EGFR (epidermal growth factor receptor) binding and EGFR mRNA *(11)*. The antiestrogenic effects of TCDD and other PCDDs appear to be proportional to the binding affinity for the AhR. This is likely to reflect binding to a xenobiotic response element of PCD complexed to the AhR, resulting in down-regulation of ER mRNA expression *(171)*.

Although DDT has been primarily associated with estrogenic activities, anti-estrogenic effects have also been reported. In the DMBA model, tumor incidence and multiplicity were decreased, and tumor latency was increased, in rats treated with DDT. However, this study used the p,p' enantiomer rather than the o,p', which has been more commonly associated with estrogenicity *(164)*.

4.3. Epidemiologic Studies

The laboratory data show fairly convincingly that the PCBs and chlorinated pesticides exhibit estrogenic activity. However, the relevance of this data to human breast cancer is difficult to ascertain for a number of reasons. Organochlorine xenoestrogens exhibit relatively low potency compared to either estradiol or the naturally occurring phytoestrogens. However, estradiol and phytoestrogens are rapidly metabolized whereas organochlorines are slowly metabolized and released from the adipose tissue in an equilibrium fashion, resulting in chronic low level stimulation. Exposures used in laboratory studies tend to be pure compounds, yet human exposures tend to be complex mixtures due to the co-contamination of many organochlorines, persistence in the environment, and bioaccumulation in the food chain. Finally, the laboratory studies focus on short-term biological effects or modification of short-term carcinogenicity, whereas humans incur long-term low level exposures. These uncertainties are not unique to the study of xenoestrogens. Because of these difficulties, however, the laboratory studies can only provide evidence of a biological mechanism but cannot determine its relevance to human breast carcinogenesis.

A number of trends in breast cancer occurrence have been cited as evidence for or against the role of xenoestrogens. However, ascribing a causal interpretation to these ecologic data is fraught with difficulty. For example, after accounting for the effect of increased mammography usage, the long-term trend of gradually increasing breast cancer incidence in the U.S. and other countries has been put forth as evidence in support of risk associated with xenoestrogens *(47)*. However, this increase has occurred during a time of changes in reproductive patterns, dietary changes, and occupational roles for women, all of which could also influence breast cancer risk. Data from Israel showed a lower breast cancer mortality rate in 1986 compared to 1976, which was ascribed to a decrease in pesticides in breast milk and cow's milk *(183)*. However, the mortality changes occurred during a time of migration of lower-risk Asian and African women *(162)*. Interpretation of the Israel data also is obscured by the fact that incidence was only recorded for the single years 1986 and 1976, rather than using average rates over five years which are subject to less random variation *(171)*. The low levels of breast cancer incidence among Japanese women, despite high body burden of organochlorines, has been cited as evidence against the xenoestrogen hypothesis *(171)*. However, other elements of the Japanese diet and their reproductive patterns are both associated with lower breast cancer risk, so the total of these effects could still overcome a small risk associated with organochlorines, if such a risk existed. The lower breast cancer risk of African American women compared to white women, despite higher body burdens of DDT is also cited as evidence against a role for xenoestrogens *(171)*. Again, African American women have reproductive patterns associated with lower risk, and risks for young African American women actually exceed those for whites *(170)*, so it also is difficult to draw conclusions from these data. In summary, examination of breast cancer incidence and mortality trends based on ecological data does not provide convincing evidence that the estrogenic effects of organochlorines increase the risk of human breast cancer.

The evidence that has drawn the most attention and controversy has been that derived from case-control studies, in which biological specimens from women with breast cancer have been compared to those of healthy women. There have been twelve case-control studies to date. Only five had reasonably adequate sample sizes *(104,115,179,193,198,199)*, and only three have been based on prospective measurements of organochlorines; i.e. measurements that were made prior to the development of breast cancer *(103,191,198)*.

Most of the studies based on retrospective measurements involved a comparison of DDE levels in breast adipose tissue from breast cancer cases and controls *(9,46,52,57,130,172,179)*. Four of these studies in adipose tissue found higher levels of DDE in cases than controls *(9,52,57,179)*, but those by Wasserman and Albert included fewer than 10 cases and 10 controls. The studies by Dewailly and Falck also found significantly higher risks associated with PCBs. The study by Dewailly was noteworthy because significant elevations in adipose tissue levels of DDE and PCB were observed for ER-positive cases compared to controls, but not for ER-negative cases compared to controls. This is consistent with *in* vitro data, wherein organochlorines induced estrogenic effects in ER-positive but not ER-negative breast tumor cells. One study found no differences in DDT, DDE or PCBs, but a significant increase in risk associated with β-HCH *(130)*. Odds ratios in these studies suggested that risk at the higher levels of exposures was three-to-tenfold higher than at lower levels. Only the studies by Unger and Mussalo-Rauhaumaa used statistical adjustment for other potential risk factors.

Two additional retrospective studies were recently published. The study by van't Veer, the largest of all the epidemiologic studies of organochlorines and breast cancer, was based on measurements made on adipose tissue from the buttocks rather than the breast. The study included 347 postmenopausal breast cancer cases and 374 controls from five European countries *(176)*. DDE levels in cases were significantly lower than among controls, with an odds ratio of 0.48 (95% C.I. 0.25, 0.95) for the highest vs the lowest quartile, adjusted for age, body mass index, age at first birth and alcohol intake. Thus, this study offered no support for excess risk associated with organochlorine exposure. The study excluded women with tumors $\geq$5 cm., and the controls appeared to be derived from both population and hospital sources. There was no discussion of the possible effects of these design elements. A study in Mexico City also found a nonsignificant decrease in risk associated with increased serum DDE levels, with OR = 0.76 (95% CI: 0.41, 1.42) for the highest vs lowest tertile *(199)*. This hospital-based study included 141 case-control pairs, with matching on age. Odds ratios were adjusted for important risk factors, including lactation. Blood samples were collected from 1994-1996, and samples from cases were collected prior to any treatment. Although DDT is still used in Mexico, DDE levels in study subjects were similar to those found in studies from the United States.

All of the retrospective studies, except the studies by van't Veer and Lopez-Carillo, were limited by small sample sizes. Adjustment for confounding factors was either absent, or did not consider all of the relevant confounders. In particular, few studies performed adjustment for factors that could be directly or indirectly correlated with organochlorine exposure, such as reproductive factors (other than parity), body mass index, and the duration of lactation. The latter is particularly interesting. Lactation may be a significant confounding factor because lipid-rich breast milk is the main route of excretion of organochlorines *(51,151)*, but breast feeding has been shown to be a protective factor against breast cancer *(26,122,131)*. It is important to note, however, that breast feeding would not be a confounding factor if the reduction in risk associated with lactation was actually a result of reduction in the organochlorine body burden through excretion in milk. Furthermore, only the study by Dewailly differentiated between women with ER-positive or ER-negative breast tumors. If organochlorines reflect estrogenic effects only in ER-positive tumors, then even minor shifts in the number of women with ER-negative tumors could markedly effect the results in these small studies. Finally, because organochlorines were sampled retrospectively, i.e., after the diagnosis of breast cancer, it is possible that metabolic changes related to disease could confound the observed associations. Increased metabolic activity in cancerous breasts could mobilize fat stores, resulting in decreased levels of organochlorines measured in adipose tissue (but increased levels in blood). This could be relevant to the study by Dewailly if ER-negative tumors were more advanced than ER-positive tumors.

The three methodologically strongest studies to date were based on serum measurements of DDE and PCBs in stored blood that had been collected from women without known breast cancer. Wolff and colleagues identified 58 women who were diagnosed with breast cancer within six months after attending a mammography screening clinic, and matched these to 171 women who did not develop breast cancer. Risks increased with increasing level of DDE or PCB exposure. A statistically significant trend in risk was observed with increasing DDE exposure, $p = 0.035$. The odds ratio for the highest vs the lowest decile of DDE exposure was 4.08 (95% C.I. 1.49, 11.20), adjusted for family history, duration of lactation, and age at first full-term pregnancy. A similar level of risk was observed for PCBs, although the overall trend did not attain statistical significance ($p = 0.16$). Importantly, adjustment for lactation increased the risk estimates for DDE by 38%, suggesting an important confounding role for this variable *(191)*. There are two important issues that complicate interpretation of this study. Because cases were diagnosed within six months of donating their blood sample, the samples are not a true indication of organochlorine levels prior to disease. Thus, the potential mobilization of organochlorines from adipose tissue into blood represents a potential bias that could have spuriously elevated the observed risk. However, it also is possible that the presence of subclinical tumor could reduce circulating lipids, thus reducing blood levels of organochlorines *(190)*. If this were true, the observed risks would be underestimates. The second issue concerns the time period when blood was collected, 1985–1991. This was during a period when body burdens of organochlorines in the US had been dropping for nearly two decades, so it is possible that levels measured in the study do not accurately reflect long-term exposure during the period of greatest risk. However, although levels of DDE were significantly lower than those in the study by Krieger (where samples were collected from 1964–1969), levels of PCBs were significantly higher *(103)*.

A second nested case-control study based on prospective blood collection examined the effect of DDE and PCB among white, African American, and Asian women. The study was based on healthy women members of a large insurance group who underwent a health examination during the years 1964–1969. In each ethnic group, 50 cases were matched to 50 controls, with matching criteria of age at the time of blood sampling, race, year of the examination, year of joining the insurance group and follow-up time after the examination. Cases included women diagnosed six months or more after the examination. Among white women the odds ratio for the highest vs the lowest tertile was 2.38 (95% C.I. 0.54, 10.64). Among African American women the same comparison yielded an odds ratio of 3.85 (95% C.I. 0.93, 16.05). Neither of the risks were statistically significant. No elevation of risk was seen for Asian women. When the cutpoints to derive the tertiles were made specific for the distribution of exposure within each ethnic group, the odds ratios for white and African American women decreased to 2.03 and 2.16 respectively. No increase in risk was observed for PCBs, but among white women, a statistically significant decrease was apparent, OR = 0.17 (95% C.I. 0.03, 0.89), based on the ethnic-specific cutpoints. All of these risks were adjusted for body mass index, age at menarche, parity and menopausal status *(103)*. The study was widely interpreted as evidence against the association with organochlorines. However, if data for white and African American women had been combined, the risk estimates may have achieved statistical significance.

The study has a number of notable strengths, including the long time period between blood sampling and cancer diagnosis (average 14 years), and collection of samples during a time when exposure to DDT and PCBs had not been reduced. The study also has some potential limitations. Inability to adjust for lactation may have confounded the observed risks with a bias toward no association. If the effect of lactation was similar to that observed in the Wolff study, that would probably be sufficient to explain the nonsignificant findings in white and African American women. However, Krieger was able to adjust for parity, which may incorporate some of the effect of lactation, and this adjustment did not alter observed risks. The ER status of tumors was not considered, and ER-negative tumors are more common among African American women *(170)*. Although the observed risks were somewhat higher for African American women, this does not rule out confounding by ER status because serum DDE levels were also higher in African Americans. The authors raised the possibility that, because the DDE levels were much higher than those observed in the study of Wolff et al. (40% had levels exceeding the highest quintile found by Wolff et al.), it was possible that a threshold of risk was exceeded so that a dose-response would not be detected. Evidence against such an obscuring effect was the fact that DDE levels were similar to those observed in other studies to cause suppression of lactation, suggesting that levels were not too high to capture a dose-response relationship had it existed *(103)*.

The largest nested case-control study to date included 236 cases and 236 matched controls, for whom blood had been prospectively collected as part of the Nurse's Health Study *(198)*. Cases included women diagnosed two-to-three years after blood sampling. Controls were matched to cases on birth year, menopausal status, timing of blood sampling, fasting status at blood sampling and postmenopausal hormone use. Risk of breast cancer was reduced for subjects in the highest vs lowest quintiles of plasma DDE, RR = 0.72 (95% CI: 0.37, 1.40), and for the highest vs lowest quintiles of plasma PCBs, RR = 0.66 (95% CI: 0.32, 1.37). All comparisons were adjusted for other risk factors (including lactation), but differed little from the unadjusted estimates. Risk was also reduced for women with the highest quintiles of both DDE and PCB compared to those in the lowest quintile for both compounds, RR = 0.43 (95% CI: 0.13, 1.44). None of these comparisons were statistically significant and there was no evidence of a dose-response.

The large sample size of the study and prospective blood collection are significant strengths, as is the fact that DDE and PCBs were analysed by the same laboratory used in the studies by Wolff and Krieger. Although blood samples were collected a relatively short time prior to diagnosis of the cases, it is unlikely that subclinical tumors two-three years prior to diagnosis would have major effects on circulating organochlorine levels. Because samples were collected during a time of reduced exposure to these compounds, however, it is possible that plasma levels did not reflect exposure during the period of highest risk.

4.4. Summary of the Effects of Environmental Estrogens

There has been increasing concern that exposure to environmental contaminants may be responsible for a long-term trend of steadily increasing breast cancer incidence rates. Part of the rationale for this concern relates to the lack of obvious risk factors identified in 50% or more of women newly diagnosed with breast cancer. This search for environmental risk factors converged with increasing data from the laboratory showing that chlorinated pesticides like DDT, the PCBs, and the PCDs were able to induce some of the biological effects of estrogens. Because of their widespread exposure, bioaccumulation in the food chain, and persistence in human adipose tissue, these compounds have the potential to produce chronic low-level estrogenic stimulation. The laboratory data have shown quite convincingly that many of these organochlorines behave as weak estrogens, while others (notably the PCDs) exhibit potentially antiestrogenic effects. However, the leap from demonstration of estrogenicity to establishing a causal role in breast carcinogenesis has proven to be very difficult.

The biological activity of these xenoestrogens is orders of magnitude weaker than that of estradiol, exogenous replacement estrogens, and naturally occurring phytoestrogens *(200)*. Even allowing for the possibility of large synergistic effects for combinations of xenoestrogens (which is how these exposures occur in the environment and food), the activity is still weaker than other estrogens to which women are routinely exposed. Despite this lower activity, a significant biological effect may still be plausible because, unlike natural and synthetic estrogens, xenoestrogens are long-acting due to their slow metabolism and bioaccumulation. The fact that pesticide exposure in women has been observed in association with altered lactation patterns *(151)*, at a time when endogenous estrogen levels are high, suggests that biological effects are likely. Because of their persistence in the environment, and the occurrence of some organochlorines as contaminant by-products in the production of others, the exposures that humans encounter are much more complex than those studied in the laboratory. These mixtures may have other effects relevant to carcinogenesis in addition to estrogenicity. A recent study has shown that pesticides and PCBs inhibit gap junctional communication in normal breast epithelial cells *(97)*. DDT and PCBs have been shown to induce cytochrome p450 enzymes, which can alter metabolism of steroid hormones *(140)*. If these compounds also bind to the AhR receptor (as do the PCDs) or a similar xenobiotic receptor, altered signal transduction could also affect processes such as growth and differentiation *(93)*.

The picture is not clarified by the epidemiologic data. The earlier studies were small, did not adjust for relevant confounding factors, and did not provide many details about the cases. If any measurements were made on cases who had already undergone treatment, it is possible that levels of organochlorines could have been affected. Wolff has recently shown that serum DDE and PCB levels increase after chemotherapy *(189)*.

It is not clear whether this effect would result in increased or decreased adipose tissue levels; either is plausible. Dewailly and colleagues showed the importance of considering the ER status of the tumor *(52)*, a factor that was not considered in any other studies. Lactation was an important confounder in the study of Wolff and colleagues *(191)*, and has only been evaluated in two other studies *(115,198)*.

Three studies were of reasonable size, employed adjustment for most confounding factors and used prediagnostic blood samples. The original interpretation for two of these studies may be subject to uncertainty because of the use of blood samples from subclinical cases *(191)*, and the possibility of a significant risk elevation for African American and white women combined *(103)*. There are no major sources of uncertainty for the third study, which showed statistically nonsignificant decreases in risk with higher levels of DDE or PCBs *(198)*. Two other retrospective studies employed adequate sample size and adjustment for most confounding factors, and also showed that risk decreased with increasing exposure *(176,199)*.

Thus, the epidemiologic data are largely unsupportive of the hypothesis of increased risk, despite suggestive results from some studies. A more convincing answer can only come from a larger nested case-control study with adequate latency between blood collection and diagnosis, a broad range of exposures, adjustment for all relevant confounding factors and consideration of the ER status of tumors. Whether such a study can be done with samples obtained during a period of high exposure is uncertain. Additional studies in humans to show whether sampling in the presence of subclinical or clinical disease raises or lowers serum levels also would be important. Such a study would require serial samples on cases nested within a cohort, but could probably be done with a relatively small sample. If the direction of artifacts from sampling in the presence of disease can be predicted, this may allow more valid case-control studies to be conducted. Such studies are necessary even in the face of declining use of these xenoestrogens in industrialized nations because these compounds are still common in developing nations. Furthermore, the effects of other organochlorines that are still in widespread use (such as methoxychlor and other pesticides) have not been well studied.

5. CONCLUDING COMMENTS AND FUTURE DIRECTIONS

We have chosen to focus on one common link among selected nutritional components, pesticides and pollutants, i.e., their possible estrogenicity. For the phytoestrogens, estrogenicity and exposure are sufficient in some populations to provide a physiologically relevant exposure. Thus, they are likely to be able to compete effectively with the endogenous estrogens. For the soy isoflavones there already is direct evidence for this, e.g., the ability of soy consumption to alter menstrual cycling in humans *(30,115)* and to produce estrogenic effects in the breast *(138)*. In marked contrast, the relative affinities of the environmental estrogens is significantly lower, as is the apparent relative exposure in human populations. The issue of whether the cumulative exposure, or the concentration of free compound at the receptor (the key determinant of biological response) remains open for these estrogens.

From a purely pharmacologic perspective, it is difficult to envisage the exposure to environmental estrogens significantly impacting existing breast neoplasms in adults through interactions with the ER. However, as we have observed in rodents, *in utero* exposures need only be modest to produce long term effects on the susceptibility of an offspring's mammary glands to carcinogenesis. If the same is true for the environmental estrogens, an effect on individuals exposed *in utero* is not untenable.

The final word on the potential roles of phytoestrogens and environmental estrogens is likely to be several years distant. Clearly, more and better epidemiologic studies are required. If these must include estimates of *in utero* exposures on subsequent risk, initial studies will be limited to retrospective designs or studies using surrogate end-point biomarkers. While generally considered more definitive, data from prospective studies may take over thirty years, just to determine effects on the incidence of pre-menopausal breast cancer.

ACKNOWLEDGMENTS

This work was supported in part by American Cancer Society CN-80420 (L. A. Hilakivi-Clarke), the Cancer Research Foundation of America (L. A. Hilakivi-Clarke) and PHS P50-CA58185 (R. Clarke, B. Trock) P30-CA51008 (R. Clark) and R01-CA/AG58022 (R. Clarke).

REFERENCES

1. Adami, H.-O., L. Lipworth, and L. Titus-Ernstoff. 1995. Organochlorine compounds and estrogen-related cancers in women. *Cancer Causes Control* **6**: 551–566.
2. Adams, L. M., J. R. Trout, and R. A. Karmali. 1990. Effect of n-3 fatty acids on spontaneous and experimental metastasis of rat mammary tumor 13762. *Br. J. Cancer* **61**: 290–291.
3. Adlercreutz, C. H., B. R. Goldin, S. L. Gorbach, K. A. V. Hockerstedt, S. Watanabe, E. Hamalainen, et al. 1996. Soybean phytoestrogen intake and cancer risk. *J. Nutr.* **125**: 757S–770S.
4. Adlercreutz, H. 1991. Diet and sex hormone metabolism, in *Nutrition, Toxicity, and Cancer* (Rowland, I. R., ed.), CRC, Boca Raton, FL, pp. 137–195.
5. Adlercreutz, H., S. L. Gorbach, B. R. Goldin, M. N. Woods, J. T. Dwyer, and E. Hamalainen. 1994. Estrogen metabolism and excretion in oriental and caucasian women. *J. Natl. Cancer Inst.* **86**: 1076–1082.
6. Adlercreutz, H., K. Hockerstedt, C. Bannwart, S. Bloigu, E. Hamalainen, T. Fotsis, and A. Ollus. 1987. Effect of dietary components, including lignans and phytoestrogens, on enterohepatic circulation and liver metablism of estrogens and on sex hormone binding globuline (SHBG). *J. Steroid Biochem.* **27**: 1135–1144.
7. Adlercreutz, H., Y. Mousavi, J. Clark, K. Hockerstedt, E. Hamalainen, K. Wahala, T. Makela, and T. Hase. 1992. Dietary phytoestrogens and cancer: in vitro and in vivo studies. *J. Steroid Biochem. Mol. Biol.* **41**: 331–337.
8. Akiyama, T., J. Ishida, S. Nakagawa, H. Ogawa, S. Watanabe, N. Itou, M. Shibata, and Y. Fukami. 1987. Genistein, a specific inhibitor of tyrosine-specific protein kinase. *J. Biol. Chem.* **262**: 5592–5595.
9. Albert, L., O. Hernandez-Roman, and R. Reyes. 1974. Chlorinated hydrocarbon residue concentrations in neoplastic human breast tissue, non-malignant breast tumor tissue and adjacent adipose tissues, International Congress of Peptides 5, Chemistry. IUPAC, Kyoto, Japan.
10. Arnold, S. F., D. M. Klotz, and B. M. Collins. 1996. Synergistic activation of estrogen receptor with combinations of environmental chemicals. *Science* **272**: 1489–1492.
11. Astroff, B., C. Rowlands, and R. Dickerson. 1990. 2,3,7,8-Tetrachlorodibenzo-p-dioxin inhibition of 17β-estradiol-induced-increases in rat uterine epidermal growth factor receptor binding activity and gene expression. *Mol. Cell Endocrinol.* **72**: 247–252.

12. Azzi, A., D. Boscoboinik, and C. Hensey. 1992. The protein kinase C family. *Eur. J. Biochem.* **208:** 547–557.

13. Baird, D. D., D. M. Umbach, L. Lansdell, C. L. Hughes, K. D. R. Setchell, C. R. Weinberg, A. F. Haney, A. J. Wilcox, and J. A. McLachlan. 1995. Dietary intervention study to assess estrogenity of dietary soy among postmenopausal women. *J. Clin. Endocrinol. Metabol.* **80:** 1685–1690.

14. Barnes, S. 1995. Effect of genistein on in vitro and in vivo models of cancer. *J. Nutr.* **125:** 777S–783S.

15. Barnes, S., G. Peterson, C. Grubbs, and K. Setchell. 1994. Potential role of dietary isoflavones in the prevention of cancer, in *Diet and Cancer: Markers, Prevention, and Treatment* (Jacobs, M. M., ed.), Plenum, New York, pp. 135–147.

16. Barrett-Connor, E. and N. J. Friedlander. 1993. Dietary fat, calories, and the risk of breast cancer in postmenopausal women: a prospective population-based study. *J. Am. Coll. Nutr.* **12:** 390–399.

17. Bennett, F. C. and D. M. Ingram. 1990. Diet and female sex hormone concentrations: an intervention study for the type of fat consumed. *Am. J. Clin. Nutr.* **52:** 808–812.

18. Biegel, L. and S. Safe. 1990. Effects of 2,3,7,8-tetrachlorodibenzo-p-dioxin-(TCCD) on cell growth and the secretion of the estrogen-induced 34-,52-, and 160-kDa proteins in human breast cancer cells. *J. Steriod Biochem.* **37:** 725–729.

19. Borgeson, C. E., L. Pardini, R. Pardini, and R. C. Reitz. 1989. Effects of dietary fish oil on human mammary carcinoma and on lipid-metabolizing enzymes. *Lipids* **24:** 290–295.

20. Boyd, N. F., M. Cousins, G. Lockwood, and D. Tritchler. 1990. The feasibility of testing experimentally the dietary fat-breast cancer hypothesis. *Br. J. Cancer* **62:** 878–881.

21. Boyd, N. F., G. A. Lockwood, C. V. Greenberg, L. J. Martin, and D. L. Tritchler. 1997. Effects of a low-fat high-carbohydrate diet on plasma sex hormones in premenopausal women: results from a randomized controlled trial. *Br. J. Cancer* **76:** 127–135.

22. Boyd, N. F., L. J. Martin, M. Noffel, G. A. Lockwood, and D. L. Tritchler. 1993. A meta-analysis of studies of dietary at and breast cancer risk. *Br. J. Cancer* **68:** 627–636.

23. Bruning, P. F. and J. M. G. Bonfrer. 1990. Possible relevance of steroid availability and breast cancer. *Ann. NY Acad. Sci.* 257–264.

24. Buckman, D. K., R. S. Chapkin, and K. L. Erickson. 1990. Modulation of mouse mammary tumor growth and linoleate-enhanged metastasis by oleate. *J. Nutr.* **120:** 148–157.

25. Burgess, L. W., P. E. Nelson, and T. A. Toussoun. 1982. Characterization, geographic distribution and ecology of Fusarium crookwellense sp. nov. *Trans. Br. Mycol. Soc.* **79:** 497–505.

26. Byers, T., S. Graham, and T. Rzepka. 1985. Lactation and breast cancer. *Am. J. Epidemiol.* **121:** 664–674.

27. Carroll, K. K. 1975. Experimental evidence of dietary factors and hormone-dependent cancers. *Cancer Res.* **35:** 3374–3383.

28. Carroll, K. K. 1991. Dietary fats and cancer. *Am. J. Clin. Nutr.* **53:** 1064–1067.

29. Carroll, K. K. 1993. Nutrition and cancer:fat, in *Nutrition, Toxicity and Cancer*, pp. 439–453.

30. Cassidy, A., S. Bingham, and K. D. R. Setchell. 1994. Biological effects of a diet of soy protein rich in isoflavones on the menstrual cycle of premenopausal women. *Am. J. Clin. Nutr.* **60:** 333–340.

31. Caygill, C. P. J., A. Charlett, and M. J. Hill. 1996. Fat, fish, fish oil and cancer. *Br. J. Cancer* **74:** 159–164.

32. Chan, P. C., K. A. Ferguson, and T. L. Dao. 1983. Effects of different dietary fats on mammary carcinogenesis. *Cancer Res.* **43:** 1079–1083.

33. Chan, P. C., J. F. Head, L. A. Cohen, and E. L. Wynder. 1977. Influence of dietary fat on the induction of mammary tumors by nitrosomethylurea: associated hormone changes

and differences between Sprague-Dawley and F344 rats. *J. Natl. Cancer Inst.* **59:** 1279–1283.

34. Choe, M., E. S. Kris, R. Luthra, J. Copenhaver, J. C. Pelling, T. E. Donnelly, and D. E. Birt. 1992. Protein kinase C is activated and diacylglycerol is elevated in epidermal cells from SENCAR mice fed high fat diets. *J. Nutr.* **122:** 2322–2329.

35. Clarke, R. 1996. Human breast cancer cell line xenografts as models of breast cancer: the immunobiologies of recipient mice and the characteristics of several tumorigenic cell lines. *Breast Cancer Res. Treat.* **39:** 69–86.

36. Clarke, R. 1997. Animal models of breast cancer: experimental design and their use in nutrition and psychosocial research. *Breast Cancer Res. Treat.* **46:** 117–133.

37. Clarke, R. and N. Brunner. 1996. Acquired estrogen independence and antiestrogen resistance in breast cancer: estrogen receptor-driven phenotypes. *Trends Endocrinol. Metab.* **7:** 25–35.

38. Clarke, R., N. Brünner, B. S. Katzenellenbogen, E. W. Thompson, M. J. Norman, C. Koppi, S. Paik, M. E. Lippman, and R. B. Dickson. 1989. Progression from hormone dependent to hormone independent growth in MCF-7 human breast cancer cells. *Proc. Natl. Acad. Sci. USA* **86:** 3649–3653.

39. Clarke, R., R. B. Dickson, and M. E. Lippman. 1992. Hormonal aspects of breast cancer. Growth factors, drugs and stromal interactions. *Crit. Rev. Oncol. Hematol.* **12:** 1–23.

40. Clarke, R., L. Hilakivi-Clarke, E. Cho, M. James, and F. Leonessa. 1996. Estrogens, phytoestrogens and breast cancer. *Adv. Exp. Med. Biol.* **401:** 63–86.

41. Clarke, R. and M. E. Lippman. 1992. *Antiestrogens resistance: mechanisms and reversal.* Marcel Dekker, New York. 501–536.

42. Clinton, S. K., P. S. Li, A. L. Mulloy, P. B. Imrey, S. Nandkumar, and W. J. Visek. 1995. The combined effects of dietary fat and estrogen on survival, 7,12-dimethylbenz(a)anthracene-induced breast cancer and prolactin metabolism in rats. *J. Nutr.* **125:** 1192–1204.

43. Constantino, A., K. Kiguchi, and E. Huberman. 1990. Induction of differentiation and strand breakage in human HL-60 and K-562 leukemia cells by genistein. *Cancer Res.* **50:** 2618–2624.

44. Coward, L., N. C. Barnes, K. D. R. Setchell, and S. Barnes. 1993. Genistein, daidzein, and their beta-glycoside conjugates: antitumor isoflavones in soybean foods from American and Asian diets. *J. Agr. Food Chem.* **41:** 1961–1967.

45. Crane, P. S., S. U. Rhee, and D. J. Seel. 1970. Experience with 1,079 cases on cancer of the stomach seen in Korea from 1962 to 1968. *Am. J. Surg.* **120:** 747–751.

46. Davies, J. E., A. Barquet, and C. Morgade. 1974. Epidemiologic studies of DDT and dieldrin residues and their relationship to human carcinogenesis. Recent advances in assessment of health effects of environmental pollution. *WHO CEC USEPA Int. Symp. Proc.* **11:** 695–702.

47. Davis, D. L., H. L. Bradlow, M. Wolff, T. Woodruff, D. G. Hoel, and H. Anton-Culver. 1993. Medical hypothesis:xenoestrogens as preventable causes of breast cancer. *Environ. Health Perspect.* **101:** 372–377.

48. Dees, C., M. Askari, and J. S. Foster. 1997. DDT mimicks estradiol stimulation of breast cancer cells to enter the cell cycle. *Mol. Carcinogenesis* **18:** 107–114.

49. Dekker, L. V. and P. J. Parker. 1994. Protein kinase C—a question of specificity. *Trends Biochem. Sci.* **19:** 73–77.

50. Depue, R. H., L. Bernstein, R. K. Ross, H. L. Judd, and B. E. Henderson. 1987. Hyperemesis gravidarum in relation to estradiol levels, pregnancy outcome, amd other maternal factors: a seroepidemiologic study. *Am. J. Obstet. Gynecol.* **156:** 1137–1141.

51. Dewailly, E., P. Ayotte, and J. Brisson. 1994. Protective effect of breast feeding on breast cancer and body burden of carcinogenic organochlorines. *J. Natl. Cancer Inst.* **86:** 80.

52. Dewailly, E., S. Dodin, and R. Verrault. 1994. High organochlorine body burden in women with estrogen receptor positive breast cancer. *J. Natl. Cancer Inst.* **86:** 232–234.

53. Dunn, J. E. J. 1975. Cancer epidemiology in populations of the United States—with emphasis on Hawaii and California—and Japan. *Cancer Res.* **35:** 3240–3245.

54. Dwyer, J. T., B. R. Goldin, N. Saul, L. Gualtieri, S. Barakat, and H. Adlercreutz. 1994. Tofu and soy drinks contain phytoestrogens. *J. Am. Diet Assoc.* **94:** 739–743.

55. Ekbom, A., D. Trichopoulos, H. O. Adami, C. C. Hsieh, and S. J. Lan. 1992. Evidence of prenatal influences on breast cancer risk. *Lancet* **340:** 1015–1018.

56. Enger, S. M., R. K. Ross, B. Henderson, and L. Bernstein. 1997. Breastfeeding history, pregnancy experience and risk of breast cancer. *Br. J. Cancer* **76:** 118–123.

57. Falck, F. Y., A. Ricci, and M. Wolff. 1992. Pesticides and polychlorinated biphenyl residues in human breast lipids and their relation to breast cancer. *Arch. Environ. Health* **47:** 143–146.

58. Fay, M. P. and L. S. Freedman. 1997. Analysis of dietary fats and mammary neoplasms in rodent experiments. *Breast Cancer Res. Treat.* **46:** 215–223.

59. Folman, Y. and G. S. Pope. 1966. The interaction in the immature mouse of potent oestrogens with coumestrol, genistein and other utero-vaginotriphic compounds of low potency. *J. Endocrinol.* **34:** 215–225.

60. Folman, Y. and G. S. Pope. 1969. Effect of norethisterone acetate, dimethylstilbestrol, genistein and coumestrol on uptake of [3H]oestradiol by uterus, vagina, and skeletal muscle of immature mice. *J. Endocrinol.* **44:** 213

61. Fotsis, T., M. Pepper, H. Adlercreutz, G. Fleischmann, T. Hase, R. Montesano, and L. Schweigerer. 1993. Genistein, a dietary-derived inhibitor of in vitro angiogenesis. *Proc. Natl. Acad. Sci. USA* **90:** 2690–2694.

62. Freedman, L. S., C. K. Clifford, and M. Messina. 1990. Analysis of dietary fat, calories, body weight, and the development of mammary tumors in rats and mice: a review. *Cancer Res.* **50:** 5710–5719.

63. Frisch, R. E. 1990. *Adipose Tissue and Reproduction.* Karger, Basel.

64. Gellert, R. J. 1978. Uterotrophic activation of PCBs and induction of precocious reproductive aging in neonatally treated female rats. *Environ. Res.* **16:** 123–130.

65. Giovanucci, E., E. B. Rimm, G. A. Colditz, M. J. Sternpfer, A. Ascherio, C. C. Chute, and W. C. Willett. 1993. A prospective study of dietary fat and risk of prostate cancer. *J. Natl. Cancer Inst.* **85:** 1571–1579.

66. Golinski, P., R. F. Vesonder, D. Latus-Zietkiewicz, and J. Perkowski. 1988. Formation of fusarenone X, nivalenol, zearalenone, α-trans-zearalenol, β-trans-zearalenol, and fusarin C by fusarium crookwellense. *Appl. Environ. Microbiol.* **54:** 2147–2148.

67. Gridley, D. S., J. D. Kettering, J. M. Slater, and R. L. Nutter. 1983. Modifications of spontaneous mammary tumors in mice fed different sources of protein, fat and carbohydrate. *Cancer Lett.* **19:** 133–146.

68. Hagler, W. M., K. Tyczkowska, and P. B. Hamilton. 1984. Simultaneous occurrence of deoxynivalenol, zearalenone, and aflatoxin in 1982 scabby wheat from the Midwestern United States. *Appl. Environ. Microbiol.* **47:** 151–154.

69. Haslam, S. Z. and K. A. Nummy. 1992. The ontogeny and cellular distribution of estrogen receptors in normal mouse mammary gland. *J. Steroid. Biochem. Molec. Biol.* **42:** 589–595.

70. Hawrylewicz, E. J., H. H. Huang, and W. H. Blair. 1991. Dietary soybean isolate and methionine supplementation affect mammary tumor progression in rats. *J. Nutr.* **121:** 1693–1698.

71. Henderson, B. E. and L. Bernstein. 1996. Endogenous and exogenous hormonal factors, in *Diseases of the Breast* (Harris, J. R., M. E. Lippman, M. Morrow, and S. Hellman, eds.), Lippincott, Philadelphia, pp. 185–200.

72. Hidy, P. H. and R. S. Baldwin. 1976. Method of preventing pregnancy with lactone derivates. U. S. Pat June 22, 3,966,274

73. Hilakivi-Clarke, L. A. 1997. Mechanisms of high maternal fat intake during pregnancy on increased breast cancer risk in female rodent offspring. *Breast Cancer Res. Treat.* **46:** 119–214.

74. Hilakivi-Clarke, L., R. Clarke, I. Onojafe, M. Raygada, E. Cho, and M. E. Lippman. 1997. A maternal diet high in n-6 polyunsaturated fats alters mammary gland development, puberty onset, and breast cancer risk among female rat offspring. *Proc. Natl. Acad. Sci. USA* **94:** 9372–9377.

75. Hilakivi-Clarke, L., I. Onojafe, M. Raygada, E. Cho, R. Clarke, and M. Lippman. 1996. High-fat diet during pregnancy increases breast cancer risk in rats. *J. Natl. Cancer Inst.* **88:** 1821–1827.

76. Hilakivi-Clarke, L. A., M. Raygada, A. Stoica, and M.-B. Martin. 1998. Consumption of a high-fat diet during pregnancy alters estrogen receptor content, protein kinase C activity and morphology of mammary gland in the mother and her female offspring. *Cancer Res.* **58:** 654–660.

77. Hirano, T., K. Oka, and M. Akiba. 1989. Antiproliferative effects of synthetic and naturally occurring flavoids on tumor cells of the human breast carcinoma cell line, ZR-75-1. *Res. Comm. Chem. Path. Pharm.* **64:** 69–78.

78. Hirayama, T. 1982. Relationship of soybean paste soup intake to gastric cancer risk. *Nutr. Cancer* **3:** 223–233.

79. Hirohata, T., T. Shigematsu, A. M. Y. Nomura, Y. Nomura, A. Horie, and I. Hirohata. 1985. Occurrence of breast cancer in relation to diet and reproductive history: a case-control study in Fukuoka, Japan. *Natl. Cancer Inst. Monogr.* **69:** 187–190.

80. Hirose, K., K. Takima, N. Hamajima, M. Inoue, T. Takezaki, T. Kuroisha, M. Yoshida, and A. Tokudome. 1995. A large scale, hospital-based, case-control study of risk factors of breast cancer according to menopausal status. *Jpn. J. Cancer Res.* **86:** 146–154.

81. Hoel, D. G., D. L. Davis, and A. B. Miller. 1992. Trends in cancer mortality in 15 industrialized countries. *J. Natl. Cancer Inst.* **84:** 313–320.

82. Holm, L.-E., E. Nordevang, M. L. Hjalmar, E. Lidbrink, E. Callmer, and B. Nilsson. 1993. Treatment failure and dietary habits in women with breast cancer. *J. Natl. Cancer Inst.* **85:** 32–36.

83. Hoshiyama, Y. and T. Sasaba. 1992. A case-control study of stomach cancer and its relation to diet, cigarettes, and alcohol consumption in Saitama Prefecture, Japan. *Cancer Causes Control* **3:** 441–448.

84. Howe, G. R. 1992. High-fat diets and breast cancer risk. The epidemiological evidence. *JAMA* **268:** 2080–2081.

85. Howe, G. R., C. M. Friedenreich, M. Jain, and A. B. Miller. 1991. A cohort study of fat intake and risk of breast cancer. *J. Natl. Cancer Inst.* **83:** 336–340.

86. Howe, G. R., T. Hirohata, T. G. Hislop, J. M. Iscovich, J. M. Yuan, K. Katsoyanni, F. Lubin, E. Marubini, B. Modan, and T. Rohan. 1990. Dietary factors and risk of breast cancer: combined analysis of 12 case-control studies. *J. Natl. Cancer Inst.* **82:** 561–569.

87. Howell, D. E. 1948. A case of DDT storage in human fat. *Proc. Oklahoma Acad. Sci.* **29:** 31–32.

88. Hsieh, C., M. Pavia, M. Lambe, S. J. Lan, G. A. Colditz, A. Ekbom, H. O. Adami, D. Trichopoulos, and W. C. Willett. 1994. Dual effect of parity on breast cancer risk. *Eur. J. Cancer* **30A:** 969–973.

89. Hsueh, A. M., R. Shipley, and H. A. Park. 1992. Quality of dietary protein during initiation and promotion of chemical carcinogenesis in rats, in *Dietary Proteins: How They Alleviate Disease and Promote Better Health* (Liepa, G. U., D. C. Beitz, A. C.

Beynin, and M. A. Gorman, eds.), Amercian Oil Chemistry Society, Champaign, IL, pp. 151–162.

90. Hu, J., Y. Liu, Y. Yu, T. Zhao, and S. Liu. 1991. Diet and cancer of the colon and rectum: a case-control study in China. *Int. J. Epidemiol.* **20:** 362–367.

91. Hug, H. and T. F. Sarre. 1993. Protein kinase C isoenzymes:divergence in signal transduction. *Biochem J.* **291:** 329–343.

92. Hulka, B. S. and A. T. Stark. 1995. Breast cancer: cause and prevention. *Lancet* **346:** 883–887.

93. Hunter, D. J. and K. T. Kelsey. 1993. Pesticide residues and breast cancer: the harvest of a silent spring? (Editorial). *J. Natl. Cancer Inst.* **85:** 598–599.

94. Hunter, D. J., D. Spiegelman, H. O. Adami, L. Beeson, P. A. van den Brandt, A. R. Folsom, G. E. Fraser, R. A. Goldbohm, S. Graham, G. R. Howe, L. H. Kushi, J. R. Marshall, A. McDermott, A. B. Miller, F. E. Speizer, A. Wolk, S. Yuan, and W. Willett. 1996. Cohort studies of fat intake and the risk of breast cancer—a pooled analysis. *N. Engl. J. Med.* **334:** 356–361.

95. Ip, C. and M. M. Ip. 1981. Serum estrogens and estrogen responsiveness in 7,12-dimethylbenz(a) anthracene-induced mammary tumors as influenced by dietary fat. *J. Natl. Cancer Inst.* **66:** 291–295.

96. Jurkowski, J. J. and W. T. Cave. 1985. Dietary effects of menhaden oil on the growth and membrane lipid composition of rat mammary tumors. *J. Natl. Cancer Inst.* **74:** 1145–1150.

97. Kang, K. S., M. R. Wilson, and T. Hayashi. 1996. Inhibition of gap junctional intercellular communication in normal human breast epithelial cells after treatment with pesticides, PCBs, and PBBs, alone or in mixtures. *Environ. Health Perspect.* **104:** 192–200.

98. Kellis, J. T. J. and L. E. Vickery. 1984. Inhibition of human estrogen synthetase (aromatase) by flavones. *Science* **225:** 1032–1034.

99. Knabbe, C., M. E. Lippman, L. M. Wakefield, K. C. Flanders, R. Derynck, and R. B. Dickson. 1987. Evidence that transforming growth factor-beta is a hormonally regulated negative growth. *Cell* **48:** 417–428.

100. Kohlmeier, L., J. Rehm, and H. Hoffmeister. 1990. Lifestyle and trends in worldwide breast cancer rates. *Ann. NY Acad. Sci.* **609:** 259–268.

101. Kolonel, L. N., M. W. Hinds, and J. H. Hankin. 1980. Cancer patterns among migrant and native born japanese in Hawaii in relation to smoking, drinking and dietary habits, in *Genetic and Environmental Factors in Experimental and Human Cancer* (Gelboin, H. V., B. MacMahon, T. Matsushima, et al., eds.), Japan Science Society, Tokyo, pp. 327–340.

102. Korach, K. S., P. Sarver, and K. Chae. 1988. Estrogen receptor-binding activity of polychlorinated biphenyls: conformationally restricted structural probes. *Mol. Pharmacol.* **33:** 120–127.

103. Kreiger, N., M. Wolff, and R. A. Hiatt. 1994. Breast cancer and serum organochlorines: a prospective study among white, black, and Asian women. *J. Natl. Cancer Inst.* **86:** 589–599.

104. Kuiper, G. G. J. M., B. Carlsson, K. Grandien, E. Enmark, J. Haggblad, S. Nilsson, and J. A. Gustafsson. 1997. Comparison of the ligand binding specificity and transcript tissue distribution of estrogen receptors alpha and beta. *Endocrinology* **138:** 863–870.

105. Kuiper, G. G. J. M., E. Enmark, M. Pelto-Huikko, S. Nilsson, and J. A. Gustafsson. 1996. Cloning of a novel estrogen receptor expressed in rat prostate and ovary. *Proc. Natl. Acad. Sci. USA* **93:** 5925–5930.

106. Kuiper-Goodman, T. 1990. Uncertainties in the risk assessment of three mycotoxins: aflatoxin, ochratoxin, and zearalenone. *Cancer J. Physiol. Pharm.* **68:** 1017–1024.

107. Kupfer, D. and W. H. Bulger. 1977. Interaction of o,p'-DDT with the estrogen-binding protein (EBP) in human mammary and uterine tumors. *Res. Commun. Chem. Path. Pharmacol.* **16:** 451–462.

108. Kushi, L. H., T. A. Sellers, J. G. Potter, C. L. Nelson, R. G. Munger, S. A. Kaye, and A. R. Folsom. 1992. Dietary fat and postmenopausal breast cancer. *J. Natl. Cancer Inst.* 84**134:** 1092–1099.

109. Kutz, F. W., P. H. Wood, and D. P. Bottimore. 1991. Organochlorine pesticides and polychlorinated biphenyls in human adipose tissue. *Rev. Environ. Contamin. Toxicol.* **120:** 1–82.

110. Lamartiniere, C. A., J. B. Moore, N. M. Bown, H. Thompson, M. J. Hardin, and S. Barnes. 1995. Genistein suppresses mammary cancer in rats. *Carcinogenesis* **16:** 2833–2840.

111. Laug, E. P., F. M. Kunze, and C. S. Prickett. 1951. Occurrence of DDT in human fat and milk. *AMA Arch. Indust. Hyg. Occup. Med.* **3:** 245–246.

112. Lee, H. P., L. Gourley, S. W. Duffy, J. Esteve, J. Lee, and N. E. Day. 1991. Dietary effects on breast cancer risk in Singapore. *Lancet* **337:** 1197–1200.

113. Locke, F. B. and H. King. 1980. Cancer mortality among Japanes in the United States. *J. Natl. Cancer Inst.* **65:** 237–242.

114. Lopez-Carrillo, L., L. Torres-Arreola, and L. Torres-Sanchez. 1996. Is DDT use a public health problem in Mexico? *Environ. Health Perspect.* **104:** 584–588.

115. Lu, L.-J. W., K. E. Anderson, J. J. Grady, and M. Nagamani. 1996. Effects of soya consumption for one month on steroid hormones in premenopausal women: implications for breast cancer risk reduction. *Cancer Epid. Biom. Prev.* **5:** 63–70.

116. Luo, Y., T. Yoshizawa, and T. Katayama. 1990. Comparative study on the natural occurrence of fusarium mycotoxins (trichothecenes and zearalenone) in corn and wheat from high- and low-risk areas for human esophageal cancer in China. *Appl. Environ. Microbiol.* **56:** 3723–3726.

117. Martin, P. M., K. B. Horwitz, D. S. Ryan, and W. McGuire. 1978. Phytoestrogen interaction with estrogen receptors in human breast cancer cells. *Endocrinology* **103:** 1860–1867.

118. Mason, R. R. and G. Schulte,J. 1981. Interaction of o,p'-DDT with the estrogen binding protein (EBP) of DMBA-induced rat mammary tumors. *Res. Commun. Chem. Path. Pharmacol.* **33:** 119–128.

119. Matsukawa, Y., N. Marui, T. Sakai, Y. Satomi, M. Yoshida, K. Matsumoto, H. Nishino, and A. Aoike. 1993. Genistein arrests cell cycle progression. *Cancer Res.* **53:** 1328–1331.

120. Mayr, U., A. Butsch, and S. Schneider. 1992. Validation of two in vitro test systems for estrogenic activities with zearalenone, phytoestrogens and cereal extracts. *Toxicology* **74:** 135–149.

121. McBain, W. A. 1987. The levo enantiomer of o,p'-DDT inhibits the binding of 17 -estradiol to the estrogen receptor. *Life Sci.* **40:** 215–219.

122. McTiernan, A. and D. B. Thomas. 1986. Evidence for a protective effect of lactation on risk of breast cancer in young women. Results from a case-control study. *Am. J. Epidemio.* **124:** 353–358.

123. Menon, N. K., C. Moore, and G. A. Dhopeshwarkar. 1981. Effect of essential fatty acid deficiency on maternal, placental, and fetal rat tissues. *J. Nutr.* **111:** 1602

124. Messina, M. 1997. Isoflavone intakes by Japanese were overestimated. *Am. J. Clin. Nutr.*

125. Messina, M., V. Persky, K. D. R. Setchell, and S. Barnes. 1994. Soy intake and breast cancer: a review of the in vitro and in vivo data. *Nutr. Cancer* **21:** 113–131.

126. Michal, F., K. M. Grigor, A. Negro-Vilar, and N. E. Skakkebaek. 1993. Impact of the environment on reproductive health: executive summary. *Environmental Health* **101:** 159–167.

127. Michels, K. B., D. Trichopoulos, J. M. Robins, B. A. Rosner, J. E. Manson, D. Hunter, G. A. Colditz, S. E. Hankinson, F. E. Speizer, and W. C. Willett. 1996. Birthweight as a risk factor for breast cancer. *Lancet* **348**: 1542–1546.
128. Murrill, W. B., N. M. Brown, J. X. Zhang, P. A. Manzolillo, S. Barnes, and C. A. Lamartiniere. 1996. Prepubertal genistein exposure suppresses mammary cancer and enhances gland differentiation in rats. *Carcinogenesis* **17**: 1451–1457.
129. Mussalo-Rauhamaa, H. 1991. Partitioning and levels of neutral organochlorine compounds in human serum, blood cells, and adipose and liver tissue. *Sci. Total Environ.* **103**: 159–175.
130. Mussalo-Rauhamaa, H., E. Hasanen, and H. Pyysalo. 1990. Occurrence of β-hexachloro-cyclohexane in breast cancer patients. *Cancer* **66**: 2124–2128.
131. Newcomb, P. A., B. E. Storer, and M. P. Longnecker. 1994. Lactation and a reduced risk of premenopausal breast cancer. *N. Engl. J. Med.* **330**: 81–87.
132. Nishizuka, Y. 1992. Intracellular signalling by hydrolysis of phospholipids and activation of protein kinase C. *Science* **258**: 607–614.
133. Noble, L. S., E. R. Simpson, A. Johns, and S. E. Bulun. 1996. Aromatase expression in endometriosis. *J. Clin. Endocrin Metab.* **81**: 179
134. Nomura, A., B. E. Henderson, and J. Lee. 1978. Breast cancer and diet among the Japanese in Hawaii. *Am. J. Clin. Nutr.* **31**: 2020–2025.
135. Okura, A., H. Arakawa, H. Oka, T. Yoshinari, and Y. Monden. 1988. Effect of genistein on topoisomerase activity and on the growth of (val 12) Ha-ras-transformed NIH 3T3 cells. *Biochem. Biophys. Res. Commun.* **157**: 183–189.
136. Palmiter, R. D. and E. R. Mulvihill. 1978. Estrogenic activity of the insecticide kepone on the chicken oviduct. *Science* **201**: 356–358.
137. Parkin, D. M., C. S. Muir, and S. L. Whelan. 1992. *Cancer Incidence in Five Continents.* IACR, Lyon.
138. Petrakis, N. L., S. Barnes, E. B. King, J. Lowenstein, J. Wiencke, M. M. Lee, R. Miike, M. Kirk, and L. Coward. 1996. Stimulatory influence of soy protein isolate on breast secretion in pre- and postmenopausal women. *Cancer Epidemiol. Biomark Prev.* **5**: 785–794.
139. Pike, M. C., B. E. Henderson, and J. T. Casagrande. 1981. The epidemiology of breast cancer as it relates to menarche, pregnancy, and menopause, in *Hormones and Breast Cancer* (Pike, M. C. , P. K. Siiteri, and C. W. Welsch, eds.), CSH, Cold Spring Harbor, pp. 3–17.
140. Poland, A., D. Smith, and R. Kuntzman. 1970. Effect of intensive occupational exposure to DDT on phenybutazone and cortisol metabolism in human beings. *Clin. Pharmacol. Ther.* **11**: 724–732.
141. Potter, J. D., J. R. Cerhan, T. A. Sellers, P. G. McGovern, C. Drinkard, L. R. Kushi, and A. R. Folsom. 1995. Progesterone and estrogen receptors and mammary neoplasia in the Iowa Women's Health Study: how many kinds of breast cancer are there. *J. Natl. Cancer Inst.* **85**: 32–36.
142. Prentice, R., D. Thompson, C. Clifford, S. Gorbach, B. Goldin, and D. Byar. 1990. Dietary fat reduction and plasma estradiol concentration in healthy postmenopausal women. *J. Natl. Cancer Inst.* **82**: 129–134.
143. Prentice, R. L., M. Pepe, and S. G. Self. 1989. Dietary fat and breast cancer:a quantitative assessment of the epidemiological literature and a discussion of methodological issues. *Cancer Res.* **49**: 3147–3156.
144. Pritchard, G. A., D. L. Jones, and R. E. Mansel. 1989. *Lipids* in breast carcinogenesis. *Br J Surg* **76**: 1069–1073.
145. Ralston, A. T. 1978. Effect of zearalanol on weaning weight of male calves. *J. Anim. Sci.* **47**: 1203–1206.

146. Ramamoorthy, K., F. Wang, and I. C. Chen. 1997. Estrogenic activity of a dieldrin/toxaphene mixture in the mouse uterus, MCF-7 human breast cancer cells, and yeast-based estrogen receptor assays: No apparent synergism. *Endocrinology* **138:** 1520–1527.

147. Rao, G. A. and S. Abrahams. 1976. Enhanced growth rate of transplanted mammary adenocarcinoma induced in C3H mice by dietary linoleate. *J. Natl. Cancer Inst.* **56:** 431–432.

148. Read, L. D., G. L. Greene, and B. S. Katzenellenbogen. 1980. Regulation of estrogen receptor messenger ribonucleic acid and protein levels in human breast cancer cell lines by sex steroid hormones, their antagonists, and growth factors. *Mol. Endocrinol.* **3:** 295–304.

149. Reddy, B. S., B. Simi, N. Patel, C. Aliaga, and C. V. Rao. 1996. Effect of amount and types of dietary fat on intestinal bacterial 7alpha-dehydroxylase and phosphatidylinositol-specific phospholipase C and colonic mucosal diacylglycerol kinase and PKC activities during different stages of colon tumor promotion. *Cancer Res.* **56:** 2314–2320.

150. Robinson, P. E., G. A. Mack, and J. Remmers. 1990. Trends of PCB, hexachlorobenzene, and β-benzene hexachlorinde levels in the adipose tissue of the U.S. population. *Environ. Res.* **53:** 175–192.

151. Rogan, W. J., B. C. Gladen, and J. D. McKinney. 1987. Poly-chlorinated biphenyls (PCBC) and dichlorodiphenyldichloroethane (DDE) in human milk: effects on growth, morbidity, and duration of lactation. *Am. J. Public Health* **77:** 1294–1297.

152. Rogers, A. E. and M. P. Longnecker. 1988. Dietary and nutritional influences on cancer: a review of epidemiologic and experimental data. *Lab. Invest.* **59:** 729–759.

153. Rose, D. P., J. M. Connolly, R. T. Chlebowski, I. M. Buzzard, and E. L. Wynder. 1993. The effects of a low-fat dietary intervention and tamoxifen adjuvant therapy on the serum estrogen and sex hormone-binding globulin concentrations of postmenopausal breast cancer patients. *Breast Cancer Res. Treat.* **27:** 253–262.

154. Rose, D. P., J. M. Connolly, J. Rayburn, and M. Coleman. 1995. Influence of diets containing eicosapentaenoic or docosahexaenoic acid on growth and metastasis of breast cancer cells in nude mice. *J. Natl. Cancer Inst.* **87:** 587–592.

155. Russo, I. H., J. Medado, and J. Russo. 1994. Endocrine influences on the mammary gland, in *Integument and Mammary Glands* (Jones, T. C., U. Mohr, and R. D. Hunt, eds.), Springer-Verlag, Berlin, pp. 252–266.

156. Safe, S., M. Harris, and L. Biegel. 1991. Mechanism of action on TCDD as an antiestrogen in transformed human breast cancer and rodent cell lines, in *Banbury Report 35. Biological Basis for Risk Assessment of Dioxins and Related Compounds* (Gallo, M. J., R. H. Scheuplein, and K. A. van der Heijden, eds.), Cold Spring Harbor, New York, pp. 367–375.

157. Sanderson, M., M. Williams, K. E. Malone, J. L. Stanford, I. Emanuel, E. White, and J. R. Daling. 1996. Perinatal factors and risk of breast cancer. *Edidemiology* **7:** 34–37.

158. Sandoz, L. T. D. 1980. Pharmacological trials of Frideron P-1496. Sandoz Ltd.

159. Schoental, R. 1974. Role of podophyllotoxin in the bedding and dietary zearalenone on incidence of "spontaneous" tumors in laboratory animals. *Cancer Res.* **34:** 2419

160. Schoental, R. 1985. Trichothecenes, Zearalenone, and other carcinogenic metabolites of fusarium and related microfungi. *Adv. Cancer Res.* **45:** 217–290.

161. Scribner, J. D., N. K. Mottet, and M. C. Pike. 1981. DDT accelaration of mamary gland tumors induced in the male Sprague-Dawley rat by 2-acetamidophenanthrene. *Carcinogenesis* **2:** 1235–1239.

162. Shames, L. S., M. T. Munekata, and M. C. Pike. 1994. Blood levels of organochlorine residues and risk of breast cancer (letter). *J. Natl. Cancer Inst.* **86:** 1642

163. Shutt, D. A. and R. I. Cox. 1972. Steroid and phyto-estrogen binding to sheep uterine receptors in vitro. *J. Endocrinol.* **52:** 299–310.

164. Silinskas, K. C. and A. B. Okey. 1975. Protection by 1,1,1-trichloro–2,2-bis(p-chlorophenyl)ethane (DDT) against mammary tumors and leukemia during prolonged feeding of 7,12-demthlybenz[a]anthracene to female rats. *J. Natl. Cancer Inst.* **55:** 653–656.

165. Steinmetz, R., N. G. Brown, D. L. Allen, R. M. Bigsby, and N. Ben-Jonathan. 1997. The environmental estrogen bisphenol A stimulates prolactine release in vitro and in vivo. *Endocrinology* **138:** 1780–1786.

166. Steinmetz, R., P. C. M. Young, and A. Caperell-Grant. 1996. Novel estrogenic action of the pesticide residue β-hexachlorocyclohexane in human breast cancer cells. *Cancer Res.* **56:** 5403–5409.

167. Susser, M. 1990. Maternal weight gain, infant birth weigh, and diet: causal consequences. *Am. J. Clin. Nutr.* **53:** 1384

168. Sylvester, P. W., M. Russell, M. M. Ip, and C. Ip. 1986. Comparative effects of different animal and vegetable fats fed before and during carcinogen administration on mammary tumorigenesis, sexual maturation, and endocrine function. *Cancer Res.* **46:** 757–762.

169. Thomas, D. B. and M. R. Karagas. 1987. Cancer in first and second generation Americans. *Cancer Res.* **47:** 5771–5776.

170. Trock, B. J. 1996. Breast cancer in African American women: epidemiology and tumor biology. *Breast Cancer Res. Treat.* **40:** 11–24.

171. Ahlborg, U. G., L. Lipworth, and L. Titus-Ernstoff. 1995. Organochlorine compounds in relation to breast cancer, endometrial cancer, and endometriosis: an assessment of the biological and epidemiological evidence. *Crit. Rev. Toxicol.* **25:** 463–531.

172. Unger, M., H. Kiaer, and M. Blichert-Toft. 1984. Organochlorine compounds in human breast fat from deceased with and without breast cancer in a biopsy material from newly diagnosed patients undergoing breast surgery. *Environ. Res.* **34:** 24–28.

173. Utian, W. H. 1973. Comparative trial of P-1496, a new non-steroidal oestrogen analogue. *BMJ* **1:** 579–581.

174. van den Brandt, P. A., P. Van't Veer, R. A. Goldbohm, E. Dorant, A. Volovics, R. J. J. Hermus, and F. Sturmans. 1993. A prospective cohort study on dietary fat and the risk of postmenopausal breast cancer. *Cancer Res.* **53:** 75–82.

175. van der Schouw, Y. T., M. D. Al, G. Hornstra, Bulstra-Ramakers, and H. J. Huijes. 1991. Fatty acid composition of serum lipids of mothers and their babies after normal and hypertensive pregnancies. *Prostaglandind Leukot. Essent. Fatty Acids* **44:** 247–252.

176. Van't Veer, P., I. E. Lobbezoo, and J. M. Martin-Moreno. 1997. DDT and postmenopausal breast cancer in Europe: case-control study. *Br. Med. J.* **315:** 81–85.

177. Walker, B. E. 1990. Tumors in female offspring of control and diethylstilbestrol-exposed mice fed high-fat diets. *J. Natl. Cancer Inst.* **82:** 50–54.

178. Wang, X., W. Porter, and V. Krishnan. 1993. Mechanism of 2,3,7,8-tetrachlorodibenzo-p-dioxin (TCDD)-mediated decrease of the nuclear estrogen receptor in MCF-7 human breast cancer cells. *Mol. Cell Endocrinol.* **96:** 159–166.

179. Wasserman, M., D. P. Nogueira, and L. Tomatis. 1976. Organochlorine compounds in neoplastic and adjacent apparently normal breast tissue. *Bull. Environ. Contam. Toxicol.* **15:** 478–484.

180. Wei, H., L. Wei, K. Frenkel, R. Bowen, and S. Barnes. 1993. Inhibition of tumor-promoter induced hydrogen peroxide formation by genistein in vitro and in vivo. *Nutr. Cancer* **20:** 1–12.

181. Welsch, C. W. 1992. Relationship between dietary fat and experimental mammary tumorigenesis: a review and critique. *Cancer Res.* **52:** 2040–2048.

182. Welshons, W. V., C. S. Murphy, R. Koch, G. Calaf, and V. C. Jordan. 1987. Stimulation of breast cancer cells in vitro by environmental estrogens enterolactone and the phytoestrogen equol. *Breast Cancer Res. Treat.* **10:** 379–381.

183. Westin, J. B. and E. Richter. 1990. The Israeli breast-cancer anomaly. *Ann. NY Acad. Sci.* **609:** 269–279.

184. Wiggins, J. P., H. Rothenbacher, L. L. Wilson, R. J. Martin, P. J. Wangness, and J. H. Ziegler. 1979. Growth and endocrine responses of lambs to zearanol implants: effects of preimplant growth rate and breed of sire. *J. Anim. Sci.* **49:** 291–297.

185. Willett, W. C. 1989. The search for the causes of breast and colon cancer. *Nature* **388:** 339–394.

186. Willett, W. C., M. J. Stampfer, G. A. Colditz, B. A. Rosner, and F. E. Speizer. 1990. Relation of meat, fat, and fiber intake to the risk of colon cancer in a prospective study among women. *N. Eng. J. Med.* **323:** 1664–1672.

187. Williams, B. A., K. T. Mills, C. D. Burroughs, and H. A. Bern. 1989. Reproductive alterations in female C57BL/Crgl mice exposed neonatally to zearalenone, an estrogenic mycotoxin. *Cancer Lett.* **46:** 225–230.

188. Witte, J. S., G. Ursin, J. Siemiatycki, W. D. Thompson, A. Paganini-Hill, and R. W. Haile. 1997. Diet and premenopausal bilateral breast cancer: a case control study. *Breast Cancer Res. Treat.* **42:** 243–251.

189. Wolff, M. 1996. Breast cancer and environmental risk factors: epidemiological and experimental findings. *Ann. Rev. Pharmacol. Toxicol.* **36:** 573–596.

190. Wolff, M., N. Dubin, and P. G. Toniolo. 1993. Organochlorines DDT and breast cancer. *J. Natl. Cancer Inst.* **85:** 1873–1875.

191. Wolff, M., P. Toniolo, and E. Lee. 1993. Blood levels of organochlorine residues and risk of breast cancer. *J. Natl. Cancer Inst.* **85:** 648–652.

192. Wu, A. H. and M. C. Pike. 1995. Dietary soy protein and hormonal status in females. *Am. J. Clin. Nutr.* **62:** 151–152.

193. Wu, A. H., R. G. Ziegler, P. L. Horn-Ross, A. M. Y. Nomura, D. W. West, L. N. Kolonel, et al. 1996. Tofu and risk of breast cancer in Asian-Americans. *Cancer Epidemiol. Biomarkers Prev.* **5:** 901–906.

194. Yuan, J. M., Q. S. Wang, R. K. Ross, B. E. Henderson, and M. C. Yu. 1995. Diet and breast cancer in Shanghai and Tianjin, China. *Br. J. Cancer* **71:** 1353–1358.

195. Ziegler, R. G., R. N. Hoover, M. C. Pike, A. Hildesheim, A. M. Y. Nomura, D. W. West, et al. 1993. Migration patterns and breast cancer risk in Asian-American women. *J. Natl. Cancer. Inst.* **85:** 1819–1827.

196. Shekhar, P. V. M., J. Werdell, and V. S. Basrur. 1997. Environmental estrogen stimulation of growth and estrogen receptor function in preneoplastic and cancerous human breast cell lines. *J. Natl. Cancer Inst.* **89:** 1774–1782.

197. McLachan, J. A. 1997. Synergistic effect of environmental estrogens: report withdrawn. *Science* **277:** 462–463.

198. Hunter, D. J., S. E. Hankinson, F. Laden, G. A. Colditz, J. E. Manson, W. C. Willett, F. E. Speizer, and M. Wolff. 1997. Plasma organochlorine levels and the risk of breast cancer. *New Engl. J. Med.* **337:** 1253–1258.

199. López-Carillo, L., A. Blair, M. López-Cervantes, M. Cebrián, C. Rueda, R. Reyes, A. Mohar, and J. Bravo. 1997. Dichlorodiphenyltrichloroethane serum levels and breast cancer risk: A case-control study from Mexico. *Cancer Res.* **57:** 3728–3732.

200. Safe, S. 1995. Environmental and dietary estrogens and human health: Is there a problem? *Environ. Health Perspect.* **103:** 346–351.

About the Editor

Dr. Anne M. Bowcock is Associate Professor of Internal Medicine and Pediatrics and a member of the McDermott Center of Human Growth and Development at the University of Texas Southwestern Medical Center at Dallas. She obtained a Ph.D. from the University of Witwatersrand, Johannesburg, South Africa in 1984 and conducted postdoctoral training in the Department of Genetics at Stanford University until 1990. She has published extensively in the areas of human genetics and the molecular genetics of breast cancer. She has also served on and chaired many committees and grant review boards relating to the human genome project, human genetics, and breast cancer, including the American Society of Human Genetics committee on breast and ovarian cancer screening.

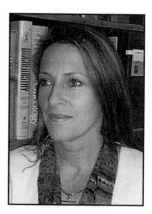

Index